I0213047

Healthcare Facilities
in Times of Radical Changes

23rd Congress of the International Federation of Hospital Engineering (IFHE)
25th Latin American Congress of Architecture and Hospital Engineering

Proceedings
edited by Romano Del Nord

October 13th-16th, 2014
UCA Puerto Madero, Buenos Aires, Argentina

Published by
TESIS Inter-University Research Centre
Systems and Technologies for Social and Healthcare Facilities
University of Florence
Italy

Scientific Editor:
Prof. Romano Del Nord
Director of TESIS Inter-University Research Centre
University of Florence

Session introductions (pp. 39, 99, 163, 253, 273, 361) and volume layout:
Francesca Nesi
Arch. PhD
University of Florence

Published by

TESIS Inter-University Research Centre "Systems and Technologies for Social and Healthcare Facilities"

Department of Architecture DIDA
University of Florence

Via San Niccolò 93
info@tesis.unifi.it
+ 39 055 275 5348
Florence 50125
Italy

ISBN 978-88-907872-6-3

First Print 2015

Foreword

The realization of the 23rd IFHE Congress, from October 13th to 16th, 2014, in Buenos Aires, Argentina, was an old wish of the Argentine Association of Hospital Architecture and Engineering (AADAIH), not only of its present members but also of earlier members, among them the fellow founders.

This Congress represented a great success for all of us and for our Latin American colleagues that accompanied and supported us. It also represented a great challenge for the International Federation, that trusted our organization and our capacity to accomplish this international congress for the first time in this part of the world.

But we relied not only on the trust of the Federation, we also received the support of the great number of registered speakers and attendants, coming from all continents from around 50 countries. To mention all countries one by one would take too long, but we can state that we had participants from nearly every Latin American country, as from North America, 15 European countries, and a significant number from Africa, Asia and Oceania.

Those five Congress days were a great opportunity for personal encounters and exchange of experiences between all professionals working in hospital architecture and engineering in different parts of the world.

The high-level scientific programme, with 72 from its 80 oral presentations, is now available for all the interested professionals, those that participated in Buenos Aires and those that could not attend. We want to express our special gratitude to Prof. Romano Del Nord and TESIS Inter-University Research Centre from the University of Florence, Italy who made possible the publication of this book.

PRESIDENT CONGRESS IFHE 2014
Arch. Luciano Monza

PRESIDENT IFHE 2014-2016
Arch. Liliana Font

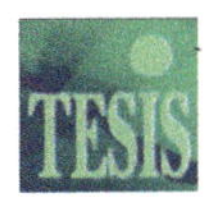

Authorities

CONGRESS PRESIDENT

Arch. Luciano Monza

ORGANIZING COMMITTEE

Arch. Alicia Preide - Academic Secretariat
Arch. Osvaldo Donato - Treasurer
Arch. José Turniansky - Latin America Coordinator
Arch. Carlos López - Commercial Exhibition Coordinator
Arch. Alberto Marjovsky - International Exhibition And Award Coordinator
Arch. Susana Kasslater - Social Events Coordinator

SCIENTIFIC COMMITTEE PRESIDENT

Arch. Liliana Font

SCIENTIFIC COMMITTEE MEMBERS

Eng. Salvador Benaim (Argentina)
Arch. Fabio Bitencourt (Brazil)
Arch. Luis Gonzalez Sterling (Spain)
Eng. Marcello Fiorenza (Italy)
Arch. Martin Fiset (Canada)
Eng. Gaston Lam (The Netherlands)
Bioeng. Barbara Mouriño (Argentina)
Prof. Eng. Arch. Yasushi Nagasawa (Japan)
Dr. Mario Rovere (Argentina)
Eng. Andy Wavell (UK)

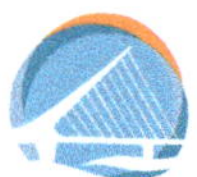

Editor's Foreword

The healthcare building sector is increasingly being hailed as the most responsive towards innovation and technologies that affect both the delivery of therapeutic care and of clinical management. The impact of such new technologies tends to radically change not only the morphology of the space for care and the physical configuration of the new hospitals but also the organizational models of the activities they are supposed to perform.

This conceptual upheaval of the core principles of the hospital of the future is, today, more and more associated the need to contain construction, operating and maintenance costs during the entire lifecycle of the facilities. This upheaval pushes the hospital engineering practitioners and researchers in healthcare technology to update their knowledge in order to foresee the potential that the market will be asked to express.

Thus, the Congresses of International Federation of Hospital Engineering (IFHE) become more and more culturally aware to compare and debate about the different approaches and solutions implemented to improve the quality of care despite the foreshadowed budgetary constraints.

The Interuniversity Research Centre TESIS of Florence has been engaged for many years in the gathering and disseminating the participants' contributions in a series of publications of the UIA-Public Health Group international seminars that are held annually in different countries.

TESIS welcomes now the opportunity offered by IFHE to publish the proceedings from the Congress held in Buenos Aires in 2014. The presented papers offer a comprehensive vision of the evolutionary dynamics that are taking place in the health sector and, at the same time, show the results of experimental and operational experiences of great interest to readers and professionals engaged in healthcare. In order to facilitate a selected reading of the contributions, the book has been structured in sections with much relevance to the iconographic part for immediate readability and consultation.

The essays analyse technical-engineering issues that are increasingly integrated with architectural ones, revealing the priority given to the different type of users and the strategic value of the user centered design. Comfort, wellbeing, safety, humanisation, sustainability and efficiency are the key words that describe the different facets and angles of the debated topics.

The innovative insights expressed in many papers are an incentive to venture more and more consciously in the world of innovation and experimentation for the benefit of the whole community.

Romano Del Nord

TESIS Inter-University Research Centre
Systems and Technologies for Social and Healthcare Facilities
University of Florence, Italy

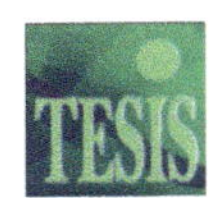

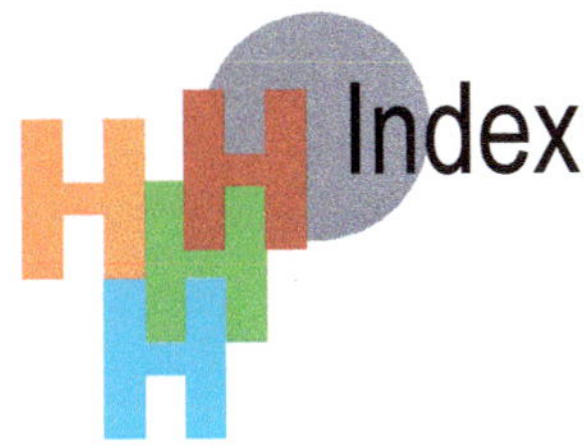

TESIS Inter-University Research Centre
Systems and Technologies for Social and Healthcare Facilities
University of Florence, Italy

TESIS

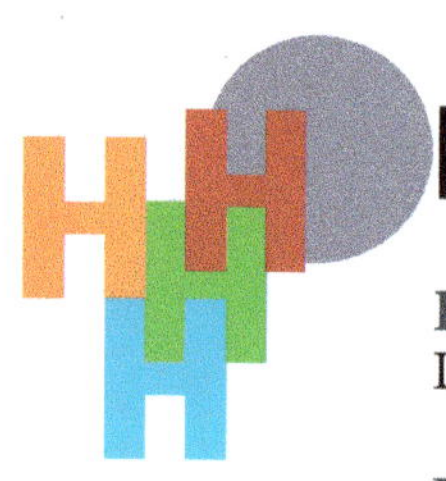

Index

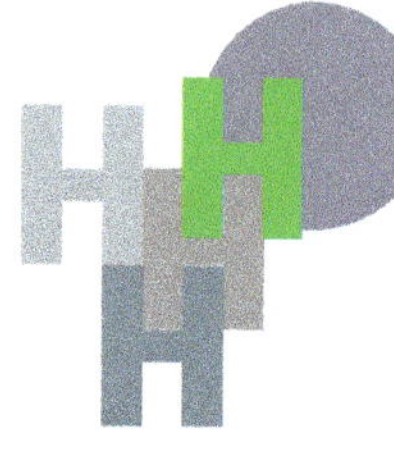

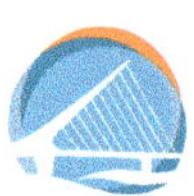

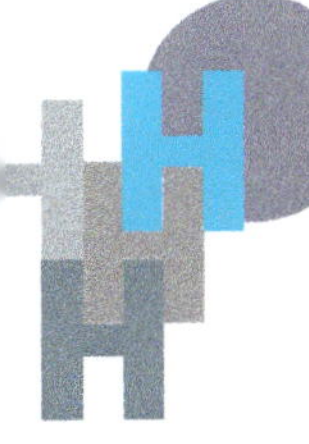

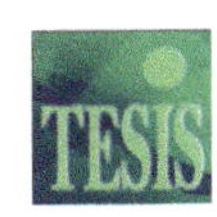
TESIS

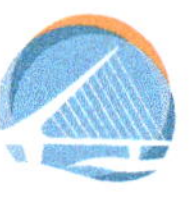

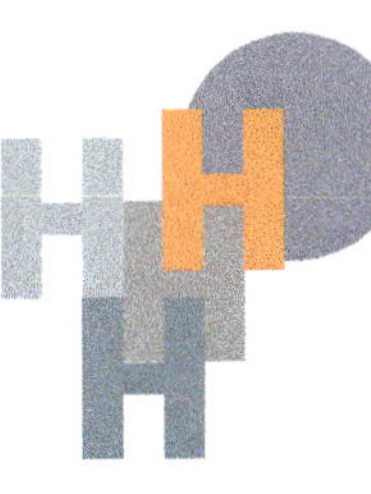

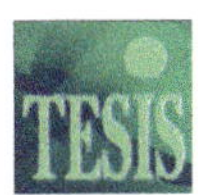
TESIS

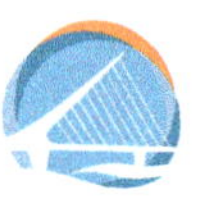

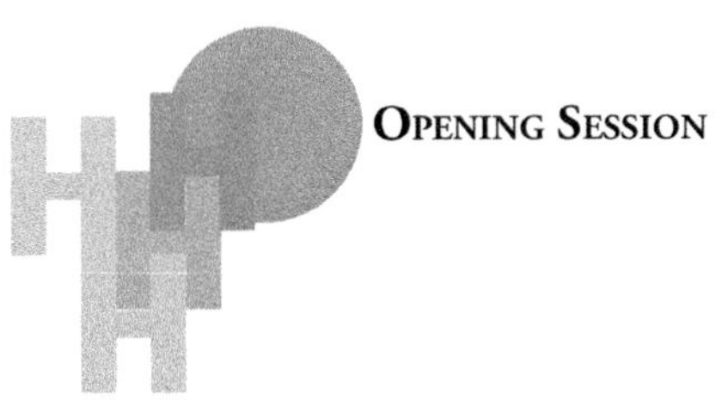

Opening Session

Redefining Health Settings Facing Demographic, Epidemiological, Technological and Political Changes, within an International Perspective

Mario Rovere

roveremarior@gmail.com
Asociación Argentina de Arquitectura e Ingeniería Hospitalaria (AADAIH), Argentina

Since the beginning of 21st century we've seen so many amazing changes that we can hardly remember, without a smile, the theory that predicted the end of history. It seems much more appropriate to quote "when I learned all the answers, the questions were changed". To have stationary or regressive population pyramids that resemble orthodox cathedrals with the silent irruption of chronicle diseases combined with extreme climatic phenomena breaking historic records and technological advances so surprising as shocking, oblige us to review all the scenarios of planning. And talking about scenarios, we adopt the theatrical metaphor to help us to understand that the stage designer is no longer behind the scene but he may become the first actor depending on the script of the play.

Therapeutic action, as long as many human activities gets intensified or neutralized accordingly with the space in which it's developed; that's the reason why we need to think in an evolution of health facilities just based in its own experiences and innovations. Social transformations of health also reach the values' system and a wide acceptance of health as a substantial social right in the construction of citizenship; in that way we find a big stimulus to search for answers towards a health infrastructure helping the universal access and a de-concentration movement of every element that may and must be placed close where population live, study, work and recreate.

Mario Rovere. *Sanitarian Doctor with Residence in International Health, Paediatrician and Honorary Member of AADAIH. He has been Director of Hospital and Health Region in the province of Salta, Director of Health Planning of Buenos Aires City, and Secretary of the National Social Policy in Argentina and Regional Consultant at HR Development OPS/OMS. Ex Former Coordinator Associated in ALAMES (Latin American Association of Social Medicine) Teacher graduated in Public Health and Social Policy for 30 years in Argentine and Latin American universities. Currently Dean Organizer of Health Department in the National University of La Matanza.*

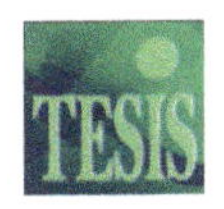

In the modern performing arts the scenographer is included as an actor. This principle is the basic idea to support this presentation where I assume that every architect, every engineer, every technician dedicated to health facilities or hospital maintenance, building or design is a colleague, is part of the health workforce, is part of the health team. A health team who now, yesterday and always, should be focusing in how to contribute with significant improvements in health services, as in health population.

That's why I like to share with all of you this reflections about new settings, new scenarios in health and in health services and systems.

The scenario approach for planning is not a new tool. It was a major instrument in the first oil international crisis (70's and 80's) and probably will be useful every time we'll need to face uncertainty, turbulence environment, instability, crisis or simply a non linear change.

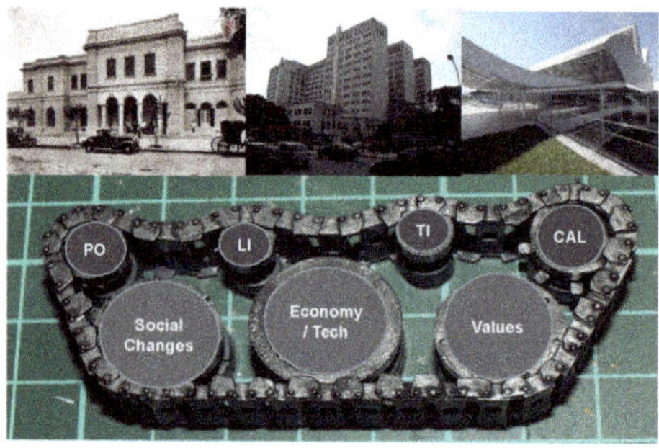

Figure 1. Scenarios.

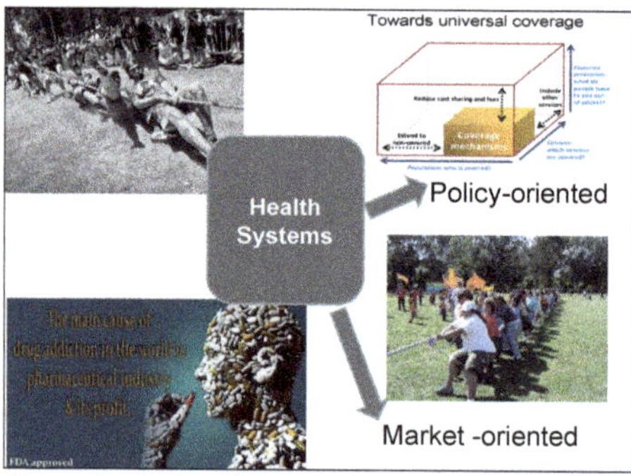

Figure 2. Political scenarios.

The strategic perspective includes scenario's approach but it let's consider health workforces, not just as "resources" but as a "social actor". In most countries health workforces represents between 1 to 3% of the population. That's why we can work with the future not just as a forecast useful to try to adjust our professional behavior to this predictable scenario. We can visualize new desirable futures in health and act as a vector to obtain it (Figure 1-2).

In a context of global health it is very important to take benefit of this opportunity to share with people from many different countries a brief analysis of what seems to be "seeds of future" in the present and some exercises of what could happen with health services and health systems in the near future.

At the same time, I'd like, too, thank to IFHE authorities for this opportunity and its trustee and I'd like to congratulate all of you for the success of this 23rd Congress in Buenos Aires City.

In a brief perspective I separate artificially political, social, economic, technological and cultural dimensions as features for shaping the future scenarios. I know that every dimension is full of rich interactions with the others but we can link it after a deeper analysis.

If we think or speculate about political scenarios the main idea is how the creative tensions between policy and market oriented could define the future of health at local and global levels.

In an extremely simplified overview these contradictory vectors could produce as an outcome more luxurious and

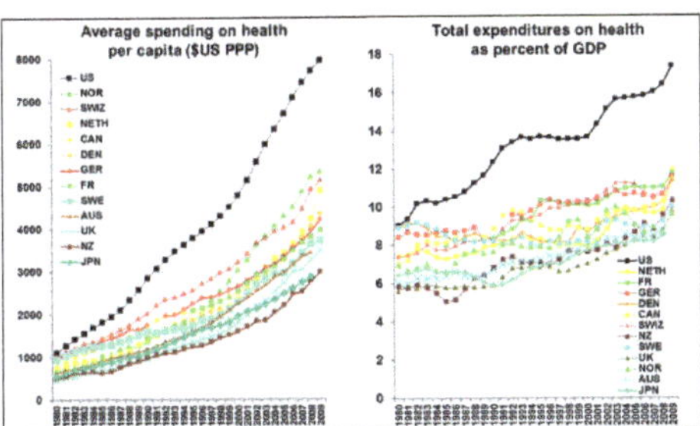

Figure 3. International comparison of spending on health, 1980 - 2009. Source: OECD Health Data 2011 (Nov. 2011).

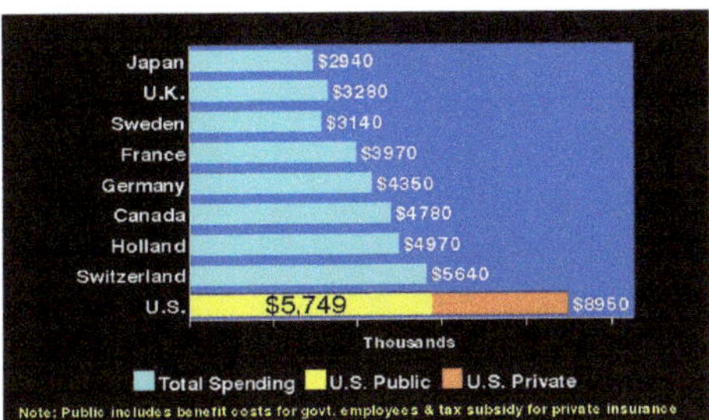

Figure 4. U.S. public spending per capita for heath is greater than total spending in other nations. Source: OECD 2013; NCHS Health Aff 2002.

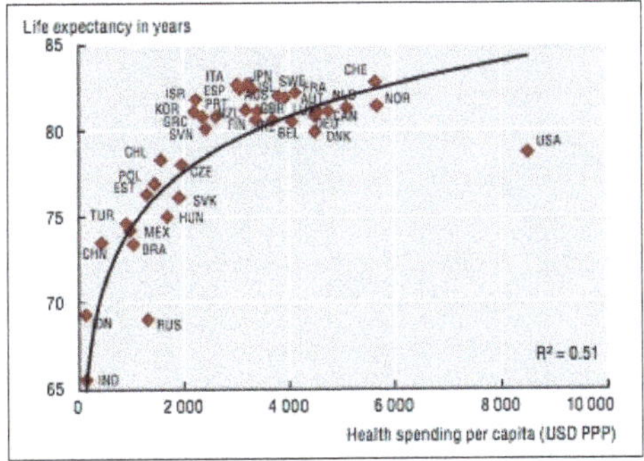

Figure 5. Efficiency. Source: OECD Health Statistics 2013.

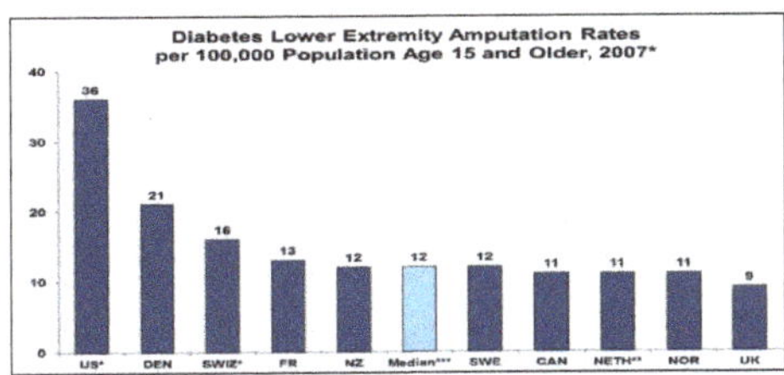

Figure 6. Effectivity. Source: OECD Heath Care Quality Indicators Data 2009.

fitted health services for less people who can afford it or reasonable health services for all the people.

However the tensions look useful to build and to sustain a creative force campus because health insurances, innovations, coverage, quality, complexity, access, delays, failures and "malapraxis" persist as components or a huge debate about the future of health system is settled in a context of more and more technologies, chronic diseases and elderly population.

The extreme arguments in this debate are exemplified in these questions:

Is the big pharma looking for the physicians mediation between producers and consumers?

Using the power of media communications and marketing techniques: Are the health technologies companies pushing patients demand?

Or is the big pharma promoting self-prescription?

Are they creating new diseases through the hypochondria? ¿are the big national health services fatally affected by bureaucracy and delays?

However, the answers are not neutral because they affected the questions of the health costs. If we compare different mix public/private we can see how USA shows an extreme level of expenditure in relatives and absolute terms.

According to IMF estimation for 2014, 88 of 190 countries in the world have a Gross Domestic Product GDP per habitant below the expenditure in health per habitant of the USA (8,900 U$A). In other terms neither using the 100 % of its wealth, these countries could afford this level of expenditure.

What is obvious for the low income

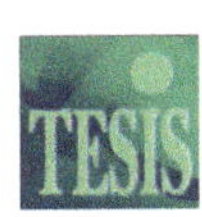

countries is at the same time a big challenge for the middle income countries, including various European ones. If the market oriented perspective prevails many of them could have in the near future a burden of costs risking its welfare systems with unpredictable social and political consequences.

What is really surprising in this matter -or at least it is less known- is the source of the huge health expenditure in USA. The relevant data is further that the main source is the public sector.

In other words the most costly and luxurious health system in the world is possible just because the state is the main fund rising (more than 60% of all sources) and whose caption capability is superior of the total caption for health expenditure of any country in the world. That's probably why the medical industrial complex (MIC), the USA internal and foreign policy and the World Bank are supporting the "universal health coverage" through insurances, no matter if they are public or private.

The main idea is that the MIC discovered the business opportunities of the health right over the idea that governments must guarantee just the nonprofit measures like prevention, it must guarantee the funds and it must abandon progressively the direct health services delivery.

That's why we are talking about "political dimension" because a debate between health coverage and health accessibility is affecting policy decisions in different levels of health government, from global to local.

The global scenario is changing because the European social welfare was since the end of the second world war a huge dyke for profit medicine and that's the main explanation for reasonable health expenditures but in the context of the European crisis the market oriented investments and the transnational health corporations are looking for weak welfare states. This is not a democratic debate, they are simply taking advantage of a strong alliance between USA, IMF, WB and the European Economic to impose these regressive reforms.

Everybody knows that its consequences will be a most costly, inefficient and stratificated health system. Most of the governments look dubitative because the experience of The "White Wave" movement in Madrid, Spain, and the Greek political situation alert for a governability crisis in the near future.

That is not just a question of efficiency; the effectiveness and the health consequences of a market oriented health system could be a major impact in health outcomes such as we can observe in an international comparison of the diabetes lower extremity amputation rates. This sensitive index shows that in the very center of the medicine scientific frontier, in USA the ratio is 4 times superior than an integrated system like UK /NHS who has a total spending in health per habitant 3 times inferior.

Most of our Latin-American countries looked at NHS in UK as a model for five decades. But this model is under attack since the Thatcher era and in recent years it suffered a new experiment for regressive reforms with such fundamentalism than the own Tories government is changing its mind and admit it. According to The Time in his cover of October 13th 2014 Tories admit that reforms was our worst mistake and it was qualified as an "unintelligible gobbledygook" (Figure 7).

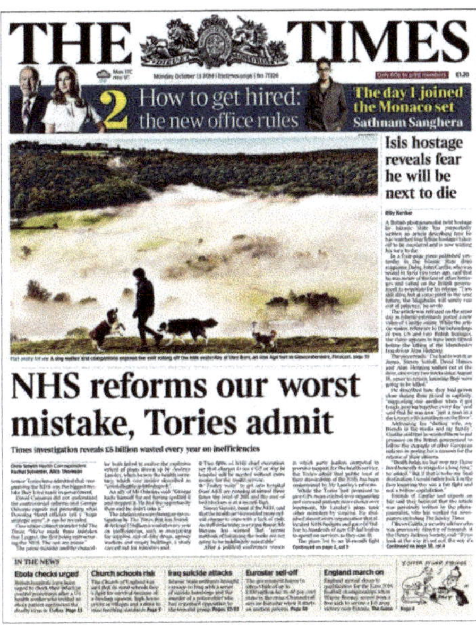

THE TIMES

How to get hired: the new office rules

The day I joined the Monaco set
Sathnam Sanghera

Isis hostage reveals fear he will be next to die

NHS reforms our worst mistake, Tories admit

Times investigation reveals £5 billion wasted every year on inefficiencies

IN THE NEWS

Ebola checks urged

Church schools risk

Iraq suicide attacks

Eurostar sell-off

England march on

Figure 7. Time cover of October 13th 2014.

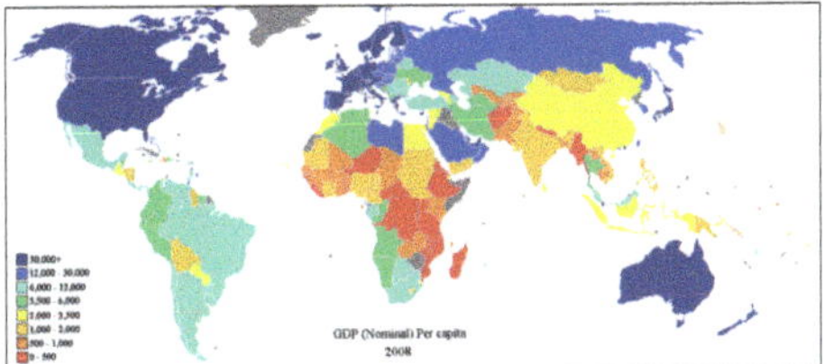

Figure 8. GDP (nominal) per capita. Source: International Monetary Fund, April 2008.

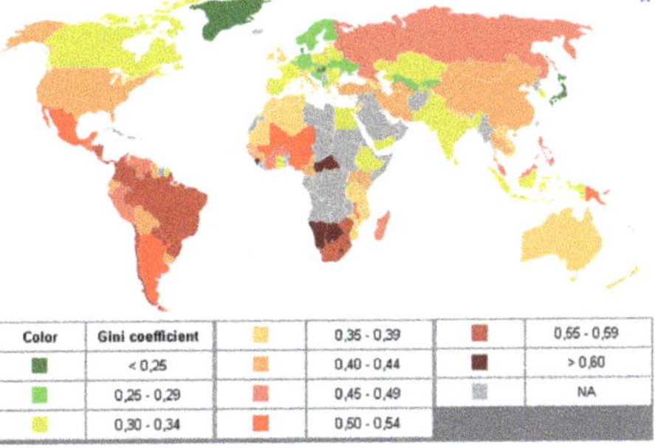

Figure 9. Social justice (GINI) is compatible with economic development.

Meanwhile many British and international analyst and observers declare than the NHS and the health rights in UK are in serious danger.

At the same time we face important changes in the social and sanitary environment.

In a demographic dimension the longevity or the increase of the age average is now a major problem in any country of the world and not just in the developed ones. The worst of it is that the mix of longevity and poorness is a very more complicated problem.

Urbanization was in focus last years when a mythic proportion changed at world level. We are talking about, since 2008, more than 50 % of the humanity population lives in cities, which produces a new huge and complex phenomenon in relation with housing, environment, poverty, land distribution, and health.

Migrations is the third social aspect we'd like to mention, because in a globalized context, more than 3 % of the world population don't live in the country where they were born. The consequences for the health services in those countries where the workforce, especially in the service areas, has a high proportion of foreign people is a big challenge to close the intercultural gap.

Mentioning Climate change let's take a look for an example of how this areas could be mixed we suffered in Argentina an example of the "perfect storm" in April 2013 in La Plata, a quarter million habitants city, a huge storm flooded an unexpected part of the town. The main casualties and victims were elderly people because in this part of the town many middle class old citizens lived alone and they couldn't face the emergency. Many of them died as a consequence of exag-

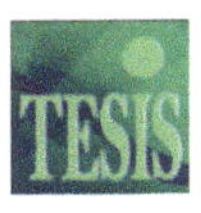

gerated security measures in houses who became a trap.
In an epidemiological dimension a mix of vaccines and antibiotics is creating a false perception that there is no menace in the horizons which we can´t afford. But just in the last two decades the world epidemiological surveillance showed a list of emergent diseases produced by new or mutated agents or by new conditions to propagate faster than ever. HIV, Multidrug-resistant tuberculosis (MDR-TB), SARS or bird flu, H1N1 or pig flu, and the recent African Ebola epidemics are just examples of why we must be alert about infectious diseases that need special health facilities to take in and to carry on patients in isolated conditions to protect them and health workers. Chronic diseases are growing without ceiling because a combination of medical advances, new technologies, longevity, and changes in life quality and life styles. In the context of emergent and chronic diseases we need to open a special space for other maladies that affect millions of people in the world but are concentrated in low income countries, in tropical areas or in poor population inside countries and cities. We are talking about neglected diseases a cluster of 17 diseases which kill more people than Malaria and tuberculosis together especially in sub-Saharan Africa. They are a medically diverse group of tropical infections which are especially common in low-income populations in developing regions of Africa, Asia, and the Americas. They are caused by a variety of pathogens such as viruses, bacteria, protozoa and helminths.
As we can observe in an international comparison we can assert: “Social justice (a lower Gini coefficient associated with a high GDP per Capita) is clearly compatible with a high economic development” and at the same time a lot of scientific evidence let’s confirm that at least in the health field “inequality is more harmful than poverty” (Figure 8-9). That’s why we must not just forecast but at the same time push to a fair social and geographic distribution of health facilities.
The success of medicine and the scientific development are producing new ways of life. Basically, because, we are not frequently “solving” problems but, in most cases we are transforming deathly and acute diseases in chronic ones. If we are looking for a good example for this we can quote the Chronic Obstructive Pulmonary Disease (Figure 10) .
In the late summer of 2014 in Buenos Aires we faced an electric supply default, it lasted more than 10 days in some parts of the city. The media showed the population protest, many people were very angry and one of the main focus was a surprising “electric dependant people” a new kind of citizen who demand the right to be served with electric power as a life-death issue.
A growing number of patients are needing concentrated oxygen not just to survive but to live with quality, comfort and dignity and they are looking for new devices and environment to obtain it.
Diabetes is another good example of how a lethal historic disorder till the first decade of XX century is actually a disease with treatments fitted for a normal life including local health facilities. Diabetes could affect at all ages since new born, usually a mother who suffer Diabetes can deliver a baby with a dangerous high weight, and the Diabetes type II has an increasing prevalence with aging (Figure 11). However, a person af-

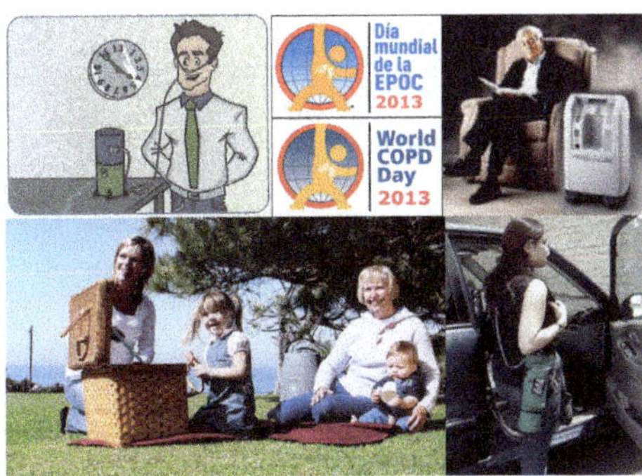

Figure 10. World COPD Day is an annual event organized by the Global Initiative for Chronic Obstructive Lung Disease (GOLD).

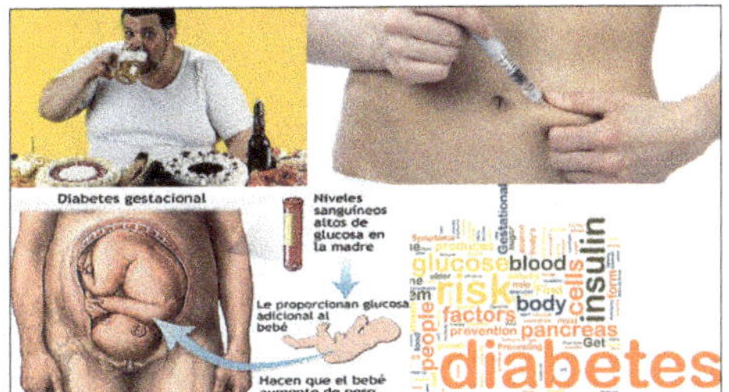

Figure 11. Diabetes.

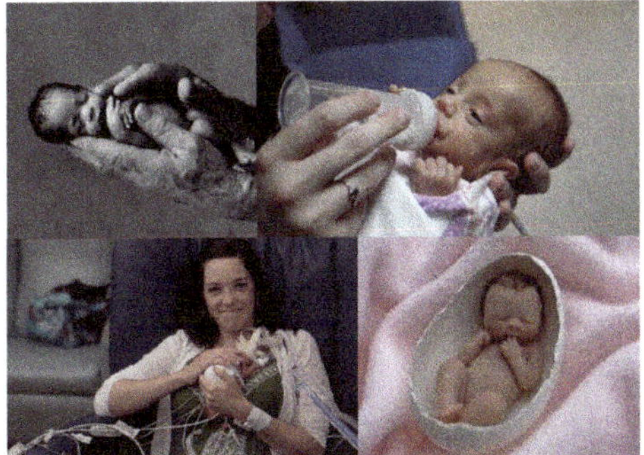

Figure 12. Premature babies.

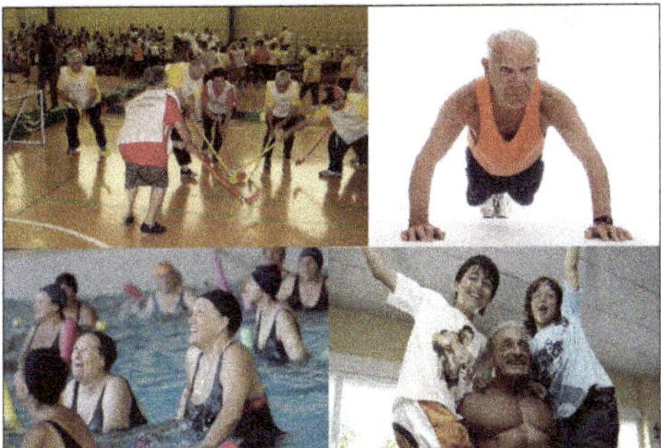

Figure 13. Healthy longevity.

fected can avoid serious complications with adequate combinations of: diet, drugs, health facilities access, and appropriate life style.

Primary health care was in the very beginning a gold strategy to face inequalities and poverty morbidity and early mortality, but in recent years it became at the same time a key instrument to face chronic diseases that need a systematic control and a professional personalized follow up. However, will provide in the near future the same professional prestige to design a network of community health centers than to project a big hospital?

And what about a very low birth weight? This is one of the best examples of how the medicine advances can at the same time create new challenges.

When a newborn weight is lower than 1500 gs or 3,4 pounds we call it "extreme low weight". 1,5 % of the newborn are in this group but the proportion is increasing because the quality of health care, and at the same time because the fertility programs produced more multiple pregnancies (Figure 12).

But if we think in a universal phenomenon transforming our health and our society there is not a better example than longevity. The life expectancy is climbing in all the world and in recent years the middle and low income countries are included in this phenomenon although they are affected by two big differences: the first one –as it was mentioned- is the obvious and explosive combination between elderly and poverty, the second one less known is that in these countries

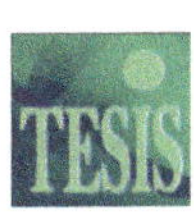

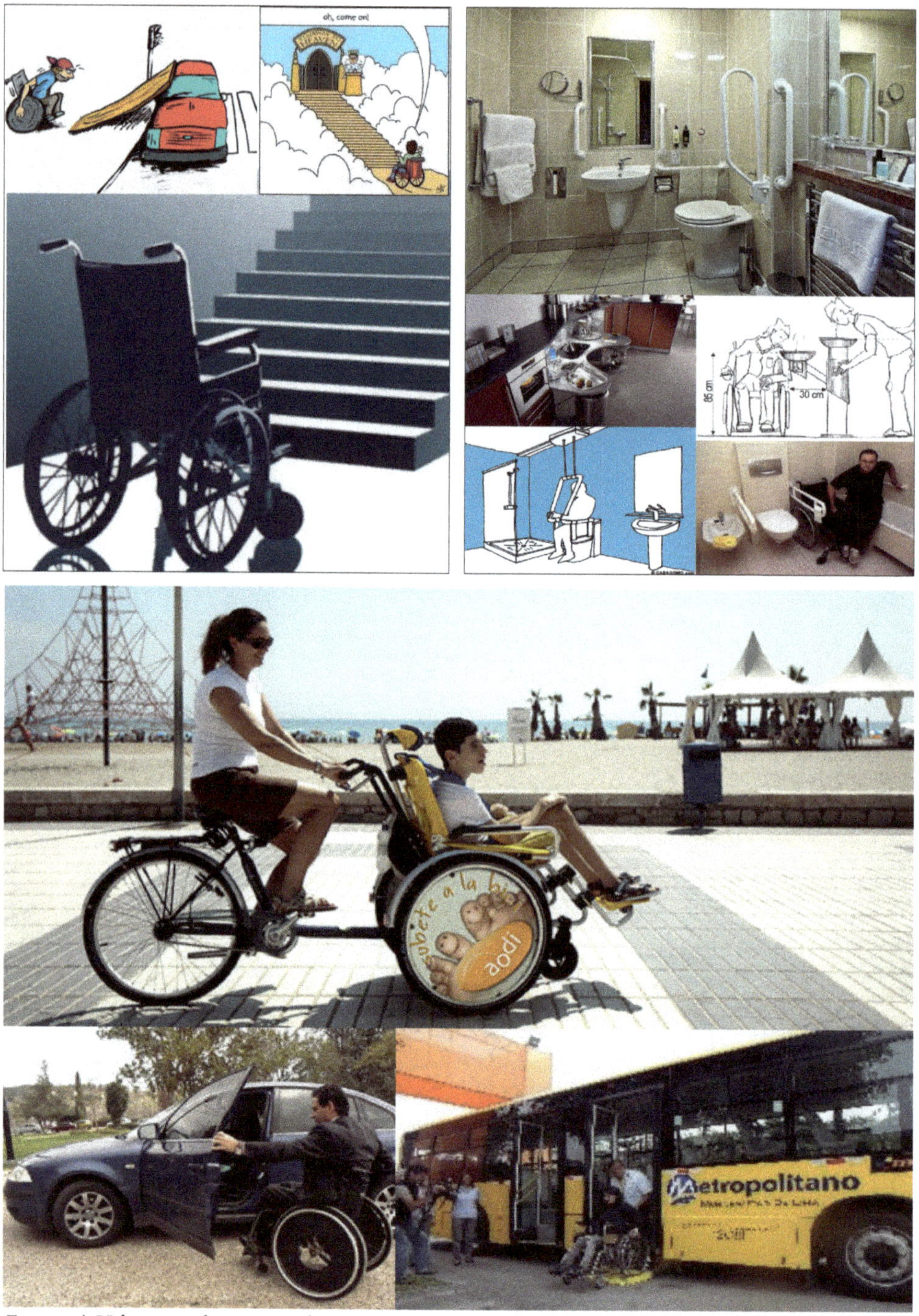

Figure 14. Urbanistic, domestic, architectural suitable designs in streets, building access, buses, health facilities, houses for disabled citizens.

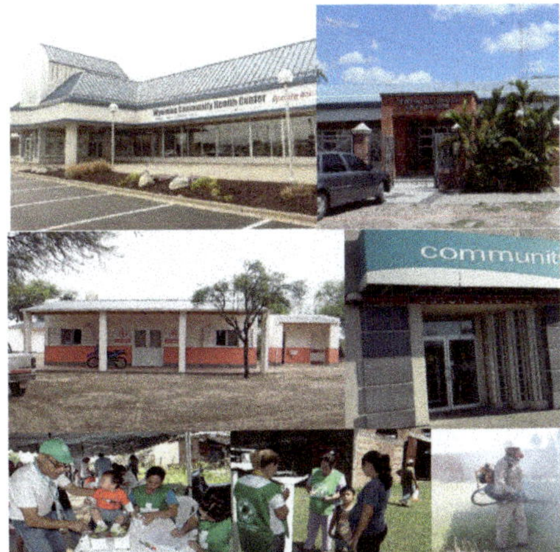

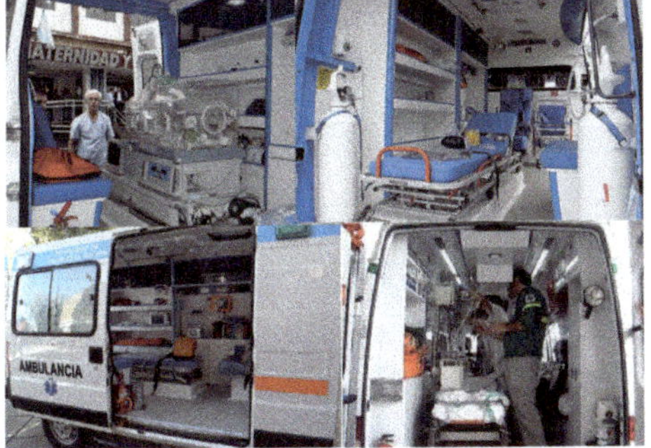

Figure 15. Community health centre and from ambulance to public and private transportation.

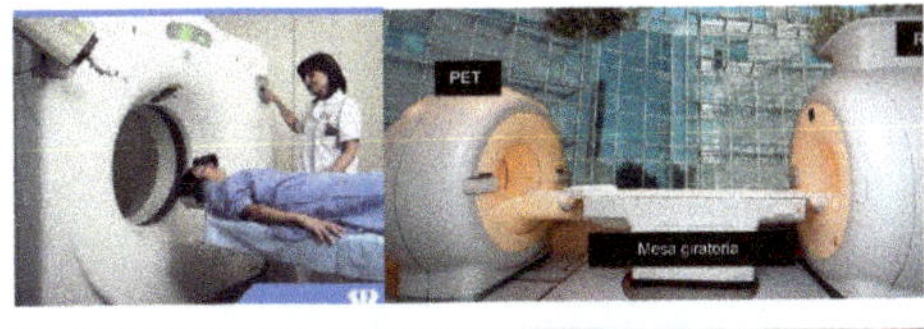

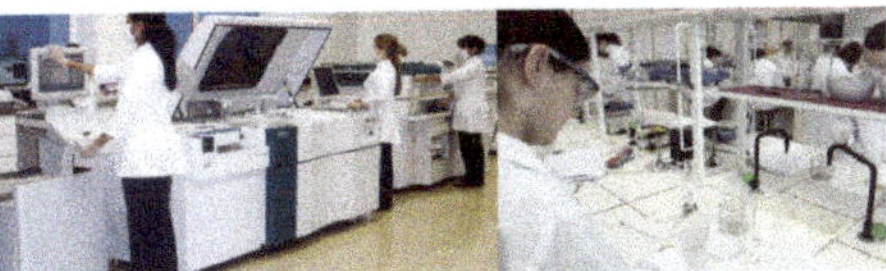

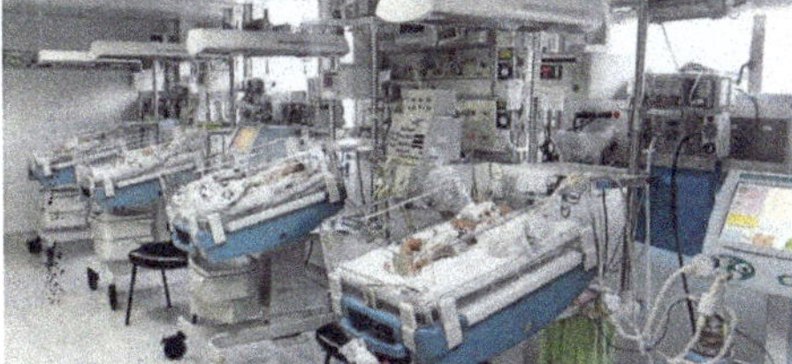

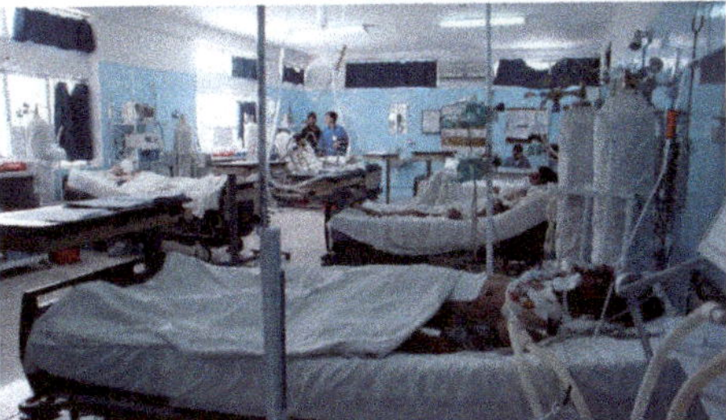

Figure 16. Technology.

the increase of elderly people is faster than in the developed one. It generates a collapse in health facilities and a challenge for services more prepared for maternal and child health problems (Figure 13).

If in the very beginning of the XXI century we are talking about differences and multiculturalism facing all kind of inequalities in race, gender, age, religious, migrants, refugees, age etc. we must focus too, in the growing disabled citizens who needs urbanistic, domestic, architectural suitable designs in streets, building access, buses, health facilities, houses. In disabling rights is common reference to use a formula if you don´t have barriers you don´t have disabilities (Figure 14).

As you can see in many of the health problems and social determinants that we mentioned, it's necessary to redefine the scope of "health facilities" since a lot of hospital architecture and engineering knowledge could be very useful to health community centers design and it can extends to public building and housing design to include people with chronic disease and affections. In the same perspective we can extent tech innovations from ambulance to public and private transportation (Figure 15-16).

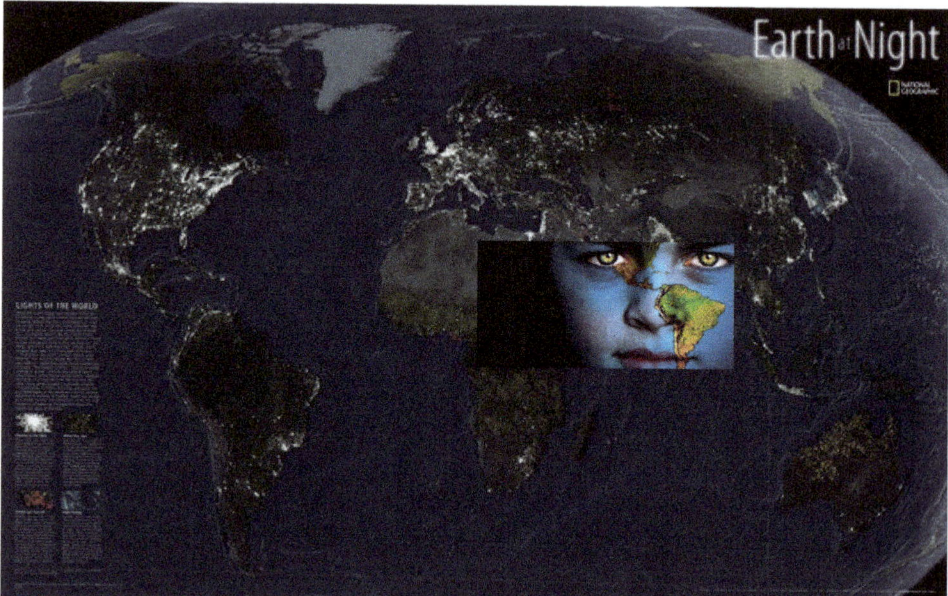

Figure 17. From a world's region that holds health as a right through the active participation of citizens we ask our "stage designers" (engineers, architects) to redouble efforts towards build together better settings to concrete this right for all.

As a brief synthesis

Probably in the next years we'll assist to a "silence revolution" that will remind us the 60's "hospitals without walls" utopia. Most of health facilities spaces, technology and "know how" could be demand for housing, streets, publics areas, and so on. Every health workers, as a professional and as a citi zen, should contribute in the next years to drive the health facilities to answer the Challenge of Health as a main component of human rights using the Equity principle as a North which means the same access to health services, the same protection for any avoidable health risk, and the same understandable information available for all to take key decisions caring our own families, communities, and ourselves.

When any proved new technology, capable to improve the "natural story of a disease", is created simultaneously a new human right has born. That means humanity, with our humble contribution, must go toward a universal coverage with real accessibility and an increasing resolution capability in Primary Health Care, including preventive to palliative care for all.

The technological advances in health technologies menace as to forget definitively the essential of the medical practices in relation with mercy, empathy and humanization: the interpersonal dimensions of quality in doctors-patients relationship.

From a world's region like Latin-America that holds health as a right through the active participation of citizens we ask our "stage designers" (engineers, architects, technicians) to redouble their efforts towards building together better settings to concrete this right for all.

A Sustainable Approach to Developing and Maintaining Healthcare Estates

Greg Markham

greg.markham@emcoruk.com
Institute of Healthcare Engineering and Estate Management (IHEEM), United Kingdom

This presentation will set out the current challenges facing the healthcare system within the United Kingdom, the predicted future pressures from population growth and ageing and quantify the financial impacts associated with these pressures. The presentation will also explore the fundamental requirements of a sustainability plan, detail the targets set within the UK for reducing emissions and outline some of the engineering solutions that have been successfully delivered across the healthcare estate and their actual benefits in terms of emissions reductions and financial savings.

Greg Markham *has been involved in Healthcare Engineering since 1990 in both the NHS and PFI sectors managing a variety of hospitals sites up to 1,000 acute beds. He gained his degree in 1996 and became a Chartered Engineer in 1998. In 2007, Greg became Chief Engineer with Carillion covering wider disciplines in addition to healthcare and this has progressed to his current role of Technical Director with EMCOR. Greg joined IHEEM in 1996 and has served the Institute in many ways and is the current President serving his two year term through to October 2014.*

UK Background

The National Health Service (NHS) was founded in 1948 by the post war Labour Government under the pioneering politician Aneurin Bevan. The key principle was, and remains Healthcare provided free at the point of delivery for all UK citizens, although this now also extends to selected EU citizens. UK population today is approximately 64 million, up from 50 million in 1948 and growing. Expectations of care have increased since the NHS was created and annual NHS spending is now around £110 billion (from <£0.5 billion in 1948 £3.5 billion inflation adjusted).

Population Pressure

Average life expectancy has risen since the NHS was created, from 65 (1950) to 80+ today with further increases forecast to 85 years within the next decade and to 90 by 2040. The retired population of the UK is predicted to outnumber those working within 20 years.

At death, the average UK citizen will have been under continuing treatment for one or more complex, chronic conditions for the last 17 years of their life. All this leads to massive cost pressures on the NHS with additional costs of £30-£50 billion per annum (30-45%) predicted by 2020.

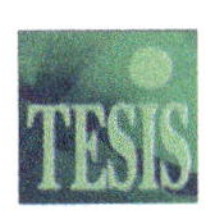

THE HEALTHCARE ESTATE

The NHS has an Estate of around 69,000 km^2 (Greater Buenos Aires 3,830 km^2) and around 16,000 buildings which costs around £7billion per year to operate. Significant renewal programme undertaken since 1997 with the PFI scheme using Private Finance to fund new hospitals (over 200) but this has faltered of late.

The NHS faces a current backlog of outstanding maintenance costs of around £4billion and many facilities are outdated and not fit for purpose.
This ageing estate is expensive to power, heat and cool - £600 million per annum emitting 3.7 million tonnes CO2. Energy costs are set to rise by 7% pa over the next 5 years.

THE PRINCIPLES OF ALL PLANS

Any plan, including sustainability plans, must include the four basic principles:

- *Plan*: this must set out what is to be achieved and in what timescale;
- *Measure/Report:* in a standard format to aid comparison, to improve something, first you need to know where you are;
- *Evaluate*: Good Corporate Citizen tool, as the plan evolves, measure progress and evaluate effectiveness;
- *Engage:* to influence people, you must engage and provide information and learning.

NHS England has formed its own Sustainability Unit SDU to address the macro issues and provide guidance (*www.sduhealth.org.uk*).

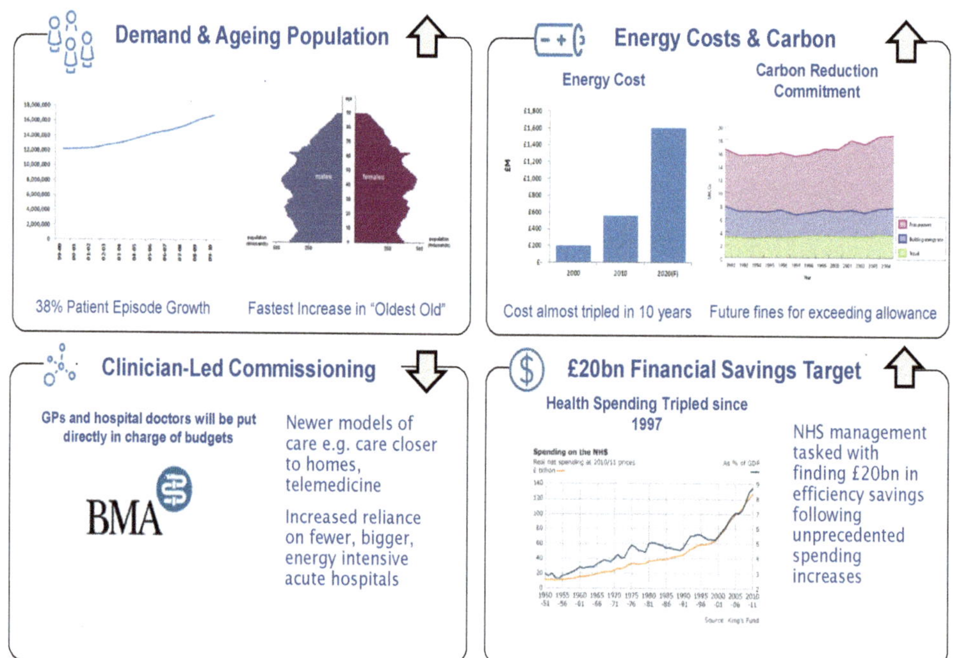

Figure 1. Challenges for the NHS: macro conditions applicable to all developed world health systems.

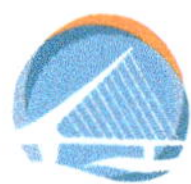

Key Areas for SDU: Leadership, Engagement and Development; Carbon Hotspots; Commissioning and Procurement; Sustainable Clinical and Care Models; Healthy, Sustainable and Resilient Communities; Metrics; Innovation, Technology and R&D; Creating Social Value.

The NHS Emissions Plan

As part of the UK Governments commitment to reducing Greenhouse Gas Emissions, the NHS adopted a carbon reduction plan: 2007 carbon emissions were set as the baseline; 10% reduction target set for 2015 (achieved already); 34% reduction by 2020; 80% reduction by 2050. All stakeholders have a part to play, users, staff and leaders but we will focus on the Role of the Engineer.

The Engineering Challenge

There is a major focus on reducing energy costs through: improved efficiency of buildings and systems; introducing renewable technologies (mainly wind & solar); extended use of Combined Heat and Power (CHP); a trend towards Energy Performance Contracting (EPC). Some 3,500 properties in the Primary Care sector have been transferred into a new, central NHS Property Services Company to rationalise and renew the estate. Technology changes quickly and even more so in Biomedical Engineering, this must be accounted for in the refurbishment.
Compliance of the ageing estate must be achieved with reducing budgets – unnecessary estate must be disposed of.
Maintenance of ever more complex equipment, dispersed throughout the estate and wider community must be achieved with less cost. The advances in tele-medicine must be accommodated and, where possible, predicted with flexibility 'built-in' to our estate. Current practices and accepted processes must be challenged at every opportunity.

Some Success Stories

The Carbon Trust's Carbon Management Program helped 49 Trusts achieve savings of 125,000 tCO2 and £ 14million p.a.
Pilgrim Hospital (Boston) installed a biomass boiler and reduced the carbon footprint of heating by 50% (6,000 tCO2 p.a.).
Rotherham Hospital committed to a Forward Commitment Procurement (FCP) to harness the benefits of ultra-efficient lighting saving an estimated 50% of energy use by lighting.
Heat Pump installation at Kings Mill Hospital in Mansfield has achieved savings of 2,000 tCO2 and £127k p.a.
Ground source heating and cooling at Churchill Hospital, Oxford has achieved savings of £150k and 1,422 tCO2 p.a.

Guy's and St Thomas

Solution

Installed a 3MW natural gas Jenbacher engine to provide heat and power at each hospital.

Results

£1.5m energy savings a year initially now over £2m a year. Over 11,000 tons of CO2 saved each year. First Trust to get Mayor of London Green 500 Platinum award. Enabled Trust to exceed its 20% emissions savings target in the first year.

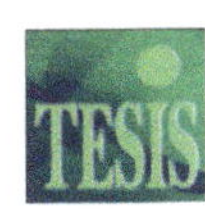

Guys & St Thomas, London
Client: G&ST Trusts
Commissioning: May 2009
2 x J620
$6MW_e$ & $5.5MW_{th}$
<3 Year Payback!
>£1.5m energy cost saving!

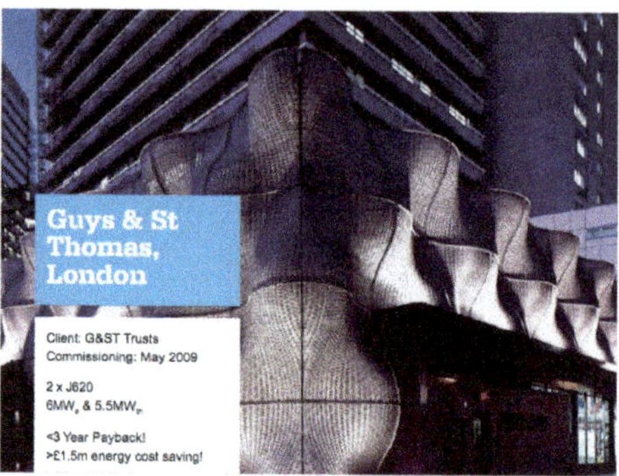

Figure 2. Guys & St Thomas, London.

CHP Benefits

Savings in primary energy usage (~45%). Reduced transportation and distribution losses across the network. Attractive life-cycle savings (freeing up revenue). Resilience of operation (high availability when maintained properly). Quick return on investment (2-5 year payback). Significant reduction in CO2 emissions (~30%). Overall efficiencies can exceed 90%. Flexible solutions to meet various applications. Finance packages available.

Succession Planning

An area often overlooked by Engineers!
The population is ageing, but so too is our workforce.
Estimates suggest >50% of Healthcare Engineers are aged over 50 years. We need to engage with the engineers of tomorrow, but expect competition. A recent report by the Gatsby Foundation suggested that UK PLC requires over 1,000,000 new engineers to sustain economic growth ambitions by 2020.
So how do we engage these engineers and attract them to Healthcare Engineering?

Once we have attracted them, how do we train them?
We need to retain knowledge and transfer this knowledge to our new recruits;
We have to recognise and identify the new skillsets required for modern engineers – IT knowledge is key along with any engineering skills. Our processes and systems have been developed and refined over many years, often as a result of tragedy – we need to ensure this learning and perspective is embedded in our future generations of engineers;
We have to create a career ladder for progression to ensure we retain our new found engineering talent!

Creating Social Value

Often the support staff in Hospital Engineering are among the lowest paid within the facility.
How do they afford housing?
What role can the NHS play?
Work is underway in Central London to utilise some of the surplus estate to invest in low cost housing to provide accommodation for the lower paid staff Project TLC.

The Role of IHEEM

Act as a source of knowledge and share best practice and case studies. IHEEM provide a comprehensive events programme covering key areas such as: energy management and carbon reduction; water hygiene practices; training for key engineering knowledge; working with the NHS to provide updates to the Health Technical Memorandum (HTM) guidance; assisting the NHS and wider UK Government with workforce planning and training.

Remodeling and Expansion of Monumental Hospitals in Urban Areas: The Approach to Sustainable Culture

Romano Del Nord

romano.delnord@unifi.it
Professor, University of Florence, Director of TESIS Inter-University Research Centre, Director of CSPE Professional Office, Italy

My paper and presentation will focus on different design experiences that emphasize the importance of social and structural interactions that the environmental and urban context intertwine and beckon for building reuse. This also means dealing with the meaning of sustainability in design context that aim to give increasing importance to the "cultural value" of hospital architecture, either historical or mainstream Modernism.
The issues of regeneration and functional integration with the city's urban fabric and services are closely related to the strategic importance of social, economic and environmental sustainability that involve topics such as: accessibility; building dimensions; urban integration; time distance; visual impact and, last but not least, cultural value.

Culture must therefore be addressed as a sustainable renewable resource. This implies that we must preserve all the buildings and monuments belonging to a specific historical period, that contribute to the tradition and cultural life of a community in terms of historical value, monumental value and landscape value.
It also means that we must preserve all the richness and complexity of Modern Architecture, bringing attention to the importance of evaluating the existing stock more in a holistic and sustainable term, rather than looking at the problem with short-sighted goals.
Cultural sustainability (the fourth dimension of the sustainable development) means preserving and improving access to the architecture which shape local and regional identity and make an important economic, social, educational and environmental contribution through its conservation (Figure 1).
It is therefore vital to implement research into new tools, methodologies and technologies able to understand the needs to support this new visions of healthcare design. For us, architects and researchers, a strategic question arises when we have to decide: how, if and which are the tools to value the memory of the past?
More and more frequently, in Europe and in Italy in particular, hospitals located in historic centres are perceived as no longer adequate to provide the services that people expect today.
The problem of 'if' and 'how' to update, is often addressed through a feasibility study that evaluates whether it is more appropriate to "delocalize" a new hospi-

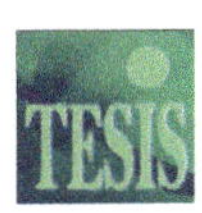

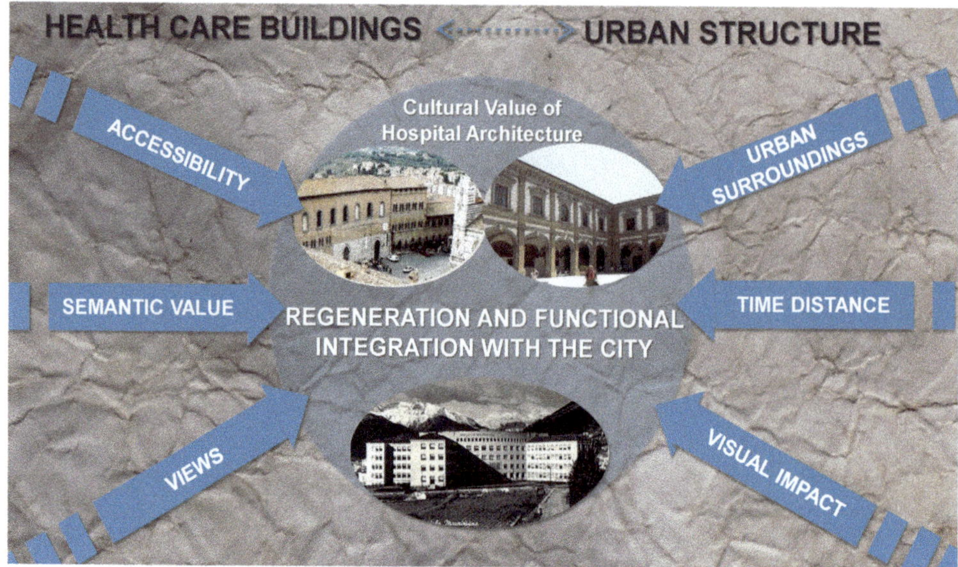

Figure 1. Global sustainability.

tal out of the city centre or to "extend, adapt & reuse" the existing hospital with permanence in the urban context.

Once established the way forward, planning options address the implementing strategies. The choice to keep a hospital in its original location implies two different strategies of expansion:

1. The first one is densifying the existing area with new infill that integrate the old buildings with the new ones.
2. The second choice addresses the same issue with a rather different approach. New independent facilities are built ex novo nearby the hospital precinct.

More and more advanced assessment methodologies are used to c ompare advantages and disadvantages of the two alternatives. Among the many parameters of "value analysis" procedures that favour the permanence in the urban context, we could list: integration of the healthcare facility with the social and public centres; sharing facilities with the Community; facilitated accessibility; regeneration of urban areas through hospital refurbishment programs; revitalization of monumental buildings (Figure 2).

The decision of permanence in the urban context brings many Community benefits, (as an extension of the Patient Central Approach) that turn the hospital reorganization in an opportunity to enhance the memory of the past or redevelop new urban areas for the benefit of the whole Community.

I would now explain how sustainability has guided three case studies in Italy that address the relationship between the hospital and the city. These case studies give answers to different fields of research such as: how to evaluate the "resilience" of the historical healthcare facilities in relation to future uses; which are the fields to orientate technology research to facilitate the integra-

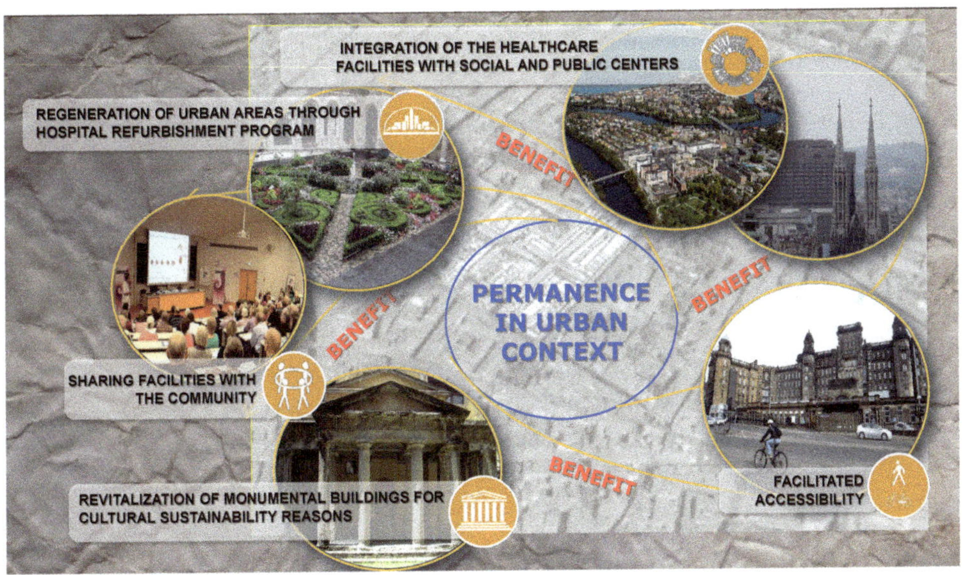

Figure 2. Permanence in urban context: when and why.

tion between the old and the new; how to evaluate "permeability" of historical healthcare facilities in relation to the principles of economic, social and environmental sustainability.

Among the reasons for selective the following three case studies, I would like to mention: the importance of "knowledge" as a prerequisite for taking appropriate decision on the intended use; the necessary "knowledge" has requested strong "interdisciplinary" measures from historical data (texts, archives, etc.) to archaeological excavations to structural surveys, etc.; sociological research on the role of public service for the benefit of the community and the redevelopment of urban areas; the strategic importance of the Feasibility Study and of its instrumental contents about how to achieve the multidimensional expected goals; the significant contribution offered by the "Community participation" in the decision making process (Figure 3).

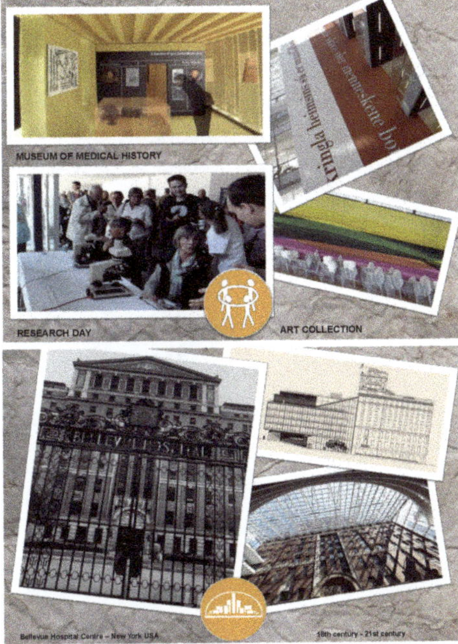

Figure 3. Benefit of permanence in urban context: sharing facilities with the community (above); maintaining the historical façade, adding a new ambulatory care facility in a new space, Bellevue Hospital Centre – New York USA (below).

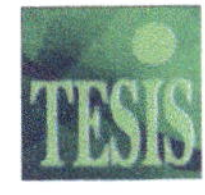

Case Study 1: Santa Maria della Scala Hospital, Siena

Sustainability is about keeping our past alive and, most of all, accessible to all. The case study of the hospital of Santa Maria della Scala is an excellent example of an adaptive reuse of a whole city block that has evolved through the centuries as "a city within a city" generating its own urban system.

The uniqueness of Santa Maria della Scala lies on a number of elements, such as: the strategic urban role of this hospital, the oldest in the history and development of the city of Siena (Figure 4); the wealth of historical memory integrated into the heritage and still visible today; the concept of a new space through which enhance and transmit the memory of the past to future generations; the technical and technological innovations used to maximize the embedded historical value.

Santa Maria della Scala was built opposite the Duomo and it is probably the oldest hospital in Europe that was kept working from the middle Ages to the XX century when it was finally turned into a museum. It is important to learn the story of S.M. della Scala's development to fully appreciate its contemporary use.

Its origins date back to the Middle Ages (Figure 5). The archives report that its construction started in the 11th century and that kept the original configuration till 1257. The birth of the hospital and its first century of life was accomplished by the will of the Episcopal Church of Siena: the heart of the ecclesial community, but also the episcopal seat in which the urban community recognizes its own identity and highest expression of its policy initiatives.

The real estate expansion and the transformation of the structure of the church in its duties is carried within the building-block through the creation of specific environments used for a myriad of various activities connected with the hospital. In conjunction with the acquisition of new properties, the church brings to completion the reconstruction of buildings acquired, located in Vallepiatta di Sopra, in a single building complex. This process is done in stages to exhaust the entire building's potential. In the 14th century the complex started to grow again. The political analysis of society and the economy of the first half of the fourteenth century

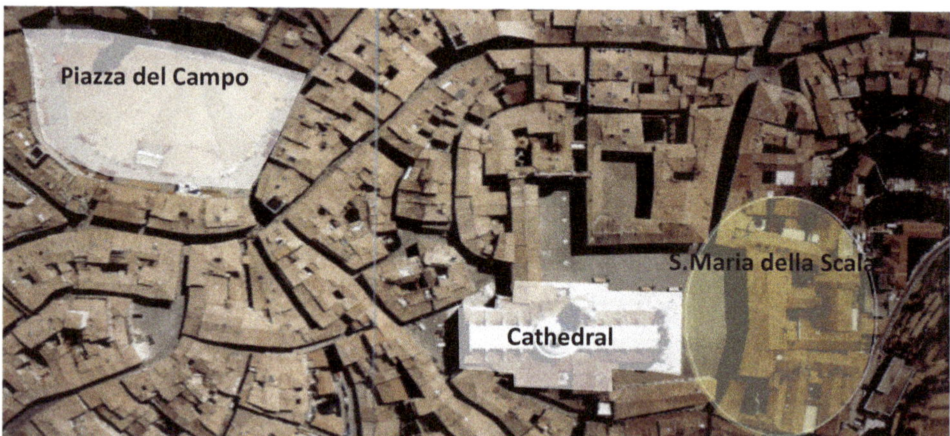

Figure 4. Siena: aerial view of the historical urban settlement as it has been preserved today.

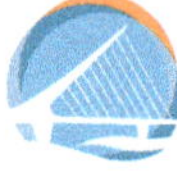

explain the motivation which led to its expansion. When the bank encounters difficulties in the international market and there are clear limits of its productive powers, Siena begins to invest in the 'public realm' in various forms. Money is made available to finance large public works, such as the city hospital and Santa Maria della Scala forms the ideal retreat for the wealth produced in previous years. Therefore, it is appropriated for the government to provide finances to the hospital for the building of a new shelter to provide accommodation and care for the poor and the sick. The Welfare Building becomes an impressive block that occupies an entire hill slope with its different floors, its large roofs and numerous windows, with its garden and its cemetery.

In the first half of the thirteenth century, the building consists of several separate structures together: a shelter, in which is housed equally poor and sick pilgrims of both sexes; a refectory; a portico that hosts administrative functions such as drafting documents, offering ceremonies; several houses already owned by the hospital in which lived family members of the hospital staff (Figure 6).

Through the 20th century, Santa Maria della Scala retained its healthcare function: the old shelter was used as wards and the other rooms as out-patients clinics, stressing the resilience of its architecture.

At the beginning of 2000, the new demands of modern healthcare made it impractical to keep the hospital in the historical centre. The Municipality took the decision to delocalize it and build "Le Scotte Hospital" while, at the same time, transform the old Santa Maria della Scala into a Museum that would keep history alive for the future generations. Thanks to this operation, the wealth of historical memory integrated into the heritage has become visible and accessible to today's citizens and visitors.

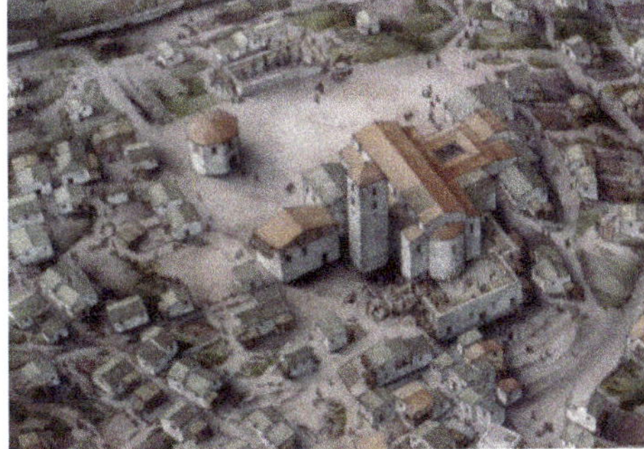

Figure 5. The origins (1090 – 1257).

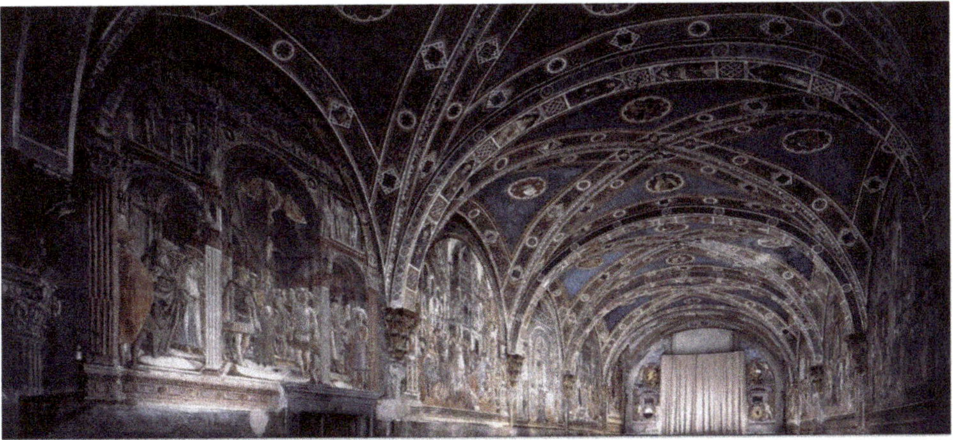

Figure 6. The shelter, the vaulted ceiling with paintings by Domenico di Bartolo.

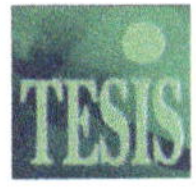

CASE STUDY 2 - SANTA MARIA NUOVA HOSPITAL, FLORENCE

Another excellent example of cultural sustainability is Santa Maria Nuova hospital, the oldest hospital in Florence, that dates back to the 13th century. Recently refurbished, it offers a high quality of care to all the residents in the historical centre (Figure 7).

The characteristics of this intervention are multifaceted and comprise issues such as: the role of care delivered in an urban context over the centuries by a hospital surrounded by the most important historical monuments in the city of Florence (Figure 8); the scientific character of technical investigations at the base of the Feasibility Study; the emphasis given to the interdependence of artistic development, hospital reuse and social rehabilitation of the urban core; the restoration of the works of art as part of the restoration of the hospital; the uniqueness of the new use as a "hospital-museum" (Figure 9).

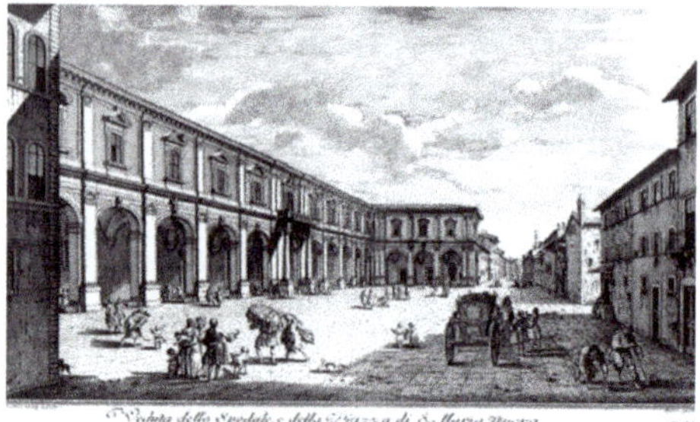

Figure 7. Santa Maria Nuova Hospital, Florence.

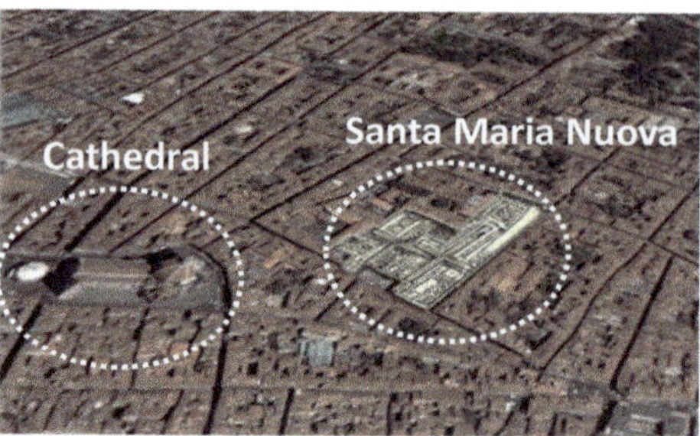

Figure 8. Florence: urban context.

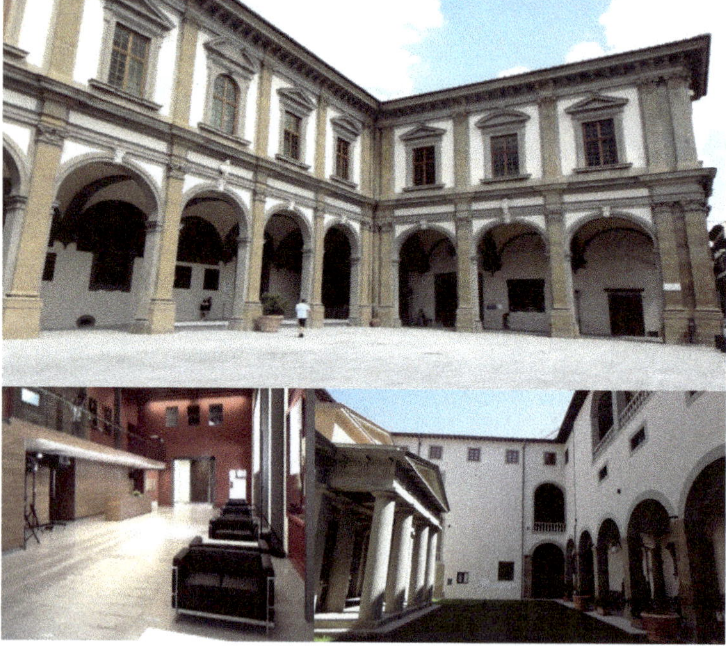

Figure 9. The regeneration of the 13° century hospital in the historic centre of Florence reiterates the value of heritage for the Community's sustainable future (above), The entrance of the Museum (below, left); the interior portico (below, right).

Case study 3 - Parini Hospital, Aosta

The Parini Hospital's case study emphasizes the importance of social and structural interactions that the environmental and urban context intertwine and beckon for building reuse: a condition that sparkles a whole set of multi-disciplinary connections and strategic decisions that affect both the healthcare, the social and the urban systems.

This scenario of decision-making assessments is the framework of this case, in which the final decision was based on an evaluation process that involved extensive participation and even a "referendum" extended to all local citizens. The pivotal problem underlying the final decision concerned the way such large scale expansion would have affected the city of Aosta and, above all, its hospital services network.

The Mauriziano Hospital is a 1940's building of mainstream modern Italian architecture. It was built in the same location of the demolished 18th century hospital. So, both from an architectural and urban point of view, the Hospital is charged with historical references and connections. The Parini Hospital today is nestled in the city and surrounded by the public parking and the modern road system. The hospital is the centre of the mobility network both at the scale of the local and regional road system. It is also strongly integrated in the urban core as a landmark for the Communityn (Figure 10).

During the years, the hospital has grown with uncontrolled expansions but without a proper planning vision. This situation has caused at least 4 kind of problems: cluttered the hospital area, changed the original architectural image of the hospital, limited pedestrian acces-

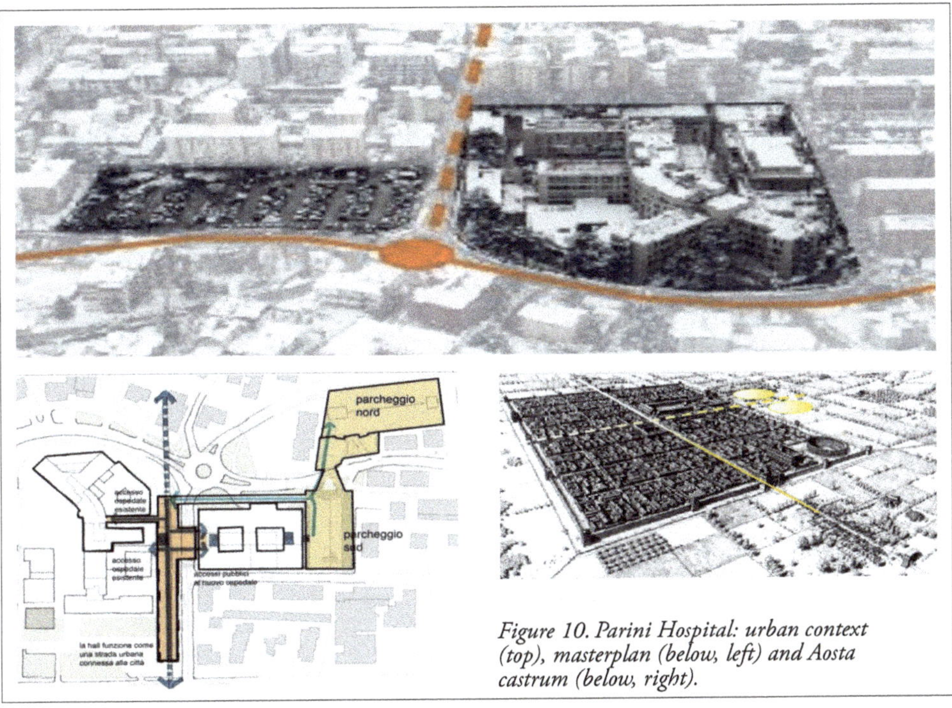

Figure 10. Parini Hospital: urban context (top), masterplan (below, left) and Aosta castrum (below, right).

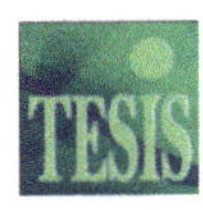

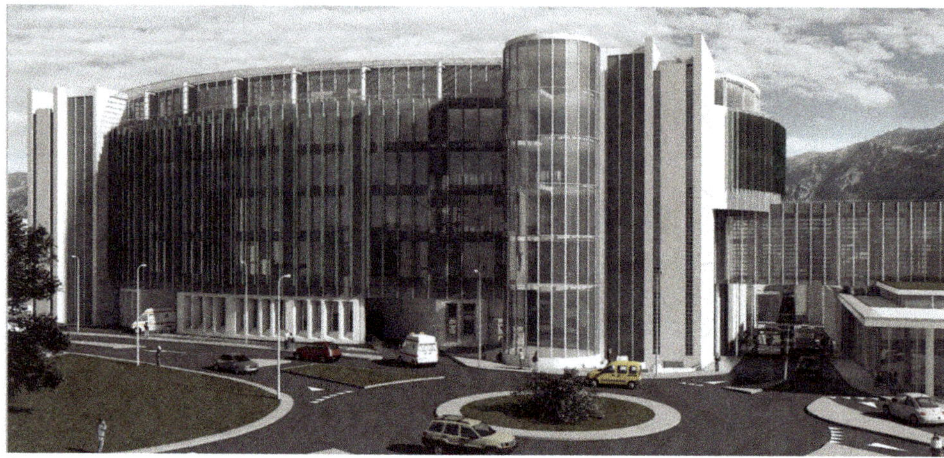

Figure 11. Parini Hospital, the new emergency entrance.

sibility to the hospital precinct, limited his social appeal.

The Hospital is axially placed along the historic road and it is the center point of a hierarchy of routes: pedestrian, mechanized, fast flowing as well as being fully integrated with local services, mobility and transport. The Client's Masterplan included: an extensive renovation of the existing Mauriziano hospital, a new expansion for the critical and emergency department, a car park underneath the new hospital. The Masterplan did not take into account that the proposed reorganization implied a critical extensive refurbishment of the old Mauriziano Hospital and, above all, closing the historical axis of viale Ginevra, disrupting the existing road system. The proposed project principles reorganized these masterplan's shortfalls and proposed a three hub layout divided for intensity of care. The three hubs house: the high intensity, the low intensity and Mother and Child centre. An important consequence of this arrangement is that it allows to keep Viale Ginevra open, restating the hospital as a pivotal urban and social node. The old Mauriziano Hopital works as 12H-Hospital with day hospital, clinics, support services. The new Parini Hospital operates as the 24H-Hospital.

The city services - such as shops, caffetteria, pharmacist, newsagent - are brought inside the hospital and housed in the "hospital street" that is conceived as an urban thoroughfare with activities and services for the Community (Figure11).

In conclusion, we must be increasingly aware that our "historical and cultural heritage" has limited resources that, once destroyed or damaged, cannot be replaced any more. It is therefore fundamental to develop different design approaches that span from urban redevelopment, through adaptive reuse, to refurbishment with a new use or type of care focus.

Choosing the appropriate approach in response to the typological potentials of each facility is a central theme involving aspects of multifaceted sustainability, that means considering not only energy matters, but also apparently far apart topics, such as the enhancement of cultural identity and of human and economic resources for a cost value national health service.

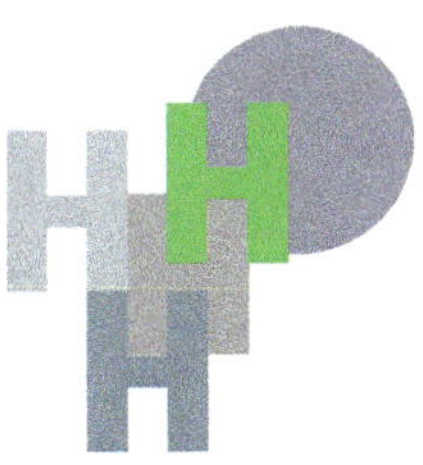

Sustainable Design, Architecture and Engineering

Session Introduction

The hospital presents a series of issues related to the sustainability of the choices made at different stages of the design phase, from planning to use, involving several management aspects such as building and design services, maintenance, medical equipment, patient care and staff satisfaction.

These issues are common throughout the world and therefore the exchange and sharing of knowledge should be encouraged through a network of experts on this subject consisting of architects, engineers, academics and scientists.

Designers and planners should know how to optimize the site's resources in an attempt to exploit the characteristics of the site to reduce energy consumption and encourage the use of local materials, orienting the building in order to maximize the collection of solar energy and take advantage of natural ventilation.

All measures taken to promote natural light in the different hospital environments should be accompanied and balanced by an assessment of the cooling solutions. Any decisions related to energy cost reduction should not compromise health, comfort, or staff efficiency in the hospital.

Specifically, in order to make choices concerning the reduction of energy consumption in hospitals, it is necessary to observe how the equipment is used and which control and savings strategies can be adopted while maintaining high quality treatment. It is also necessary to consider the possibility of using integrated systems for storing and distributing the energy produced, focusing on methods and possible layouts.

The sustainability of the design choices affects the building and the whole urban area where the complex is located, and the concept of sustainability must be extended to also consider how the hospital is integrated with the city through the incorporation of leisure, sports and recreational facilities.

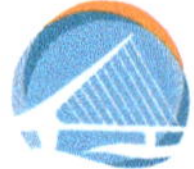

Green Hospitals Worldwide, Global Green and Healthy Hospitals - A Global Network Accelerating Sustainability in Health Care

Scott Slotterback[1], Javier Sartorio[2], Maria Della Rodolfa[3], Humberto da Mata[4]

sslotterback@hcwh.org, javier.sartorio@gmail.com, mariadellarodolfa@saludsindanio.org
[1]Policy Director, Global Green and Healthy Hospitals Health Care Without Harm
[2]Architect, Partner of AFS Architects and Professor, University of Buenos Aires
[3]Head of Programs for Salud sin Daño / Health Care without Harm Latin America
[4]Utility Engineering Manager, Hospital Sírio-Libanês, Brazil

Do you have a difficult health care sustainability problem to resolve when you are designing, building a hospital or managing a hospital's operations? Imagine posing your problem to a community of health care sustainability experts - architects, engineers, academics and scientists- from around the world. Imagine them helping you solve your problem and hospitals working on similar issues offering you examples of how they addressed them. You are imagining the Global Green and Healthy Hospitals (GGHH) network and its online global community GGHH Connect.

At a moment when the twin crises of public health and the environment are merging and building on one another, we need to come together and help each other resolve these challenges by reducing the environmental footprint of our health care institutions. GGHH is providing the tools and resources needed to facilitate these changes.

This distinguished panel will illustrate how this international network of health care providers, hospitals, health ministries, health systems and sustainability experts are joining forces to rapidly accelerate a comprehensive ten-part sustainability agenda by collaboratively engaging the health sector to promote sustainability in hospitals on every continent.

***Scott Slotterback** co-leads GGHH and authored numerous sustainability case studies, white papers, articles, and presentations and co-authored the Green Guide for Healthcare.*

***Javier Sartorio**, Architect with expertise in Sustainable Architecture. Partner of AFS Architects, specialized in Healthcare design since 1970, and Professor in the University of Buenos Aires.*

***Maria Della Rodolfa** Medical Doctor Degree granted by the University of Buenos Aires. Since 2005 Head of Programs for Salud sin Daño /Health Care Without Harm Latin America.*

***Humberto da Mata**, Utility Engineering Manager at Hospital Sírio-Libanês. He is a Mechanical Industry Engineer and has further development in health sector management.*

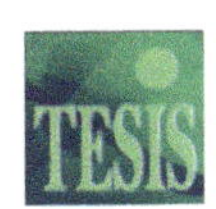

We are living in a moment in which the twin crises of public health and the environment are merging, the confluence of the two magnifying the destructive power of each. Climate change, chemical contamination, and unsustainable resource use are all exacerbating ill-health the world over. These environmental health problems are increasing pressure on, and eroding the capacity of, already thinly stretched health care systems.

Meanwhile, the health sector itself is paradoxically contributing to these very environmental health problems, even as it attempts to address their impacts. Through the products and technologies it deploys, the resources it consumes, the waste it generates and the buildings it constructs and operates, the health sector is a significant source of pollution around the world, and therefore an unintentional contributor to trends that undermine public health. Yet the converse is also true. While there is a confluence of crises, there is also a growing convergence of solutions that foster both public health and environmental sustainability, pointing the way toward a greener, healthier future.

The Global Green and Healthy Hospitals Agenda builds on the good work happening around the world, facilitating the exchange sustainability knowledge that can be replicated by thousands of hospitals and health systems in a wide range of countries and health settings.

A project of Health Care Without Harm, the Global Green and Healthy Hospitals Network (GGHH) serves as a virtual community for hospitals and health systems seeking to implement GGHH Agenda Goals by charting progress in achieving measurable outputs, while sharing best practices and finding solutions to the challenges they share.

Health Care leaders on every continent representing thousands of hospitals are participating in GGHH to dramatically accelerate their sustainability efforts. These efforts focus on 10 GGHH Agenda Goals: Energy; Water; Buildings; Waste; Leadership; Chemicals; Transportation; Food; Pharmaceuticals; Purchasing.

This paper focuses on four key goals focused on the built environment: Energy; Water; Buildings; Waste.

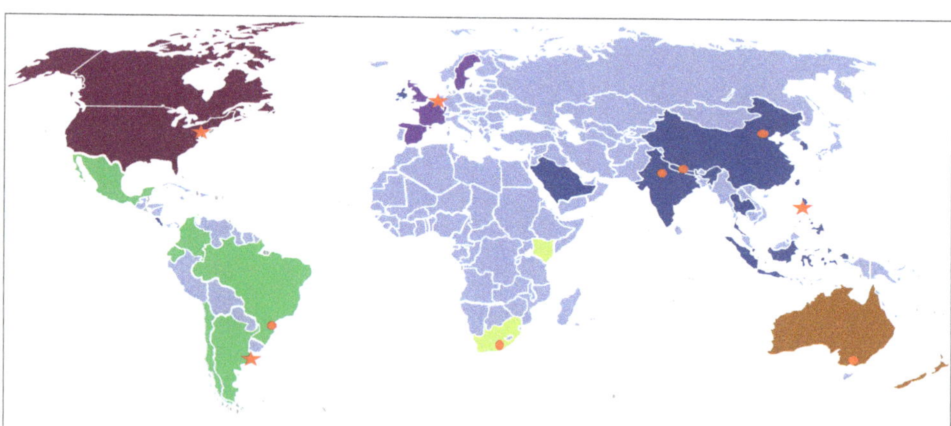

Figure 1. A worldwide community: Global Green and Healthy Hospitals (GGHH).

Energy

Most of the environmental and public health harm produced by energy consumption is from the combustion of fossil fuels, such as oil, coal and gas. The emissions generated from fossil fuel combustion are major contributors to global climate change and local health problems. GGHH members are reducing fossil fuel energy use and improving public health. They achieve this through energy efficiency improvements and renewable energy use. In addition, they expand their positive environmental impact by sharing their successes with other health systems and hospitals around the world.

An example of an innovative energy saving solution is integrated energy conservation approach used in the design of the new Sanatorio Finochietto in Argentina.

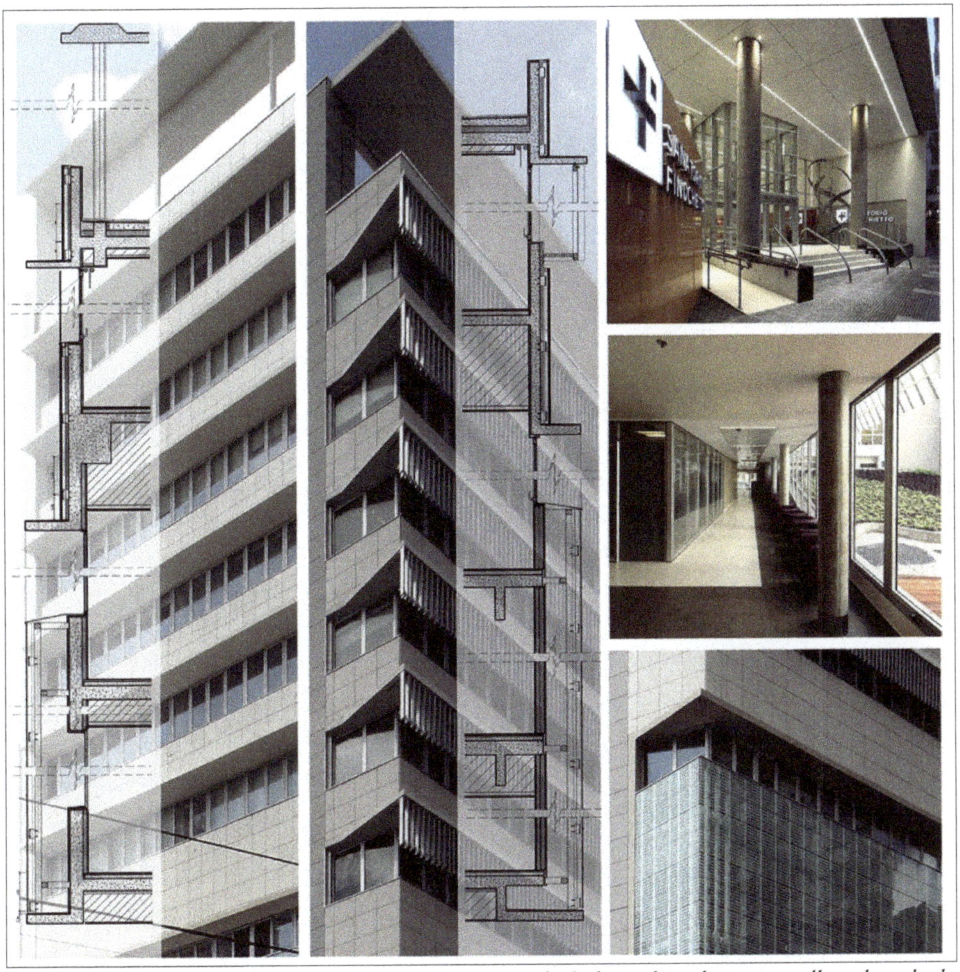

Figure 2. Sanatorio Finochietto, Buenos Aires, Argentina: thick thermal insulation in walls and sunshades and a ventilated façade system.

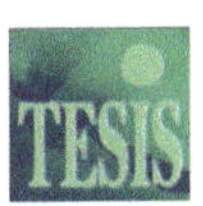

Sustainability was one of the fundamental pillars for the concept and design of the new "Sanatorio Finochietto". Both the architectural and mechanical design were central to the environmental performance of the design: a communion between comfort & humanization and efficiency & technology. The facade was designed to be responsive to site orientation and Buenos Aires climatic characteristics and solar radiation, as well as, interior spatial distribution, visual access to the exterior environment, use of natural lighting, color and warm finishes. Along with the façade, several sustainable roof gardens or green roofs, aim to achieve high levels of user comfort while optimizing the passive energy performance of the building.

The use of thick thermal insulation in walls and ceilings, air infiltration control, sealed double glazed aluminum framed windows with thermal breaks, eaves, sunshades and a ventilated facade system in sectors with direct solar exposure, work together to ensure the efficiency of the thermal shell of the building. Additionally, the air conditioning system incorporates innovative solutions such as heat recovery VRV, water condensed systems supplemented with geothermal interchange and heat exchange between the exhausts, and fresh air inlets. All artificial lighting is low energy or LED.

All facilities are supervised and controlled by a programmable and automated smart system that can be customized in order to lower energy consumption and, at the same time, ensure permanent control of the operation and maintenance expenditure.

In addition to energy conservation measures, Potable water use was minimized through dual flush toilets, robotics activated systems and reuse of condensate water and rainwater for toilet flushing.

Water

Availability of potable water is an increasing issue around the world. This lack of fresh water coupled with a lack of sanitation infrastructure is a major problem that directly impacts hospitals and health care systems.

Many GGHH member hospitals are implementing water-conserving fixtures in their new and existing facilities and developing treatment and reuse systems to significantly reduce their fresh water consumption and reduce costs.

An example of an innovative wastewater treatment and reuse system is the system developed for the Hospital Sirio-Libanes in Brazil.

The Hospital Sirio-Libanes project provides treatment for the greywater originated in the sinks, showers and urinals for reuse in the toilet bowls, cooling towers and vegetated areas of the hospital (project was implemented in the new towers constructed in the hospital).

The system employs customized technology developed exclusively for the Hospital project, using a system that separates organic material by flotation with subsequent ultrafiltration, providing ultra-filtered reusable water without suspended solids and biological material.

The project results in significant fresh water conservation and cost savings.

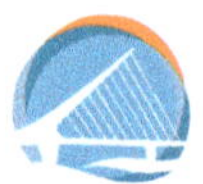

With the flow of reuse water of up to 10 m^3/h, the system is projected to save approximately 90,000 m^3 of water per year. The pay back, including cost reduction with water and sewer, will be around R$ 650,000/year (approximately US$280.000) and the financial return on investment breaks-even within 12 months. Considering that the increase in water rates and sewer at estate of São Paulo (Brazil) is always greater than the inflation associated with the cost of the system, the savings tend to be even higher over the years.

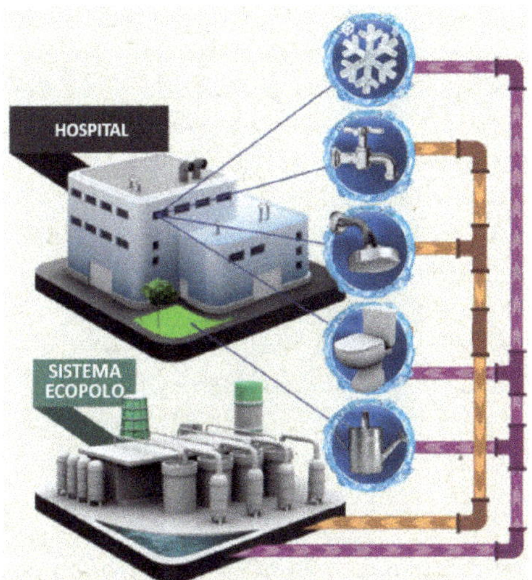

Figure 3. Treatment/reuse of greywater, Hospital Sirio-Libanes, São Paulo, Brazil.

Buildings

The built environment influences health. A host of contemporary environmental health problems - climate change, toxic pollution, biodiversity loss and more - can be linked to the production and maintenance of the built environment.

As development accelerates, the production of buildings becomes more resource intensive, stressing local and bioregional building material supplies and methodologies beyond their sustainable capacities. Buildings have a huge environmental health footprint. The UN Environment Programme estimates that global building-related activities may be responsible for up to 40 percent of carbon dioxide releases.

Site planning significantly impacts achieving a high performance building. Coordinating solar orientation of the building, and other environmental factors, with the design of the building envelope in conjunction with heating, cooling, lighting and shading systems is fundamental to optimizing passive design. It also contributes to minimizing the building's energy demand, while providing natural ventilation, daylight, shade, and thermal comfort.

The massing of the building and depth of the building footprint also has significant impacts on the effectiveness of passive systems, especially the integration of daylight. While this often can be accommodated in an office building, it is a particularly challenging in hospitals, where there are patient privacy considerations and crucial programmatic adjacencies. Due to these complexities, these factors need to be evaluated very early in the design of the hospital using in integrated team approach where the Architects and Engineers are able to openly discuss the opportunities and constraints to optimize the design.
Integrating the design of the building façade with the heating, cooling and lighting systems is essential to the success of

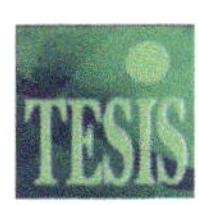

the passive systems and optimizing the buildings energy performance and the comfort of its inhabitants. By integrating building exterior envelope design and mechanical systems, hospitals can realize significant savings, like those demonstrated in the Sanatorio Finochietto project discussed in the Energy section.

Waste

The World Health Organization has published Core Principles describing safe and sustainable healthcare waste management as a public health imperative and calling on all associated with it to support and finance it adequately. A United Nations Human Rights Commission Special Rapporteur has called for "the development of a comprehensive international legal framework aimed at protecting human health and the environment from the adverse effects of improper management and disposal of hazardous medical waste." GGHH members seek to protect public health by reducing the volume and toxicity of waste produced by the health sector, while implementing the most environmentally sound waste management, recycling and disposal options.

Optimizing waste management often is largely influenced by operational protocols. However, the design of waste management systems can be particularly important when reducing the toxicity of waste. The treatment of medical waste has historically involved incineration, a significant contributor to environmental emissions. Incineration has been found to be a major contributor to carbon dioxide and dioxin emissions and a source of health risks to communities in areas where they are used. Alternative treatment technologies operate at high temperatures to sterilize the waste. These temperatures supply the necessary treatment and disinfection of infectious and medical waste without the physical and chemical changes of combustion, gasification and pyrolysis that produce such hazardous byproducts.

Conclusions

The health sector should not need to argue that delivering high quality healthcare requires a passport for waste and energy intensity. Indeed, the healthcare sector is in a pivotal position to lead the twenty-first century reintegration of environment, health, and economic prosperity. By critically reinventing the hospital as a regenerative place of healing, and participating in worldwide collaboration, the healthcare sector can signal a new relationship to healing and health and create green hospitals.

Mozambique. The Paradox of a Green Clinic in the Heart of a Coal Mine

Gonzalez Nagel, Joao Athayde Melo

ernesto.gonzalez.nagel@gmail.com

Project: Clinic for preventive examinations and emergencies within the coalmine exploitation. The project is located in the Vale coalmine in northern Mozambique. The company is questioned throughout the world for environmental damage created by coal mining. But when we read the documents and the same goals, seem dedicated to saving the environment. The documents of the company is used by the authors to justify the implementation of a project of a green building using local materials being extracted and the mine (stone, wood, coal), systems passive climatic control (orientation, building microclimate, wind control, burial buildings, water harvesting and use thereof for humidification) and Green Technology (tubes use of geothermal energy, capturing sunlight, etc.). The project tests a compact scheme differentiated circulation, minimizing the movement of technicians.

Ernesto González Nagel. *Architect, born and graduated in Rosario, Argentina, coursed a PHD in Barcelona, Spain, with 25 years of experience, 20 of those in Mozambique working mostly for the Ministry of Health. He passed for all the building processes in Mozambique, from project, to building direction, elaboration and evaluations of tender for building and service contracts, management of building supervision consultancy and planning for the Health Education Systems. His work lead to the creation of a Technical Implementation Unit for the European Union and the French Cooperation. He mapped and analyzed the health system of 5 provinces. He presented papers in two international Hospital Congresses.*

The Location

Moatize, Tete Province, northern Mozambique, southern Africa, coordinates 16°10' south, 33°43' east. 13 km from the capital of the province, the city of Tete, located on the border of the Zambezi River that crosses Africa from Angola to the Indian Ocean.

The Site

At the headquarters of an open-air coalmine, next to pre-existing management offices, and close to workshops and food hall. The existing buildings have a bad orientation in relation to the sun path, insufficient natural ventilation and natural lighting, which requires the use of an in-

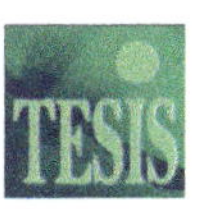

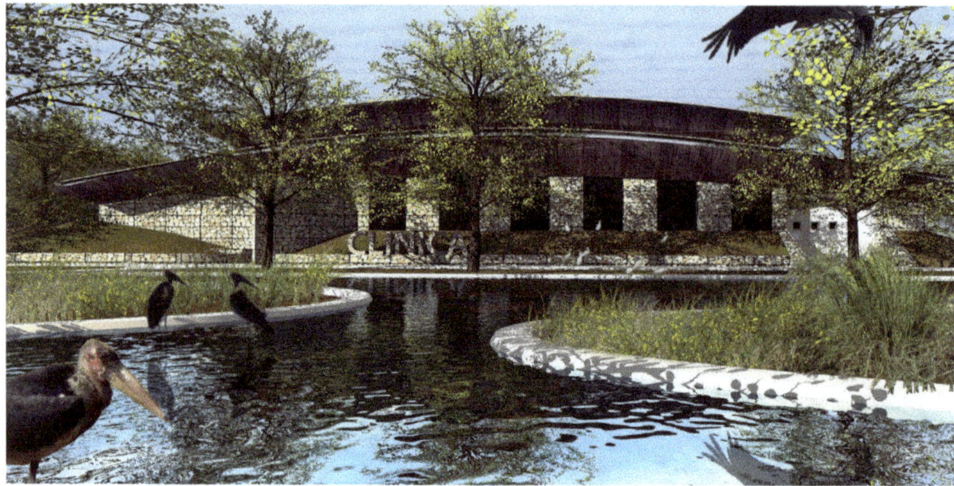

Figure 1. The clinic.

efficient air conditioning system and the use of artificial light all day long. The site lacks a proper Master Plan to organize the circulations and functions. There are no covered circulations paths for the connection of the buildings. According to a sustainability study done by the University of Maputo, it is recommended that, in Tete province, the longest façades of the buildings are along an axis almost perpendicular to north (with an inclination of 7° towards East). The prevailing winds come from the East, where the open air coal mining is located (Figure 2).

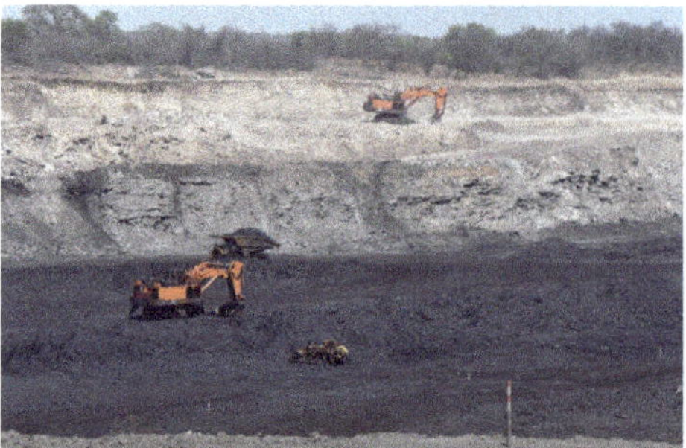

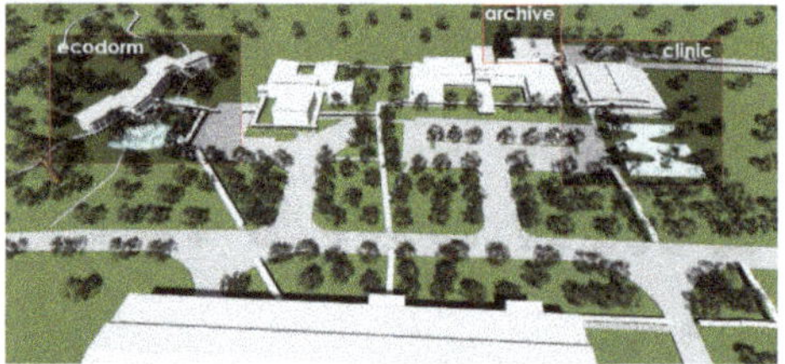

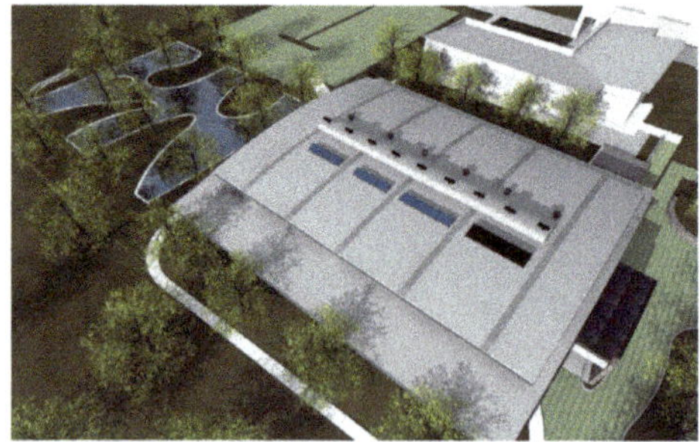

Figure 2. The site.

The Climate

Harsh dry tropical with a rainy season. Considered vulnerable to desertification. The average annual temperature is 26ºC, with average maximum of 36ºC and minimum of 15ºC. There was record maximum of 45ºC. In the rainy season it falls 620 mm in 5 months and in the dry season it only falls 48 mm. The UV index reaches to 11 in 8 months of the year.

THE CLIENT AND USER

Tete province has the largest coal reserve of the world with its 2.4 billion tons. Our client company provides for the extraction of 11 million tons/year investing 5 billion US dollars in 5 years. The marketed policy of the company sets guidelines and principles for the sustainable development action of the projects and operations, articulated with social, economic and environmental responsibility. The users are the staff of the mine, forecast of 3,000 workers (Figure 3).

THE PROGRAM

A clinic for the personnel working in the mine-oriented permanent control of lung health and hearing, areas mostly affected by this type of work. The clinic has an emergency sector to respond to possible accidents, only to stabilize the patient for evacuation to a main hospital. An area for the maintenance of the protection masks was added to the program: administration; pulmonology; otorhinolaryngology; general practice; emergencies; occupational hygiene; treatment of masks; technical services.
The program is adjusted to the final size of the compound and is not expected to grow.The projects of a dorm for personnel who work in shifts and a technical archive, where done at the same time of the clinic.

THE FUNCTIONAL PROPOSAL

There are 3 types of traffic clearly segregated: public, restricted and technical. The technical circulation is in the shape of a cross. The u-shaped public and restricted circulations embrace the cross to East and West and work simultaneously as waiting courtyards.
The consultation rooms of the linear buildings have technical access from one side and public access from the other.
The first floor has the administration and occupational hygiene.
The area of consultation lies to the east side, accessible from the existing main street and parking area. The emergency services lie to the west, accessible from a street created for this purpose (Figure 4).

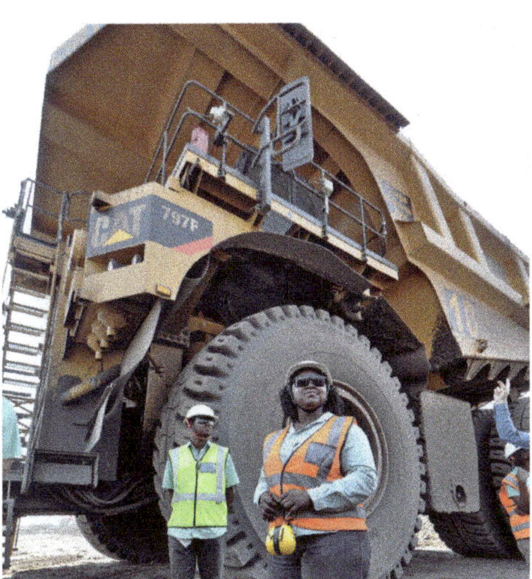

Figure 3. The client and the end users (photo António-Henrique Silva).

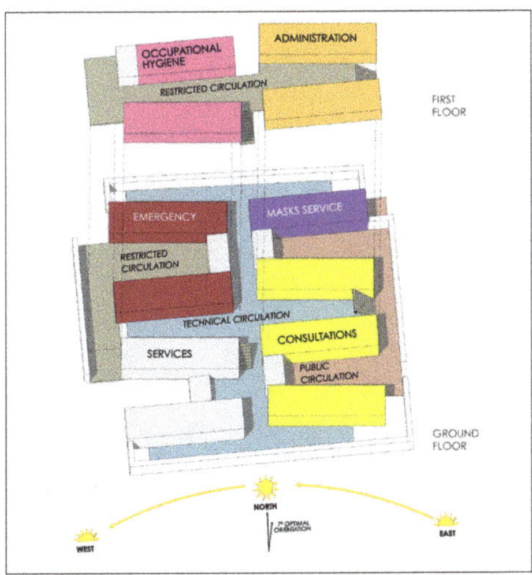

Figure 4. The functional proposal.

The Fire

To counteract the adverse climate, mostly hot and dry, it is proposed to create patios with a moist and cool microclimate.
To have a highly efficient relation to the sun path, most of the buildings are oriented along east west axis, perpendicular to the North or with a recommended tilt of 5º to the East. There's a wide roof, covering the buildings and courtyards, with some translucent parts to allow the growth of trees and leave a controlled natural light. In the patios and circulations, ponds with fountains were created to decrease the temperature with vaporization. The electrical power system combines the energy produced by photovoltaic panels and from the public grid, which is powered by the nearby Cahora Bassa dam, one of the largest in the world.
The "conventional" lighting system uses LED lamps. Besides the natural light from the windows, there´s a system that catches the sunlight on the roof and uses fiber optic to bring it to where ever it is necessary. This system allows you to control the incidence of the sun, to keep the twilight necessary to work with computer, is beneficial to the health and to grow plants within the work areas.

The Water

There´s an artificial lake located to the East, that harvests the majority of the annual rainfall, around 700,000 m3 of water. The lagoon was planned to have trees grown all around, preventing the evaporation and creating an ideal place to attract the rich local wildlife specially a wide variety of birds. The prevailing winds pass over the lagoon, which helps to cool and filter the particles of sand and coal in the air, before it passes through the clinic. The water of the lagoon feeds a cooling cascade and the ponds located in the inner courtyards (Figure 5).

The Air

The east winds spread the coal dust and dirt particles, exceeding the recommended rate for human respiration almost all year round with the exception of the rainy season. Excessive movement of air causes discomfort in dry climates (Figure 6). There´s a surrounding wall that protects the exterior covered spaces of the clinic, by directing the air up through a filter of thin braches of local timber and causing the precipitation of particles before entering the clinic area.

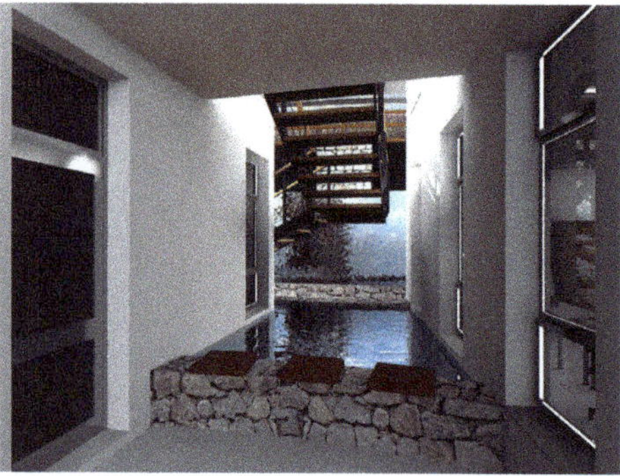

Figure 5. The water.

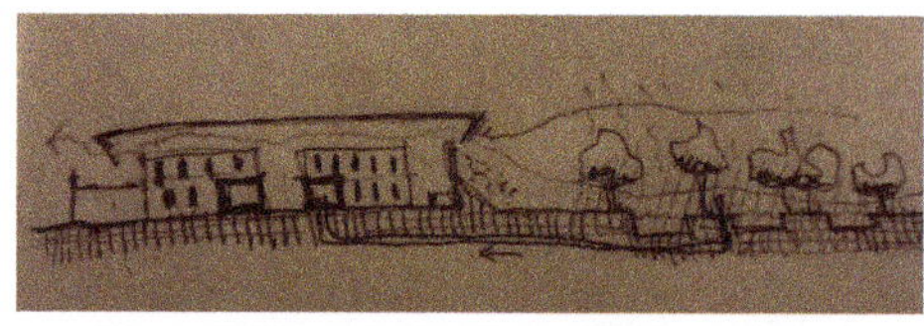

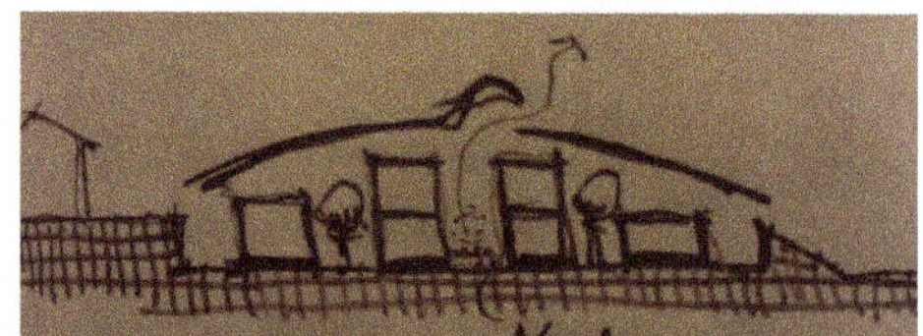

Figure 6. The air sketch.

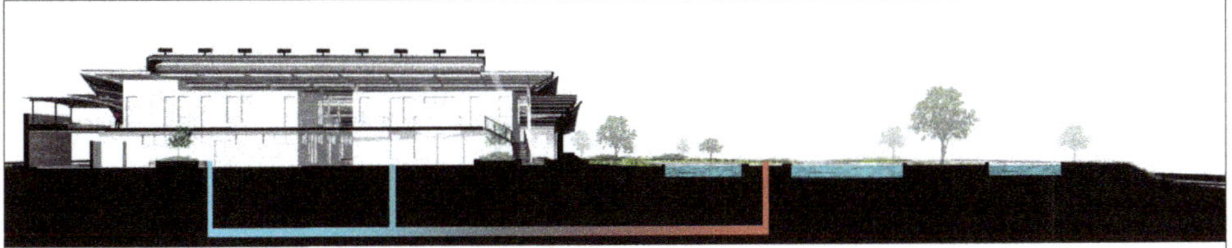

Figure 7. Clinic longitudinal section, earth pipes.

The shadow and the ponds cool down the air that ventilates the clinic. The roof that covers the courtyards and buildings has a central skylight and side openings that promote ventilation by convection, expelling the hot air up. The windows of the building go from floor to ceiling, with openings on top and bottom also promoting the convection of air, taking advantage of the air refreshed at the courtyards (Figure 8).

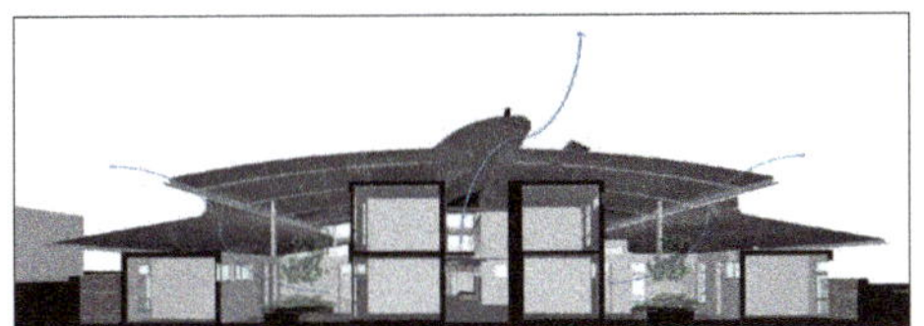

Figure 8. Clinic section, ventilation by convection.

There´s a earth pipe air cooling system that works by letting the air from the lagoon trees shadows, go to depth of 2 meters over 30 meters and naturally lower to the almost constant temperature of the earth ~15°C, and then redirect the cooled air to the buildings (Figure 7).

THE EARTH

Locally, the soil is used for the handcrafted burned brick. Stone is part of the structure and walls of most traditional buildings.

The process of open air coal mining involves the withdrawal of the extended surface of vegetation, soil and stone covering him.

These materials are used extensively in the clinic. It has stone gabions that protect the entire covered space. The walls of the buildings are made of bricks of soil-cement.

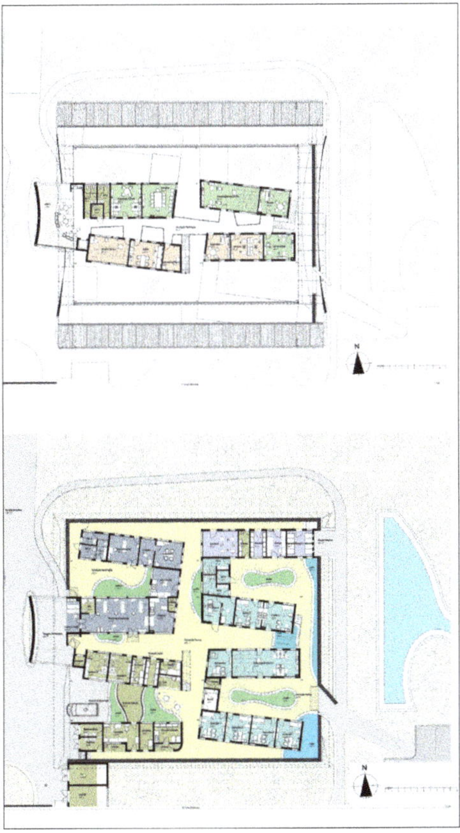

Figure 9. Plans.

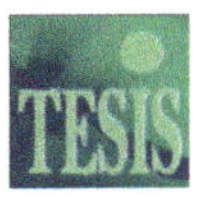

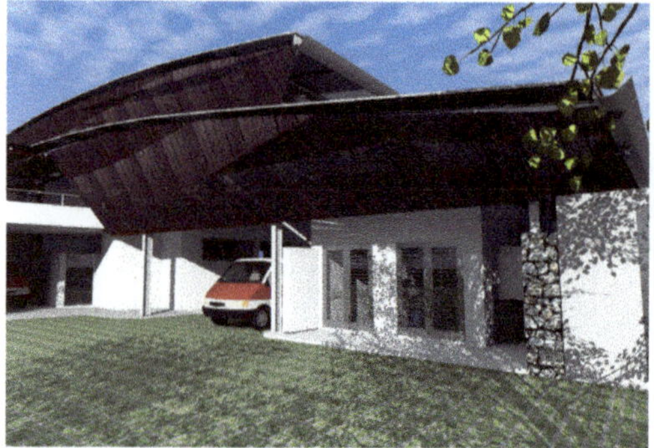

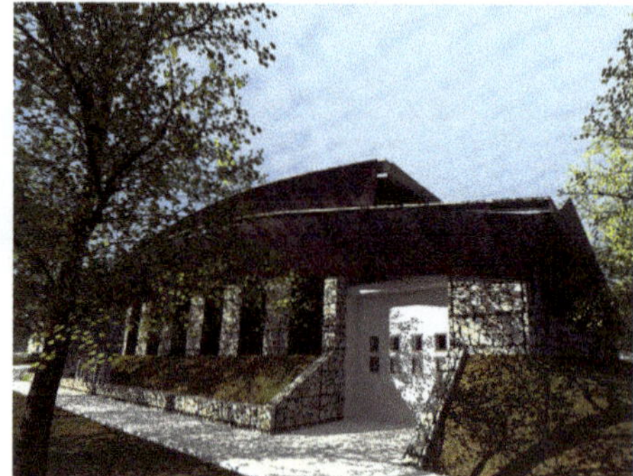

Figure 10. Emergency.

THE WOOD

Wood is traditionally used in wall structures, and also in roofs. The wood removed from the mining areas is used as a filter of air and light around the building.

THE SPACE

The clinic is located next to the administration building that was built on an artificial embankment of more than 2 meters. As a mean of passive climate control the clinic is partially dug into the embankment. A gabion wall closes all the covered outer space. Within this space, six buildings create four patios and the internal cross shaped circulation. The buildings layout of the buildings causes resistance to the undesired excessive movement of (hot) air.

The careful articulation of corridors and patios, under the shadow with water and vegetation, and where the air is more pure and fresh is used to make the clinic's space an integral instrument of preservation of health and wellbeing.

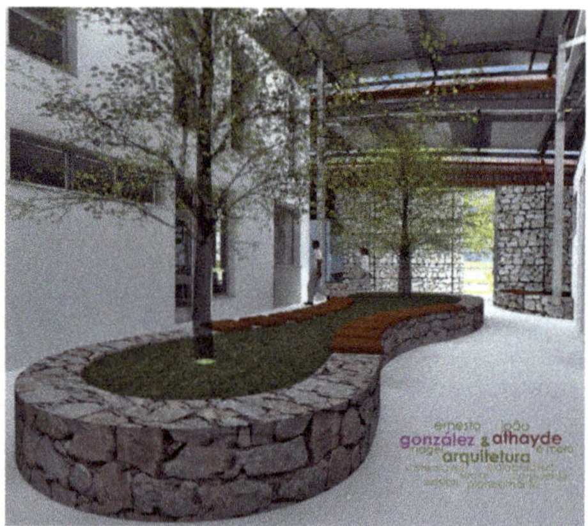

Figure 11. Patio.

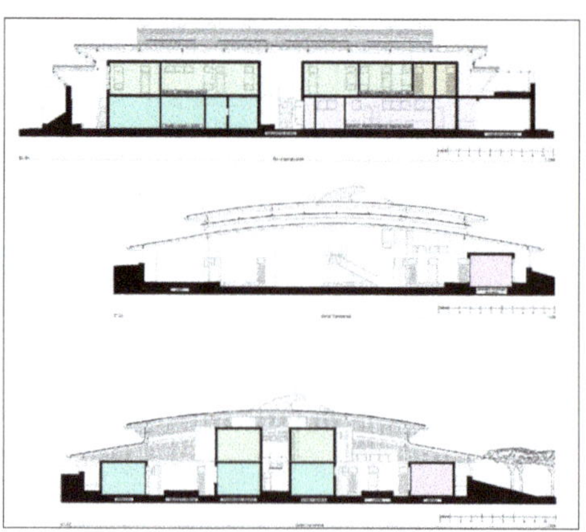

Figure 12. Sections.

Latin American Future in Hospital Design

Teresa Egozcue, Guillermo Vidal, Gabriela Pastorino, Simonetta Pozzolo

teresa.egozcue@evpp-arq.com.ar
ev+pp arquitectos – BEV s.a.

A lot has been said and written about the hospital of the future, evidence based design, use of templates, Lean and Sustainable Design, patient centered facilities, all concepts must be put in context when designing the Hospital of the Future in areas like South America, where the economies are not always blooming. That leaves us, health care designers, with a question: how do we achieve a balance and still design the Hospital of the future? Needless to say: a huge responsibility finding the equilibrium between high tech, costs, and local issues.

María Teresa Egozcue*. 1968 – School of Architecture, University of Buenos Aires. 1969/1979 – Urban regional Planning, SAP/SCA. Founder partner (1968) of ev+pp arquitectos –Egozcue Vidal + Pastorino Pozzolo-. The firm has been awarded multiple national and international prizes in public and private competitions, specializing in Health Care. National Pediatrics Hospital in Buenos Aires -104.000 m², Hospital Pedro de Elizalde–23.000 m², Centro de Imágenes moleculares de FLENI – 8.000 m². Recently a member of Triconsul, a multinational group awarded three major hospitals in Chile – 420.000 m². Egozcue twice elected President of the Consejo Professional de Arquitectura y Urbanismo CPAU–Professional Council for architecture and urbanism (2000 2004). Since 1988 has held different charges in the institution. She has been Professor at the University of Buenos Aires, School of Architecture, for more than 20 years. Currently she is a professor at the University of Belgrano.*

Introduction

In current times, hospital design needs to focus on performance initiatives that must be kept as essentials in the future. This is sometimes easier said than done. South America needs to consider a new generation of hospital design, that integrates a particular response to every site: orientation, climate, access roads, and the like. This new Design should also consider the use of template rooms, and systematize solutions in order to reduce time and costs. It must be based on a modular response with strategically located structural elements, vertical cores and shafts. At the same time, flexibility, expandable uses, growth are

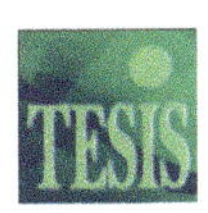

issues which must be taken into consideration, for they allow the hospital to be reconfigured according to local models, thus respecting the future users, both medical and patients. Last but not least, energy efficient buildings must be thought of and designed to allow for a better use of natural resources and a safer and better planet.

Hospitals do not only provide health care, they hold within programs related to research and development, education and training, thus changing cities, defining traffic flows, and walking paths. They may change inside, grow, expand, but it is unlikely that they will change location, at least in the short term. Our responsibility as health care designers is not only to the hospital, but to the city and its inhabitants. We need to consider all the parties whose life will in different ways be touched by our actions.

Project's efficiency, effectiveness, relevance, impact and sustainability. As planners and health care designers, these are some of the basic issues that need to be addressed. Achieving all of them will depend on costs, time and the ability of the designers to include them in designs which are more often lead by financial issues than anything else.

Local Environments and Security

Natural light, orientation, views towards open green areas, every location has a different perspective and a local flavor that has to be part of the equation when deciding on orientation and other energy saving issues.

Unbelievable though it may sound, Public Hospitals in South America tend to be subject to vandalism. Therefore, every effort made to generate clinical areas that can be segregated from the public is welcome. The concept is hard to understand for other cultures but it is a strong issue in these latitudes. Patients, visitors and staff are all part of the same hospital environment.

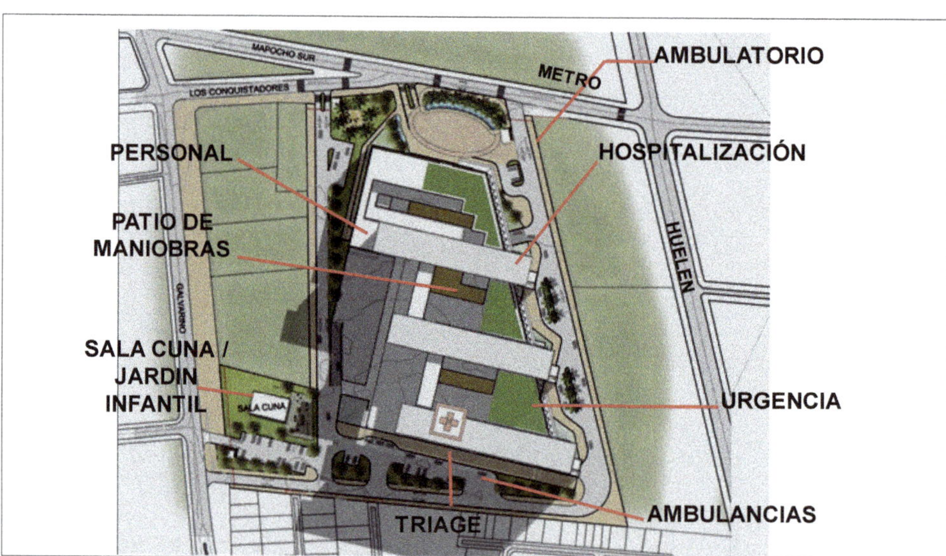

Figure 1. Context, Felix Bulnes - HFB, Chile.

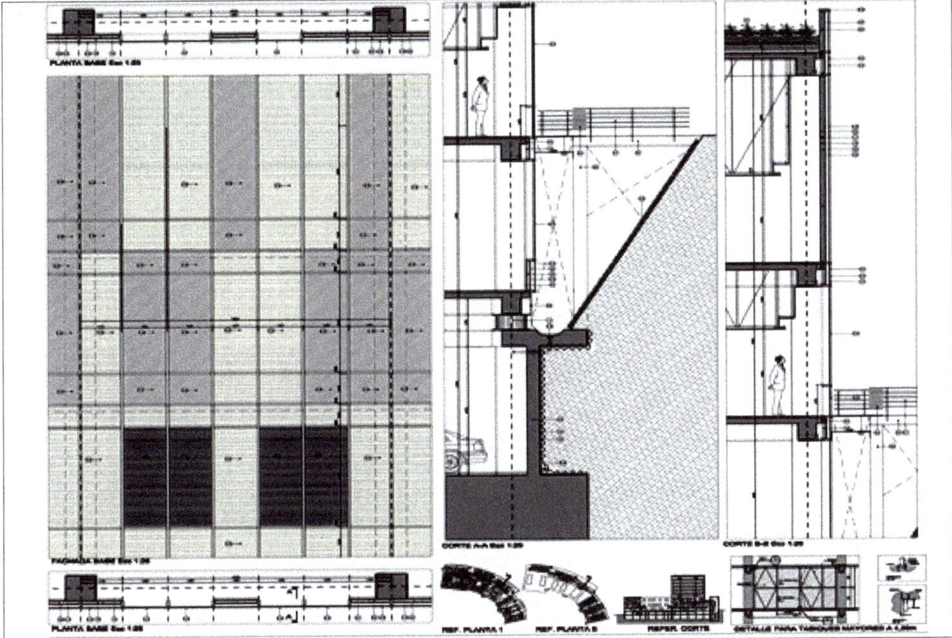

Figure 2. Scantlings, Sótero del Río - HSR, Chile.

Sustainable Design

Employing local materials, energy and water resources efficiently, and minimizing building and surrounding impacts are only some of the issues that need to be considered when designing the Hospital of the Future.

Some concepts have been around for a while, but in South America they have only been put into practice in the last years. Everything is new in Public operated hospitals, and therefore, there are a number of barriers that need to be pulled down, in order to move forward.

Green, efficient and sustainable buildings are all new concepts that people relate to conceptually, but are difficult to comprehend sometimes.

Value Engineering

For the past years, an effort has been made by all designers to reduce unnecessary costs, allowing for more cost / efficient buildings, which can provide the same services with reduced costs and functioning structures. Constructions, maintenance, operation, replacement are all items considered in the value engineering process and they all add to a better building with an enhanced life span.

Modular Buildings

The infrastructure should also walk side by side with new techniques. Larger bays, and floor to floor heights, easily adaptation to new infrastructure, flexibility. Modularity has always been the key to successful hospital design. Today,

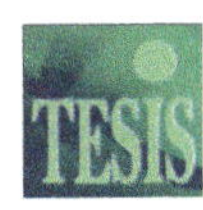

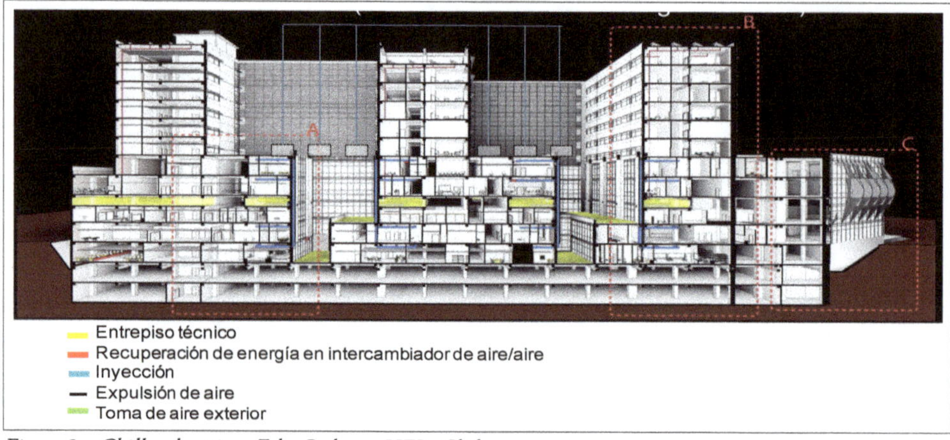

Figure 3. Chillers location, Felix Bulnes - HFB, Chile.

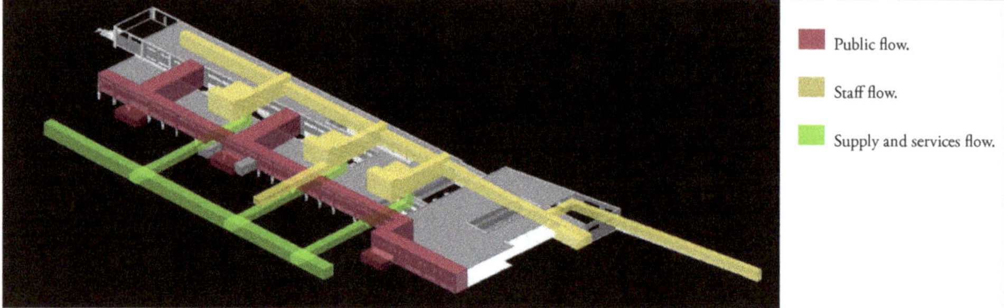

Figure 4. Flexibility circulation flows, Fleni – Centro de Imágenes Moleculares.

more than ever, it is the key that provides for future changes and adaptation. D&T areas can expand or change into other areas, provided modularity has been properly applied.

Flexibility

Between critical beds and ambulatory care. Not only the Hospital of the Future in South America will have to be prepared to accommodate both modalities, health care providers, nurses and doctors should be prepared as well. A change in infrastructure will have to be accompanied by a change in treatment types, and those changes should necessarily come from the different Ministries in charge.

Patient Rooms

It is still a local custom in South America to develop patient rooms for 3 or even 4 patients. In the last years this tendency has been dropping, changing into 2 or 1 patient bed. This issue is of course strictly connected to financing flows, and although evidence based design shows that individual rooms are much better, it is a huge economic difference changing to individual patient rooms. This is one of the challenges designers face.

Technology

Since most large scale hospitals in South America are Public, it is not always possible to define the technology at an early stage during the design phase. Governments are usually not able to consider this option: either they lack the funding or the ability to understand the complexity of the issue. Therefore as designers we need to make our best effort to provide for spaces and support for different models of the same equipment, knowing that by the time it is acquired, the design will be almost ready.

Template Design

More and more rooms must be considered as flexible as possible allowing from template rooms. These are spaces that are repetitive such as patient rooms, ORs, ambulatory care boxes, and others, that because they are repetitive efforts must be made to turn them into "templates".

Evidence Based Design

Case studies will be presented comparing results from a Children´s hospital designed in the 70s and one designed in the same city (Buenos Aires) and built in 2008. Not only for patients is the evidence based design useful. Improved staff recruitment, retention and performance of staff can also be measured in buildings with neat working environments. These environments must be able to stay friendly in the long run, at a logical cost.

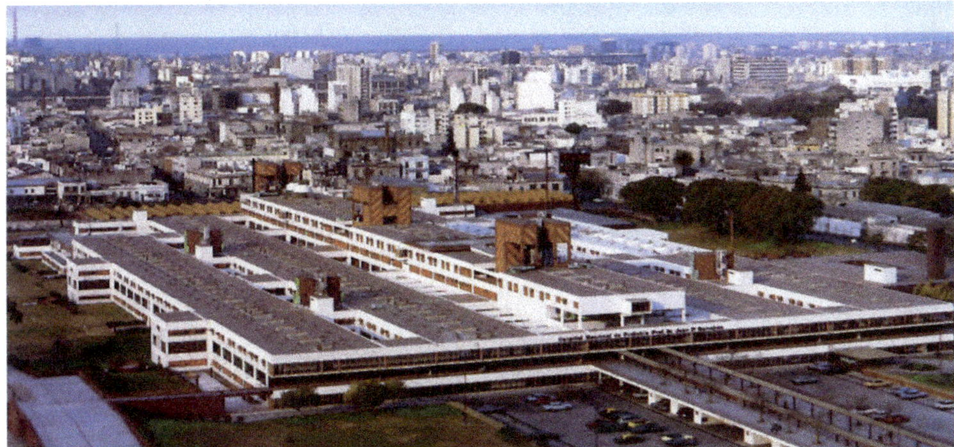

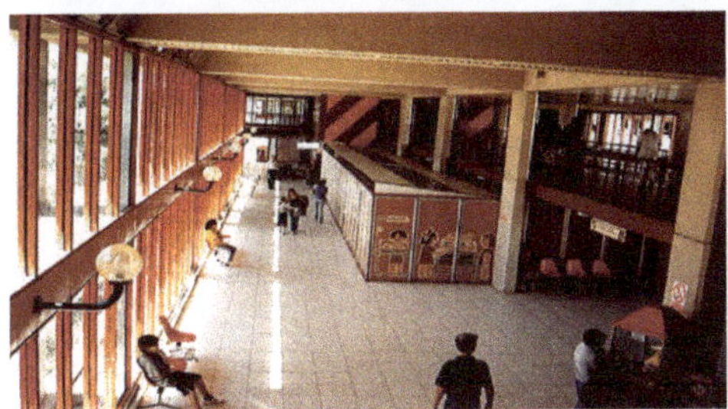

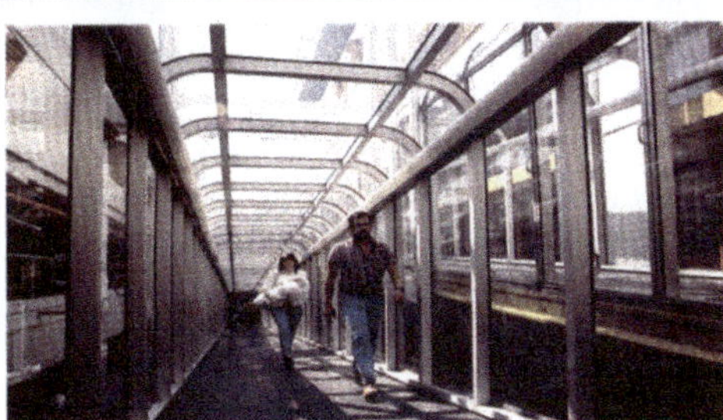

Figure 5. Hospital Nacional De Pediatria Dr. Juan P. Garrahan, Argentina.

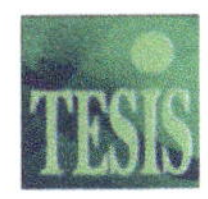

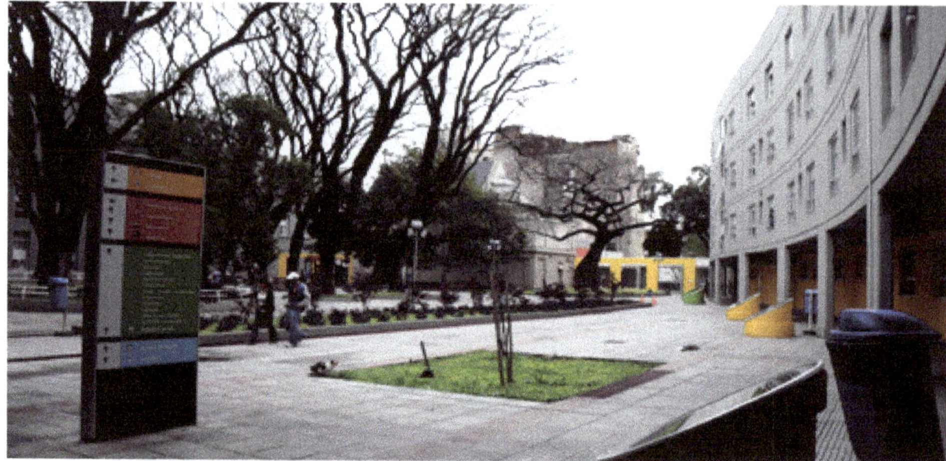

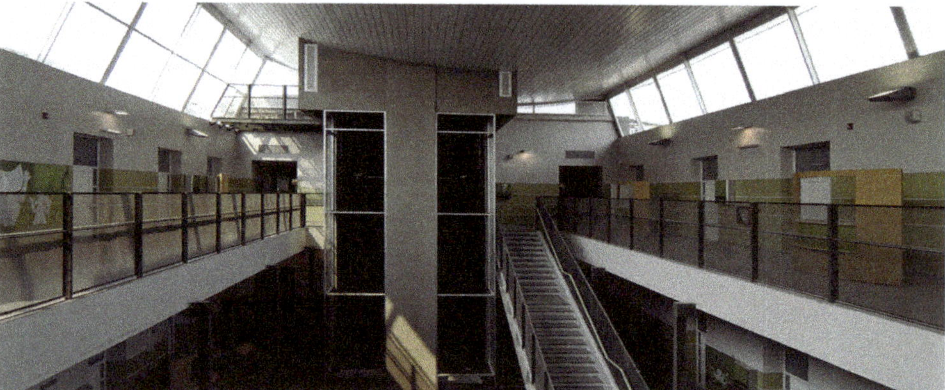

Figure 6. Evidence Based Design: Hospital General Dr. Pedro de Elizalde, Argentina.

Lean Design

Based on a waste free operational process, it is nowadays an important issue to be considered. Capital investments also impact on the hospital, allowing for positive practice environments to develop.

Concrete examples

Projects in Chile and Argentina of Figures 1-7 show the similarities and differences, context, scale and operating methodology.

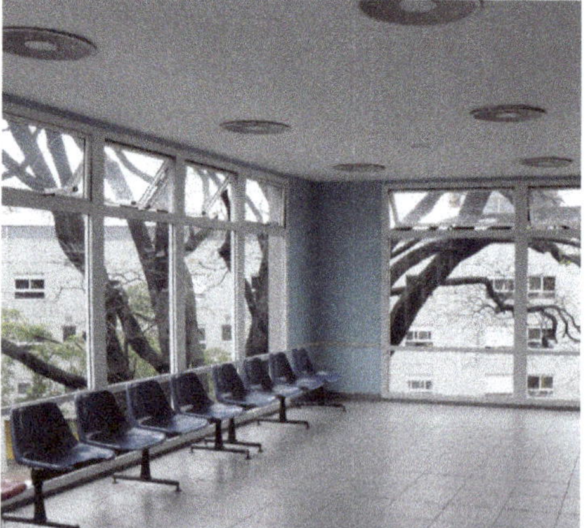

Figure 7. Vegetation and natural light: Hospital General Dr. Pedro de Elizalde, Argentina.

Regional Vision of a Local Hospital
New High Complexity Health Center Sunchales Santa Fe

Esteban Urruty, Alberto Marjovsky

estebanurruty@gmail.com
Marjovsklу-Urruty Arquitectos

This new High Complexity Health Center (CRAC Atilra) presents a new concept through a program that goes beyond the purely medical use since it integrates the hospital into the city through leisure, sports, health care and recreation units.

Esteban Roberto Urruty, *FADU, UBA. Study Partner Marjovsky-Urruty Architects. Former Professor of Design School at FADU- UBA. To deliver he has intensive experience as a presenter at Seminars and Conferences around the world and in Argentina. He is specialized in healthcare architecture since 1974 until now. Awards in different competitions and published in magazines, newspapers and books.*

Description of the Concept

The new Center CRAC Atilra is a project based on 4 pillars:
- family involvement;
- synergy between high complexity and humanized spaces;
- prevention and health education;
- integration with the community.

A health care hospital integrated into a sports centre provides a place to continue being physically active, overcoming a sense of confinement which sometimes have health center, as the patient establishes social bonds. This center would also prove useful for both hospital staff and visitors.

This kind of spaces are usually integrated as therapeutic gardens, sports medicine areas, fitness rehabilitation, occupational therapy, social spaces, sports and recovery zones.

Consequently, this integration of social and leisure spaces brings about an improvement in the quality of the patients care, together with the inclusion of their families and the reduction of waiting time which is the biggest hassles.

The whole project is based on this sort of duality: an amalgamation of sophisticated resources for the patients and the humanization of spaces.

This is a distinguishing feature and is achieved by placing the user - patient at the centre of all management policies and also the projective constitution of each service.

TESIS Inter-University Research Centre
Systems and Technologies for Social and Healthcare Facilities
University of Florence, Italy

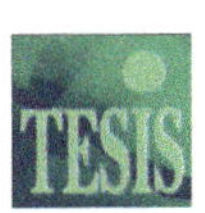

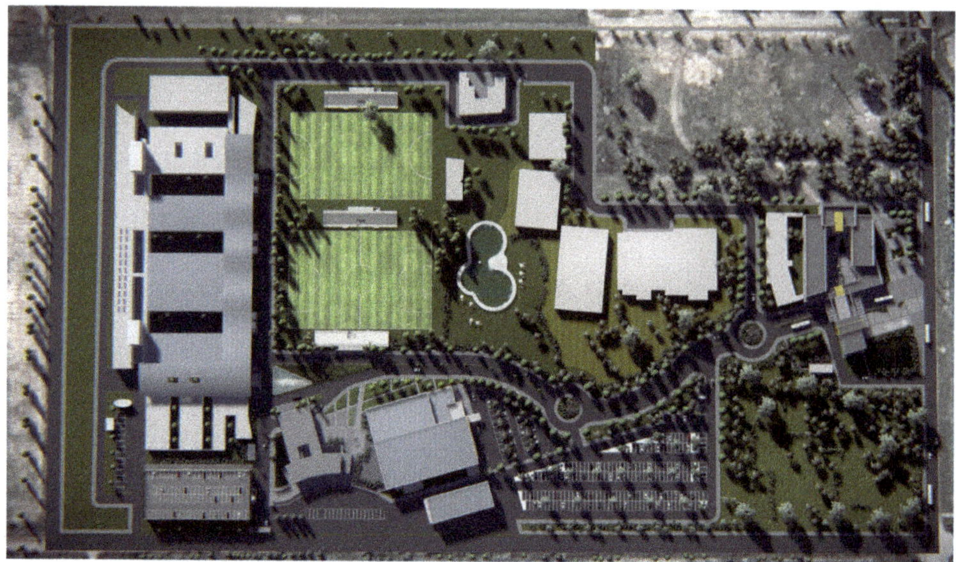

Figure 1. Complex aerial view, Center CRAC Atilra.

The party adopted is that of a "Systemic Hospital". This concept that emerges from the old "Pavilion Hospital" which may allow a clearer and a more efficient circulation and access to the different areas in the hospital.

The main advantage is that it will be possible to achieve a clearer differentiation of the areas together with a distinct separation between public and medical/ technical services. This will facilitate the user orientation inside the hospital by avoiding uncomfortable circulatory crosslink's. Additionally, this will result in the staff working more comfortably and efficiently.

A horizontal organization project was adopted following the concept of "Evolutionary Hospital" that allows a flexible architecture that can adapt to rapid changes in technology and medical practices.

The use of technical mezzanines located on the areas of greatest complexity giving a guarantee of efficiency and enables the hospital to changes.

In this project, the image is looked especially through the study of facades and cuts, reinterpreting the image of the Dairy Factory: tanks, chimneys and roofing felt recreate it. The choice of shapes, materials and colours emerges as modern thinking with contemporary styles and materials and technologies found in the region.

The idea of the Hospital placed back on the site as part of a collection of buildings dedicated to sports, cultural, commercial and institutional activities, is related to the boulevard with street access which connects directly to the city and thus forms part of a whole preventing an isolated building in the countryside

During the last 10 years there were great changes in the field of Health due to incorporation of new technologies and change of health care paradigms mak-

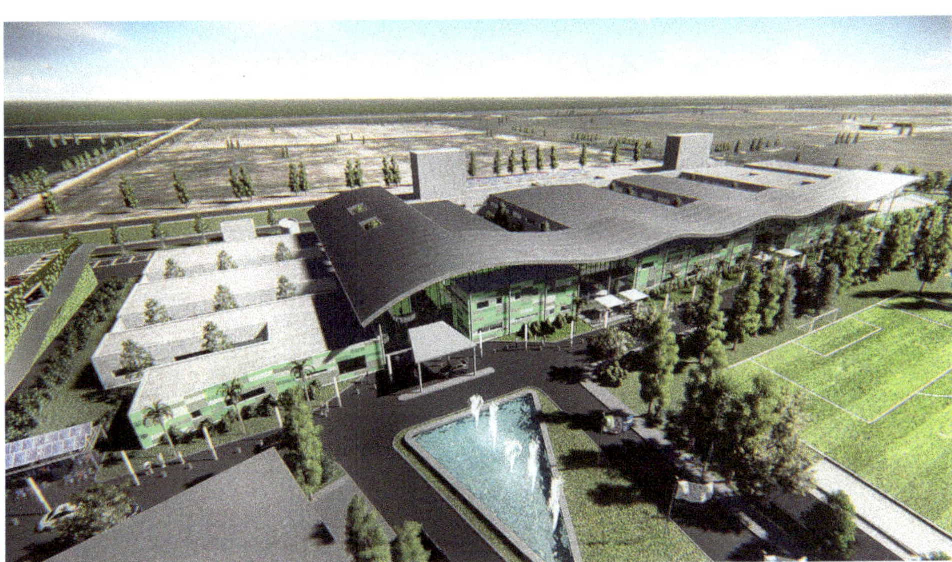

Figure 2. Principal CRAC Atilra.

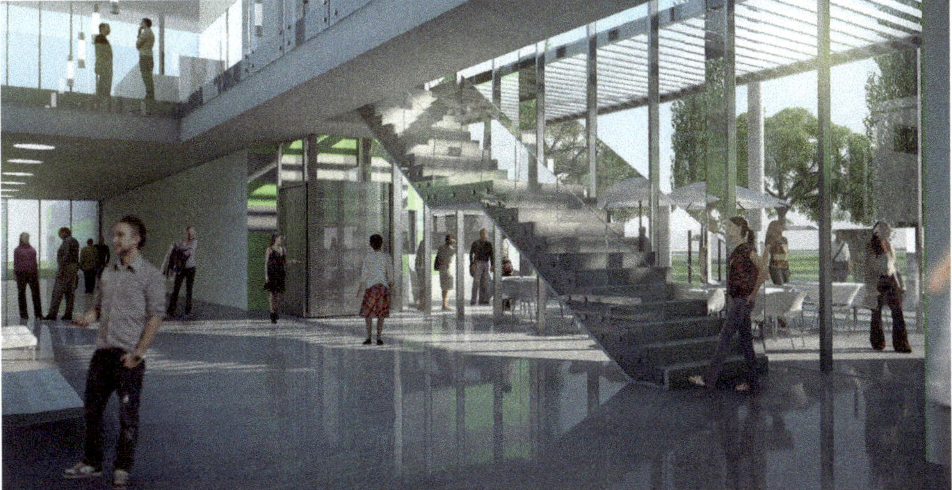

Figure 3. Interior street.

ing an impact on the design of hospital spaces.

As the chinese american arquitect Andrew Tang says: “There is a physician interested in having a well-designed environment and rearrange spaces to create a situation that also heal and reduce anxiety. Improving the patient environment creates a better place to heal. Being physically and visually exposed to nature reduces stress. Begin to appear glazed streets and courts. Become claustrophobic waiting rooms with wi-fi, bars, and shopping areas. It takes away the drama appears Hospital and spatial experience.”

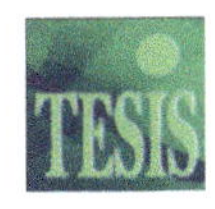

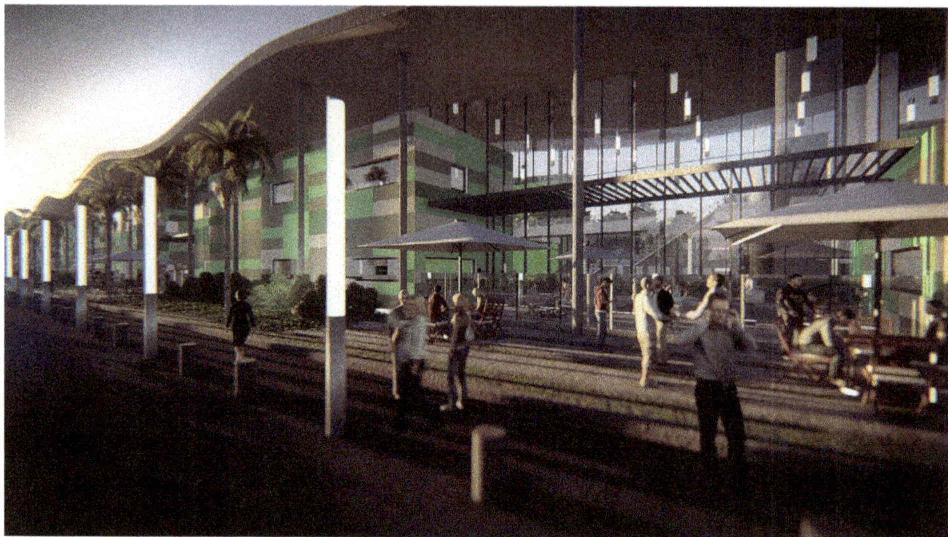

Figure 4. Front Street.

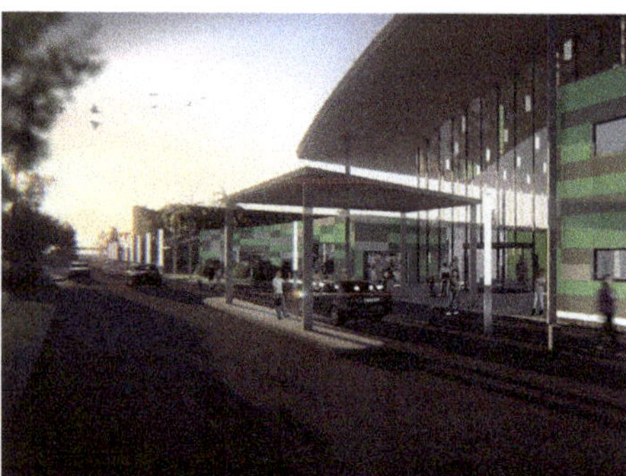

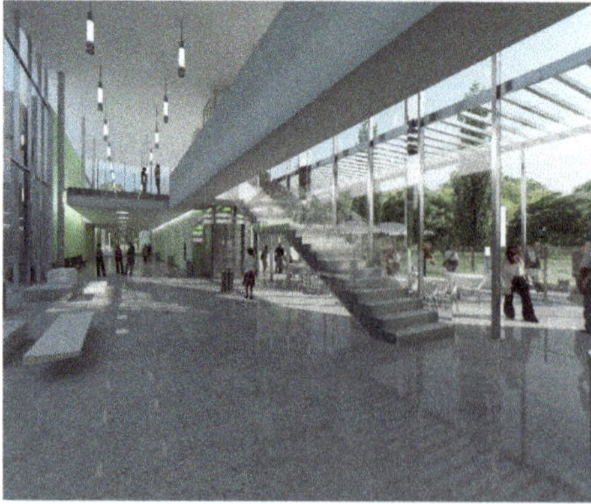

Figure 5. Integration between indoor and outdoor environments.

Taking these concepts, the idea of the great street covered as an integrating activity space and spatial relations, medical and non-medical .The large central space, brings together most of outpatient waits, sectored by specialty, with courtyards that create a rich interior -exterior, green relative to the field.

The contribution of light and outdoors is along the entire project in his capacity as integrating elements and healing time.
Mezzanines, courtyards, high ceilings, views from balcony, reinforce this idea of green indoor and outdoor integration. This project has been carefully maintained the "sustainability" and bioclimatic conditions in its architecture. For this purpose a study of technical advice in sustainable architecture was hired

Which trends foreshadowed 20 years ago, today are "assumptions of design".

The Sustainable Design of the New Sanatorio Finochietto, Comfort, Safety & Technology for the Human and Environmental Healthcare

Javier Sartorio

info@afs-arq.com.ar / javier.sartorio@afs-arq.com.ar
Estudio AFS Arquitectos

One of the main objectives in the design and construction of the New Finochietto Sanatorium was to apply sustainability criteria at all levels, from the conception of the business, programming, building and services design, function and operation, maintenance, medical equipment, patient care and staff satisfaction, among others. The architectural design was instrumental in integrating the different requirements in a consistent and successful proposal. It is the aim of this presentation to describe those design decisions, construction solutions and non-traditional thermo-mechanical, sanitary and electrical installation systems that were incorporated during the development of the project of this new health care building, with the purpose of optimizing energy efficiency, enhancing user comfort, and reducing environmental impact and consumption of non-renewable natural resources. Also, some problems or difficulties are mentioned that were encountered during the process, which can be further explored in future projects to provide new methods or solutions for the development of buildings of similar or better features in the local environment.

Javier Sartorio. *Architect, graduated from the University of Buenos Aires in 1995. With Posgraduate studies in Bioclimatic Design, Solar Architecture and Sustainability. Member of "Centro de Investigación Hábitat y Energía" and professor at undergraduate and graduate courses of the same University. Member from 1994 and partner from 2003 of Alvarado – Font – Sartorio Arquitectos, an architectural office with specialization in Healthcare architecture.*

Presentation

The New Finochietto Sanatorium was fully conceived as a sustainable institution. The building design is accompanied by a more general approach to sustainability that covers various aspects.

General approach

In an environment of rapid changes, it was decided to remain current for the next 20 or 30 years by means of the introduction of technology, based especially on an internal network of

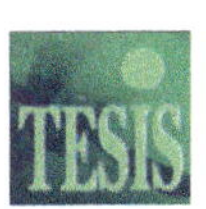

high capacity, flexibility and security. Rationality and economic viability determined the scale of the project, reaching an optimum capacity of 180 beds, and the technology was adapted to the scale and available resources. The total area per bed, less than 100 m², and the optimization of a highly functional circulatory scheme ensured high efficiency in the use of physical space.

Focused on the care of health, the whole design and the technological tools employed enhance patient safety and comfort, using unique patient identification systems, computerized preparation and supply of drugs, radio frequency systems for the control of hand washing and infection prevention on patients and newborns, and online registration on the patient's electronic medical history of parameters issued by medical equipment. Finally, care of the environment was also a priority in the configuration of building operation and maintenance strategies, including the elimination or reduction of the use of materials and equipment with toxic components such as mercury, impairing the use of disposable materials and imposing differentiated waste collection and disposal.

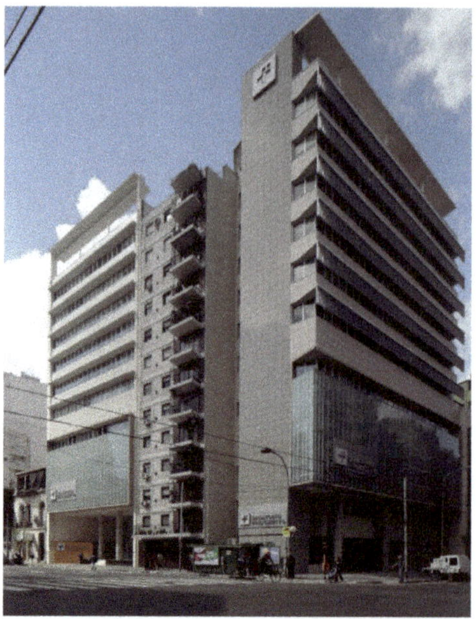

Figure 1. Main Façade, Córdoba Av. and Ecuador Street, New Sanatorio Finochietto - Buenos Aires.

Architectural and bioclimatic design

A primary objective was to reduce the undeniable impact of a health center in an urban area, while achieving a clear and safe functionality.

The new building's silhouette, 10 stories high, will assist in the creation of a friendly urban landscape, respectful of its setting by means of the volumetric conformation and the differentiated treatment and heights of its facades, significantly improving the pre-existing situation.

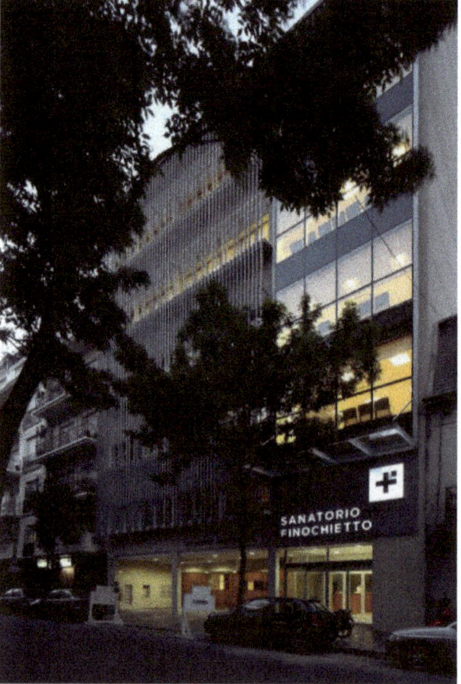

Figure 2. Outpatient entrance, Boulogne Sur Mer Street, NSF - Buenos Aires.

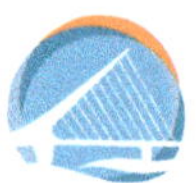

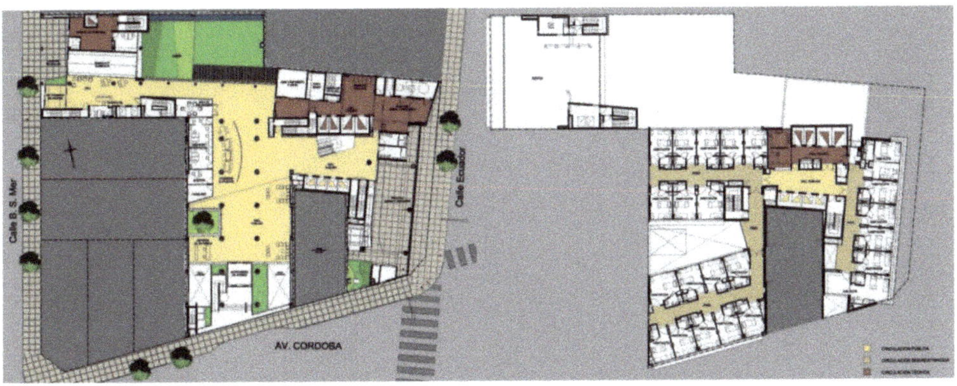

Figure 3. Ground floor plan (left) and inpatient typical floor (right), NSF - Buenos Aires.

The peculiar configuration of the site allowed for a neat differentiation between the main public access on Córdoba Avenue and the secondary entrances to the Outpatient Department on Boulogne sur Mer Street, or the ambulance, staff and suppliers access on both lateral streets.

Based on the strategic placement of the vertical circulation cores, a double public / technical circulatory network was designed with the purpose of connecting the 16,700 m^2 built areas, ensuring the highest efficiency in the health care function, but also caring for the comfort of patients, visitors and personnel.

The design of facades according to site orientation and Buenos Aires city climatic characteristics and solar radiation, interior spatial distribution with visual access to the exterior environment, use of natural lighting, color and warm finishes, and several sustainable roof gardens or green roofs, aim to achieve high levels of user comfort while optimizing the passive energy performance of the building.

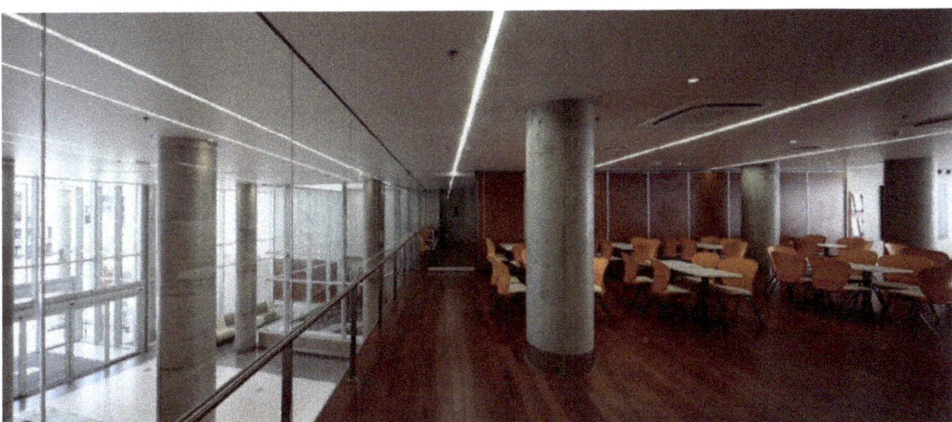

Figure 4. Main entrance hall and cafeteria with natural daylighting, NSF - Buenos Aires.

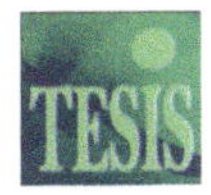

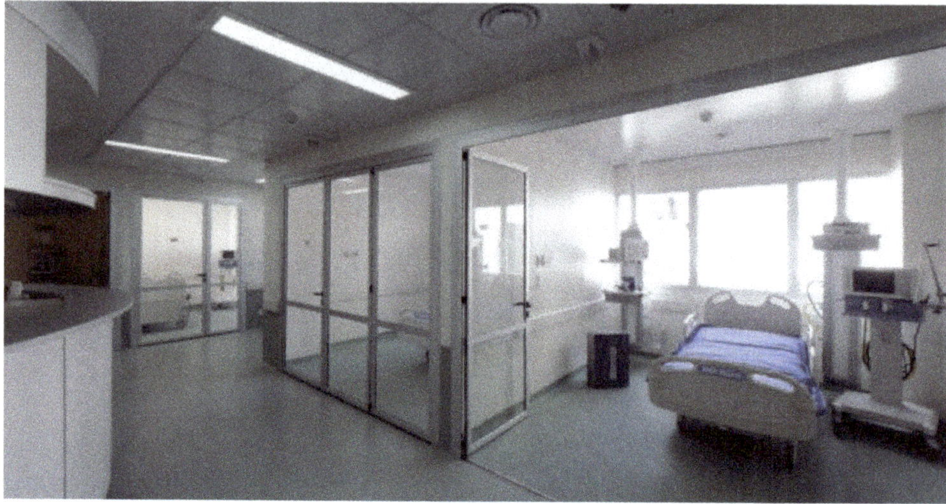

Figure 5. Intensive Care Unit with natural daylighting, NSF - Buenos Aires.

In a very dense urban environment like this, with a 100% occupation of natural terrain, it is critical to compensate the heat island effect and the building thermal mass. The use of green vegetated roofs helps to reduce this effect, simultaneously slowing the evacuation of storm water discharge and improving thermal insulation.

The use of large thicknesses of thermal insulation in walls and ceilings, air infiltration control, sealed double glazed aluminum framed windows with thermal break, eaves, sunshades and a ventilated facade system in sectors with direct sunlight, altogether ensure the shell thermal efficiency.

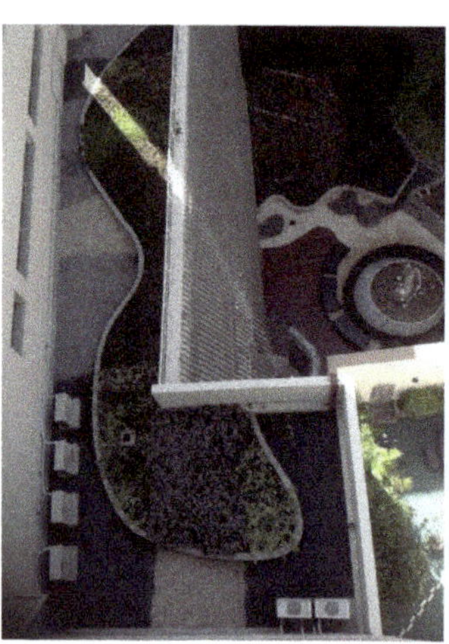

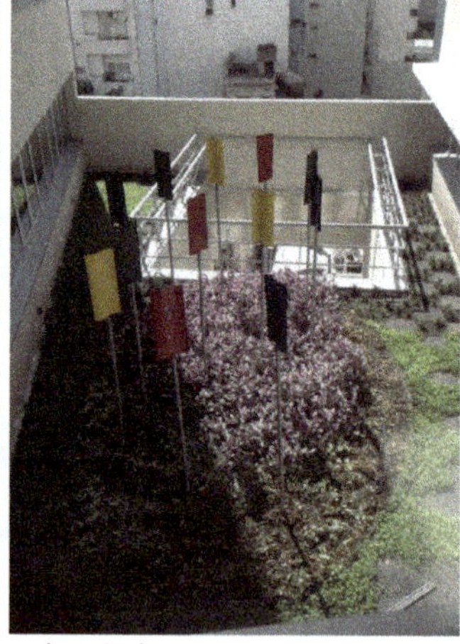

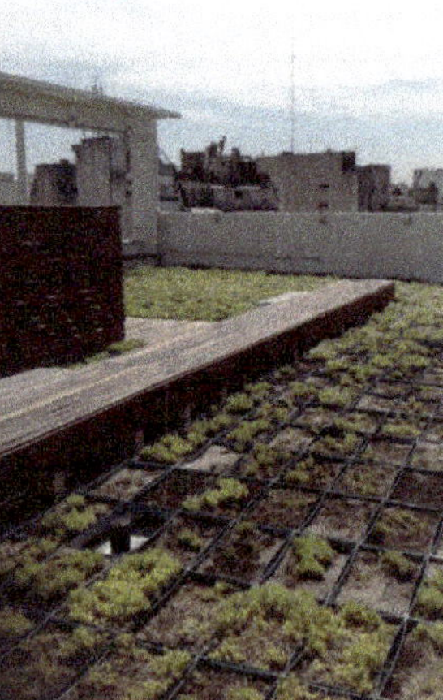

Figure 6. Roof gardens (ground floor, 2nd and 5th floor) and sustainable green roof (11th floor).

Energy efficiency - Relevant technical characteristics

All mechanical and electrical systems have been designed with the special objective of obtaining security and energy savings, and at the same time allowing permanent control of the operation and maintenance expenditure. Among the novelties introduced in this building the following should be mentioned:

- A centralized and automated control system for the entire facility, including thermo mechanical systems, lighting, power supply system, pumping systems, medical gases supply, elevators, and others;
- The adoption of an electric co-generation system which helps to reduce peak power consumption from the public service. This system runs on natural gas that has low contaminating emissions compared to other types of fuel.
- The adoption of a water condensed VRV (Variable Refrigerant Volume) high efficiency air conditioning system for all inpatient areas, improved by geothermal exchange for water cooling. In this system the volume or flow rate of refrigerant is accurately matched to the required heating or cooling loads required in each room, thereby saving energy and providing more accurate control, as an outcome of its ability to recover heat from refrigerating units and use it on heating ones, thus "moving" heat from one room to another in case there is the need to.
- The addition of three energy recovery heat-exchange machines, to reduce up to 80 % of the losses of heat (or cold) produced by the exhausts of mechanical ventilation from bathrooms and toilets. This also facilitates fresh air filtration, as it concentrates the intakes on three points where 90% filters are installed, highly improving indoor air quality.
- An intelligent control system of artificial lighting for large public spaces and external areas, and the use of LED technology to minimize energy consumption.
- Careful selection of electro and electromechanical equipment (pumps, elevators, etc.) taking into account their energy efficiency.
- Continuous monitoring of energy consumption, according to a strict calendar and hourly schedule commanded by the BMS (Building Management) system to optimize performance and avoid waste.

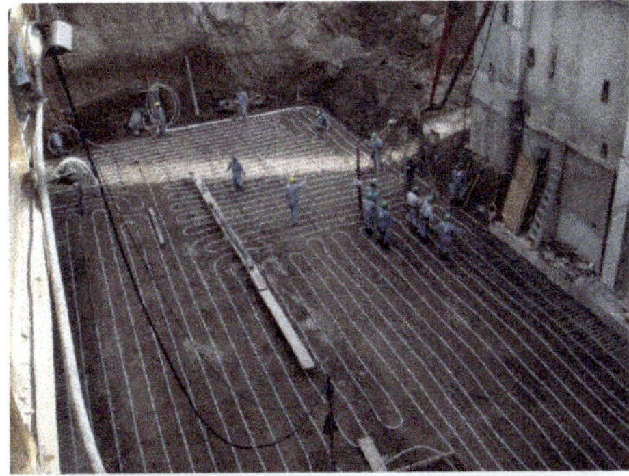

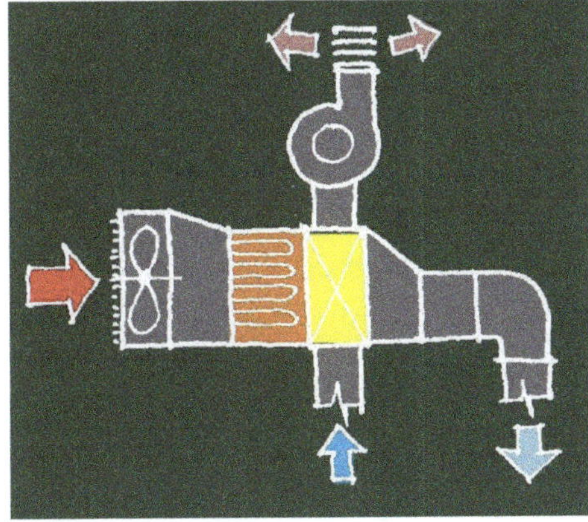

Figure 7. Geothermal exchange pipes and energy recovery heat exchange systems schematic.

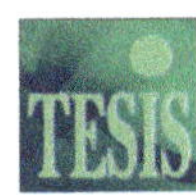

Water consumption

Potable water is one of the scarce and essential natural resources. The building includes a reduction in consumption achieved by incorporating the following actions:

- Reuse of condensate water from the HVAC system and rainwater for toilet flushing.
- Selection of low water consumption medical devices, dual flush toilets and robotics activated systems to minimize waste of potable water.
- The design of the gardens and outdoor spaces with public access contemplates the use of vegetation with very low irrigation requirement. For those terraces exclusively accessed by staff of the Institution a special system was adopted, composed of sustainable green roof trays carrying an artificial 8cm thick soil substrate and a single plant variety (Sedum), with virtually no irrigation requirement.

Choice of materials and future maintenance

Consistent with the overall objectives of the project, strong and durable materials were selected, such as acrylic exterior monochrome plasters, potentially recyclable materials as steel, aluminum and glass, and others with recycled contents such as most of the ceramic tiles and much of the plastic laminate plates with particle board backing.
The use of paint was minimized to avoid periodic maintenance or refinishing and in most cases only water based paints and adhesives were employed.
However, the local construction market has not yet developed a wide provision of low-impact materials and, for example, no acceptable alternative products were found to eventually replace current PVC coatings for floors and walls, critical in hospital buildings because of the need of easily washable continuous surfaces, resistant to bleach and other agents.

Interior walls and partitions were built with lightweight metal framing and drywall finishing, foreseeing future adaptations or functional changes.

Ease of maintenance and upgrading of facilities and services was another premise for the project. Despite the need for economizing floor space, it was possible to make all major wiring and plumbing networks accessible, both vertically and horizontally.

The third floor of the main building block became a technical core which houses VRV condensing units, hospital-type air handling units, chillers, primary and secondary pumps, the medical gases supply plant, pneumatic conveyor pump, main electrical panels and transformers, and UPS room, all of them adjacent to the main Datacenter, the Security bunker and Maintenance headquarters, ensuring quick and easy access for service, for example changing filters without disturbing medical areas.

The rest of the technical rooms were located on the 2nd basement and on the 11th floor, also easily accessible.

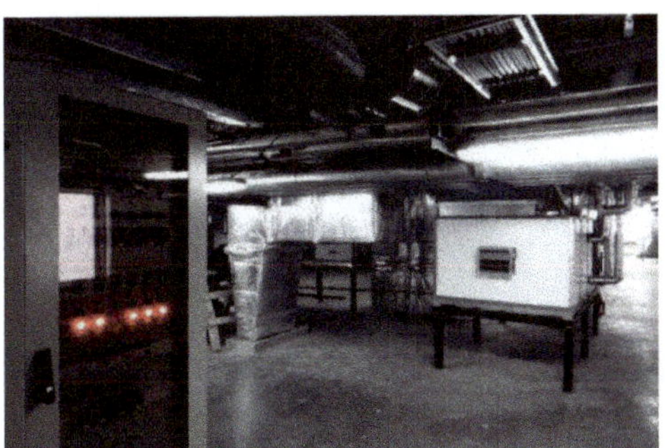
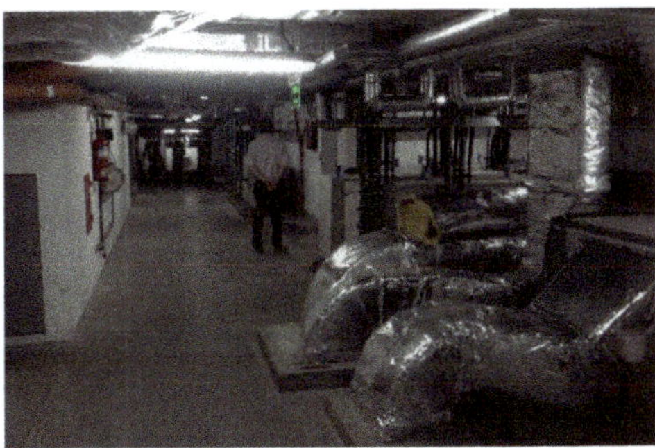
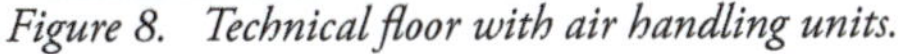

Figure 8. Technical floor with air handling units.

Design process

The design and construction took four busy years (2009 – 2013), during which the site was enlarged in a 20 percent by the incorporation of a neighboring lot and the design re-adapted to its final scope. The Sanatorium was officially inaugurated in October 2013.

At the design stage, the configuration of all functional spaces and equipment was discussed and decided by an interdisciplinary team composed of AFS Arquitectos, their specialized consultants, and representatives of the medical, nursing, administrative, technical and maintenance staff responsible for the future operation of the Institution.

The design team always sought to generate an extensive exchange of information between the members responsible for different areas, aiming to achieve better synergy and creative solutions. AFS acted as coordinator between such diverse topics as structure and civil works, mechanical and electrical installations of all kinds, medical equipment, furniture, decoration, etc.

Another aspect that deserved special attention and in some cases fell short of our expectations was the overall integration of the mechanical and electrical installations. Not enough experience exists yet in our milieu of coordinated or joint work between consultants and/or installation companies of different headings. Combined solutions as, for example, electro-thermal co-generation was not implemented mainly for this reason, the initial idea of the project having been to reduce or replace the use of boilers for hot water generation. Even the design and installation of the centralized control system had several drawbacks due to lack of availability or exchange of information.

Many of the design decisions, especially in the realm of mechanical and electrical installations, involved complex processes of feasibility and cost - benefit analyses, and some of them were conditioned by undesired external constraints. For example, the use of cooling towers for the condensation phase of HVAC systems was a compromise, since the City regulations do not allow to exploit the geothermal capacity of the groundwater table. Instead, during the course of the works, the City approved the use of systems of rainwater harvesting, originally not allowed, which anyway had already been planned in the project.

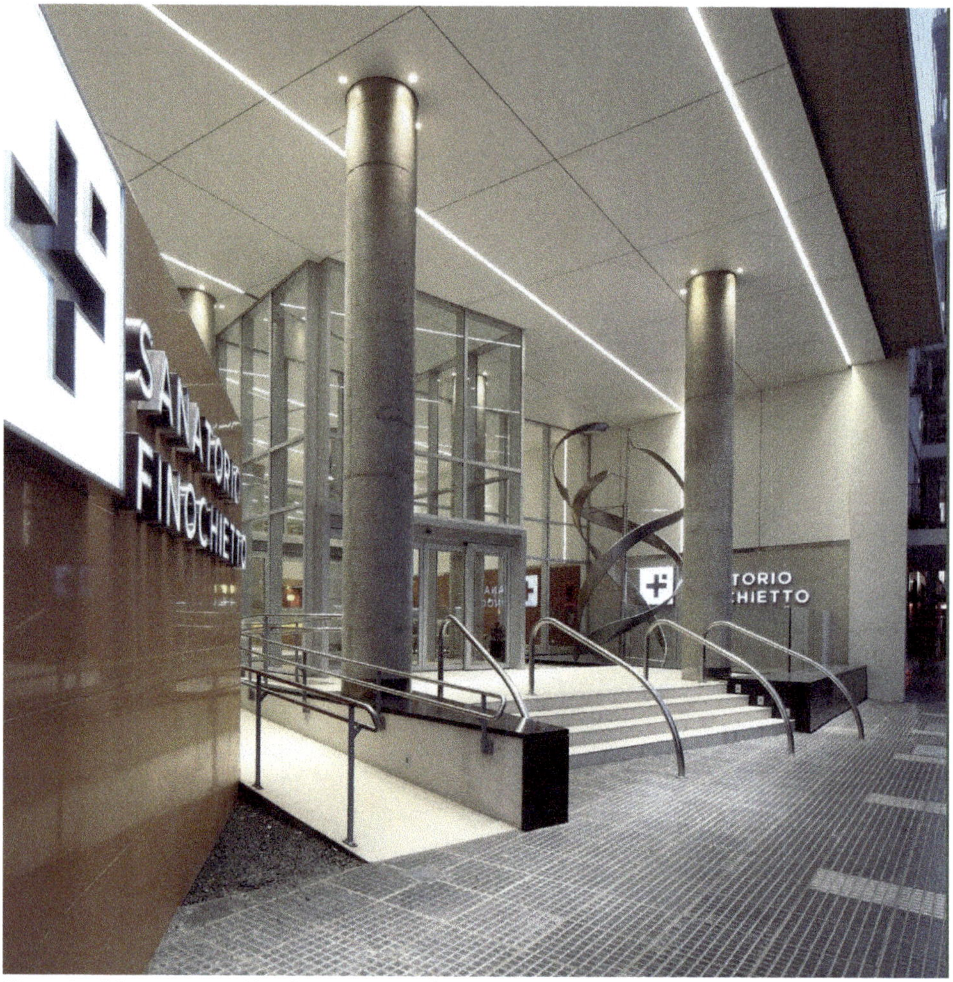

Figure 9. Main entrance, New Sanatorio Finochietto - Buenos Aires.

Conclusions

Convinced that the current broad concept of sustainability must be present in the generation and development of buildings for health, we strove with the collaboration of our client, to integrate it in this project, sometimes forcing the transformation of traditional standards, organizational culture or processes, but with the clear target of obtaining a safe, user-friendly building responsible for the environment, and hoping that this pioneering work will encourage many others to follow the way to an improved physical support for the care of a healthier population, which in turn will deliver significant returns to health care institutions in terms of enhanced organizational performance.

Raising from Destruction, the Challenge of Building in Haiti. The Example of Gonaives Hospital

Antonio Baio
M. Jean-François Laurent
antonioba@unops.org
United Nations Office for Project Services - UNOPS, Haiti

The Gonaives hospital in Haiti, the first major public hospital to be built in this country for the past 50 years, is a 10,000 sq.m, 200 beds facility with preferred mission to mother and child care, equipped for all main specialties, either in term of integrating outpatients with inwards care.
The project behind the construction of this second level hospital was designed and implemented with an integrated approach to cover as many sustainable aspects as possible.
The Hospital was conceived to resist at stronger hurricanes and earthquakes and it is equipped to continue functioning in the aftermath.
Sustainability was achieved in many terms: in financial terms, minimum standard fitting into the limited budget; in environmental terms with innovative low consumption solutions and renewable energy production (natural lighting and ventilation, photo voltaic plant, rainwater harvesting, landscaping, sewage wastes treatment, etc..); in technological terms with tailored equipment and materials; in managerial terms with a master plan matching with existing resources, and in social terms with developing the capacity of local man-power and community engagement.

Antonio Baio*. Mr Baio is an architect who combines more than 25 years of international organization work experience, development infrastructures projects. Mr. Baio is currently Project Coordinator of The Gonaives Hospital project in the UNOPS Haiti Health Unit.*

M. Jean-François Laurent*. M. Laurent is an engineer who combines 17 years of private and international organization work experience. M. Laurent is currently managing the Health Infrastructure Unit at the UNOPS office in Haiti. UNOPS Haiti Health Unit oversees a portfolio of construction projects – hospitals, maternity clinics, medicines and vaccines depots, midwife/nursing school and capacity building and maintenance support projects.*

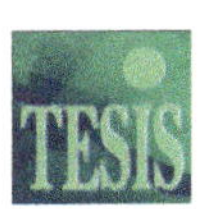

Unless expressly stated otherwise, the findings, interpretations and conclusions are those of the author and do not necessarily represent the view of UNOPS, the United Nations or its Member States.

The 2008 floods left Gonaives, including its Hospital, in ruins. The Hospital reconstruction was planned in the aftermath, but the implementation was postponed by the terrible earthquake that hit the country in 2010.

The challenge was to create a "replicable model", in a context where difficulties are still overwhelming weak resources. In this framework the design was focused on sustainability; the process being highly participative, the approach interdisciplinary and valuing appropriate technology. The project includes simple solutions, able to adapt and grow at the same rhythm of local capacity. Functionality and sustainability were guiding definition of principles on which design should be based on.

Functionality intended either for staff than for users. One entry, simple distribution, tailored space and use of colors to ensure easy perception and accustomed use by the patients and the public. Dedicated courses, rational sequence or proximity and appropriate technology to facilitate staff in providing services.

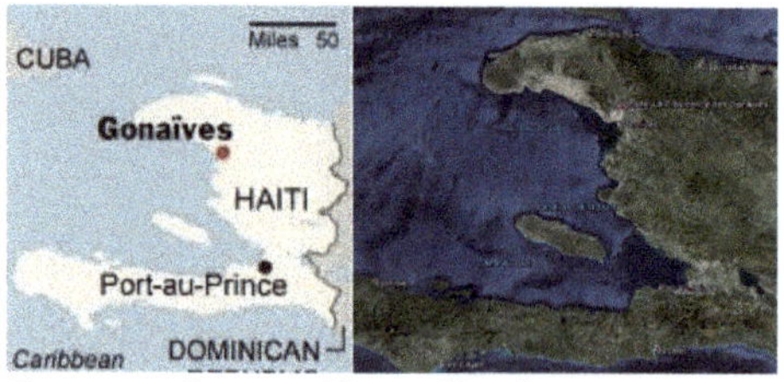

Figure 1. Gonaives Hospital localization.

Sustainability intended: in financial terms, minimum standard fitting into the limited budget; in environmental terms with innovative low consumption solutions and renewable energy production; in technological terms with tailored equipment and materials; and in managerial terms with a master plan matching with existing resources.

The pre-investment study (2009) allowed assessing the need, it gave indications on standards, aligning with national "policies", and it outlined binding conditions. At that stage the Steering Committee composed of the donor, the beneficiary (Ministry of Health) and UNOPS reviewed and adjusted the target, to match with the available budget; this procedure was intended to be replicated during the whole process.

Dedicated studies were carried out all along the process to ensure proper attention to the environment impact, including indications on how to manage the Project implementation as well as the functioning in terms of waste production and disposal. The data brought to decide upon a 200 beds, second level hospital, with preferred mission to mother and child care, being equipped for all main specialties, either in term of integrating outpatients with inwards care.

The location choice (late 2011), 4 km out of town, was dictated by the height (above sea level), to avoid un-doubtfully repeating the dramatic experience of the previous floods; it was strategically placed in the middle of the future settlement area. This implied additional efforts for creating infrastructures such as road, electricity and water distribution systems promised by the Haitian Government.

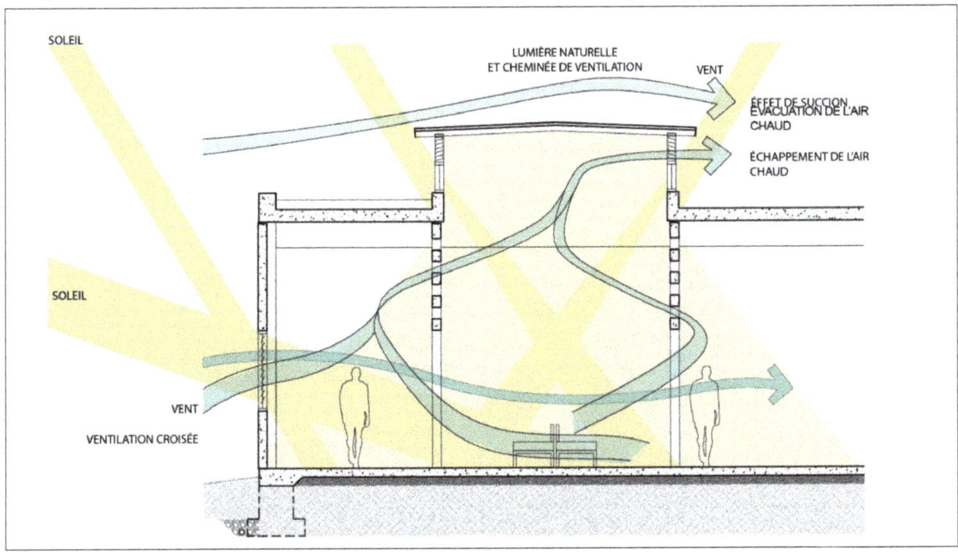

Figure 2. Room layout allow natural lighting and cross ventilation.

The design phase (first half of 2012) was a participative and interdisciplinary exercise. An important emphasis was given to the direct involvement of the Haitian Ministry of Health through its Engineering Department. This approach was implemented in order to maximize the local capacity building.

Conceptual design took into consideration common guiding principle such as: rationalized functional distribution/sequence, structural and typological modularity or disaster endurance. In addition some specific inputs were considered suitable: reinforced concrete structure; dedicated spaces adapting to cultural habits, to facilitate public perception and use; technological minimum standards, either for budget constraints than to ensure contextualization (also in terms of maintenance sustainability); environmental care, in terms of low pollution as well as sustainable solutions.

During the design phase of the hospital, special attention was paid to the reduction of energy consumption. As a result, the layouts of various rooms and windows have been deliberately conceived so as to allow a natural lighting while allowing a natural and harmonious air flow. Thus, only few specialized services would have the use of air conditioning.

Materials as well as technologies were chosen thinking at their easier maintenance, availability, durability and of course analyzing their adaptability to the hostile dusty context.
Simplicity and flexibility were transversal principles that guided all design process, ensuring that the context, in the largest sense, could absorb the Hospital as "part of" and not as a traumatizing element "fallen into". Even if "exceptional" the Hospital shall remain tailored for social and professional local level, producing "sustainable" changes and improvements.

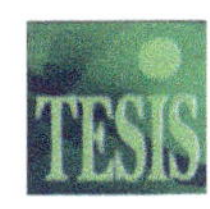

The total surface is lightly over 10,000 square meters, all placed at ground floor, 70% being closed buildings and the rest covered open spaces, for distribution or waiting. Typologically the central corridor, laid on a unique quote to facilitate displacement of wheel chairs and litters, distributes all eleven main buildings, in terms of circulation, ensuring direct access, installations, duct hosting all main networks and natural ventilation. It is connected to the entrance through the large waiting hall, where public will be limited and/or filtered.

Two others courses are lined a side: one for the patients, crossing in logical sequence all the clinical services (outpatients, lab & diagnostic, emergency, surgical, Intensive Care); and the other reserved for the staff, connecting the wards. General services and administration are located at the two extremities. Supplies arrival is gathered in a dedicated area, where all technical installations and premises are concentrated. The complex includes complementary buildings for dedicated functions. Specific social as well as organizational conditions suggested some particular functions, such as residence (part of the retention strategy for the personnel), waiting home hosting pregnant women needing exceptional care, an equipped area for visitors accompanying patients. Those are spread within the large fenced plot, without interfering with the normal Hospital functioning.

The Hospital is conceived to resist at stronger hurricanes and earthquakes and it is equipped to continue functioning in the aftermath. Large reserve of water and fuel will guarantee autonomy in case of prolonged lack of services, equipment are hooked or fixed in a way not to spoil due to shake or strong winds, wood panels are foreseen to be placed in front of all openings in order to completely close the buildings during hurricanes alerts.

The Project, thanks to extra funding made available by another donor during the implementation, could be integrated with photo voltaic plant ensuring self-production, improving sustainability, enlarging autonomy, in case of disaster.

Since portable water is a resource that exists in insufficient quantity in Haiti, "low-flow" faucets have been installed

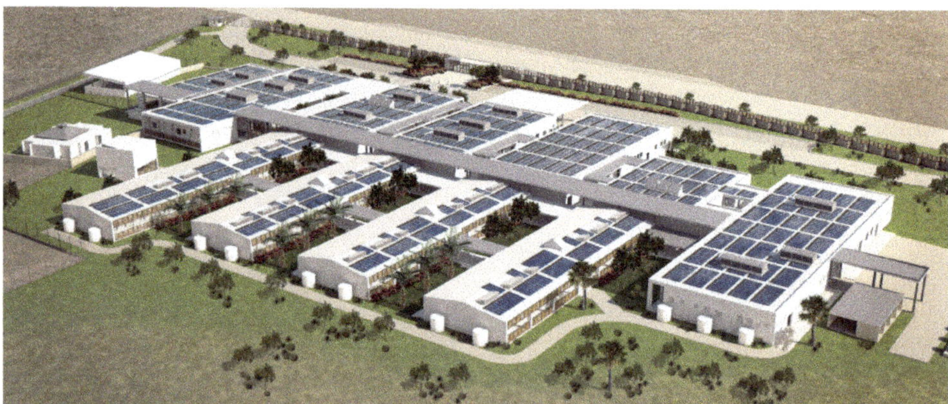

Figure 3. Gonaives Hospital project.

throughout the building. Rainwater harvesting has also been introduced in the design in order to collect gray waters for the garden watering and the sanitary drainage system.

Sewage wastes are treated within the premises; solid through strict selected collection and eventual incineration and liquid through pretreatment for special areas, septic tanks and anaerobic purifying fields.
Finally, landscaping have been promoted, thereby reducing the spread of dust while creating a shady and cool environment.

Parallel to the construction process, the definition of the equipment characteristics went on (2013), through involvement of all sector stakeholders, taking advantages of lesson learned by previous experiences, thanks to coordination and synergy with other initiatives and almost all continuously adapting to the "strengthened" capacity of the staff.
The design was never conceived as a closed package, being continuously updated. Inputs or feedback came from the equipment specifications as well as from the definition of functioning protocols (refined during the Master Plan redaction). In this process as well the participation of the staff was promoted gaining a growing involvement. This process was planned to be carried out mainly in the initial phase of the works execution; during the process, being successful, was enlarged lasting in some cases up to the final stage of the works.

A large awareness campaign and selected seminars were organized before starting the construction, in order to ensure proper information to the public, to the staff and potential stakeholders.

Lack of previous experiences and references for the construction and equipment of one of the largest health facility in Haiti imposed cautiousness measures, such as pre-qualification (for the construction) or lots split (for the equipment). While the construction contract was awarded to an international consortium, local resources were intensively utilized with on-site training and capacity building approach. The construction generated a significant income generating opportunity in the extremely weak job market of the area.

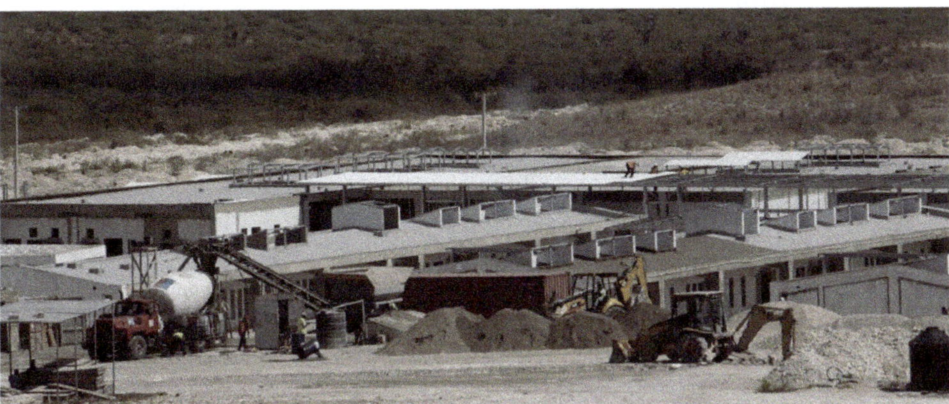

Figure 4. Gonaives Hospital construction site.

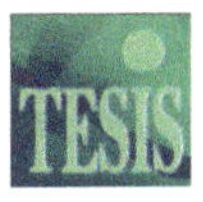

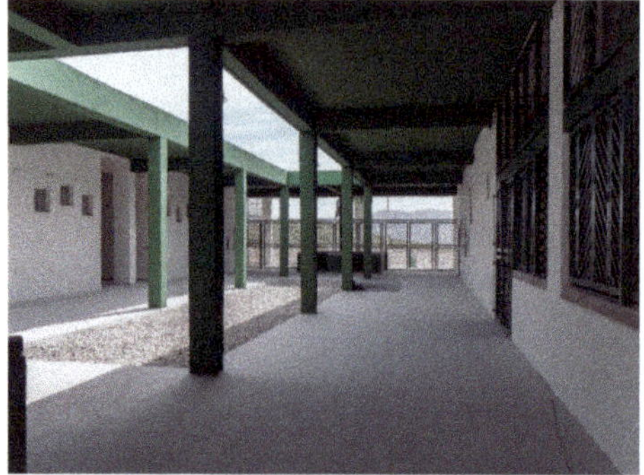

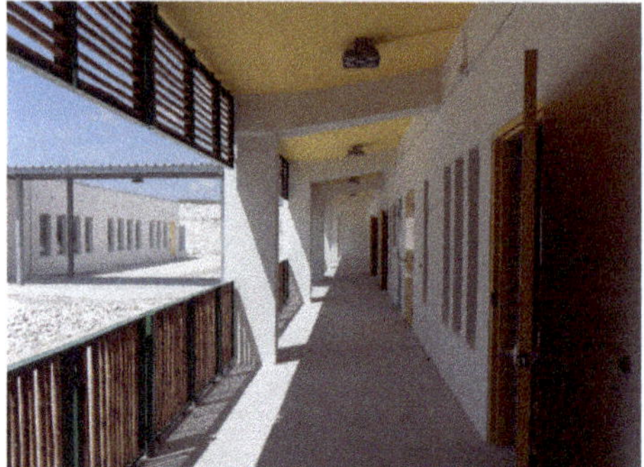

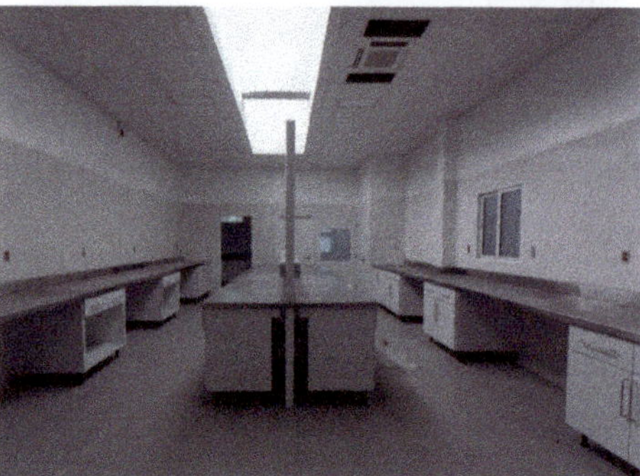

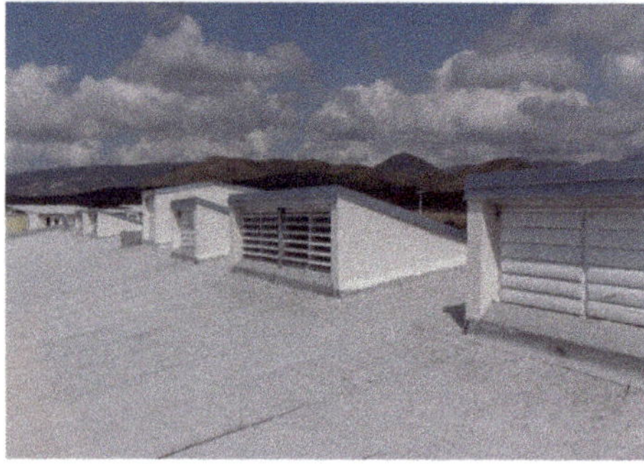

Figure 5. Simplicity and flexibility were transversal principles that guided all design process.

Contracts award for the supply and installation of medical equipment have also been very complex, needing several rounds of tenders, due to emerging status of this particular market. Local representations for technical support are however increasing and should facilitate in the near future the maintenance and customer services.

Construction process, lasting almost two years (beginning 2013 to late 2014) was a built along experience. The hospital is the biggest building ever built in Gonaives and the second large hospital built in the last 50 years in Haiti. Given the poor international experience of the general Contractor and considering the constraints of the context, the setting up the site was long and toilsome. All stages, from the concrete production up to the more sophisticated installations, were step by step approached.

The site management was carefully carried out, strictly respecting environment criteria, making the hospital the first ever (and still unique) "case" implementing selected garbage collection and disposal.

Supply of materials, from the aggregate to the technological equipments, was involving an extensive use of logistics resources, huge coordination efforts and a grueling process of technical verification. Keeping adequate quality control, to ensure high technical level of works, was a continuous dare. Planning was monitored strictly, through operational schedules, trying to avoid or limit delays (finally resulting within 10%).

The Ministry of Health Engineering Department was constantly involved, supported to get acquainted of all the process; they were assisting at all steps either for material approval than process quality control, in order of being enabled to take over the facilities with all needed case knowledge.

A Departmental Committee was created, organized, supported and followed to accompany the process, chaired by the local Authorities, including representatives of the social society, potential stakeholders and international institution. The Committee, within the responsibility of the Government, was considering all aspects related to social impacts and sustainability, from the garbage collection to the new settlement policies for the Hospital environment.

Handing over was conceived as a long process; it started during the work execution and continuing up to the opening. Tests were accompanied or followed by training sessions; data are recorded and registered to link with the management system.

In addition to the difficulties arisen by the peripheral location, the equipment installation phase was facing the challenge given by the lack of available resources able to guarantee the correct functioning. Despite well advanced planning, the issue remains one of the most relevant critical point to ensure a correct hospital functioning.

Intense and long organizational work was (and still is) carried out, aimed to strengthen the managerial and operational capacity of the, insufficient and mainly unskilled, hospital medical, administrative and support staff.

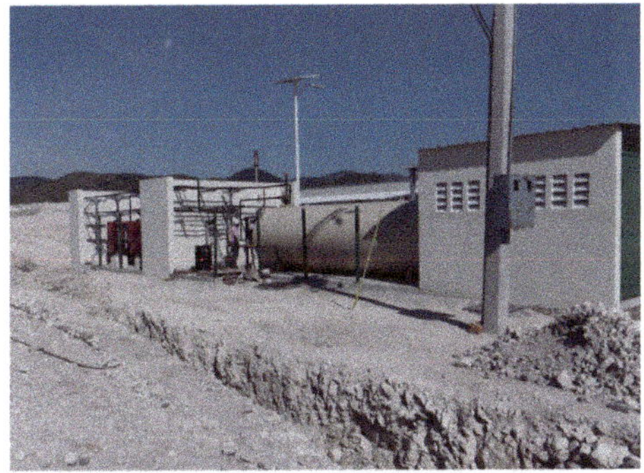

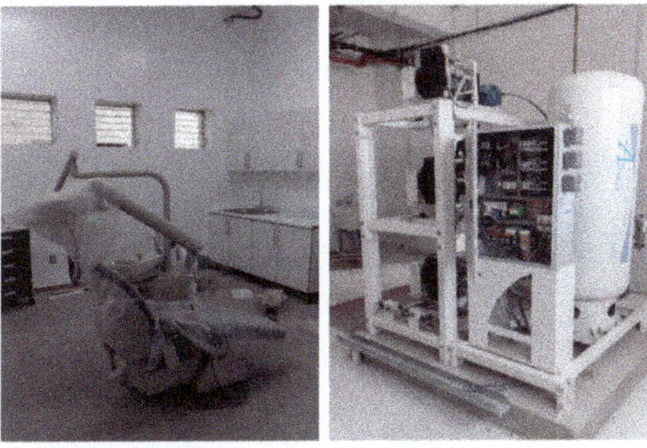

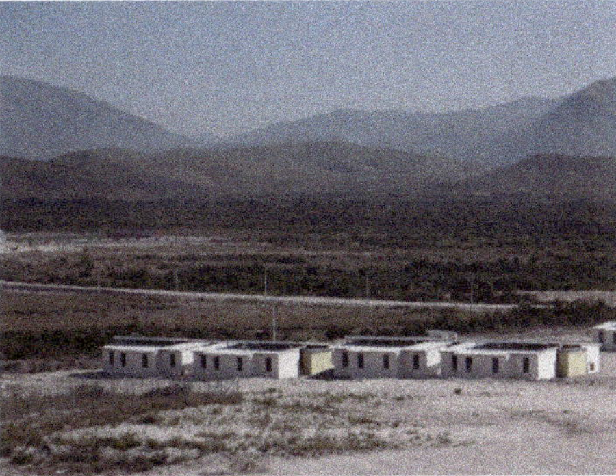

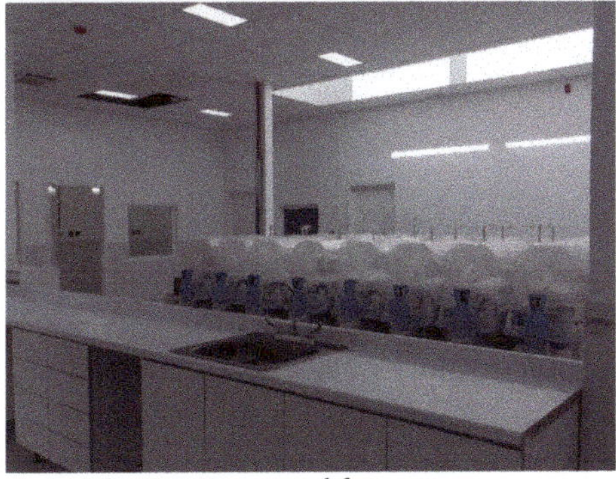

Figure 6. Equipment and functioning.

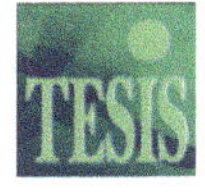

In the initial phase the Project was concentrated in assessing and understanding the real situation, resulted in poor –either in number than in technical capacity- human resources available. As mentioned, the technical assistance has been tailored for social and professional local level. The model should be replicable, meaning somehow to limit at changes and improvements resulting "sustainable".

Along with dedicated training, the Project allowed producing a strategic Hospital Master Plan. It was drafted from the bottom, with a deep involvement of all institutional levels. It is conceived to grow in a middle term span, five years, being initially tailored to match with limitation still characterizing the context.

Dedicated team worked along almost all the process to ensure a fair and smooth transfer, in order to guarantee set up in function in a shorter time possible. The structure will initially work at around 25 % of its potential capacity, growing gradually in line with demand as well as strengthen capacity.

Simulation took places numerously to familiarize with new protocols and to weaken changes resistance -that between the staff was initially strong-. The period to absorb –by the staff and by the Institutions- the new facilities, equipments and tools, implies an operational follow up, characterized mainly by the on the job training.

One of the main results expected by this final stage is to set up a maintenance service. The service organization include the provision of a software (on which equipment inventory and installations data have been registered), recruitment and training of the staff, connection to specialized networks, negotiation with suppliers and market coordination.

Benefits of an Environmental Management System in the Management of a Hospital: Experience of the Past 11 Years

Francois Bester

francois.bester@mediclinic.co.za
Environmental Systems Manager
Mediclinic Southern Africa

ISO14001 is an Environmental Management System (EMS) that encourages good business practices to limit the environmental impacts the business has on its surroundings. Well managed companies do this every day as environmental (resources and waste) management and it is integrated in their day to day operations. Many businesses already do most of what is required in an EMS without realising it.

In November 2002, eight hospitals from within the Mediclinic Group have decided to lead the way to a better and more sustainable environment in the Healthcare industry and have been awarded an ISO14001 international certification. Since 2008 an additional 31 hospitals have been added to the international certificate of the Mediclinic Group.

ISO14001 uses a systematic approach based on the following principle: Plan, Do, Check and Act.

***Francois Bester** is the Group Environmental Systems Manager at Mediclinic Corporate Office. Over the past 24 years Francois has gained experience in all aspects of Safety, Health, and Environment legislation in South Africa. He is providing specialist Safety Health Environment support to all the hospitals within this group. He joined the group in 2001 and his responsibilities include legal compliance, implementation of the ISO 14001:2004 system, developing planned maintenance procedures, advising and monitoring new and amended legislation and influencing the hospital environment. He obtained a National Higher Diploma in Mechanical Engineering in 1990 at the Central University of Technology (SA). He is a national council member of the South African Federation of Hospital Engineering (SAFHE).*

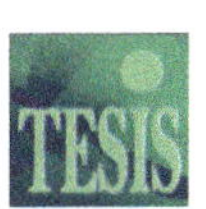

Controlling our Environmental Aspects means developing and documenting good practice in our work procedures, training of employees and setting goals to find other ways to make sure that our processes are less wasteful or unavoidable wastes are treated and managed in a responsible way. All of these above actions are the responsibility of hospital management.

Setting out on the path of environmental awareness and responsibility 11 years ago, it was not possible to foresee all the benefits the implementation of the EMS would bring. This paper will take a look at the EMS; how applicable it is on the hospital industry, the implementation thereof and derived benefits. It will also specifically show how EMS eases the burden of managing a hospital. The EMS also assists in the management of energy, water and gases consumption. EMS also actively assists in emergency preparedness and disaster management at hospitals.

Since actively communicating the benefits of an EMS system since 2007, the other two major private hospital groups in South Africa also started to implement the EMS. In 2013 the National Department of Health promulgated legislation that all public and private hospitals must implement similar environmental management systems.

Carbon Disclosure Project 2013

Our overall electricity consumption in terms of kWh used decrease despite growth in our business in terms of increased bed days sold, full-time employees, square meterage and operational beds.

This was achieved through initiatives with regards to improved operational efficiency of technical installations and behaviour change of staff within the group.

Electricity consumption decrease by 3 million kWh, this is a reduction of 2% in total electricity consumption although there was an increase of 3.6% in bed days sold.

The electricity consumption per bed day sold decrease by 5.4% to 85 kWh.

The total electricity consumption for the financial year 2012/2013 was 149/146 MWh.

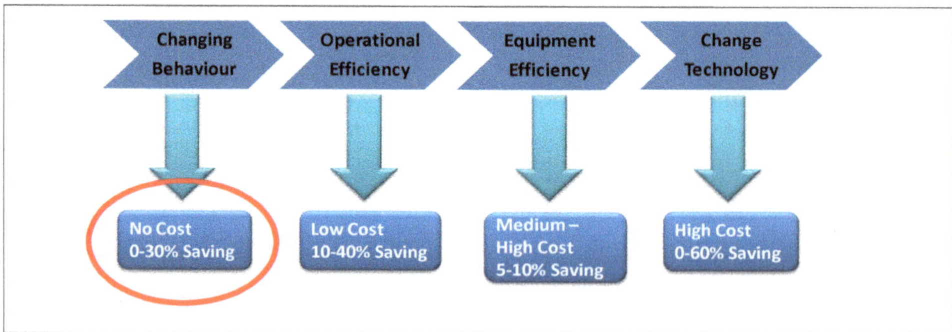

Figure 1. Human behaviour and cost saving.

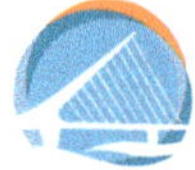

Hospital Towards Zero CO_2 Emissions

Marcello Fiorenza

m.fiorenza@asl.rieti.it
Eng., Head of the Technical Division of the ASL (Local Health Authority), Province of Rieti, Italy

The Hospital San Camillo De Lellis was built in the period 1969-1973. The Hospital is located in the city of Rieti, Lazio Region, in the central part of Italy, about 70 km from Rome, at the foot of the chain of the Apennines. It is in a climatic zone classified E, with 2,324 degree days. The total area is about 56,000 square meters, its volume is approximately 191,000 cubic meters. It is formed by a central body that is divided into wings of different heights. The glass surfaces are around the 7.000 m^2*.*
Currently, the number of beds is 405, of which about 15 per day hospital. And 'ongoing restructuring and functional building, as well as the adaptation to the seismic and fire protection and units plant. In this logic has been introduced the concept of optimization of energy consumption because the present energy production plants have been realized at the end of 1990's and their capacity is still able to cover the needs of the hospital, which, hovever are quickly rising because of the growth of the energy request occurred during these last years. The situation is particularly critical form the cooling energy point of view.

Birth: 12.02.1950 in Messina ITALY. 11.24.1977: Master's Degree in Mechanical Engineering c/o Roma University "La Sapienza". 1978-1992: Several working technical experience before and as facility manager from 1987 to 1992 in Texas Instruments Company in Italy. From 1993 to now: Facility manager of Technical Division of Rieti Local Health Authority in Italy. In 2006, founder member and scientific secretary of SIAIS (Società Italiana dell'Architettura e dell'Ingegneria per la Sanità). Building Director of new hospital in south of Rome. Teacher at Rome University - 2^ level master.

Aim: optimization of energy consumption aimed at reducing CO_2 emissions into the atmosphere.
Method: in this context, the realization of a new trigeneration plant, photovoltaic system and biomas heating system will help to increase the energy sources of the hospital, producing contemporarily thermal energy, cooling energy and electrical energy.
Results: the hospital didn't reach the goal of zero carbon emissions.
Conclusions: to reach the goal of zero carbon emission it is necessary that all RES technology known.

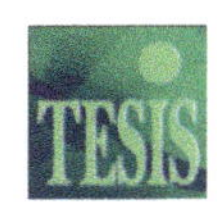

Reason for partecipating in Renewable Energy Systems (RES) Hospitals:

- the interest in the issues of the appropriate use of energy and the use of renewable sources for hospitals leads people to seek solutions made difficult by a structure made in the not yet open to the energy factors.
- contribute to the objective of spreading the culture of energy efficiency and renewable energy sources, with the widening of the environmental issues, in particular to the need for the health, reduction of greenhouse gas emissions.
- make an effort with the administrative management planning is also useful as an address to search for sources of funding.
- cooperate in the development of the guidelines, the project aims to produce and disseminate, in order to maximize the actual impact, at least in the reality of the country.
- continue the comparison with other similar problems in a wider European context.

At the moment, the hospital needs a great amount of:

- thermal energy for heating, air treatment, sanitary hot water and sterilization;
- cooling energy for conditioning and air treatment;
- electrical energy for lighting and powered systems.

The present energy production plants have been realized at the end of 1990's and their capacity is still able to cover the needs of the hospital, which, however are quickly rising because of the growth of the energy request occurred during these last years.

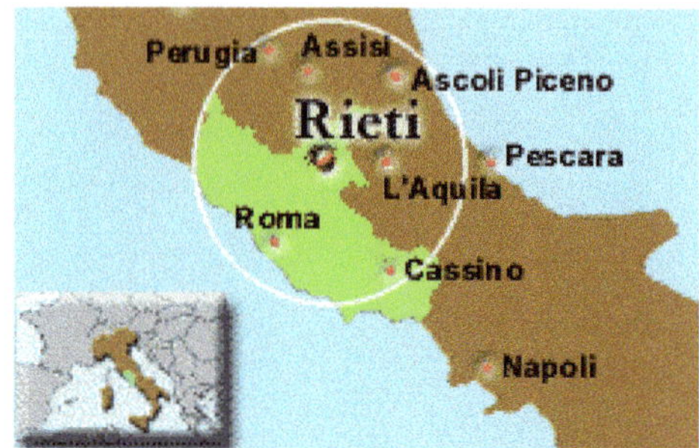

Figure 1. Rieti is a small city in the geographic center of Italy.

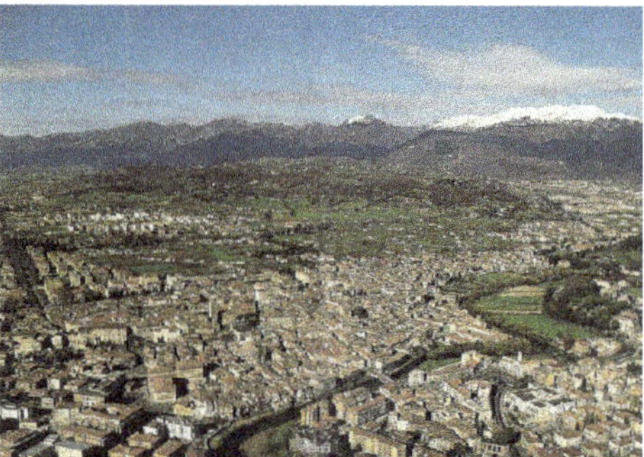

Figure 2. Rieti aerial view.

General Hospital	National Public Health System
Start of service year	1973
Restructuring	Several and ongoing
Climatic Zone	E
Degrees Day	2.324
Are	56.000 mq
Volume	191.000 mc
Typology	Two connected Blocks "H" shaped Hospital
Population Served	160,000
Beds Day Hospital	364 15
Tech. Management	Building &Plant Manager Energy manager
Measurement, Monitoring and Reporting Systems	Telecontrol Telemanagement Johnson Controls Metasys

Figure 3. Brief description of the Rieti Hospital.

Climate class (Ref. DPR 412/93)	Class E
Total conditioned surface (m^2)	56.000
Total conditioned volume (m^3)	191.000
Total glass surfaces (m^2)	About 7.000
Consumptions	
Natural gas (Scu.m./year)	1.631.068
Electrical energy (kWh/year)	8.023.855
Water (m^3/year)	70.655

Figure 4. Present Energy situation.

The situation is particularly critical form the cooling energy point of view. In this context, the realization of a new trigeneration plant will help to increase the energy sources of the hospital, producing contemporarily thermal energy, cooling energy and electrical energy.

The new trigeneration plant consists of a gas powered, internal combustion engine with:

- an alternator for the conversion of mechanical energy into electrical energy;
- heat exchangers for the recovery of heat from the internal circuits of the engine and from the exhausts and the production of hot water having a maximum temperature of 93 °C;
- an absorption chiller, for the conversion of thermal energy, recovered by the cogeneration plant, into cooling energy; it is combined with a cooling tower for the removal of heat from the condenser.

The maximum electrical power which can be produced is about 800 KW. It is expected that all the electricity produced by the alternator is absorbed by the hospital. Anyway, if the engine should produce electricity exceeding the needs of the hospital, it could be sent into the local electrical grid.

The maximum heat power recovered by the cogenerator is about 856 KW. It will be used to produce hot water at the maximum temperature of 93 °C. The hot water obtained will be used to contribute to satisfy the thermal needs for heating, sanitary hot water, air treatment, within the one produced by the present boilers.

During summer or in general when the heat demand should be lower than the recovery from the cogenerator, the recovered heat will be used in the absorption chiller to produce cooling energy, within the present electrical chillers.

Wood Biomass Plant. Wood biomass represents a copious renewable energy source in the disctrict of Rieti, which is rich of mountains and forests. This obviously makes it an energy source of particular interest. The type of plant which has been thought about is micro gas turbine with external combustion, feeded by woodchips.

Micro gas turbine. This type of plant offers several advantages compared to the other types employing the same energy source, such as the high efficiency, the small dimensions and the complete absence of powders in the exhausts. The plant consists of a gas turbine, feeded by hot air, which is produced in a woodchips boiler.

Photovoltaic Plant. Another suitable technology that could contribute to the reduction of carbon dioxide emissions of the hospital is the photovoltaic. A project, which would create about 575 car parkings, covered with solar panel roofs, is in progress at the moment. According to this project, the electrical

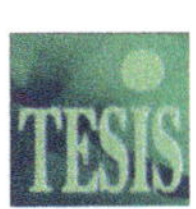

Summary:			
Present primary energy	2.846	Toe (tons of oil equivalent)	
Future primary energy	2.613	Toe	
Savings	**233**	**Toe**	**8,2%**

Figure 5. Summary.

Photovoltaic	It is under examination a project submitted to the Hospital by the adjacent Consortium for Industrial Development of the Rieti Province. It involves the Extension of the present Hospital parking area, providing it with photovoltaic panels roof. The energy that will be produced, will be made available for Hospital use.
Biomass	Considering the location of the hospital, close to the Apennines chain of mountains and the availability of good road infrastructures, a plan for the use of the biomasses coming from the nearby woods is been studied with the collaboration of the local University to determine the economic feasibility, in consideration of the quantity and type of wood available. The result is expected to be positive.

Figure 6. Energy from RES.

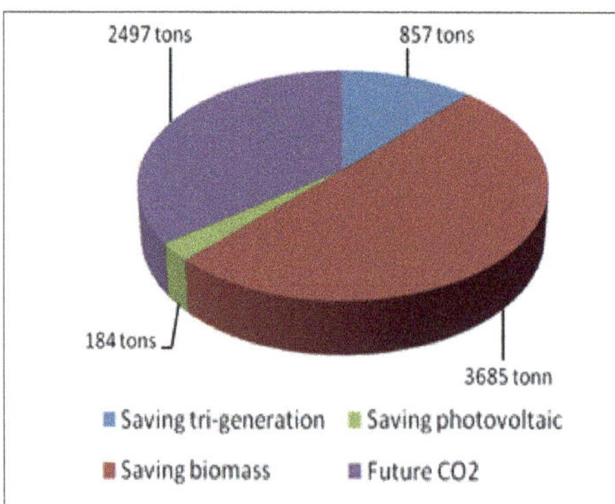

Figure 7. CO_2 emissions balance with biomass plant and PV plant.

energy produced by the PV modules could be completely absorbed by the hospital. The total surface of solar panel would be about 3.100 sqm, with a total installed power of about 300 kW. Installing the modules southward, with an inclination of 30° to the horizontal, the forecasted energy production would be about 360.000 kWh/year. As the Figure 7 shows, the total saving in CO2 emissions would be about 4.726 tons/year, equal to about 65% of the total present value. As already said, this means that, even if the hospital would realize all these projects, it wouldn't reach the goal of getting zero carbon emissions. In fact, to get this goal, the plants sizes should be so big to make the plants not compatible with energetic and technical characteristics of the hospital. Moreover, because of the very high costs of biomass plants and photovoltaic plants, even with government incentives, the business plans of these investments are not profitable.

Roadmap towards a Zero Emissions Hospital

The Rieti San Camillo de Lellis Hospital has great location advantages with regard to RES possibilities. On the other hand, its major constraint for reaching the objective of Zero Carbon emissions is its own physical facility. Constructed between the end of the sixties and the beginning of the seventies, the quality of the construction has required continuous interventions, without obviously reaching a satisfactory level of improvement also under the energy efficiency point of view. The radical policy decision of getting a new structure doesn't seem realistic for a good number of years.

Efficient Lighting in Hospitals to Minimize Cooling

Janne Grindheim M.Sc[1], Biljana Obradovic Architect[1],
Trond Thorgeir Harsem M.Sc[1,2]

janne.grindheim@norconsult.com
[1]Norconsult AS, Norway
[2]Oslo and Akershus University College of Applied Sciences, Norway

Increased focus on energy costs and environment has motivated research into more energy efficient technologies and designs for more energy-efficient lighting. We claim that these improvements will also reduce the internal cooling demand. This paper has a technical focus on energy efficient lighting in hospitals, but we emphasize that human factors and the impact on light quality must also be carefully considered when reducing lighting's energy demand for electricity and cooling.
The paper presents possible solutions of lighting design for achieving energy-efficient lighting in hospitals in general. These solutions are demonstrated using examples from several different typical hospital areas and room types. The requirements for lighting in hospitals vary greatly depending on the activities in each area or room.
Our solutions for lighting systems in different typical areas and rooms in a hospital are shown to give significant energy savings for lighting electricity and cooling energy without compromising health, comfort, or staff efficiency in hospitals.

Janne Grindheim*, Vice president - Head of Electrical Installations Commercial Buildings in Norconsult, Sandvika.*
M.Sc in Electrical Power Engineering, The Norwegian University of Science and Technology (NTNU), Faculty of Electrical Engineering and Telecommunication.
Key member of an ongoing research project funded by The Research Council of Norway to examine energy design of new hospital buildings, known as "Low Energy Hospitals" project. The main goal of the project is to discover and describe a collection of best-practices which can achieve a 50% reduction of the total delivered energy to new hospitals.
Main assignment for Grindheim in this project have been within disciplines as lighting and integrated systems, as well as assisted the project manager for working out guidelines in all technical systems (HVAC, Lighting and medical equipment).

Development

Buildings account for about 40 % of national energy consumption, and hospitals represent about 6 % of the total energy consumption in public buildings. Hospitals are the building category with the highest specific energy consumption. A large university hospital needs twice as much energy per square meter than a

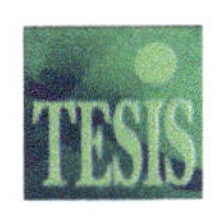

typical office building. Large university hospitals recently built in Norway have annual energy consumption between 400-500 kWh/m^2.

The authors are key members in a part of a large research project funded by The Research Council of Norway to examine energy design of new hospital buildings, known as "Low Energy Hospitals" project (www.lavenergisykehus.no). The main goal of the project is to discover and describe a collection of best-practices which can achieve a 50 % reduction of the total delivered energy to new hospitals.

A breakdown of energy consumption in a typical large hospital is shown in Figure 1. The "Other" category in this Figure represents electricity consumption by medical and office equipment.
In this paper we propose some best-practice designs and product technologies for more energy-efficient lighting in hospital, with particular focus on evaluating and reducing the lighting-induced cooling load in various hospital areas. We will also discuss human factors and evaluate the impact on light quality when reducing lighting's energy demand for electricity and cooling.

In the "Low energy hospitals" project we studied hospitals built in Norway over the last 10-15 years, looking for examples of typical and best practice with respect to energy performance. We examined buildings and building-related technical installations, and also the performance and role of medical equipment and activity patterns. We wanted to understand real hospital operations so that we could evaluate current requirements and design practice. We chose a range of hospital type and size, because energy performance can vary significantly.
Using the latest product technologies for light sources, different systems for optics and reflectors in the lighting fixture, and shading to minimise glare, we designed energy-efficient and task-effective lighting solutions for several different areas in a hospital.
Our design methodology began with identification of the actual lighting requirements for the different areas before starting detail planning. The next stage

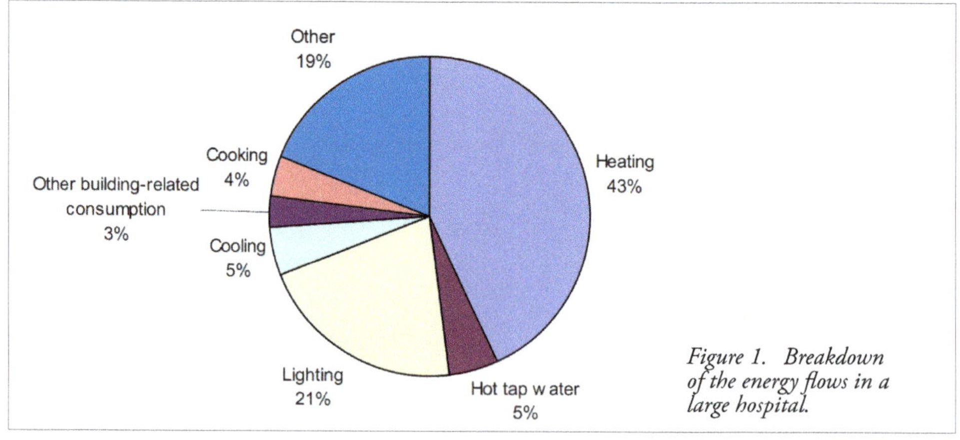

Figure 1. Breakdown of the energy flows in a large hospital.

we set the technical criteria for high system performance, but checking that our system also met regulatory requirements. Calculations show that this combination of design with new developments in fixtures, light sources and shading reduces energy consumption significantly over standard practice. In the future we would like to verify actual performance of the installed systems and analyse the cost/benefits of installing even more detectors for presence and motion in different areas.

As mentioned above, we must take into consideration the varying needs in different hospital areas in order to optimise the lighting design. This approach can be illustrated by *a patient room* in a hospital bed ward. The lighting requirements in patient rooms are different during normal stay, relaxation, examination, cleaning and recovery. It is possible to install dimmers and achieve different sequences of the light depending of the use and needs to this specific area. The lighting systems exploit opportunities from the varying activity levels and, used correctly, will provide a significant reduction in energy costs.

Also in surgical *operating rooms* there will be different needs depending of the type procedure being performed. Many procedures have very different clinical requirements for the kinds of medical equipment and other installations, the use of x-rays and monitors, the number of staff, and their task locations. All of these different cases must be considered when planning the optimal lighting system for an all-purpose operating room, including also the cases for cleaning and preparation of the rooms before doctors and other medical personnel, and the patient, arrive.

These two examples show the very different types of rooms and working conditions for health professionals in hospitals. Between these two extremes there are many other types of rooms / areas, each with varying working conditions to consider, from the perspectives of employees, patients and visitors. Each of these conditions must be treated as a separate design case. Our design methodology depends on close cooperation with hospital personnel, especially within the surgery department, to achieve optimal solutions for lighting control.

To achieve our energy reduction goal, it is important to know which lighting systems are candidates for control integration. A more integrated system will reduce energy consumption by allowing a coordination of the lighting supply to more closely match the actual demands of the space, without over-illumination. An optimal energy-efficient lighting system has the necessary automation to adapt to the current needs of the users, considering their task efficiency as well as psychological aspects of lighting, which are especially important for health care.

Previous studies have shown that replacing existing lighting system with more efficient luminaires, and adapting lighting levels by means of variable dimming controlled by daylight and presence detection, gives reduced energy consumption. The extent of this reduction depends on the room type and usage pattern.

Our literature review, however, showed relatively fewer studies of the impact of lighting system improvements on cooling loads including thermal and fan loads. Both thermal and electrical energy consumption for different lighting system so-

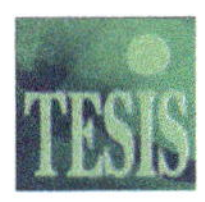

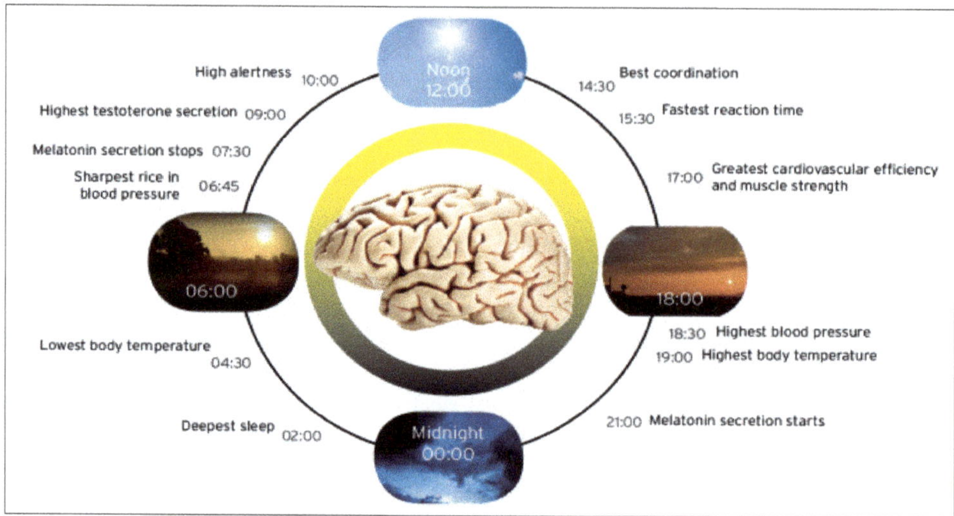

Figure 2. Planning criterias: quality parameters; energy efficient technologies; daylight; control; LCC.

lutions in this study were evaluated using a dynamic model for whole building energy and indoor climate, running in the Simien software package.

Our proposed solutions make use of a different colour temperature for artificial lighting. In northern Europe we would like to use a "warmer" light then in the southern Europe, to partially compensate for climate differences. Norway has traditionally used lamps with 2700-3000 K in offices and homes, while in southern latitudes 4000 K is normal in office lighting. This colour temperature feels more fresh and cold to users in southern climates, but in the north we prefer lighting with a warmer, more sheltered psychological effect. An increasing number of studies have established the link between daylight and health outcomes, as well as lighting and task efficiency; this research is particularly relevant to hospital settings, and has been used to guide our designs for technical lighting systems and installations in the various hospital areas.

LCC (life cycle costs) calculation is an important part of planning the light systems. Assessment of different light sources and the armature (as luminaire efficiency), together with maintenance is an important factor of achieving best solutions for different lighting systems. By using new technologies as example LED and detectors for presence and motion, and also luminaires controlled by daylight when possible, significant energy savings will be reached.

This paper will review the most important recent discoveries made in this research field, and provide a useful summary of best practice designs to guide those who want to specify, engineer and procure hospital lighting systems which reduce whole-building energy consumption.

Keywords: energy-efficient lightdesign, human factors, different behaviour and needs for different functional areas, light source, armature, detectors (presence, motion), control, impact on cooling, LCC.

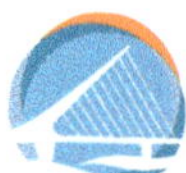

Monitoring Equipment to Reduce Energy Consumption in Hospitals

Tarald Rohde[1], Robert Martinez[2]

Tarald.Rohde@sintef.no
[1]cand.oecon, SINTEF, Norway
[2]B.Eng. (Mech.) Norconsult, Norway

The paper is the latest result from the Low Energy Hospital research project financed by the Norwegian Research Council and the partners. The partners are Norconsult, Siemens, GK, Saap project, Nordic architects, Oslo and Akershus university of applied science and the South East Hospital region in Norway and SINTEF.
The project started in 2010 and will end in April 2014. The goal is to describe the ways in which new Norwegian hospitals could be designed for half the energy consumption compared to the situation in 2010. There are several ongoing Norwegian research projects studying how to make buildings more energy-effective. The Low Energy Hospital project concentrates on hospitals; what are the specific characteristics of hospitals that designers should take into account when aiming for low energy consumption? This part of the study is on equipment. It has proven to be a difficult task to get an overview of all equipment in a hospital and how this equipment is used. This effort will hopefully fill the gaps in our understanding of how users and their equipment affect the energy balance in hospitals, and make it possible to suggest ways in which designers and equipment suppliers can help optimize energy performance, while maintaining quality in the delivery of health services.

Tarald Rohde *is a senior consultant in SINTEF, the largest independent research/consultant firm in Norway. He is working in the Department of Technology and Society. He has been working with health service related topics since 1980, covering research, the Ministry of Health, Chief Economist of a large hospital, planning the New National Hospital of Norway with among other topics being responsible for the medical technical equipment.*
Robert Martinez *is consultant at Norconsult, one of Norway's largest engineering companies, working with energy planning.*

Developement

Hospital designers and engineers are typically not aware of the energy demands and usage patterns related to most hospital equipment, with the exception of only a few large imaging units. The majority of hospital-specific equipment is the domain of medical professionals, not engineers or architects. In large and complex hospitals, this lack of awareness leads to problems with sizing the electrical, heating and cooling needs, and missed opportuni-

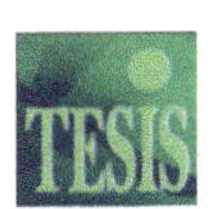

ties for storing and recycling of waste heat. A literature survey in the first phase of the research project showed a large variation in assumptions about energy and power to lighting and equipment, and that many engineers were using standard values similar to other building types.

Questionnaires were distributed to key personnel at the hospitals involved in the study, and their response was very valuable to the project. The main source of energy consumption data came from Akershus university hospital (Ahus) on the outskirts of Oslo. Detailed room-level equipment inventory and usage pattern data came from the country's 500 bed national hospital (Rikshospitalet), now part of Oslo University hospital.

Due to the size and complexity of a large university hospital, it was decided to focus our efforts on the following areas:

- the radiology department;
- operation 1 with 8 surgical units;
- the ICU for the thorax department, 11 beds;
- one bed ward, the Heart medicine department;
- the laboratory of biomedical chemistry;
- the surgical outpatient and day treatment department.

An earlier report[1] from this research project concludes that the time of activity and the intensity of that activity vary very much in a hospital. Most of the area is in use ordinary office hours during the first five days of a week. Only a smaller fraction is in full use 24/7. The project registered how many percent of the day staff that was on duty evenings, nights and in weekends. Finding the staff at bed wards was reduced to 20/30 % in the evening and to 10/15 % at night. For radiology the evening shift was 18 % of the dayshift, at night it was close to zero and in the daytime on weekends it was 7 %. For the laboratory of Medical biochemistry it is 7 % in evenings, 3 % at nights and 13 % on daytime in weekends.

Table 1 shows when the equipment in to of the studied departments were in use.

Table 2 shows the number of equipment in the hospital.

Table 3 describes the user profile of the equipment at the different departments.

The table shows that it has been some difficulties connected to find out how different equipments are turned off. The sum of different ways of doing that should be 100 % and are not, particularly not for the ICU. The reason is that some answers are connected to the equipment used at the time of registration. The main conclusion will although be that most equipment must be turned off manually by the users. Almost none is turned off automatically after a specific time of not being in activity and quite a small portion goes to stand by.

Table 4 shows the energy use per net square meter in the departments studied.

[1] *Rohde, Tarald, Brukstid for areal i sykehus, SINTEF notat, 06.07.2011*

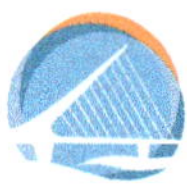

		Weekdays			Weekends		
	24/7	**Daytime**	**Afternoon**	**Night**	**Daytime**	**Afternoon**	**Night**
Medical biochemistry	40,2 %	38,50 %	10 %	10 %	2,10 %	0,80 %	0 %
Radiology		93,50 %	25,80 %	22,60 %	38,70 %	25,80 %	3,20 %

Table 1. When is the MTE in use, registration 2013.

	All hospital	**Departments studied**	**Studied as percent of all**
Medical technical equipment	18 678	930	5,0 %
Decontaminators	295	85	28,8 %
Autoclaves	70	17	24,3 %
Ventilated benches	320	46	14,4 %
ICT	11 411	2 236	19,6 %

Table 2. The number of equipment registered for the hospital and for the departments studied.

	Surgical outpatient department	**ICU, thorax**	**Cardiology ward**	**Radiology**	**Laboratory of medical biochemistry**	**Operation department, thorax**
Equipment used when registered	24,5 %	32,3 %	2,6 %	51,5 %	76,2 %	
Turns off manually after use	93,1 %	1,6 %	68,4 %	29,9 %	30,1 %	
Turns off automatically	2,0 %	0,0 %	0,0 %	7,2 %	2,9 %	
Turns to stand by	0,0 %	17,7 %	0,0 %	14,2 %	15,1 %	
On battery, loading	4,9 %	9,7 %	18,4 %	0,9 %	0,4 %	6,5 %
Must always be turned on	0,0 %	19,4 %	0,0 %	1,5 %	39,3 %	3,2 %
Not using energy	0,0 %	1,6 %	0,0 %	63,1 %	0,0 %	45,2 %
Runs 24 hours 7 days a week	0,0 %	1,6 %		0,0 %	40,2 %	
Component of other equipment		14,5 %		7,9 %		

Table 3. The use of medical technical equipment in six departments at the National hospital in Oslo, 2013.

Switchboard number	**Room number**	**Department**	**Equipment W/m²**	**Light W/m²**	**SUM W/m²**	**sum without BDS W/m²**
D202	**D2.2901**	Radiology	20	12	32	24
D203	**D3.2901**	Radiology	101	8	109	18
D104	**D4.1901**	Outpatient surgical	12	13	25	25
D108	**D4.1926**	Outpatient surgical	23	18	41	41
D406	**D2.4926**	Surgical suits west	32	8	41	41
D405	**D1.4926**	ICU	18	7	25	25
D402	**D2.4901**	Surgical suits east	51	13	64	64
C301	**C1.3901a**	Cardiology ward	12	8	20	20
B202	**B2.2901a**	Biochemical chemistry	45	-	45	45
SUM			**36**	**9**	**45**	**33**

Table 4. Effect intensity in W/m² based on measurement done in our selected departments.

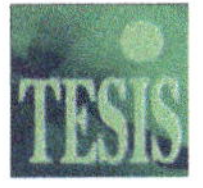

The study is about to finish so the conclusion is not absolute yet. What we can say is:
Most equipment that can be turned off is turned off when not in use.
Much energy is used when the equipment is not in use. The reason for that is that it takes a long time to make it ready for use after it has turned off. This is a challenge for the industry producing equipment that can be programmed to turn itself off and then be turned on again in due time to work when that is needed.
More complicated is equipment that also have to be calibrated to give the right answers, typically analyzing devices in the biomedical chemist laboratory.

As other projects in this study it is revealed that the activity in a hospital is varying a great deal. That is a challenge for the system delivering electric energy and the thermal systems bringing heat and cooling to where the equipment is used. This particular profile is even present in the ICU that is running 24 hours 7 days a week, but where the number of patients needing respiratory helps varies, and where the number of pumps could vary from zero to 15 for a single patient. In the hospitals studied the grids for electric and thermal energy is not congruent and light is connected to the same grid as equipment. That makes it more difficult to monitor the use of energy in an efficient way.

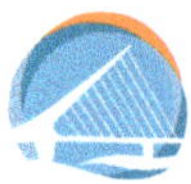

Saving Potensial with Combining Heating, Cooling and Thermal Storage

Trond Thorgeir Harsem, M.Sc[1,2], Janne Grindheim, M.Sc[1], Bent A. Børresen, PhD[1]

tth@norconsult.no
[1]Norconsult, Norway
[2]Oslo and Akershus University Collage of applied sciences, Norway

---

Increased focus on energy costs and environment has motivated research into more energy efficient technologies. In the "low energy hospitals" project we studied hospitals built in Norway over the last 10-15 years, looking for examples of typical and best practice with respect to energy performance.
Conversion and utilization of surplus heat sources represent well known technologies and are under constant development. In large building complexes there is a potential for coordinated production, storage, and distribution of energy.
Through our study new methods are developed for operation of interacting simulating models. These methods provide tools to step into optimization of combinations of integrated energy systems. The main issues focus on hydraulic water flow and storage systems as a basis. The layout is important not only with regards to utilize the energy quality, i.e. the temperature. In addition, control strategies are shown to have a highly relevant impact on the possible savings. Some details of new hydraulic layout and control design will be described and discussed in the paper.

***Trond Thorgeir Harsem**, M.Sc at Norconsult AS / Associate Professor - Oslo University College. He is educated at The Norwegian University of Science and Technology (NTNU), Faculty of Mechanical engineering. Extensive experience in research and development with respect to new as well as old technology, primarily within system design, data programming and bus technology within automation in buildings. Has developed several special programmes within climate, effect and energy consumption of buildings and glazed atria. Harsem is the project manager of an ongoing research project funded by The Research Council of Norway to examine energy design of new hospital buildings, known as "Low Energy Hospitals" project. The main goal of the project is to discover and describe a collection of best-practices which can achieve a 50% reduction of the total delivered energy to new hospitals. In this project Harsem also has been responsible for system-technical solutions within the HVAC area by applying simulation models, heat centrals, heat pumps and system solutions as well as system integration of automation solutions by applying communication bus.*

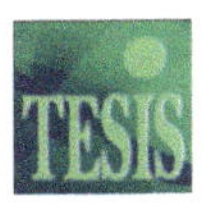

Developement

Buildings account for about 40 % of national energy consumption, and hospitals represent about 6 % of the total energy consumption in public buildings. Hospitals are the building category with the highest specific energy consumption. A large university hospital needs twice as much energy per square meter than a typical office building. Large university hospitals recently built in Norway have annual energy consumption between 400-500 kWh/m^2.

The authors are key members in a part of a large research project funded by The Research Council of Norway to examine energy design of new hospital buildings, known as "Low Energy Hospitals" project (*www.lavenergisykehus.no*). The main goal of the project is to discover and describe a collection of best-practices which can achieve a 50 % reduction of the total delivered energy to new hospitals.

A breakdown of energy consumption in a typical large hospital is shown in Figure 1. The "Other" category in this Figure represents electricity consumption by medical and office equipment.

In this paper we focus on our research where we have developed new methods for operation of interacting simulating models which provide us with tools to optimize the combinations of integrated energy systems.
Conversion and utilization of surplus heat sources represent well known technologies and are under constant development. In large building complexes there is a potential for coordinated production, storage, and distribution of energy. Building complexes with highest potential for reduced energy are buildings working with surplus heat/cool. Typically found, are large hospitals, shopping centers and schools. These can normally be included in combinations with other nearby buildings. Also, Smart Grids and an increasing number of Plus Houses will demand more reliable interaction tools in order to optimize surplus heating and, or, cooling. Development of tools for optimal energy interaction in building complexes during different time periods represents a major step forward. Hospitals are normally built up with different department with very different behavior of cooling and heating.
A hospital consists of very different types of rooms and working conditions for health professionals in hospitals.

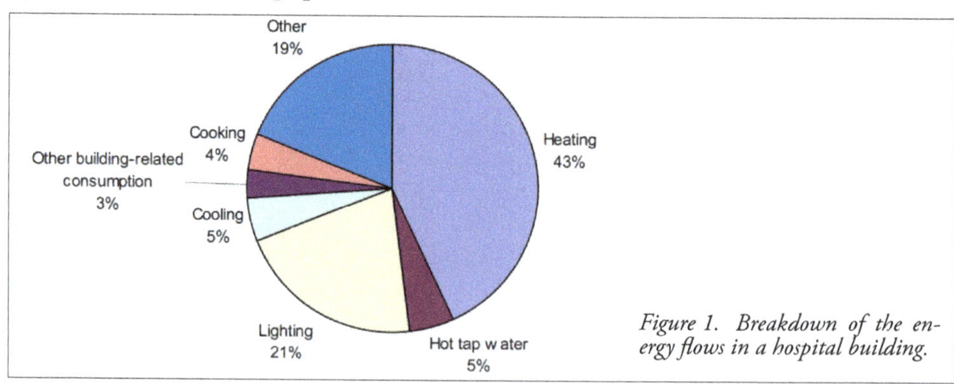

Figure 1. Breakdown of the energy flows in a hospital building.

Each area is with varying working conditions to consider, from the perspectives of employees, patients and visitors. Each of these conditions must be treated as a separate design case. Our design methodology depends on close cooperation with hospital personnel, especially within the surgery department, to achieve optimal solutions for technical installations.
As a model for our project we have built a reference hospital. The reference hospital has been divided in 10 different departments as listed: 1. Bed ward; 2. Public area; 3. Day treatment area; 4. Surgical Operation area; 5. Office and administration area; 6. Polyclinic area; 7. Imaging area; 8. Lab area; 9. Patient hotel; 10. Acute area.

As mentioned above every area has different use and internal loads. For simulation we are using the simulation model developed in the study. The approach is to vary the heating and cooling system layout, including the pipeline connections and couplings. Further, the design temperatures for radiators, cooling coils and heat pumps were varied. And at last we varied the outdoor temperature compensation curves.
The optimization process at this stage of the project has been performed as a manual approach. The model set up has been formed to perform high speed calculations so the high number of simulations can be run within a short time.

Results from the preliminary simulations in our model, with all the different departments included, are listed in the table below (table 1). In this study we have simulated the hydraulic system for radiators and ventilation coils in serial connection (Figure 2 and 3). Our research have concluded with a saving potential between 10-30% for this special connection, and from worse, to may be the best, up to 50% saving potential for energy delivery to heating.

No	ALTERNATIVE SYSTEM INPUT	SYSTEM COP	SAVINGS (%)
1	Reference 80/60 °C – heat pump	2,31	0
2	Reduced return temperature ventilation coil 40 °C	2,44	5
3	Reduced return temperature ventilation coil 30 °C	2,48	7
4	Reduced return temperature ventilation coil 25 °C	2,50	8
5	Dimension temperature ventilation coil 45/25 °C	2,54	9
6	Return temperature radiator 50 °C	2,78	17
7	Return temperature radiator 45 °C	2,86	19
8	Return temperature radiator 65/45 °C	2,82	18
9	Dimension system temperature 70/50 °C	3,68	37
10	Reduced condensation temperature heat pump from 53 to 50 °C	3,20	28
11	Dimension system temperature: 60/40 °C	4,17	45
12	Return temperature radiator 55/35 °C	4,17	45
13	Improved heat pump A++	4,81	52
14	Change the evaporation temperature from 8 to 10 °C	5,13	56

Table 1. Results from preliminary simulations.

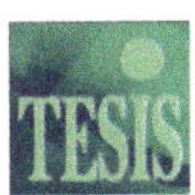

We hereby shortly explain the simulations in the table above:

- *Simulation n°1:* reference value with dimension temperature for both radiatorsystem and ventilation coil to 80/60 °C - no savings.
- *Simulation n° 2-4:* show at reduction of the saving with lower temperature for return temperature ventilation coil and series connection radiator and ventilation coil (se figure 1) for each department. Here we simulate dimension temperature return from 40 to 25 °C.
- *Simulation n° 5:* in this simulation we reduce the dimension supply temperature for the ventilation coil to 45 °C.
Simulation n° 6-7: this simulation we reduce the dimension return temperature from the radiator system to 50 and 45 °C.
- *Simulation n° 8:* this simulation we reduce the dimension supply temperature for the radiator system to 65 °C.
- *Simulation n° 9:* this simulation we reduce the system temperature for dimension condition to 70 °C (supply).
- *Simulation n° 10*: in the reference no 1 the design condensation temperature for the heatpump are reduced from 53 to 50 °C.
- *Simulation n° 11-12:* reducing the system supply temperature to 60°C, and the dimension temperature for the radiator system 55/35 °C.
- *Simulation n° 13*: in this simulation we have improved the heatpump to a A++.
- *Simulation n° 14:* evaporation temperature increase from 8 til 10 °C.

The result shown in table 1 indicates that the potential of energy savings is significant with introducing serial connection. The reference used is based on the standard design from existing hospitals of today, i.e. heating design temperatures of 80 oC / 60 oC. The heating system is equipped with a standard heat pump. Simple adjustments show a heat saving potential lying between 10 and 30 %. In the future we would like to verify actual performance of the installed systems and analyse the cost parameters.

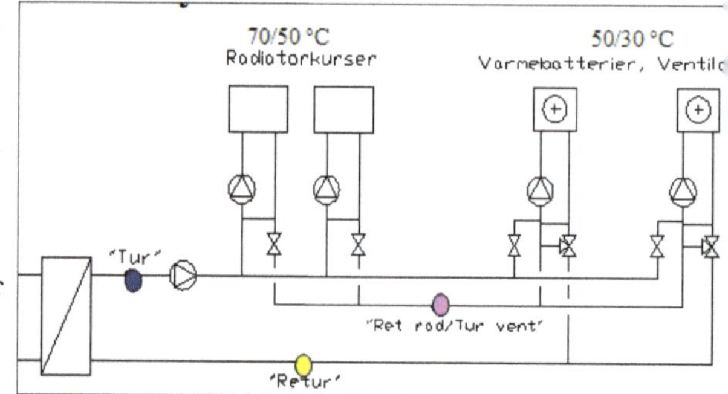

Figure 2. System outline 70/30 °C: serial connection - schematically showns.

Equivalent we have done simulations were the evaporation temperature has been changed from 8 to 10 °C, and the preliminary results shows an extra energy saving for 3,6 %.

This paper will review the most important recent discoveries made in this research field, and provide a useful simulation model to guide those who want to specify, engineer and procure hospital heating and cooling systems which reduce whole-building energy consumption.

Keywords: *Energy-efficient building and technical solutions, human factors, different behaviour and needs for different functional areas, heating, cooling, energy savings.*

Millenium Development Goals, their Progress and Effects on Future Worldwide Healthcare Development

Harry Waugh

callharry@me.com
Institute of Healthcare Engineering & Estate Management

In the year 2000 the United Nations, at The Millennium Summit, embarked on a project that should ultimately have a major impact on Healthcare on a global scale. The eight Millennium Development Goals (MDGs) were derived from the Millennium Declaration adopted by all United Nations Member States in 2000. Through the Declaration, world leaders forged a commitment to combat poverty, hunger and disease, provide education to all children and equal opportunities to both women and men, protect the environment, establish a global partnership for development, and to achieve these goals by 2015. A high level summary of the goals follows:

1. *to eradicate extreme poverty and hunger;*
2. *to achieve universal primary education;*
3. *to promote gender equality and empowering women;*
4. *to reduce child mortality rates;*
5. *to improve maternal health;*
6. *to combat HIV/AIDS, malaria, and other diseases;*
7. *to ensure environmental sustainability;*
8. *to develop a global partnership for development.*

Each goal has specific targets with corresponding timescales and progress is measured in 9 areas over Africa, Asia, Latin America, Oceana and The Caucasus. With the completion of the project now in sight it would be useful to assess success or otherwise and identify achievement and failures.

Harry Waugh. *Working life started in industry before moving into the Health Service in a technical and managerial capacity for 38 years going from Assistant Engineer through to Deputy Estates Director before specialising in Energy and Environment twenty-five years ago. Harry joined the Institute of Hospital Engineer in 1971 and was upgraded to Fellow in 1993 He spent 13 years as a Member of Council and was Chair of International Affairs for three of those and has become a Trustee of the Institute. As of August 2009 and retiral he formed Call Harry, an independent company dealing in Energy & Carbon Reduction Management.*

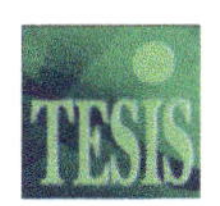

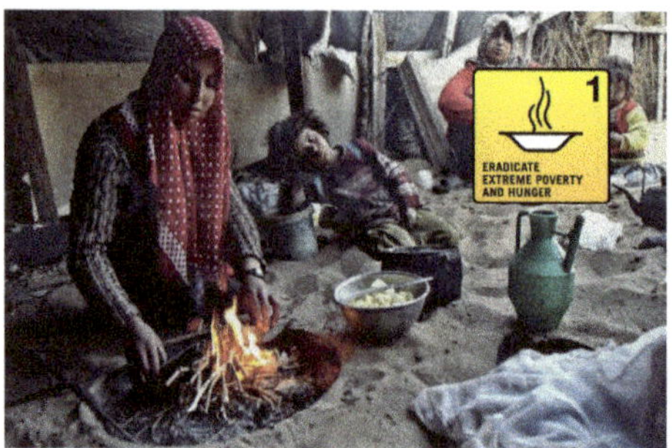

Figure 1. Eradicate extreme poverty and hunger.

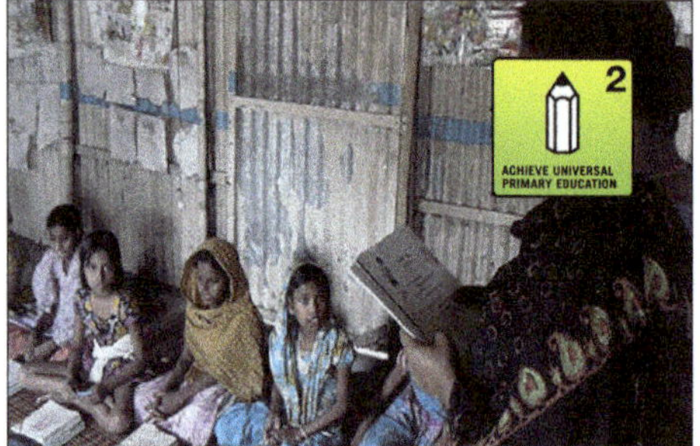

Figure 2. Achieve universal primary education.

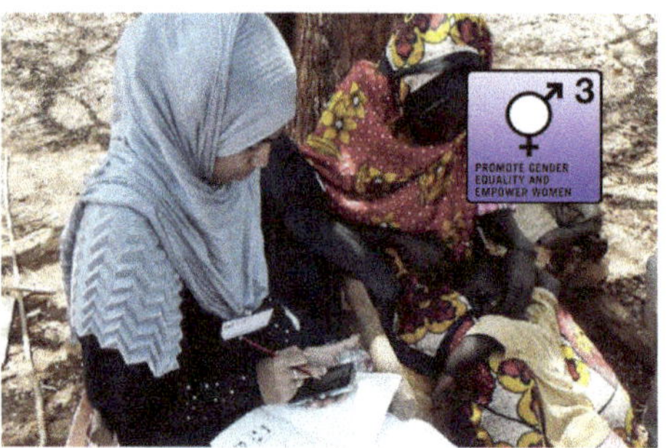

Figure 3. Promote gender equality and empowering women.

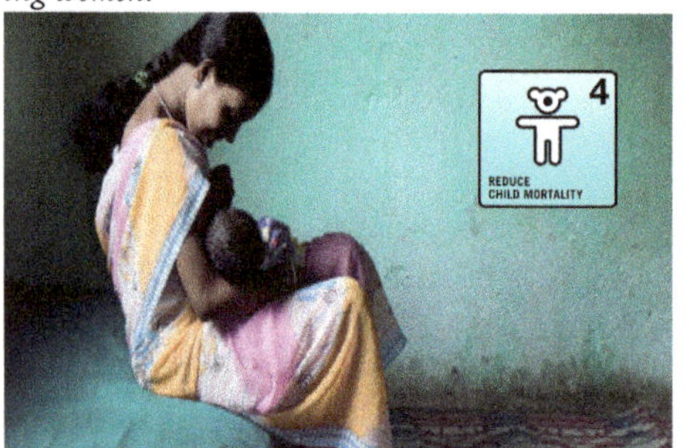

Figure 4. Reduce child mortality.

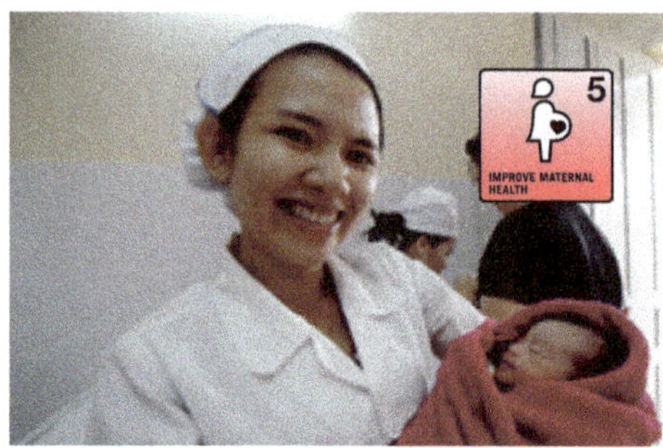

Figure 5. Improve maternal health.

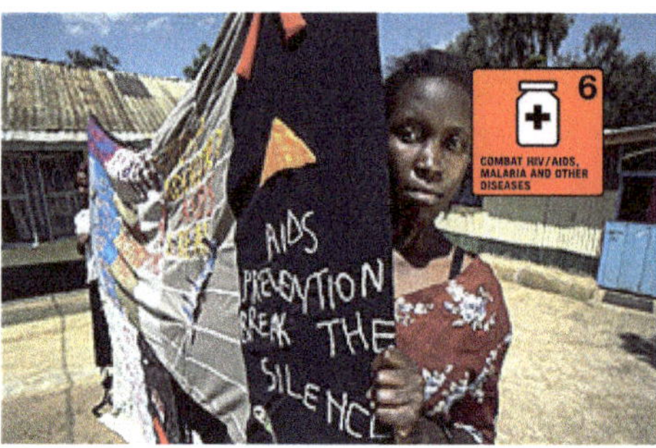

Figure 6. Combat HIV/AIDS, malaria, and other diseases.

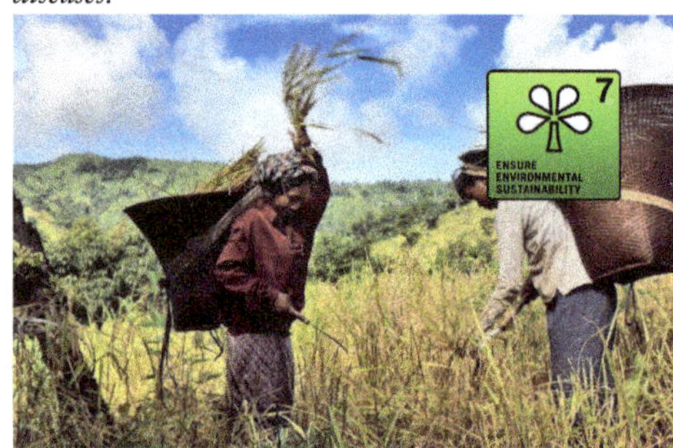

Figure 7. Ensure environmental sustainability.

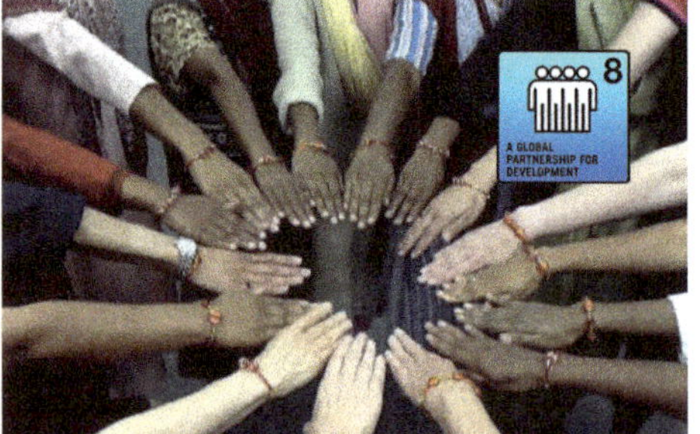

Figure 8. Develop a global partnership for development.

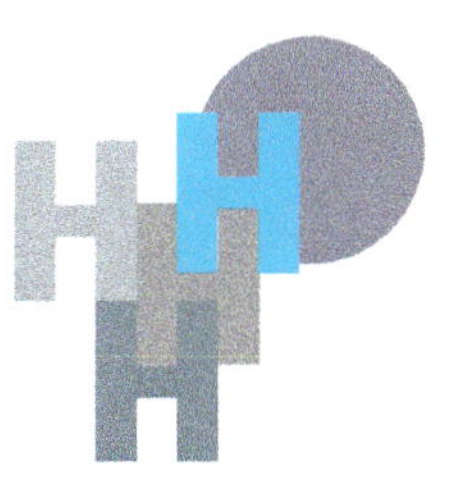

Technology, Biomedical Equipment, Connectivity, Standardization and Safety

Session Introduction

Safety in hospitals is extremely complex and requires the work of multidisciplinary teams in which each member offers specialized contributions to issues ranging from waste management, electrical installations and equipment, up to the use of ICT.
Technology has become increasingly predominant in therapeutic procedures, as evidenced by the necessary presence of instruments for analysis and treatment (for example, Radio Frequency Identification, RFID technology and all the equipment found in radiotherapy treatment areas).
Moreover, the use of tools produced by innovative technologies can play a decisive role in managing risks related to the intrinsic characteristics of the space, such as the use of new generation software-driven smart automated Ultraviolet Germicidal Irradiation (UVGI) devices, or the use of materials that favour noise control and thus prevent communication interference, which can generate medical errors.
An important aspect for safety in hospital environments is the staff's knowledge of the characteristics and state of the space, thus in this regard, to ensure greater security in the use of the facilities, it is appropriate to propose room standardization based on the hygiene and electrical safety classes.

In the design process the use of BIM technology for the 3D visualization of environments and to continuously edit their changing requirements imposed by technological, therapeutic, and legislative developments is essential.
The use of information communication technology tools in the efficient management of the future paperless hospital, improving internal communication between staff members and doctor-patient dialogue, will play a decisive role in reducing the risk of human error during treatment and also allow staff to communicate with patients even when they are in distant locations.
The complexity and specificities of each of these aspects make it necessary to review the education plans offered by universities in order to turn out professionals capable of operating in the world of technology, biomedical equipment, and the construction and management of hospitals.

The Complex Relationship between Medical Assistance, Technology and Architecture, the Future in the Oncological Field. CNAO Pavia, Italy

S. Melissa Godínez de León

simego22@gmail.com
Msc. Arch., Università degli Studi di Ferrara, Facoltà Scienze dell'Ingegneria, Italy

Thanks to the different researches in the field of oncology, we can see a new concept of spaces in the radiotherapy treatment area. This new technique was worked by the multidisciplinary team composed of doctors, oncologist, physicist, engineers and epidemiologist. In the whole world, the researchers have been working to improve and refine the treatment techniques with electromagnetic waves and currently hadrons. The new technology is already used in Japan, USA, Germany, China, France and Italy.

This article is to present the work of the Fondazione Centro Nazionale di Adroterapia Oncologica (CNAO) located in Pavia, Italy. The government from Italy released the law 388 on December 23th 2000. The article 92 of this law, named the CNAO, as an entity of research. During the same year, the Ministry of Health gave to CNAO, the authorization for the design, construction and operation of the building designated as the Oncological Hadrontherapy Center of the country. The construction of the center was finished in 2009.

***Melissa Godínez** is a Guatemalan architect. She has worked in health infrastructure projects since 2005. In 2009 she participated at the Index Hospital Safety course conducted by the Pan-American Health Organization, and, on the same year, she obtained a Master Degree in "Architettura per la Salute" in a program directed by Sapienza of Rome University and San Carlos of Guatemala University. On 2011 she obtained the specialization in Organization and Management of Health Structures at Bologna's University. During the last five years, she has worked as a designer and consultant for the Inclusive Health Institute, the Spanish Red Cross in Guatemala and KOIKA.*

Introduction

In the last century, the new medical process has had a great impact in the utilization of the diagnosis and treatment spaces and also in the form to construct them. The architecture and the engineering had to go hand in hand with these new medical processes. One clear example in how technology has influenced the diagnosis spaces is the discovery of X-rays by the Professor Roentgen in 1895. Another example is the change that resulted in the hospital's facilities for using gas anesthetics inside the area of surgery. At the beginning of the 20th century, we

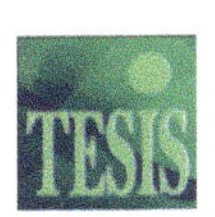

can tell that the implementation of the elevator in the buildings has changed the type of building from horizontal to tower, and recently, we can see the resizing of the surgical wards by the implementation of laser noninvasive surgery.

The examples mentioned and other events in the medical assistance, has changed the use of the spaces inside the hospitals, clinics, and treatment centers. Obviously, there is a direct relationship between technology and the transformation of the highly complex environments intended to diagnosis and cure.

At the oncological field the scientists and specialists have used several methods to combat cancer, some invasive and other noninvasive. We can name: the chemotherapy, surgery, radiotherapy (conventional, using X-rays). And right now, there is an innovative method of treatment that eradicates cancer from its molecular composition, and it is known as Hadrontherapy. With this technique, the tumors are eradicated using the precision like a tool. Around the world Hadrontherapy is now being used. Japan has opened two centers; there is one in Germany, two centers in France, China and one in Italy.

How does Hadrontherapy Work?

This method uses protons (ions of hydrogen), ions of carbon and neutrons, called hadrons. This is why the technique was called Hadrontherapy. The Hadrons are accelerated particles stronger than electrons. The acceleration is caused by a sincrotone that is just a magnetic field that attracts or repels the ions. It works different from the electromagnetic waves, because the Hadrons go to one specific point in the body of the patient, and that's because the main feature in this method is the accuracy.

Their electrical charge ionizes the molecules of the tissue, leaving the great part of its energy density in the last few centimeters of the path. The stop point is called "Bragg Peak". The accelerated protons and ions are able to destroy tumors located as far as 250 mm under the skin. This process is less invasive than the convectional radiotherapy. It has to be considerated that Hadrontherapy is 2 to 3 times more expensive than the utilization of X-rays.
At this point the question is: why invest in an oncological high level of specialization when there are so many problems

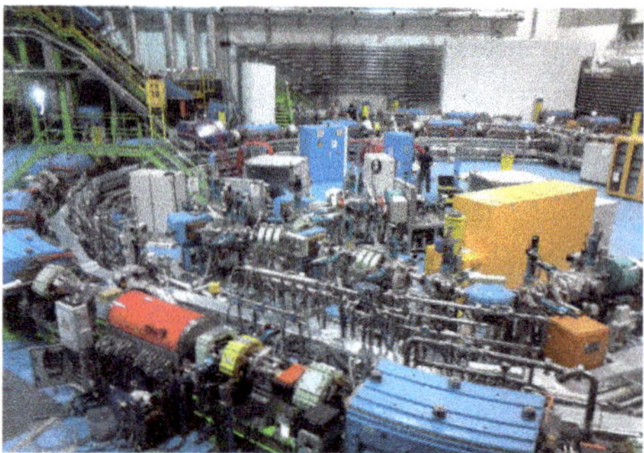

Figure 1. The Synchrotron has a diameter 25 m.

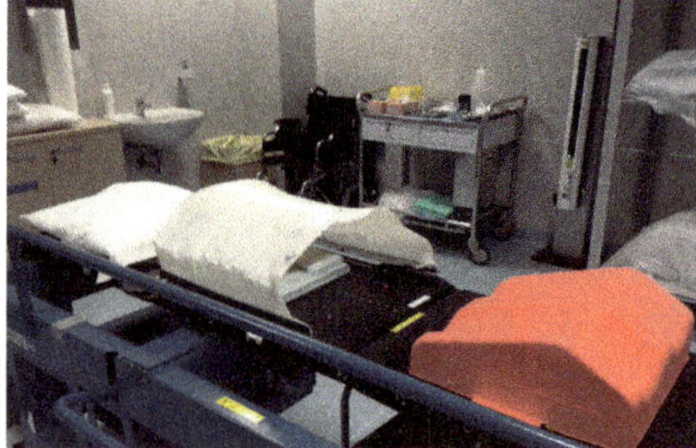

Figure 2. Treatment rooms.

to solve? To answer the question we have to see the epidemiological evolution of cancer during the latest 20 years, and also, the number of the oncological cases around the world. According to experts in AIRC (Associazione Italiana per la Ricerca Sul Cancro) almost 70% of the tumors could be prevented or diagnosed early. Some numbers in Italy can tell us the importance of developing hadron-therapy in the country:

- The incidence: the statistics presented in 2013 tell that in one year there were 364.000 new cases of tumors. 56% among men, 44% among women. The most common types of cancer are: colon cancer, breast cancer, prostate cancer and in the fourth place: lung cancer.
- The mortality: in Italy 2012, there were about 175.000 deaths because of some kind of cancer.
- The survival: The average survival at five years after diagnosis of a malignant tumor is 52% among men and 61% among women.

THE MAIN STRUCTURE IN ITALY: CNAO

The Center was born in 1991, with the publication of Ugo Amaldi e Giampi ero Tosi. The publication motivated the research and then the construction of one accelerator. In 1995 the Sincrotone was built. But it was until 2005 when the CNAO begins its construction. The structure was inaugurated on February 15th, 2010. On this date, the clinical testing phase began. The goal is to give treatment to 3000 patients in one year.

The Italian Ministry of Health approved to CNAO for treat the following pathologies: Chordomas and chondrosarcomas of the

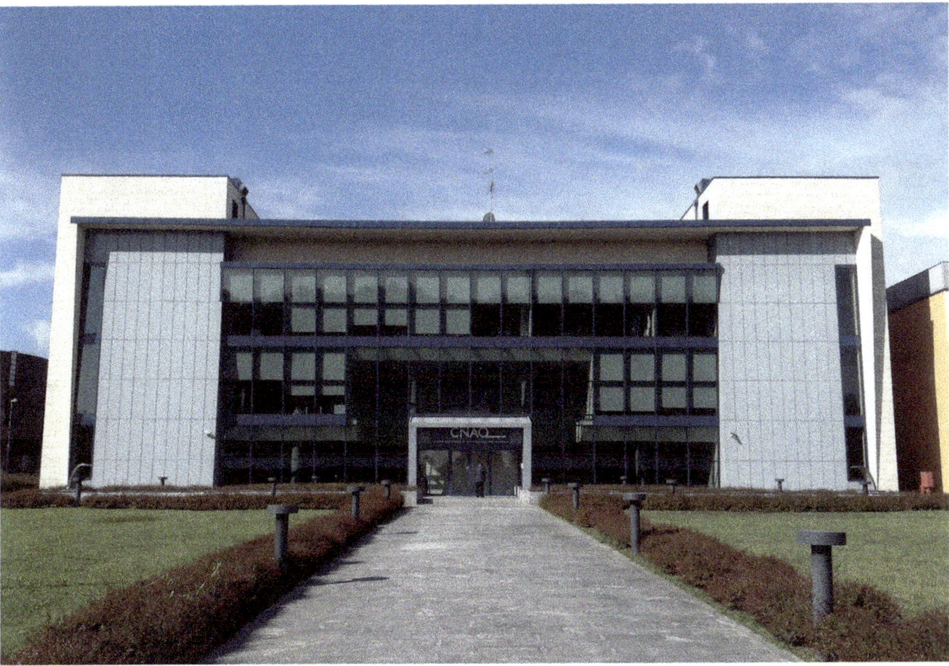

Figure 3. CNAO.

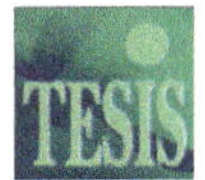

skull base and spine; adenoid cystic carcinoma of the salivary glands; sarcomas of the head and neck; sarcomas of the spine and pelvic area; malignant melanoma of the upper aerodigestive; cancer of the prostate and intracranial meningiomas.

The Heart of the Building: The Sincrotone

The Sincrotone is the accelerator which has the task of transforming the particles. It's the product of the research in physics and energy realized by: INFN (Istituto Nazionale di Fisica Nucleare) CERN (Switzerland), GSI (Germany), LPSC (France) and the Pavia's University. The heart of the building is a structure shaped like a donut, 80 meters long with a diameter of 25 meters; it has two areas inside the circumference. The particles have been accelerated and move 30.000 km in half second.

Conclusions

The implemented technology at the oncological field is changing the space structure. The architects and engineers have to work in a multidisciplinary team. The challenge of engineering is to provide a space with functional requirements of its activities, but trying to get a balance between functionality and aesthetics. An environment should be "pleasant and safe" for patients and health workers.

References

CNAO (Fondazione Centro Nazionale di Adroterapia Oncologia)
INFN (Istituto Nazionale di Fisica Nucleare)
CERN (Organisation Européenne Pour la Recherche Nucléaire)
GSI Gesellschaft für Schwerionenforschung (Compañia para la Investigación de Iones Pesados)
LPSC (Laboratoire du Physique Subatomic et de Cosmologie)

http://www.cnao.it/index.php/it/le-sale-trattamento.html

http://www.salute.gov.it/ricercaSanitaria/paginaInternaMenuRicercaSanitaria.jsp?id=810&menu=specializzazione

http://www.scienzainrete.it/contenuto/articolo/Le-conquiste-dell'adroterapia

http://archade.fr/english/comment-soigner-lhadrontherapie/

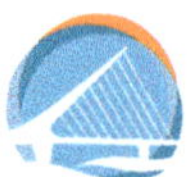

Hospitals of the Future, Paperless, Reduced Noise

Marilita Giuliano[1], Rita Comando[2], Ezequiel Pombo[3], Matias Martinez[4], Sergio Lopez[5]

giuliano.marilita@knauf.com.ar
[1]Architect, Member of the AdAA, IRAM Acoustics and Fire Subcommittee, INCOSE Technical Committee
[2]Architect, Member of the AADAIH, SCA First Vice President, CAM
[3]M.M.O., Member of the CPIC Engineering College
[4]Graduate diploma in Environmental Health; Member of "Salud sin daño" (No Health Damage) NGO
[5]Acoustic Technician. Member of the AdAA (Acoustics Association of Argentina)

Institutions/Business: Knauf AMF[1,3] CAM[2], Dr. Juan Fernandez General Acute Care Hospital, G.C.B.A[4], Acoustic Diffusers[5]

The current trend in hospital design is to incorporate new technologies to manage a paperless hospital, highlighting the implementation of computerized patient case report forms and related aspects.
However, there are other needs that have not mostly been considered in Argentina. An invisible factor is noise, as well as noise control and elimination in the different areas of the hospital. According to various studies conducted in different parts of the world, noise induces an increased risk of medical errors, contributes to staff stressing and burnout, and affects patient length of recovering. According to the World Health Organization (WHO), it interferes in speech perception including the abovementioned disorders.
The study is focused on the analysis of sound in a sensitive area of the hospital, representing other acoustically implicated equivalent areas, such as corridors and circulation areas, inpatient settings, hospital waiting rooms, neonatology. In situ measurements have been performed in accordance with international standards. Different constructive materials have been used in order to compare results on the acoustic comfort, which proved that hospital noisy areas may be improved, even in those cases where this fact has not been considered in the original project.

Marilita Giuliano. *Architect, graduated in 1990, (FADU-UBA). Current professional experience (since 2000), Knauf Argentine. Technical-Commercial Chief and Foreign Trade Representative. Conferences in International and National Seminars. Author of several technical articles. Acoustician and Member of the IRAM Acoustics and Fire Subcommittee.*
Rita Comando. *Prof. Architect, specialist in Planning of Health Physical Resources (FADU-UBA). Director of the Design and Management of the Physical Infrastructure and Health Technology Course, ISALUD University. First Vice President, SCA, Argentina. President of (AADAIH) (2006 2008). President of the XXII Congress (CAM). Author of several articles. Attendance to National, Latin American and International Conferences. Advisor in Health Building Architecture and Maintenance.*

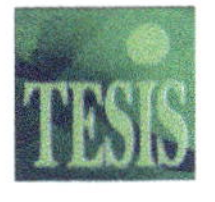

Abbreviations

AADAIH, Argentine Association of Architecture and Hospital Engineering; AdAA, Acoustics Association of Argentina; CAM, Argentine Maintenance Committee; FADU, School of Architecture and Urbanism; GCBA, Buenos Aires City Government; INCOSE, Dry Construction Institute; IRAM, Argentine Normalization and Certification Institute; SCA, Central Society of Architects, Argentina; UBA, University of Buenos Aires, Argentina.

Description

In the healthcare field, the objective is presently to attain a paperless hospital. Based on the progress in the implementation of new Information and Communication Technologies (ICT's), the digital hospital is increasingly expanding as a paperless hospital. A paperless hospital ensures the importance, integrity, confidentiality, and availability of information, orchestrating a continuous electronic interconnection within and without the service. However, this is not enough to achieve a high quality healthcare delivery and ensure patient safety.

There are additional factors to keep working on. This paper focuses onto an invisible factor, which has far-reaching health consequences: noise. Hospital design architecture still continues to minimizing the importance of an adequate acoustic comfort, both in public and private institutions. Paradoxically, noise gained rather than decreased, both day and night, in worldwide hospitals.

Sound, as well as light, is a basic source of energy and has a powerful sensorial effect onto the human being: body, soul, and spirit. Culturally-defined pleasant sounds may contribute to feelings of welfare and peace. They are positive and curative. On the opposite side, unpleasant noise may be disturbing and stressful. Intense sounds may be severely harmful for health. And just as other senses suffer from fatigue when subjected to a continuous barrage, a continuous exposure to noise (defined as undesirable) will cause ear fatigue, while the mind will be attempting to minimize this intrusion. Every single day, hospitals have a great number of people walking through, traveling down corridors, generating noise and affecting the patient and the healthcare team. Constant noise for several hours causes discomfort and generates an important problem, which in parallel may cause stress and distraction. No doubt this fact affects daily work and causes accident proneness and healthcare error, which may put the patient safety at risk. Humming of people, even though quietly, children crying, medicine and housekeeping service carts, wheeled stretchers, and every other sort of noise may be heard. Noise may also difficult the patient understanding of indications. Night-time environmental noise is usually exceeding normal standards for the patient rest. Hardly ever, room doors are closed for various reasons, and this noise, amplified by a lack of acoustic absorption, travels along long distances and pervades the patient rooms.

With reference to hospitals, this study is based on the World Health Organiza-

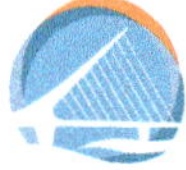

tion (WHO) Guidelines for Community Noise Recommendations (1999). Concerning environmental noise level, the WHO guidelines only present values suggested for use in internal areas. Regarding internal healthcare wards within the inpatient settings, the recommended maximum value (Maximum Level Measured - L_{max}) is 40 dB.

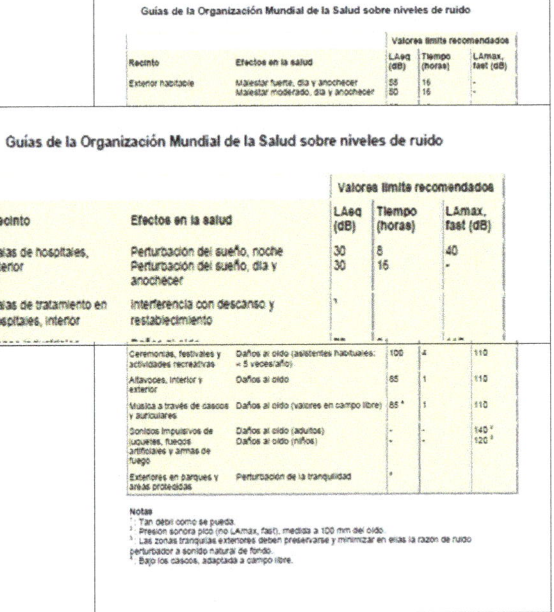

Guías de la Organización Mundial de la Salud sobre niveles de ruido

Guías de la Organización Mundial de la Salud sobre niveles de ruido

Recinto	Efectos en la salud	Valores límite recomendados LAeq (dB)	Tiempo (horas)	LAmax, fast (dB)
Exterior habitable	Malestar fuerte, día y anochecer Malestar moderado, día y anochecer	55 50	16 16	- -
Salas de hospitales, interior	Perturbación del sueño, noche Perturbación del sueño, día y anochecer	30 30	8 16	40 -
Salas de tratamiento en hospitales, interior	Interferencia con descanso y restablecimiento	[1]		
Ceremonias, festivales y actividades recreativas	Daños al oído (asistentes habituales: < 5 veces/año)	100	4	110
Altavoces, interior y exterior	Daños al oído	85	1	110
Música a través de cascos y auriculares	Daños al oído (valores en campo libre)	85 [4]	1	110
Sonidos impulsivos de juguetes, fuegos artificiales y armas de fuego	Daños al oído (adultos) Daños al oído (niños)	- -	- -	140 [2] 120 [2]
Exteriores en parques y áreas protegidas	Perturbación de la tranquilidad	[3]		

Notas
[1]: Tan débil como se pueda.
[2]: Presión sonora pico (no LAmax, fast), medida a 100 mm del oído.
[3]: Las zonas tranquilas exteriores deben preservarse y minimizar en ellas la razón de ruido perturbador a sonido natural de fondo.
[4]: Bajo los cascos, adaptada a campo libre.

Figure 1. Guidelines for Community Noise Recommendations (WHO, 1999).

As per the "Interference of Speech Perception" the WHO suggests that <1 sec Reverberation Time (RT_{60}) is necessary for a good oral communication. For sensitive groups (elderly, patients) a RT_{60} (<0.6 sec) is recommended.

Field research has been conducted. The objective of this survey was to develop a local record in order to compare these results with the standards implemented in Europe and the USA.

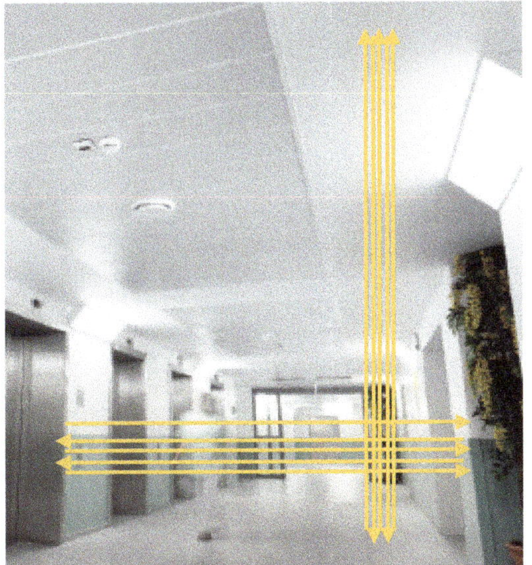

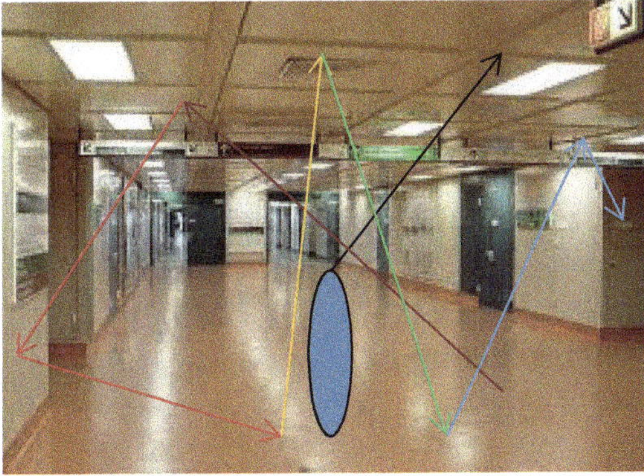

Figure 2. Reverberation time, RT60 - Geometry and volume.

In a hospital, primarily in general areas, we were limited to the project and could not make important changes in its shape or volume. We were focused on at least the acoustic absorption, understood as the absorption of an excessive reverberation in a particular space.

As to the materials, each one has a different alpha(α) or NRC (Noise Reduction Coefficient) absorption index, which may vary between 0 and 1 (maximum). Both

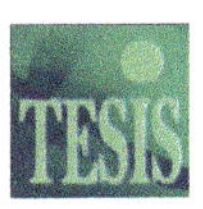

indexes show the percentage of sound absorbed by a material. These indexes vary according to the different frequencies. Therefore, a laboratory evaluation is necessary in order to obtain a single index for each material. There are two standardized approaches to the absorption analysis. While the alpha (α) index is a European index per EN ISO 11654 Regulation, the Noise Reduction Coefficient (NRC) is an American index according to the ASTM 423 Regulations. Both give a clear idea of the overall performance of material, as regards the proportion of sound absorbed. Alpha index is more accurate, and is used by acoustic experts for their calculations.

The NRC is commonly used in the commercial market. Both indexes are similar and their values may even coincide, but there is no mathematical connection between them.

Every material has a certain degree of sound absorption and sound reflectivity. It is usually understood that a material works as an acoustic absorbent material when the alpha index or NRC is greater than 0.50. As for spaces, the most significant parameter to determine whether the acoustic characteristics are suitable for the activity to be developed in a special space is the Reverberation Time (RT). The RT depends on the proportion of absorbent and reflective materials and the volume of the premises to be studied. Subjectively, the RT is defined as the time a sound is prolonged in a room after the source generating the sound stops, until the sound vanishes or becomes inaudible when absorbed by the walls, ceilings, furniture, people, &c. Technically, the time required for the sound to decay by 60 dB is usually measured in seconds and afterwards compared to an initial value.

Intrahospital infections require a special attention as far as hygiene and housekeeping services concern. Therefore, materials used in floors and walls are usually smooth and highly polished. Both floors and walls are usually lined with very low or virtually nil alpha index or NRC materials, with a very low sound absorption. Ceramics, porcelanatos, or even linoleums, for floors and walls have very low or insufficient absorption values, ranging about 0.02 (NRC).

Acoustic ceiling tiles are the best option for sound absorption, so as to compensate other materials with a very low absorption. These are continuous and present a larger surface, as compared to the other wall surfaces. On account of their characteristics, absorbent materials cannot be exposed to circulation purposes, wheeled stretchers, &c.

The enclosure analyzed in this study is approximately 970 square feet (90 m^2) and 12,360 cubic feet (350 m^3). It is important to mention that four other enclosures are coupled to the premises objective of this study, since they are attached to the hospital main entrance and other circulation areas. The original ceiling material consisted of removable plasterboard tiles 6.5 mm thick, painted with a non absorbent material, NRC = 0.05 (reflective material).

These original plasterboard tiles have been removed and replaced with new high sound absorption (mineral fiber) tiles. The existing metal framing for removable ceilings have been preserved for reinstallation.The replacement of plasterboard tiles had low impact in the hospital daily activity. The work was carried out with all the due skills and care, in accordance with good practices.

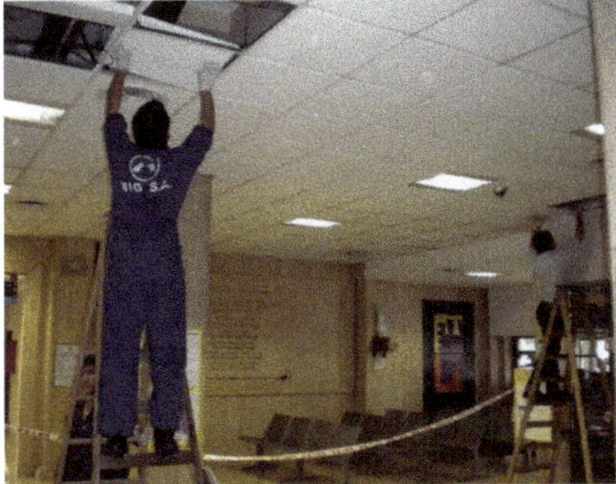

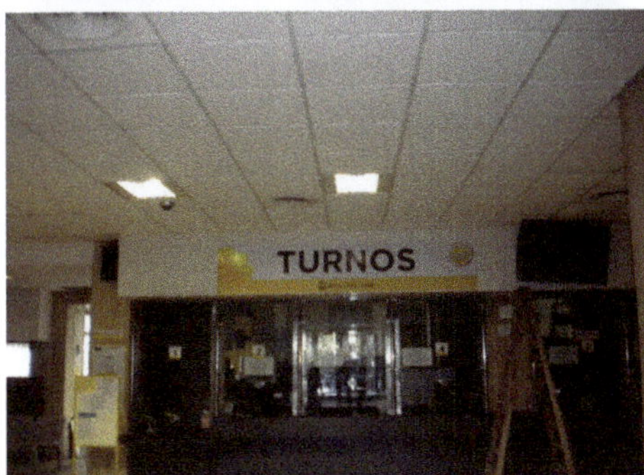

Figure 3. Job on site Hospital Fernandez: acustic modification.

Our goal was to approach the WHO recommended standards. Therefore, reverberation measures were performed in the premises and several materials were tested. The Reverberation Time (RT_{60}) and environmental impact (LAeq index) were measured both before and after the replacement of the sound absorbent material at every stage.

Highly absorbent 19 mm thick fiber mineral tiles with rebated edges were chosen. Technical characteristics of tiles were: NRC = 0.90 per ASTM C 423 regulations; α = 0.90 per EN ISO 11654; 100% humidity resistance and washable finish; included Hygena (bactericidal and fungistatic) treatment.

Being a hospital, materials chosen for sound absorption should especially meet safety fire requirements. Fire Classification of tiles used was "Re: Non-combustible", tested by INTI laboratories, according to IRAM 11910/1 Regulations.

The first RT_{60} control (Measurement #1) without any acoustic material, RT_{60} demonstrated to be too high for the space: RT_{mid} = 2.27 sec (1000 Hz). There was too much noise, people talking, difficult speech and loudspeakers messages comprehension. In order to solve the problem, the volume used to be increased, worsening the initial acoustic conditions.

With the different materials tested, the sensitively measured RT_{60} was reduced to RT_{mid} = 0.74 sec (1000 Hz) (Measurement #4, Figure 4, Table 1).

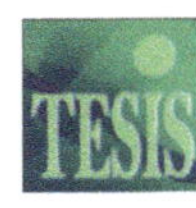

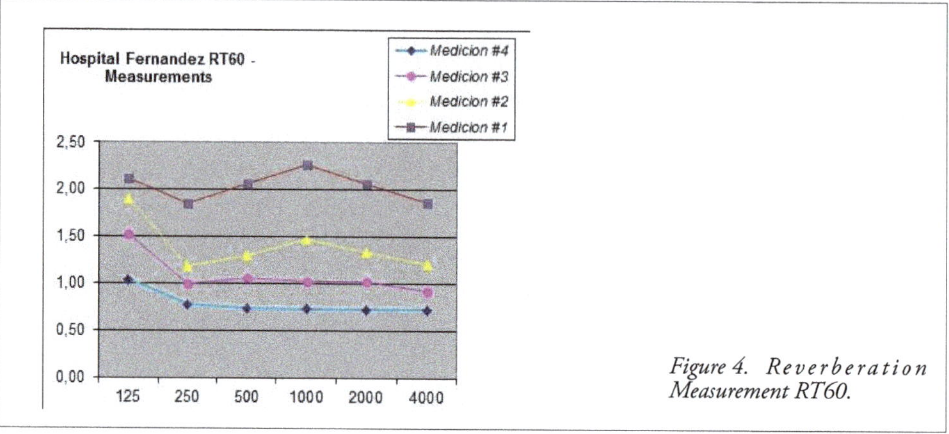

Figure 4. Reverberation Measurement RT60.

RT_{60} (sec)	125	250	500	1000	2000	4000
Measurement #1	2.11	1.85	2.07	2.27	2.07	1.87
Measurement #2	1.90	1.20	1.30	1,49	1.34	1.22
Measurement #3	1.53	1.00	1.07	1.03	1.02	0.93
Measurement #4	1.04	0.78	0.74	0.74	0.73	0.72

Table 1. Reverberation Measurements.

After the installation of acoustic mineral fiber tiles, excellent acoustic efficiency was observed. Indexes (500 Hz frequency) were compared. Improvement was over expectations.

It is important to note that statistical data is the result of observation of the same variable at different times of day, since sources of noise use to differ.

CONCLUSIONS

The main objective of this survey was to become aware and describe the problems of noise in health organizations, so as to help professionals to improve future design processes, by developing a project that may balance conditions of sound absorption, diffusion, and reflection.
The secondary objective was to demonstrate that the existing buildings can be effectively improved with minimal constructive interventions. In our case, we started by assuming that we were in front of a difficult project from the acoustic point of view. However, a simple and effective work could be done, reaching values quite close to those recommended by the WHO Reverberation Time Guidelines.

It is important to mention that a complementary work must be done on noise sources, such as, behavior changes in staff and patients, use of cell phones or beepers, maintenance of cart and stretcher bearing. This work is just an example of the results that can be achieved with a good acoustic project. However, other measures may be taken to optimize further acoustic comfort.

The Importance of Building Structures in the Waste Management of Healthcare Facilities. The Case Study of Hospital "El Cruce"

Carla Figliolo[1], María Albornoz[2], Ricardo Otero[2], Germán Marengo[1], Déborah González[1] y Luis Couyoupetrou[1]

carla.figliolo@gmail.com

[1]Universidad Nacional Arturo Jauretche (UNAJ)

[2]Hospital de Alta Complejidad El Cruce (HEC)

Waste management (WM) in healthcare facilities is a complex challenge for old facilities and newly built hospitals because there are no estimated future considerations and generally in the instance of the layout, specialists in WM are not involved. Wastes in a healthcare center are not only bio-hazardous, also hazardous chemicals, radioactive and common comparable to household waste; all must be incorporated into a waste management system. Hospital El Cruce (HEC) is a health facility following to continue its growth in infrastructure and provision of services. This growth must also be accompanied by the ability to adapt WM for all activities taking place in it. For this challenge National University Arturo Jauretche (UNAJ) was convened to accompany the growth process of the hospital with respect to the management of their wastes. The UNAJ experts began the work according with the methodology proposed by Figliolo (1) and WM assessment of Madero et al. (2). An adequacy plan for WM was formulated and was carried on. Even it is difficult to establish a system of WM and to fully comply with all requirements of the regulations when the deficiencies are matters of infrastructure, other logistic resources exist that can help to solve them.

Carla Figliolo *is biologist, with a master in environmental management for companies and a master in environmental studies. She is specialized in hazardous waste management and in policies and environmental management tools. She is the Coordinator of the Unidad de Investigación y Desarrollo Ambiental de la Secretaría de Ambiente y Desarrollo Sustentable de Argentina and professor at Universidad de Ciencias Empresariales y Sociales and Universidad Nacional Arturo Jauretche, also for posgraduate courses at ADDAIH with Universidad Nacional de La Matanza (UNLaM) and at Universidad ISALUD. She in an international speaker and has publications related with healthcare waste management and hazardous waste.*

Presentation

Waste management in healthcare facilities is a complex challenge for both old infrastructure facilities - some over a hundred years – and newly built modern hospitals. In the old hospitals, because the wastes were not even taken into consideration, they did not constitute a problematic issue and currently, because bearing in mind that wastes will be generated, there are no estimated future considerations and generally in the instance of the layout of any facility,

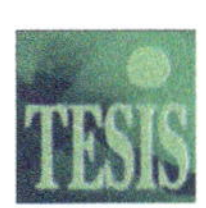

specialists in the field are not involved. Wastes in a healthcare center are not only bio-hazardous, pathogenic or infectious wastes according to the different denominations; to them it must be added hazardous chemicals and radioactive wastes, and common comparable to household waste; all must be incorporated into a system of waste management.

Hospital El Cruce (HEC), is a High Complexity health facility built five years ago, following to continue its growth in infrastructure and provision of services. This growth must also be accompanied by the ability to adapt the management of all activities taking place in it.

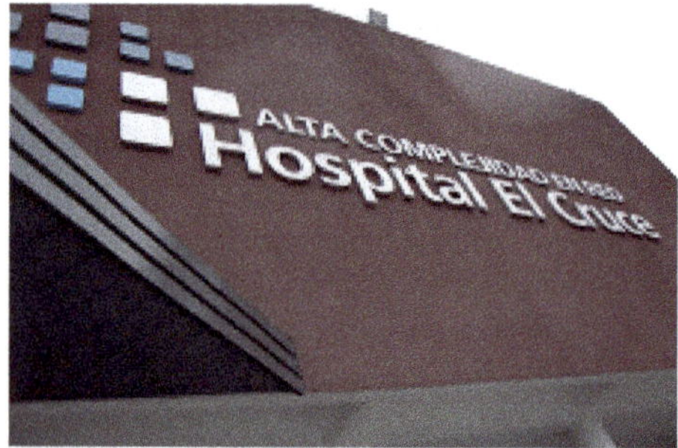

Figure 1. Hospital El Cruce (HEC), Florencio Varela Buenos Aires – Argentina.

Waste management is one of the basic requirements of environmental management and of the general policy of the hospital and is an international commitment with the Global Green and Healthy Hospitals Network. Thus in late 2013 experts in Environmental Management from the National University Arturo Jauretche (UNAJ) were convened to accompany the growth process of the hospital with respect to the management of their healthcare wastes (HCW). The team from the UNAJ began the work according with the "Methodological Proposal for Carrying out HCW Management Studies and Follow-ups" proposed by Figliolo[1] which basically includes an initial diagnosis, a first training workshop to show waste management status of the establishment and to organize follow-up work on the basis of waste management criteria. It also includes the assessment according to *Madero et al.*[2], through the "Weighted Matrix to Assess Waste Management in Health Centers with Inpatient Facilities". This diagnosis allowed identification of critical points in the waste management, rate the waste management in 3.84 on a scale of 6 according to the assessment matrix[2], check the criteria on which can scale the score and formulate the Adequacy Plan of Waste Management. As a last step of diagnosis it was held a result communication workshop aimed to the entire hospital staff. The formulation of the Adequacy Plan was developed based on a quality process management and had a pre-filing by the expert group from the UNAJ and then agreed with the Waste Management Committee created as the starting point of adequacy. The Waste Management Committee was formed

---

[1] Figliolo, Carla. Propuesta Metodológica para realizar Estudios y Seguimientos de Gestión de Residuos de Establecimientos de Salud (RES). Unidad de Investigación y Desarrollo Ambiental. Secretaría de Ambiente y Desarrollo Sustentable de la Nación. Argentina. Available at http://www.ambiente.gob.ar/default.asp?IdArticulo=10807 (last accessed April 23, 2014).

[2] Madero, Martín M., Ruggiero María Constanza, Risso Antonella, Catania Alejandro y Carla Figliolo. 2011. Nueva Matriz Ponderada de Evaluación de Gestión de Residuos de Establecimientos de Salud con Internación. Unidad de Investigación y Desarrollo Ambiental. Secretaría de Ambiente y Desarrollo Sustentable de la Nación. Argentina. Avalilable at http://www.ambiente.gov.ar/default.asp?IdArticulo=11132 (last accessed April 23, 2014).

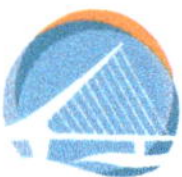

with representatives from different areas, including General Services, Health and Safety, Architecture, Nursing, Cleansing and Quality.

The main components of this adequacy plan were:

- to issue Waste Management committee by a regulation adopted by the executive director of the hospital;
- conduct a comprehensive study of waste generation to ensure the complete classification of waste from the HEC;
- assist in implementation of the draft final waste storage;
- establish the management of hazardous chemicals waste according to the generation study;
- implement a comprehensive training plan;
- incorporate signage waste management and adapting containers, - General monitoring of waste management and monitoring the indicator $Kg.bed^{-1}.day^{-1}$;
- establish the registers recording the generated waste;
- establish a procedure for annual audit in accordance with audit planning of the Hospital;
- develop and adapt Standards Procedures of waste management;
- achieve certificates of bio-contaminated waste with reliable information;
- generate a record of the chemicals used;
- assist in the recruitment of a hazardous chemical waste transporter and operator (treatment) enabled by the environmental authority;
- check the effluent management plant operations for the handling liquids of laboratory;
- generate a registration system for common recyclable waste;
- develop performance indicators;
- conduct annual management reports
– analyze the best alternatives for the treatment of bio-contaminated waste (cost - benefit study).

From the Adequacy Plan for Waste Management of High Complexity Hospital El Cruce there were several activities planned according to the requirements. As a first instance it was performed a survey of places and use of containers according to colors and volume; the reorganization and reallocation of containers was made as requested and added signage to start the communication process and training of all the staff of the areas under the new management procedures. In accordance to this, a waste brochure for the external communication of the waste management and for the families of patients being attended at the hospital was developed. The Hospital, as a member of the "Global Green and Healthy Hospitals Network", should also promote the separation of recyclable common waste, to incorporate them into recycling circuits, so work was held by the separation of these waste in general external and internal areas and administrative areas, waiting rooms and patient admissions, with a graphic communication campaign for proper separation.

One of the main challenges to comply with the requirements of the adequacy plan emerged from the infrastructure, as still being a new hospital there are still facility deficiencies that do not allow proper waste management, particularly with respect to intermediate and final storage areas of waste. The assess matrix for waste management used has a set of criteria that corresponds to infrastructure and supplies and in it, all intermediate and final storage of waste are evaluated. A hospital must have intermediate

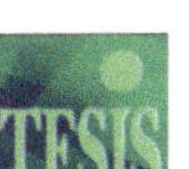

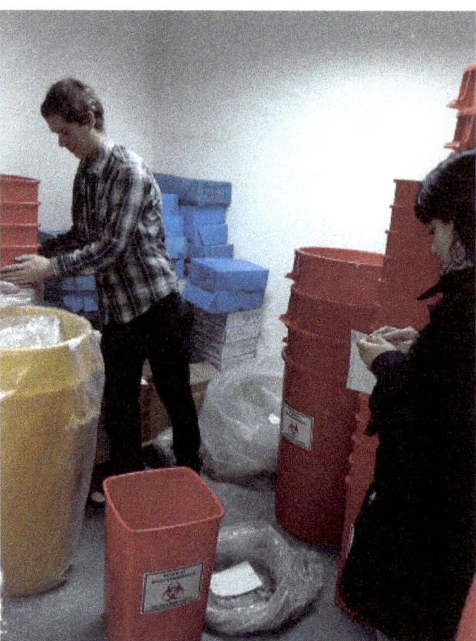

Figure 2. Storage of bio-contaminated, chemical hazardous waste.

storage for waste, in all areas of services for both bio-contaminated and common waste, and also in certain areas of hazardous chemicals generation have a proper facility for the containment until collection. The hospital El Cruce had to adapt intermediate storage areas for all purposes, since it does not have exclusive places as indicated by the law n° 11.347 (Buenos Aires) for pathogenic medical wastes, and its regulations. Thus, were destined exclusive identified trolleys for common and bio-contaminated waste respectively and all general storage areas were identified with the appropriate signage. These actions were accompanied by a change in logistics, given the need to exclude waste collectors from sensitive areas of the hospital as a principle of bio-security and infection control, who only pass through the external aisles of hospital services.

Hospital El Cruce has a final storage area for bio-contaminated waste consistent with the requirements of applicable law, but the growth in activity, number of beds and future services, was not foresaw for the final storage of waste, and is now evident the lack of place. The facility has no final storage area for hazardous chemical waste and also has not planned the storage with restricted access for common waste.

Based on these shortcomings, the Waste Management Committee requested the Hospital manager to evaluate the medium-term possibility of building a comprehensive center for final storage of waste, with exclusive areas for bio-contaminated , chemical hazardous waste , common undifferentiated (municipal) and recyclable. Regarding this issue is ongoing a new project generation. As an intermediate step to solve this issue it was decided to build a new storage area for flammable substances and use the old storage area of flammables to establish a storage for hazardous chemical wastes since both share the same safety requirements.

Even it is difficult to establish a system of waste management and to fully comply with all requirements of the regulations when the deficiencies are matters of infrastructure, other logistic resources exist that can help to solve them. The Adequacy plan has been generated in a process of continuous improvement and under the convention between the UNAJ and the HEC, and with a one year specific development agreement, is intended to leave capacity building to continue adjusting the variables of the waste management within the quality management system that the facility has.

Protection against Hospital Acquired Infections Using Advanced Ultraviolet Disinfection Technology

Normand Brais

nbrais@bma.ca
P.Eng, Ph.D, Sanuvox Technologies Inc.

Ultraviolet Germicidal Irradiation (UVGI) has been widely accepted for over 50 years and recognized as a superior alternative to chemicals for the disinfection of drinking water. UVGI is today a well mastered cost effective disinfection technology that unlike antibiotics does not create any new resistant strains and as such creates no undesirable side effect. It has proven capable of deactivating all kinds of microorganisms by dimerization of the thymine pairs of their DNA or RNA. This paper explains and demystifies the fundamentals behind a new generation of software-driven smart automated UVGI devices and how they could be used to complete the sterilization process of operating rooms, patient rooms and hospital bathrooms. Automated systems have been widely adopted in other areas of healthcare to mitigate human errors. When commenting on the future of nosocomial infection control in 1998, Dr Robert Weinstein wrote: "Given the choice of improving technology or improving human behavior, technology is the better choice."

Normand Brais *is a professional engineer that holds a PhD in Nuclear Engineering from Polytechnique of Montreal. He has founded several technological companies in fields as various as atmospheric pollution, biomass combustion, water treatment, photonics, and air/surface disinfection.*
In 1995 he founded Sanuvox Technologies, which is now a worldwide leader in air and surface disinfection for hospitals and buildings using germicidal UV irradiation.
Dr. Brais is an active board member of Univalor, a non-profit organization whose mission is to guide university professors in the commercialization of breakthrough technology. He is also President of the Polytechnique Alumni Foundation and serves as Treasurer for the United Nations Association in Canada Greater Montreal.

Introduction

It is now recognized that contaminated surfaces have been utterly underestimated as a reservoir of nosocomial infections [1-3]. Some recent studies have clearly indicated that admission to a room previously occupied by a patient with Clostridium difficile, vancomycin-resistant enterococci (VRE), meticillin-resistant Staphylococcus aureus (MRSA), Acinetobacter baumannii

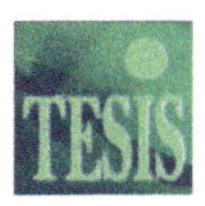

and Pseudomonas aeruginosa increases the infection probability for subsequent occupants by a factor of two or more[1,4-8]. Such statistics points to the fact that current cleaning and disinfection following the discharge of patients is far from being adequate and needs major improvement. The emergence rate of epidemic strain of C.-Difficile and other multidrug-resistant Gram-negative bacteria that can also survive on surfaces is a further motivation to improve hospital disinfection processes [9,10].

Current cleaning and disinfection using conventional methods relies heavily on a human operator to appropriately select and use a suitable agent and spread it to all target surfaces with a sufficient concentration and contact time. Any improvement of these conventional methods requires the modification of human action and behaviour, which is in practice extremely challenging, to say the least.

The use of new automated room disinfection systems based on the well-known germicidal properties of special ultraviolet light sources provides an alternative approach, which almost removes or greatly reduces reliance on the operator's ability [11-14]. Automated systems have been adopted widely in many other areas of healthcare to alleviate human error.

Indeed, commenting on the future of nosocomial infection control in 1998, Dr Robert Weinstein wrote: 'Given the choice of improving technology or improving human behavior, technology is the better choice [15].

Limitations of conventional cleaning and disinfection

Conventional cleaning and disinfection is actually accomplished by a human operator using all kinds of liquid detergent products. Several microbiological studies have shown that such conventional disinfection procedure rarely succeeds at eradicating pathogens from surfaces [17-20]. Problems associated with both 'product' and 'procedure' contribute to this, in particular, the reliance on the operator to repeatedly ensure adequate selection, concentration, distribution and contact time of the disinfectant. For example, a wide assessment of conventional cleaning in 36 hospitals using fluorescent markers has shown that less than 50% of high-risk objects in hospital rooms were disinfected after patient discharge [21].

As we all know, improving human behaviour is quite difficult but many valuable initiatives are often taken. Those include routine microbiological analysis of surface hygiene, the use of fluorescent markers or ATP assays to monitor the cleaning efficiency, provide feedback of cleaning performance and pursue educational training [5,11,16,21-23].
Monitoring and feedback can somehow improve the frequency of surfaces that are cleaned and reduce the level of environmental contamination [5,21,24,25,26-28]. However, no studies have evaluated the practical sustainability of those improvement initiatives. In fact, recent evidence indicates that simply changing the location of fluorescent dye spots has significantly reduced the proportion of cleaned surfaces from a level 90% down to about only 60%.

Summary of problems associated with actual conventional disinfection:

- Infectiveness of cleaning products against some pathogens; for example, many frequently used hospital disinfectants are not effective against C.-Difficile spores and norovirus [30,33,35].
- Toxicity to staff and/or the environment [30,31].
- Damage to hospital materials and equipment [30].
- Potential for biocide/antibiotic cross-resistance [32].
- Problems with cleaning/disinfection procedures include: Adequate distribution of the active agent, given the challenges of the complex hospital environment [21].
- Ensuring correct contact time for the microbial reduction achieved in vitro.[35]
- Repeatability of the process depends on the operator [21].
- Designation of responsibility for various items, particularly complex portable medical equipment [36].
- Compliance with protocols/policies from a sometime poorly paid, poorly motivated workforce [37].
- Inadequate training and education of personnel [37].
- Improper formulation/concentration of the disinfectant [32,38].
- Contamination of cleaning equipment [38,39].

Ultraviolet Germicidal Irradiation Technology

Ultraviolet Germicidal Irradiation (UVGI) has been widely accepted for over 50 years and recognized as a complement to chemicals for the disinfection of drinking water. UVGI is today a well mastered cost effective disinfection technology that unlike antibiotics does not create any new resistant strains and as such creates no undesirable side effect. There has been no sign of adaptability of any microbes to UVGI even after almost half a century of use. The same thing cannot be said of chemical cleaners and for antibiotics!
Germicidal UV or UV-C has proven capable of deactivating all kinds of microorganisms by dimerization of the thymine pairs of their DNA or RNA.
The operating principle for surface decontamination is to deliver a specific dose of 254 nm wavelength light that has a deleterious effect on DNA. The germicidal UV dose is defined as the product of UV light intensity in microwatt/cm^2 multiplied by the exposure time in seconds. The resulting dose is thus expressed in microjoule/cm^2. Because of its important use in water disinfection for over 50 years, the UV susceptibility of a wide variety of microorganisms has been sampled and measured and there have been thus far no signs of emergence of resistance from any bacterial strains.

When used as a single unit, the device is generally placed in the centre of the room and frequently touched mobile items are arranged close to the device for optimal exposure. Because just like any other light, UV travels in straight lines, it is evidently not as effective in shadow areas out of direct line of sight.

For the above reason, some early UV devices manufacturers have recommend multiple cycles from different locations.34 This is not practical as it not only doubles and triples the disinfection cycle time but also requires an operator intervention and attendance between each move.

But akin to any lighting system, the use of two, three or more emission sources strategically placed to eliminate shadow zones is a much more effective strategy to keep the cycle time low. Also, the additive property of the superimposed UV fields emitted by each UV unit increases the overall intensity and hence contributes to reducing the disinfection cycle time.

Disinfection efficacy of UVGI

Disinfection levels of 6 Log (i.e 99.9999% or 1 survival per million) on C.Diff and MRSA have been achieved in lab tests.

The fact is that knowing the UV susceptibility constants of C. Diff, MRSA, VRE, KLEB, etc., it is relatively easy to determine the required UV intensity to reach a preset target disinfection level.
Measurement of the UV intensity field emitted as a function of the distance from a UV disinfection unit can be easily performed and then the required cycle time can be computed to deliver the desired UV dosage for a target disinfection level.
For example, given the tabulated UV susceptibility of the target bio-contaminants and the UV intensity, the required cycle times to reach 99.9999% disinfection i.e. 6 Log can be computed as in Table 1.

As shown in the table below, providing an adequately sized powerful pair of UVGI units, a disinfection cycle of 15 minutes is possible at distances up to 10 feet (3 m) away. If the maximum distance from the units is less than 5 ft (1.5 m), then only 5 minutes of disinfection time is required.

Not only a dual unit disinfection system minimizes shadow areas, but it also provides an enhanced overall irradiation field that allows for faster sterilization cycle. When tested in the lab, it showed >99.999% disinfection of C.-Difficile, VRE, and MRSA after only 5 minutes of exposure. In the case of very large rooms, three or four units can be used simultaneously to keep the cycle time short.

The complete disinfection cycle is fully automated and operated by wireless communication by using any smart phone or computer tablet such as ipad.
For safety, the units are equipped with eight (8) wide-range infrared motion sensors that will cause the units to shut down in the event someone would walk into a room undergoing a disinfection cycle.
The units have a built-in downloadable data logger that records each and every sterilization cycle performed at any given time and location.

Disinfection target :	**ASPETIX TANDEM DISINFECTION PERFORMANCE CHART**						
99,9999%	**Distance =**	**5 ft**	**6 ft**	**7 ft**	**8 ft**	**9 ft**	**10 ft**
	UV output in mW/cm2 =	1314	999	778	620	504	417
C.diff	*Exposure time required in Minutes :*	*4,6*	*6,0*	*7,7*	*9,7*	*11,9*	*14,4*
MRSA	*Exposure time required in Minutes :*	*1,2*	*1,6*	*2,1*	*2,6*	*3,2*	*3,8*
VRE	*Exposure time required in Minutes :*	*0,4*	*0,6*	*0,7*	*0,9*	*1,1*	*1,3*
Klebsiella pneumoniae	*Exposure time required in Minutes :*	*0,3*	*0,4*	*0,5*	*0,7*	*0,8*	*1,0*

Table 1. Aspetix tandem disinfection performance chart.

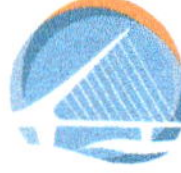

CONCLUSIONS

Given that conventional disinfection methods have inherent limitations that may be overcome through the use of a UVGI disinfection system. Strong evidence now exists that the level of terminal disinfection of clinical areas used by patients with pathogens associated with transmission from the environment should be increased in order to prevent environment-borne transmission between patients, and it is in this situation where new automated UVGI technology are most strongly indicated.

There are now clear evidences that automated UVGI technology is an effective adjunct to conventional methods of terminal disinfection, and that it can reduce transmission in endemic and epidemic settings. Just like it did so well for drinking water around the world in the last 30 years, it is likely that UVGI technology will become a cornerstone to raise the level of hospital infection control in the near future.

REFERENCES

1.Otter JA, Yezli S, French GL. The role played by contaminated surfaces in the transmission of nosocomial pathogens. *Infect Control Hosp Epidemiol* 2011;32:687e699.

2. Maki DG, Alvarado CJ, Hassemer CA, Zilz MA. Relation of the inanimate hospital environment to endemic nosocomial infection. *N Engl J Med* 1982;307:1562e1566.

3. Weber DJ, Rutala WA, Miller MB, Huslage K, Sickbert-Bennett E. Role of hospital surfaces in the transmission of emerging health care-associated pathogens: norovirus, Clostridium difficile, and Acinetobacter species. *Am J Infect Control* 2010;38:S25 e S33.

4. Shaughnessy MK, Micielli RL, De-Pestel DD, et al. Evaluation of hospital room assignment and acquisition of Clostridium difficile infection. *Infect Control Hosp Epidemiol* 2011;32:201 e 206.

5. Datta R, Platt R, Yokoe DS, Huang SS. Environmental cleaning intervention and risk of acquiring multidrug-resistant organisms from prior room occupants. *Arch Intern Med* 2011;171:491 e 494.

6. Huang SS, Datta R, Platt R. Risk of acquiring antibiotic-resistant bacteria from prior room occupants. *Arch Intern Med* 2006;166:1945 e 1951.

7. Drees M, Snydman D, Schmid C, et al. Prior environmental contamination increases the risk of acquisition of vancomycinresistant enterococci. *Clin Infect Dis* 2008; 46:678 e 685.

8. Nseir S, Blazejewski C, Lubret R, Wallet F, Courcol R, Durocher A. Risk of acquiring multidrug-resistant Gram-negative bacilli from prior room occupants in the *ICU. Clin Microbiol Infect* 2011;17:1201 e 1208.

9. Peleg AY, Hooper DC. Hospital-acquired infections due to gramnegative bacteria. *N Engl J Med* 2010;362:1804 e 1813.

10. Dubberke ER, Reske KA, Noble-Wang J, et al. Prevalence of Clostridium difficile environmental contamination and strain variability in multiple health care facilities. *Am J Infect Control* 2007;35:315 e 318.

11. Rutala WA, Weber DJ. Are room decontamination units needed to prevent transmission of environmental pathogens? *Infect Control Hosp Epidemiol* 2011;32:743 e 747.

12. Davies A, Pottage T, Bennett A, Walker J. Gaseous and air decontamination technologies for Clostridium difficile in the healthcare environment. *J Hosp Infect* 2011;77:199 e 203.

13. Falagas ME, Thomaidis PC, Kotsantis IK, Sgouros K, Samonis G, Karageorgopoulos DE. Airborne hydrogen peroxide for disinfection of the hospital environment and infection control: a systematic review. *J Hosp Infect* 2011;78:171 177.

14. Byrns G, Fuller TP. The risks and benefits of chemical fumigation in the health care environment. *J Occup Environ Hyg* 2011;8:104 e 112.

15. Weinstein RA. Nosocomial infection update. *Emerg Infect Dis* 1998;4:416 e 420.

16. Dancer SJ. How do we assess hospital cleaning? A proposal for microbiological standards for surface hygiene in hospitals. *J Hosp Infect* 2004;56:10 e 15.

17. French GL, Otter JA, Shannon KP, Adams NM, Watling D, Parks MJ. Tackling contamination of the hospital environment by methicillin-resistant Staphylococcus aureus (MRSA): a comparison between conventional terminal cleaning and hydrogen peroxide vapour decontamination. *J Hosp Infect* 2004;57:31 e 37.

18. Byers KE, Durbin LJ, Simonton BM, Anglim AM, Adal KA, Farr BM. Disinfection of hospital rooms contaminated with vancomycinresistant Enterococcus faecium. *Infect Control Hosp Epidemiol* 1998;19:261 e 264.

19. Manian FA, Griesenauer S, Senkel D, et al. Isolation of Acinetobacter baumannii complex and methicillin-resistant Staphylococcus aureus from hospital rooms following terminal cleaning and disinfection: can we do better? I*nfect Control Hosp Epidemiol* 2011;32:667 e 672.

20. Wilcox MH, Fawley WN, Wigglesworth N, Parnell P, Verity P, Freeman J. Comparison of the effect of detergent versus hypochlorite cleaning on environmental contamination and incidence of Clostridium difficile infection. *J Hosp Infect* 2003;54:109 e 114.

21. Carling PC, Parry MM, Rupp ME, Po JL, Dick B, Von Beheren S. Improving cleaning of the environment surrounding patients in 36 acute care hospitals. *Infect Control Hosp Epidemiol* 2008;29:1035 e 1041.

22. Mulvey D, Redding P, Robertson C, et al. Finding a benchmark for moni-

toring hospital cleanliness. *J Hosp Infect* 2011;77:25 e 30.

23. Boyce JM, Havill NL, Dumigan DG, Golebiewski M, Balogun O, Rizvani R. Monitoring the effectiveness of hospital cleaning practices by use of an adenosine triphosphate bioluminescence assay. *Infect Control Hosp Epidemiol* 2009;30:678 e 684.

24. Carling PC, Briggs JL, Perkins J, Highlander D. Improved cleaning of patient rooms using a new targeting method. *Clin Infect Dis* 2006;42:385 e 388.

25. Goodman ER, Platt R, Bass R, Onderdonk AB, Yokoe DS, Huang SS. Impact of an environmental cleaning intervention on the presence of methicillin-resistant Staphylococcus aureus and vancomycin-resistant enterococci on surfaces in intensive care unit rooms. *Infect Control Hosp Epidemiol* 2008;29:593 e 599.

26. Eckstein BC, Adams DA, Eckstein EC, et al. Reduction of Clostridium difficile and vancomycin-resistant Enterococcus contamination of environmental surfaces after an intervention to improve cleaning methods. *BMC Infect Dis* 2007;7:61.

27. Dancer SJ, White LF, Lamb J, Girvan EK, Robertson C. Measuring the effect of enhanced cleaning in a UK hospital: a prospective cross-over study. *BMC Med* 2009;7:28.

28. Hayden MK, Bonten MJ, Blom DW, Lyle EA, van de Vijver DA, Weinstein RA. Reduction in acquisition of vancomycin-resistant enterococcus after enforcement of routine environmental cleaning measures. *Clin Infect Dis* 2006;42:1552 e 1560.

29. Jeanes A, Rao G, Osman M, Merrick P. Eradication of persistent environmental MRSA. *J Hosp Infect* 2005;61:85 e 86.

30. Dettenkofer M, Block C. Hospital disinfection: efficacy and safety issues. *Curr Opin Infect Dis* 2005;18:320 e 325.

31. Mirabelli MC, Zock JP, Plana E, et al. Occupational risk factors for asthma among nurses and related healthcare professionals in an international study. *Occup Environ Med* 2007;64:474 e 479.

32. Meyer B, Cookson B. Does microbial resistance or adaptation to biocides create a hazard in infection prevention and control? *J Hosp Infect* 2010;76:200 e 205.

33. Humphreys PN. Testing standards for sporicides. *J Hosp Infect* 2011;77:193 e 198.

34. Boyce JM, Havill NL, Moore BA. Terminal decontamination of patient rooms using an automated mobile UV light unit. *Infect Control Hosp Epidemiol* 2011;32:737 e 742.

35. Fraise A. Currently available sporicides for use in healthcare, and their limitations. *J Hosp Infect* 2011;77:210 e 212.

36. Havill NL, Havill HL, Mangione E, Dumigan DG, Boyce JM. Cleanliness of portable medical equipment disinfected

by nursing staff. *Am J Infect Control* 2011;39:602 e 604.

37. Dancer SJ. Mopping up hospital infection. *J Hosp Infect* 1999;43:85 e 100.

38. Weber DJ, Rutala WA, Sickbert-Bennett EE. Outbreaks associated with contaminated antiseptics and disinfectants. *Antimicrob Agents Chemother* 2007;51:4217 e 4224.

39. Werry C, Lawrence JM, Sanderson PJ. Contamination of detergent cleaning solutions during hospital cleaning. *J Hosp Infect* 1988;11:44 e 49.

Preliminary Study of RFID Technologies for Healthcare Applications

G. Borelli [1], F.V. Caredda[2], A. Fanti C, G. Gatto[3], G. Mazzarella[3], P.F. Orrù B, A. Serpi[3], I. L. Spano[3], E. Tanzi[3], A. Volpi[4], F. Zedda[5]

gianlucaborelli@aob.it, vale_caredda@tiscali.it, alessandro.fanti@diee.unica.it, gatto@diee.unica.it, mazzarel@diee.unica.it, pforru@unica.it, alessandro.serpi@diee.unica.it, ivan.spano@diee.unica.it, enricotanzi@hotmail.com, andrea.volpi@unipr.it, francescozedda@gmail.com

[1]AOB, Azienda Ospedaliera Brotzu, Piazza Ricchi 1, 09121, Cagliari – Italy
[2]CINSA, Centro Interdipartimentale di Ingegneria e Scienze Ambientali, Via S. Giorgio 12, 09124, Cagliari – Italy
[3]DIEE, Dipartimento di Ingegneria Elettrica ed elettronica, University of Cagliari, Piazza d'Armi, 09123, Cagliari – Italy
[4]Dipartimento di Ingegneria Industriale, University of Parma, Via G.P. Usberti 181A, 43124, Parma – Italy
[5]DIMCM, Dipartimento di Ingegneria Meccanica, Chimica e dei Materiali, University of Cagliari, Piazza d'Armi, 09123, Cagliari – Italy

This paper describe the feasibility analysis of Radio Frequency Identification (RFID) applications in Transfusion Medicine, with the aim of improving patient safety and blood inventory management processes.
In the first part of the paper, a reverse engineering of present processes (AS IS Model) was performed, then an RFID-based processes re-engineering has been designed (To Be Model). Then a Return on Safety assessment was performed via FMECA and KPI design. Two RFID technologies were considered, HF (13,56 MHz) and UHF (865-868 MHz), and an economic assessment was performed in order to evaluate the investment sustainability of the two technologies, showing the suitability of the UHF option.
The second part of the paper regards the experimental analysis of EMC immunity of an IMD against RFID sources in an Electromagnetic Anechoic Chamber. For each RFID technology considered the Electromagnetic Compatibility test, within the Electromagnetic Anechoic Chamber, was performed in order to evaluate the radiated emission and radiated immunity. In particular the RFID interference was measured in order to evaluate the coexistent between the RFID system and the medical devices in hospital environment.

__Gianluca Borelli__ was born in Cagliari in 1967. Since 1997 he is Chief Engineer and Head of the Facility Operations at Brotzu Hospital in Cagliari. He developed several Healthcare projects for Italian Hospitals. He is member of the board of S.I.A.I.S. (Società Italiana dell'Architettura e dell'Ingegneria per la Sanità).

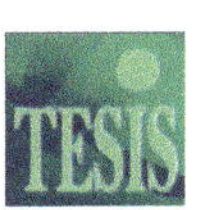

Introduction

Clinical Risk reduction, safety and quality improving of Healthcare system services are nowadays a priority and Transfusion medicine is one of the most interesting areas with high intervention potential. Regarding the clinical risk, the most serious transfusion risks are: virus infection and hemolytic reaction.

Since the early nineties, thanks to the introduction of new compulsory tests, virus transmission incidence has been lowered. On the other hand, acute hemolytic reaction due to transfusion of ABO conflicting blood, today still represents the most serious potential adverse event with deadly consequences for patients in about 10% of cases [1].

Due to high complexity of transfusion process, probability of human errors is still the most dangerous. Recent international studies reveal that pre-analytical and clinical errors, which include incorrect ABO bedside testing and mistaken or missing patient identity check, represent about 80% of total adverse events [2]. This problem is very significant in countries with a large request of blood components, as the territory of the application of our study, Sardinia Island. This study is applied in the most important Healthcare facility of Sardinia Island, the Brotzu Hospital (AOB), where blood request is about 64 packed red blood cells units/1000 inhabitants, while national average (Italy) is 42 blood cells units/1000 inhabitants. Due to the huge demand, almost 50'000 units per year, 60% of blood bags are imported from other Italy's regions [3].

Reengineering process management for improving patient safety is a clear need, especially regarding patient identification and blood components traceability. The target is to devise a method for reducing clinical risk in transfusion medicine with a process re-engineering application, based on introduction of Radio Frequency Identification (RFID) technology.

RFID systems can be considered an integration and evolution of barcodes, and they are currently used for assetting traceability in different sectors. Potential of RFID technology within health care environments has been assessed by several studies [4], showing positive effects on patient safety and logistics concerning patients and medical products.

Processes Analysis

The first step of the project consisted of the analysis of transfusion processes [5], which aimed to identify critical issues related to service efficiency and safety. Current processes analysis involved Blood Transfusion Centre (BTC) and two AOB Units (Neurosurgery and Transplant Unit).

Criticalities related to efficiency and effectiveness of the processes (AS IS model) were highlighted through a Return on Safety (ROS) assessment, using the Failure Mode Effects and Criticalities Analysis (FMECA) in order to suggest suitable actions for process improvement. Failure modes were identified and studied, then a Risk Priority Index (RPI) was defined and ascribed to each failure mode. According to RPI, errors were classified through a bar chart set and a variable threshold ABC analysis. FMECA and ABC analysis put in evidence that critical activities are related to patient recognition and manual operations, such as: pilot test tubes and blood

bags labelling; copying donation data from hand written paper to management software's database.
Then, an RFID-based processes re-engineering (TO-BE Model) has been designed in order to reduce criticalities and to improve Transfusion Medicine service performances. The TO BE model's RFID-enabled processes were submitted to FMECA and some Key performances Indicators (KPI) were calculated in order to highlight process performance variation within the AS IS – TO BE transition (Table 1).

In order to develop the TO BE model, two main RFID technologies were considered:

- HF (13,56 MHz): it is the currently standard approved by the FDA for transfusion medicine applications. Despite the indisputable reliability of the system, reading potentialities at medium-long range and multiple readings are limited.

- UHF (865-868 MHz): it is the currently standard for worldwide commercial logistic and it is characterized by several advantages compared to HF technology, such as: low cost, high performance in terms of multiple reading and reading distances.

ECONOMIC ANALYSIS

In order to evaluate the investment sustainability of the two technologies, an economic assessment was performed [6]. The analysis has been made considering the application of RFID for the whole AOB and all the blood components (red blood cells, platelets, plasma). Traditional financial indicators for investment evaluation, such as Net Present Value (NPV) and Pay Back Period (PBP) were calculated.
Main plant costs were related to: hardware and software purchasing; network infrastructure adaptation or realization; personnel training. Main operating costs were related to tag purchasing. The difference between the plant cost installation was almost limited, UHF costs are about 1.5% higher than HF, while UHF tags average cost is about 30-40% lower than HF tag cost, so this difference greatly affects the technology choice. Maintenance costs were calculated as a fraction (1% - 2%) of each item cost.
Cash revenues only, due to ceasing expenses (productivity improvement and wasted blood units reduction), were considered for the analysis, while other kind of benefits such as image return, legal disputes missed costs etc. were ignored.

Macro Process	Average RPI [%]	Number of activities [%]	Peak RPI [%]	Cycle Time [%]
Blood Component Request	-73.2	-31.2	-75.0	-13.3
Blood Transfusion	-67.4	+30.0	-55.6	+0.8
Blood Donation	-81.8	+100.0	-70.4	+9.1
Whole Blood check-in	-77.3	+4.3	-62.5	-66.7
Blood Component assignation	-26.4	-33.3	-25.0	-2.3
Blood components check-out	-63.7	+50.0	-33.3	+6.3
Total	**-67.6**	**-3.8**	**-60.2**	**-0.8**

Table 1. KPI variation within AS-IS and TO-BE models.Preliminary RFID characterization in the RF Anechoic Chamber.

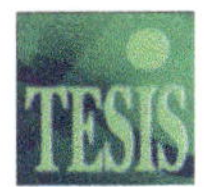

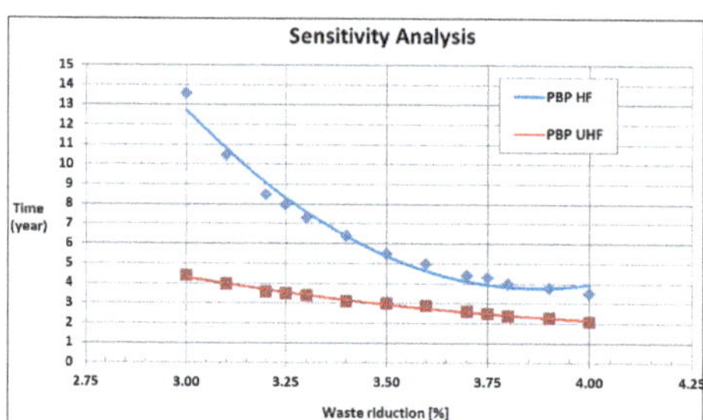

Figure 1. Pay Back Period for HF and UHF technologies.

Due to the high unit cost of blood components, waste reduction is the key parameter which substantially conditions positive cash flows trend. Therefore, it was decided to perform a sensitivity analysis estimating a range between 3% and 4%.

The results showed us that UHF technology is rather more convenient (Figure 1). The sensitivity analysis pointed out that the two Pay Back Periods, related to the different technology, are comparable just in case project implementation allows a waste reduction higher than 3.5% (3.5-5 years for HF, 2-3 years for UHF). Assuming waste reduction values below the 3.5% threshold, the payback time difference between the two technologies increases dramatically (5-13 years for HF, 3-5 years for UHF).

For the reasons mentioned above, the UHF technology was chosen for the subsequent step: laboratory analysis of the systems to implement in the AOB. EMC of Implantable Medical Device versus RFID signals.

The recent development of RFID technologies and, consequently, the increased use of intentional radio frequency (RF) sources, makes electromagnetic interference (EMI) a growing problem. In fact, when an electronic device is exposed to RF signals, they may prevent it to correctly operate, causing malfunction. In this context, EMI issues in hospital environment are particularly critical for Implantable Medical Devices (IMDs). Therefore, the evaluation of IMD electromagnetic susceptibility to RFID devices has become fundamental [7].

EMI issues are particularly critical for medical equipment, such as heart monitors, heart pumps, glucose monitors and Implantable Medical Devices (IMDs), such as pacemakers (PMKs) and Implantable Cardiac Defibrillator (ICDs) [8]. IMDs are generally used for people, whose spontaneous heartbeat is not sufficient to ensure normal living conditions, having to suppress dangerous arrhythmias, such as bradycardia, tachyarrhythmia and fibrillation. These are detected by an accurate measure of the cardiac signal, which consists in transducing the heartbeat in a series of electrical pulses. Thus, IMDs deliver the most appropriate therapy based on the frequency and amplitude of the measured cardiac signal. In this context, EMI immunity of IMDs against RFID signals is experiencing an increasing attention from researchers all around the world, as confirmed by many papers in the literature that deal with electromagnetic interactions between IMDs and RFID devices [9]. It is worth noting that RFID devices have to pass several tests before they are on the market. These tests are performed by manufacturers directly in accredited EMC laboratories, in accordance with international standards, but they do not take into account the work environment (such as hospital rooms), where a number of EMI sources may be present. In this paper, an electromagnetic characterization of the hospital environment is carried out in order to determine its level of EMI. In the first step, we have preliminary characterized the reader in RF anechoic chamber in absence of any EMI source, reflection and interference,

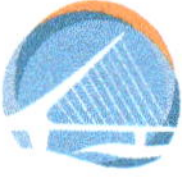

whose results are reported in Table 2. In the second stage, we have characterized the blood transfusion center. Measurements have been performed using a reader placed at the height of one meter from the floor. The corresponding results are reported in Table 3.
The measurement of the immunity and electromagnetic compatibility between RFID and IMD devices, compliance with the international standards, is then performed in the third stage.

	Distance = 0.5 m	Distance = 1 m
Degrees	E [V/m]	E [V/m]
0	0,66	0,85
30	0,75	0,30
60	0,66	0,46
90	0,63	0,00
120	0,55	0,00
150	0,53	0,00
180	0,81	0,00
210	0,61	0,00
240	0,48	0,00
270	0,51	0,00
300	0,75	0,26
330	0,99	0,45

Table 2. Preliminary RFID characterization in the RF Anechoic Chamber.

Reader Distance [m]	E [V/m]
0	1,18
2	0,60
3	0,52
1	0,56
2	0,02
2,64	0,34
5	0,25

Table 3. EMC characterization of the transfusion center.

Experimental setup - Test Methods

The experimental tests are carried out in the RF anechoic chamber shown in Figure 2 (4m x 7,9m x 2,6m), which guarantees a correct management of EMI generation, shielding against external EMI sources at the same time. In fact, it is a shielded room, whose walls, floor and ceiling are covered with appropriate materials (polyurethane pyramids and/or ferrite tiles) that scatter or absorb the incident electromagnetic energy, in order to simulate the free space. Furthermore, it consists of an outer casing of galvanized steel, which is an efficient external EMI shield. Therefore, the RF anechoic chamber allows EMC testing in accordance with international standards, thereby ensuring their reliability.

Immunity test

The tests are performed in accordance with the schematic representation shown in Figure 3. In particular, the RFID system (reader, antennas and tag [10]) is placed inside the RF anechoic chamber. Then, a bi-log antenna (Schaffner CBL6143) is properly aligned and placed 3 m away from the front surface. Both the bi-log antenna and the RFID system are linked to their corresponding external equipment through appropriate shielded cables. In particular, the bi-log antenna is connected to an EMI signal generator (Rhode & Schwarz SML03) by means of a directional coupler and an amplifier (Schaffner CBA9433). In addition, the directional coupler allows the coupling of the bi-log antenna with a power meter (Rhode & Schwarz NRVD) in order to monitor the power levels of the generated EMI signals.

Emission test

The tests have been performed with reference to the schematic representation shown in Figure 4. In particular, the RFID system (reader, antennas and tag) is placed inside the RF anechoic chamber, about 1m far from the Human Body Model (HBM). In this case the HBM is linked to its corresponding external equipment through appropriate shielded cables. The HBM is directly

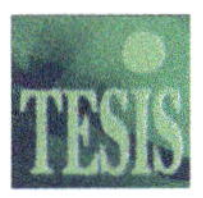

Figure 2. A sight of the RF Anechoic Chamber.

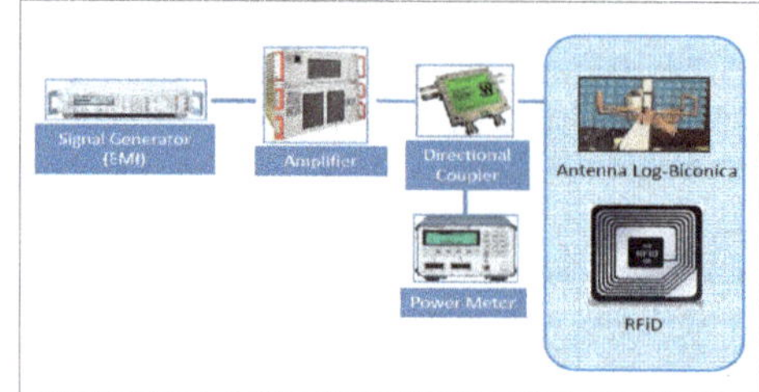

Figure 3. Experimental setup of Immunity tests.

coupled to a multi-channel IO board (NI USB 6211), which provides the heartbeat signal to the ICD and acquires its pacing pulses at the same time. These data are accurately elaborated by means of a specific software program, which is developed in the Labview environment.

REFERENCES

1. De Sanctis Lucentini E., Marconi M., Bevilacqua L., et al., *Risk Management in Sanità. Il problema degli errori.* Ministero della Salute Commissione tecnica sul rischio clinico, Roma, 2004.
2. Ahrens N., Pruss A., Kiesewetter H., et al., Failure of bedside ABO testing is still the most common cause of incorrect blood transfusion in the Barcode era. *Transfusion and Apheresis Science*, No.33, pp. 25-29, 2005.
3. Istituto Superiore della Sanità. Centro Nazionale Sangue. *Il Sistema Trasfusionale in Italia: organizzazione nazionale, nuove politiche e prospettive.*
4. Van der Togt, R., Bakker, P.J.M., Jaspers, M.W.M., 2011. Framework for performance and data quality assessment of Radio Frequency IDentification (RFID) systems in health care settings. *Journal of Biomedical Informatics*, 44, 372–383A.
5. Borelli G., Orrù P.F., Zedda F., Safety and logistics performance evaluation of a RFID system in a Blood Transfusion Center. *International Journal of Mechanics and Control*, ISSN 1590-8844.
6. G. Borelli G., Orrù P.F., F. Zedda. Economic assessment for a RFID application in transfusion medicine. *14th International Conference on Harbor, Maritime & Multimodal Logistics Modelling and Simulation*, Wien, 2012.
7. S. Futatsumori, T. Hikage, T. Nojima, B. Koike, H. Fujimoto, T. Toyoshima, "A Novel Assessment Methodology for the EMI Occurrence in Implantable Medical Devices Based Upon Magnetic Flux Distribution of RFID reader/writers", in *Proc. IEEE International Symposium on Electromagnetic Compatibility (EMC 2007), Honolulu (USA)*, July 9-13, 2007, 6 pp.
8. T. Hikage, Y. Kawamura, T. Nojima, "Numerical Estimation Methodology for RFID/Active Implantable Medical Device-EMI based upon FDTD Analysis", in *Proc. XXXth URSI General Assembly and Scientific Symposium, Instabul (Turkey)*, Aug. 13-20, 2011, 4 pp.
9. S. Futatsumori, T. Hikage, T. Nojima, B. Koike, H. Fujimoto, T. Toyoshima, "A Novel Method of Mitigating EMI on Implantable Medical Devices: Experimental Validation for UHF RFID reader/writers", in *Proc. IEEE International Symposium on Electromagnetic Compatibility (EMC 2009), Austin (USA)*, Aug. 17-21, 2009, pp. 197-202.
10. http://www.motorolasolutions.com/XU-EN/Product+Lines/Psion

Core Telehealth - Province of Mendoza. A Strategy for Integration

Osvaldo Garcia, María Susana Bresca,
Nadia Carrasco, Raúl Zangrandi

osvaldoedgarcia@gmail.com

Ministry of Health - Province of Mendoza, Argentina

Clearly the impact of Information Technology and Communication (ICT) has been emerging in today's society, abruptly changing our habits, our ways of relating and our traditional ways of working.

While many sectors of society are participating in this global phenomenon, the acceptance and inclusion of these technologies has been mixed, probably in relation to old paradigms that complicate implementation whichever branch of activity concerned.

Public health is just beginning to find their place in this new communication scenario. Without a doubt the possibility of incorporating ICT to practice medicine brings an added value that increases their efficiency and productivity in the medical act, but also improves accessibility to health system, transcending time and geographical boundaries and mainly covering the gap is generated in remote and inaccessible places by the lack of timely, permanent Human Resources, lack of accessible physical resources, to the detriment of the health of the people those remote areas.

Today telemedicine should not be understood simply as a technology, but as a new organizational system for the medical profession.

***Osvaldo Garcia** Electrical and Electronic Engineer, graduated from the Faculty of Engineering of the University of Mendoza in 1982. Responsible for developing of the Single Health Record (RUS) in 1994. Between 1996 and 1999 he participated Hospitals Informatization Project Guillermo Rawson and Marcial Quiroga - Province of San Juan. From 1994 to 2007 directed the Department of Technology Management of Diego Paroissien Hospital.*

From 2008 to 2013 Director of Information Technology, Ministry of Health of Mendoza. Responsible Manager ICT by Mendoza before the SISA. He currently serves as Responsible for Core TeleSalud Virtual Campus and the School of Public Health, Ministry of Health of Mendoza. Founder member of Provincial Telehealth Network. Professor in the Department of TeleMedicine and Director, Institute of Bioinformatics and TeleHealth.

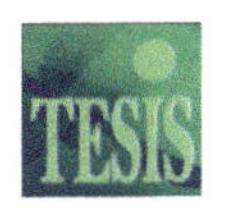

Mendoza is located in west-central Argentina. It borders with the Republic of Chile, with strong trade exchanges through international Cristo Redentor, which is used by all the countries of MERCOSUR.

Constitutes, together with San Juan, San Luis and La Rioja, New Cuyo Region, to which reference is in production and services in general and health services in particular.

Mendoza has an area of 148,827 km^2 and a population of 1.7 million peoples, 95% of which are concentrated in less than 4% of the territory. The population density is 10.6 peoples per km^2.
Human settlements have been deployed around three irrigation oasis: the North, where it extends the "Gran Mendoza" which concentrates 62.5% of the population, the South and the Centre.

The concentration of the population corresponds to the presence of road infrastructure and services in relation to the productive activities of the oasis and the needs of the population. The resident upland, however, people must assume deficiencies in the road network and a strong dependence on equipment and services, in many cases, long distances from urban centers. Meanwhile, West provincial departments, identified with large potential for development for housing resources, have deficits in infrastructure and services.
About 20% of Mendoza's population lives in rural areas.

Unemployment (4.9%) and homelessness in rural households (9.45%) exceeds that of urban.

Health coverage for those living in rural areas is lower than that of urban population. The rural population without coverage was 64% (Census 2001) and while changes are recorded, the gap remains.
In rural areas, either Oasis or dry the illiteracy rate is 7.3%. Are the inhabitants of the departments of Lavalle Malargüe and those most affected by this problem.
The rurality index varies greatly by departments. However, highly urbanized departments have a significant number of people in small towns, which conditions their access to services
The population of rural areas must travel, on average, the following distances to access basic services: health centers / hospitals: 31 km; payphone: 27 km; schools: 18 km; stop collective: 97 km.

The application of telemedicine represents a new way of organizing and providing health services for the benefit of patients and medical professionals in remote areas and the health system in general. The use of telemedicine makes distances and times between primary and hospital care are shortened.
Examples are as different modes of delivery as tele-education, Second Opinion, and interventions of various medical specialties as telestroke, teleophthalmology, teledermatology and teleradiology, the silhouetted today as the big areas where more progress has been made in partnership between primary care and specialized care.
Through telemedicine avoiding unnecessary travel, waiting times are shorter in the care and diagnosis and treatment speeding distance from specialized centers, adding fairness to the medical act in population concentrations away from major urban centers.

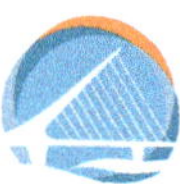

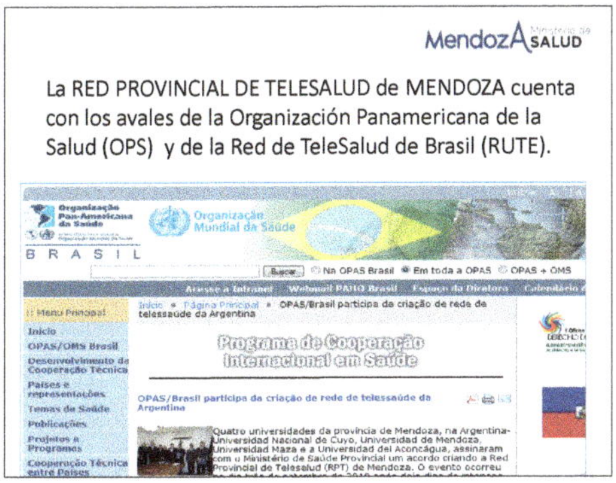

Figure 1. Provincial Telehealth Network-Mendoza.

Asynchronous applications, such as using email to transfer images or patient consultations via web, or synchronous, such as the use of videoconferencing for interdepartmental or review patients in real time are the most used in the different centers of reference worldwide.

Particularly in the Province of Mendoza kick start incorporating TeleMedicine gave it the creation of the "Provincial Red Telehealth" by Ministerial Resolution N° 399, August 2010, which brings together specialists from Public, Private areas, Universities Technology Center and the Province.
The Provincial Telehealth Network-Mendoza is currently working for the creating agency policies and technologies to standardize, regulate and promote the gradual incorporation of Telehealth around the provincial level.
It has been identified and added to their teams new members with a deep commitment to Public Health, who are betting that the incorporation of TeleSalud produce a noticeable improvement in the quality of processes, both management and care, and at all levels.

It has also been made in integrating with other experiences of implementing similar technologies, in order to exchange experiences and leverage the knowledge of who made art in this topic.

Initial activities performed immediately, jointly by the Information Technology and the Science and Technical Research Ministry, an activity that allowed the generation of 40 nodes TeleSalud distributed throughout the province.

The nodes consist of a multimedia equipment that allow the transfer of voice, video and data (presentations, videos etc..), Which was supplemented by an agreement with the National Academy of Medicine that allows us to access your collaborative platform "Elluminate" with 40 simultaneous connections.

The recent addition of the delegations of the Provincial Social Work (OSEP), in all departments of our province complements and gives integrity to the network.

This teleeducation technology platform is currently operational with a team of professionals dedicated to the management, organization and delivery of training courses in different disciplines, allowing classes to assist health staff need no longer move to the capital of Mendoza as traditionally done, and in some cases even leaving your workplace to attend training.

It also allows training in every way, where any node can become Moderator and share from their knowledge and experience.

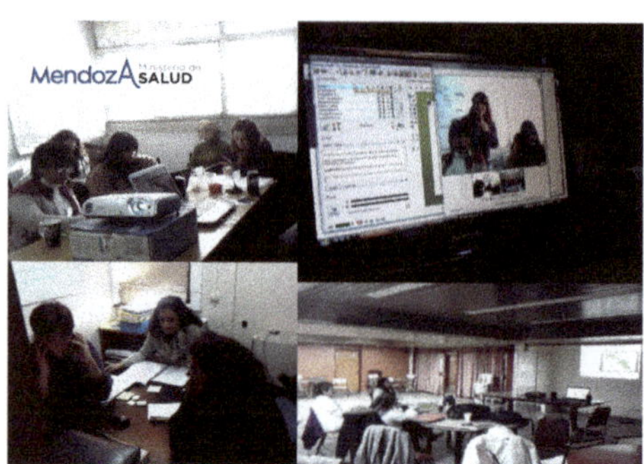

Figure 2. Teleeducation technology platform.

The learning process has been accelerated as participants are interconnected through the best technology of Voice over IP based on the implementation of the new Red Wan Government, allowing 2-way audio, an interactive whiteboard, and video.
Around 900 participants have been trained in different disciplines, without having to travel to take their classes.

The technical staff of the Center for Telehealth then gave his second step, dedicated to the study and implementation of a pilot second opinion, which was contacted by a technological link the ER Hospital Malargue to the Intensive Care Unit Hospital San Rafael, thus allowing interconsultations among professionals ensure a broader vision in diagnosis of patient and ensure the ability to transfer the same to the ICU if the patient requires.

Currently working on the technical specifications for Mental Health in Telehealth Project , which will result in the development and evaluation of a pilot controlled situation modeling to generate attention for the development of the different procedural guidelines of a virtual office in headquarters of Mental Health.
Work in identifying the personnel involved , the definition of legal issues, the estimation of supply and demand for virtual consultations, procedures and Guides in the impact assessment tools.

Simultaneously to the process of incorporating technology into health, working heavily in awareness of Health Professional of the importance of ICT in the sector, which has created the Seminar III Chair in Bioinformatics Career medicine, University of Mendoza, and are in the process of creating the Institute of bioinformatics and TeleSalud at that same university.

On March 17 this year, the Ministry gave its inaugural step of the School of Public Health, Agency, under the Ministry of Health and will canalize the entire health team training in completely virtual, using platforms in asynchronous mode virtual campus, which will complement our Provincial telehealth Network.

I think the exposure of these experiences, share them with those working on similar projects, as well as the comments and concerns of the participants, may allow, interdisciplinary and regional joint work that will surely make these new disciplines and practices are placed ICT-assisted increasingly available to all professionals who conduct their business in public, and generally in those remote, inaccessible and isolation that makes what rural doctors call "loneliness diagnosis" have a mitigating from rational use of all ICTs that are within our reach.

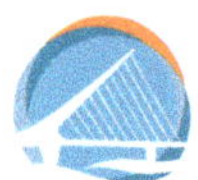

Hybrid Operating Rooms in Modular Construction

Juan Franco Mendieta

info@ht-ag.de
Manager for the Spanish-speaking world, HT Labor + Hospitaltechnik AG

Hybrid ORs are complex intervention rooms with specific requirements and challenges concerning planning, construction and workflow.
Specific requirements in terms of the building and technology have to be considered. Furthermore, continuing progress of technology (innovation), planning, and project management are important aspects to accommodate these requirements and for successful implementation. Particularly in the planning phase, the visualization of the room or unit with all clinical devices supports to establish the best workflow.
The construction preparation and especially the room size are influenced by various aspects. Flexible positioning of the walls, radiation protection up to 40 mm Pb, rapid installation, and easy exchange of single wall panels are only a few advantages a modular room system can provide. Workflow aspects, e.g. concerning visualization or lighting scenarios, are of high importance. The lighting can be easily controlled via an intuitive and hygienic touch screen. In day-to-day work, a room control based on a flexible software solution saves time and money in case of required changes.
3D planning is becoming an integral part for complex intervention rooms. To show the benefits of modular construction, the practical example INO Bern is presented.

Juan Franco Mendieta*. Since 2010 Manager for the Spanish-speaking world at HT Labor + Hospitaltechnik AG, Heideck, Germany. 2003 – 2009 Area Manager for Portugal, Spain and Latin America at Trumpf-Kreutzer Medizin Systeme GmbH. 2000 – 2003 Product Manager at Leica Microsystems, Nussloch, Germany. 1997 – 2000 Head of Department Latin America at Marquet AG, Rastatt, Germany. 1993 – 1997 International Support at BAUM Products GmbH, Wiesenbach, Germany. 1992 – 1993 Support Engineer at O.R. Industrial Computers, Augsburg, Germany. 1991 – 1992 Product Engineer at TEAC, Herrsching, Germany. 1989 – 1990 Service and Application Engineer at Optrotech, Munich, Germany. 1988 Diploma in Electrical Engineering. Until 1987 Academic studies in Electrical Engineering at "Universidad Centroamericana" in Nicaragua and University of Karlsruhe in Germany.*

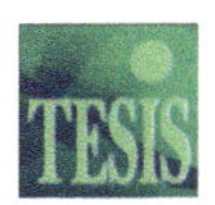

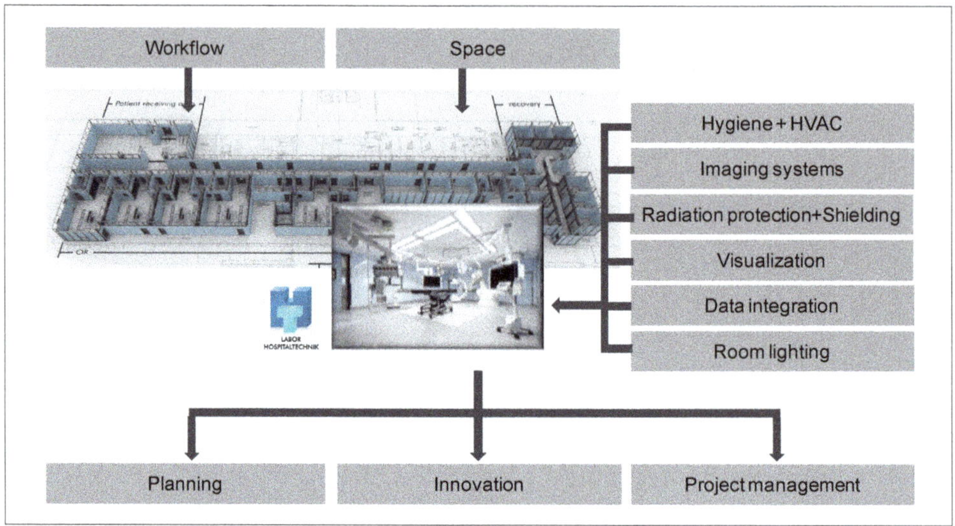

Figure 1. Engineering: Requirements + Challenges.

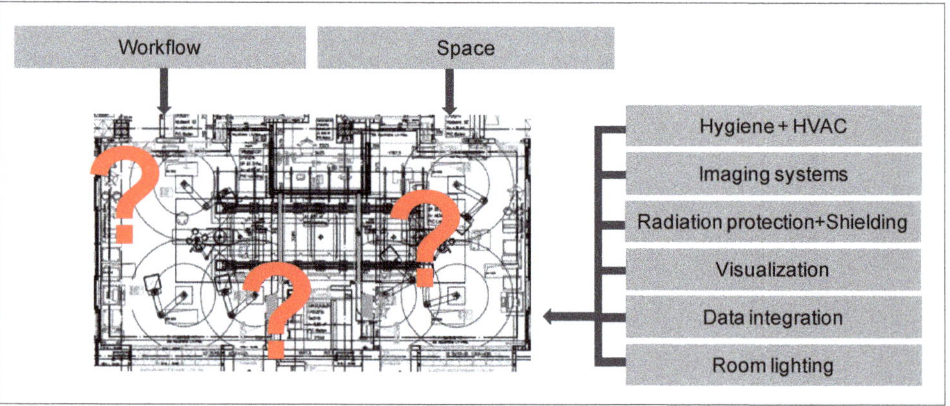

Figure 2. 2D Planning: high concentration of technical building services and medical technology in wall, ceiling and floor; demanding construction requirements for statics, radiation protection, noise protection, fire protection and hygiene; high investment costs; requirements for flexible systems/modules for wall, ceiling and floor.

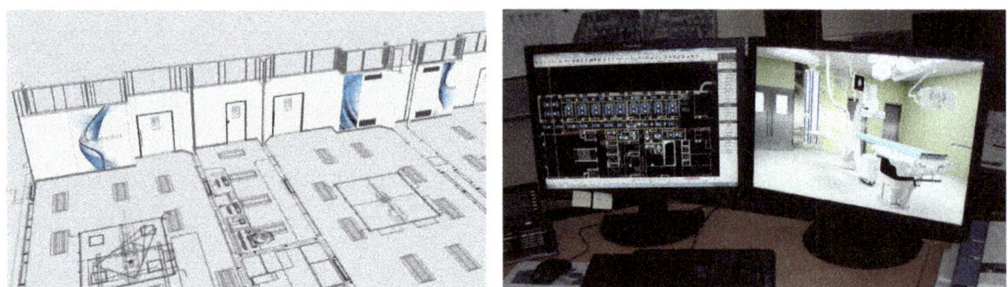

Figure 3. 3D Project Planning and Project Management. Advantages 3D Planning: demonstration of glide paths, cruising radiuses and collision risks, high planning safety and easier comprehension.

Flexibility in Hospital Building and Application by Means of Standardized Medical Room Types

P.G. Kamp*[1,3], R.L. Kooistra[1,3], H.A.H.G. Ankersmid[2], G.M. Bonnema[3]

p.kamp@zgt.nl
[1]Health Care Technology Department, ZGT Hospitals
[2]Real estate department, ZGT Hospitals
[3]Laboratory of Design, Production and Management. Department of Engineering Technology, University of Twente
*corresponding author, _presenting author

This paper presents an approach to standardization of hospital rooms. As hospitals are becoming more complex, the need for quality assurance and validation increases as well. Several sources mention the responsibility of the medical personnel for the quality and safety of the equipment with which patients are treated. The room in which patients are treated can also be seen as part of this responsibility. The hospital currently consists of hundreds of rooms with very little information available on the exact properties and state of rooms. It is thus very hard, both for medical and technical personnel, to gain insight into and be aware of the state of a medical room. This can lead to risks for the patient. In order to give this insight, we paper propose a standardization of medical rooms. Based on the hygiene and electrical safety classes, nine standard room types are defined. Additionally, rooms may have specific 'toppings' for more specialized tasks. This approach allows medical personnel to instantly acquire insight into the capabilities of a room, and the possibility of performing a certain treatment. Furthermore, maintenance requirements are clearer, there is more flexibility in room use, and it is expected that the approach will greatly simplify the planning of hospital construction projects.

***Pieter G. Kamp** received his Master's degree in Biomedical Engineering from the University of Twente in The Netherlands in 2006. He worked for two years at Simed, a Dutch company specialized in the design and construction of medical facilities worldwide, before joining the ZGT Hospital group in 2008. Currently, he is pursuing a Professional Doctorate in Engineering in Hospital Engineering at the University of Twente and the ZGT Hospitals. This education focuses on the building-related systems in hospitals and the application of Systems Engineering methods in this field.*

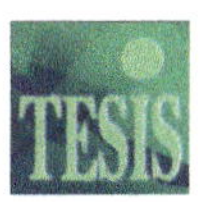

Introduction

In the Netherlands, medical personnel are responsible for making sure that the medical devices used meet their specifications. The hospital and especially the medical rooms can also be considered as a medical device [1]. However, the technical specifications of the rooms are not defined clearly.

The allowed medical treatments in a medical room are directly related to the technical specifications of that room. If these specifications are unclear, the medical personnel will not be able to determine which medical treatments are allowed. In the best case the treatment is performed in an over-classified room, costing more than strictly necessary. In the worst case, the medical treatment is performed in an under-classified room, leading to unacceptable patient risks. Furthermore, in case of (re)building a department, the specifications of the rooms needed are unclear.

Although there are a lot of regulations around the room specifications, medical personnel are unable to determine what kind of room they are in, and therefore which treatments are allowed. Experts will only give advice in their own discipline. Disciplines that are often involved are: hygiene, electrical safety, laser safety, radiation safety, occupational health and safety (OHS). This multitude of disciplines may hamper clear status information on the room.

The hospital hygienist, for example, will specify how clean a certain room must be in order to perform a certain treatment, leading to regulations for the air treatment, but the OHS will also have regulations for the air treatment. Moreover, the electrical safety regulations also state an air humidity range which provides safe working conditions. These regulations might even contradict each other, further obscuring clear status information.

In order to clarify these regulations to the medical personnel, we define standard medical room types. Each medically used room will fit in one of nine standard rooms that base on existing hygiene and electrical safety classifications.

On top of this standard nine room types, additional "toppings" are defined. So, for example, a standard room type with a laser topping will also be suitable for the use of a certain laser. The standard medical room type will have to be depicted in the room including the installed toppings.

This way, the medical personnel will be able to take responsibility for performing the medical treatment in a suitable medical room.

State-of-the-Art in Dutch Hospitals

Current hospitals in the Netherlands generally recognize the need for a flexible building configuration. The newly built Bernhoven hospital – opened in 2013 – applied the following core principles for the building: flexible, goal-oriented and with a human touch [2]. "Flexibel bouwen" [3] also emphasizes this notion, adding that these principles mainly apply to a polyclinic setting. Technologies such as Building Information Modeling (BIM) are applied to acquire information about the building and to create digital prototypes of the building. This allows for visualization of the building early in the building process, and the assessment of cost and other properties.

To a certain extent, hospitals in the

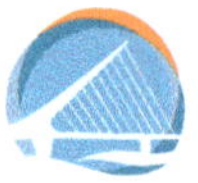

Netherlands are already implementing standardization approaches; for example, by using the same type of blood pressure sensor throughout the hospital, or by using a unified approach to risk management for all hospital technologies. Lean approaches are also increasingly common for tasks such as medical treatment and maintenance planning.

The approach we present here was designed within the ZGT hospitals group. The ZGT consists of one hospital in each of the cities of Almelo and Hengelo in the East of the Netherlands. Combined, these hospitals serve a population of around 300,000 people. The ZGT has recognized the influence that the hospital building has on the medical process. ZGT staff members published a paper [1] and, in cooperation with Twente University, started a PDEng track in Hospital Engineering.

Literature

In literature, standardization and consequent flexibility are seen as two of the main drivers of a lean organization. One of the key principles of the Toyota product development system – which may be seen as the cradle of lean thinking – is 'Utilize rigorous standardization to reduce variation, and create flexibility and predictable outcomes' [6].

When looking at health care and hospitals more specifically, De Neufville et al [7] emphasize the importance of hospital flexibility by discussing future changes in hospital care and the advantages that a flexible layout of functional rooms bring. Several sources in literature acknowledge the possible advantages of standardization within hospitals, mentioning possible gains in quality, cost and safety [8], [9].

Problem Definition

In Dutch hospitals, a typical department consists of both medical and non-medical rooms. No clear specification of the requirements of the room are shown in the room or on the outside of the room, therefore the medical personnel is unable to verify whether the room is suitable for the specific medical treatment they planned to perform. The fact that the naming looks identical (treatment room dermatology versus treatment room ENT) does not guarantee a room with equal technical specifications.

Assuming that design specifications are known, the permitted medical treatments can be defined. In order to be permitted to do the medical treatments some parameters need to be monitored. In the operating room, for example, a screen displays values such as: the pressures of medical gasses; air temperature; the relative air humidity. While active readings of the parameters can be done, the limits of the parameters are often unknown. Another problem is that not all parameters can be measured in real time [4]. The health care inspectorate in The Netherlands already obliges medical personnel to check whether medical devices meet their specification before use [5]. As the hospital and its medical rooms can be considered as medical devices [1], it is thus mandatory to be able to determine their current state. Although it is very important to verify that the medical room meets design specifications at the time of use, this paper is restricted to the design criteria and the permitted medical treatments.

When departments are upgraded or rebuilt, a clear technical specification of the desired rooms is often missing. This

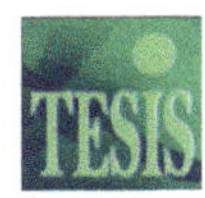

can lead to over-classified or under-classified rooms. Over-classified rooms cost more than strictly necessary, as they provide more facilities than required. Under-classified rooms on the other hand provide insufficient facilities, leading to unsafe situations while costing both time and money.

With a lack of clarity comes the disadvantage that when new rooms are created – for example by building a new hospital wing or renovating part of the hospital – there is little design information available. As a result new medical rooms are designed almost from scratch. Expensive medical rooms are built for each separate department, resulting in relatively low occupancy rates.

In summary, three key problems are defined:

- medical personnel need to be able to see to which regulations the medical room was built to or, more specifically; which medical treatments can be performed in the room:
- in order to increase the occupancy rate, we like to be able to share rooms among different departments;
- when departments are upgraded or rebuilt, a clear overview of the specifications of the required rooms is essential.

Approach Taken

To be able to deal with the three problems defined above, only the medical rooms are of interest. So rooms such as offices, hallways and storage rooms are outside the scope of this project. However, since the scope includes medical rooms throughout the entire hospital, both technical and medical information is needed to be able to determine whether the rooms meet specification and thus whether they are not either over- or under-classified. A multidisciplinary team was set up to collect all this information. This team included the first three authors of this paper, medical personnel, a building manager, and a coordinator of construction projects.

After investigating standards, laws, guidelines and recommendations, it turned out that a lot of these standards, laws, guidelines and recommendations are intended for very specific situations that do not occur in all medical rooms. For example, there are guidelines for safe working with medical lasers [edit RIVM lasers], while in most medical rooms a laser will never be used. Hygiene and electrical safety on the other hand, apply to all medical rooms. Therefore a standard grouping of medical rooms can be made with the hygiene class and the electrical safety class as a basis.

Proposition

To better define the variety of different rooms in the hospital and create a smarter and simpler system, a room standardization approach is proposed.

As stated before, the hygiene and electrical classes are the bases for standardizing the medical rooms. The electrical safety classes go from K0 / S0 to K3/ S3 [NEN 1010] the higher the number the deeper into the patients body the medical personnel is allowed to go. The S means that the room was built before 2007 after which the technically more strikt K class is introduced. Medically the same kind of treatments are allowed as long as they are numeral equal.

Hygiene classes H2 till H5 apply to medically used rooms, the higher the

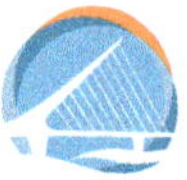

number the more strict the hygiene regulations become. The division into hygiene class is not straightforward. It depends on 6 parameters:

- Size of the incision
- Depth of the incision
- Duration of the treatment
- Implementation of materials foreign to the body
- Opening of sterile cavities
- The impact of a wound infection for the patient.

The hygiene class is determined by a hospital hygienist.
Taking the common factor of allowing deeper entry into the patient's body, a sensible combination of the hygiene and electrical safety classes can be made, as shown in Table 1. As can be seen not all possible combinations exists. The medical treatments determine which combinations are possible.

Medical Room	Hygiene class	Electrical safety class
I	H2	K0 / S0
H	H2	K1 / S1
G	H3	K1 / S1
F	H2	K2 / S2
E	H3	K2 / S2
D	H2	K3 / S3
C	H3	K3 / S3
B	H4	K3 / S3
A	H5	K3 / S3

Table 1. Overview of standard medical rooms.

Supplementing these nine standard rooms are possible specific adaptations that are required in only a few cases. These include properties such as radiation shielding or the aforementioned availability of provisions for laser application.

In order for the medical personnel to be able to work with these medical rooms, all there treatments need to be rated. The medical personnel explains how the treatment is executed and the hospital hygienist and electrical safety expert determine in which medical room the treatment can be performed. At the entrance of the medical rooms, the room classification will need to be shown (Figure 1).

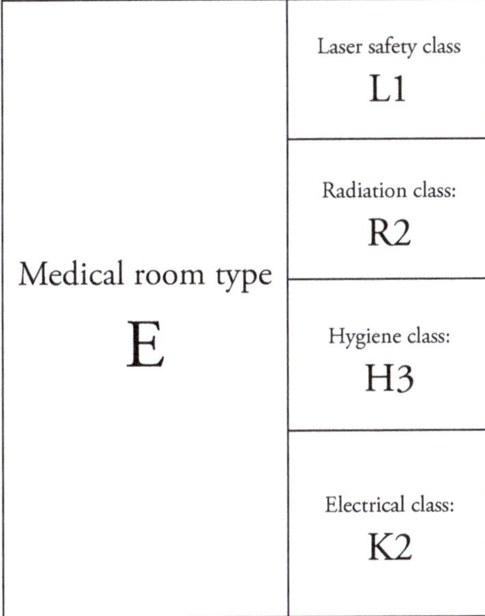

Figure 1. Room classification.

Future Extensions

The proposed approach provides an approach which is validated by input from several experts in the field, like medical personnel, a hospital hygienist and a electrical safety expert. To confirm that the proposed approach will actually work and delivers the predicted advantages, field trials will be preformed at two pilot departments.

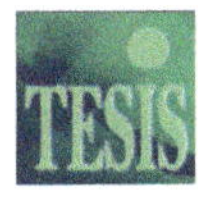

Extensions can be added to the current model. As a result of research done in parallel to the research presented in this paper [4] there are several possible directions:

- extension of the medical rooms with real-time information.
- analysis of specific technologies using the medical rooms approach. This could entail hospital infrastructure related systems such as air conditioning systems. By extending to more specific systems a general requirements overview of all rooms (both medical and non-medical) is formed.

References

1. Boeke, A.W., Lansbergen M.D.I., Adel R.J. den, and Wilden-van Lier E.C.M. van der. 2010. "Ziekenhuis is één groot apparaat." Medisch Contact, October 14, pp. 2122-2125.

2. Bouwboek Bernhoven 2008, via http://ziekenhuisbernhoven.nl/Content/

3. Scheerder R., Verweij M., 4-02-2005 "Flexibel bouwen" *Medisch Contact* p189-191

4. Kooistra Rien L., Kamp Pieter G., Bonnema G. Maarten. 2014. "The cause of complications: understanding the relation between post-operative complications and the system and processes of a hospital by means of an influence diagram". *IFHE 2014 proceeds* (pending acceptation).

5. Convenant Veilige toepassing van medische technologie in het ziekenhuis, via http://www.nfu.nl/img/pdf/NFU-11.4224_Convenant_VeiligeToepassing_MedTechn_Zh.pdf (visited march 2014).

6. Morgan James M., Liker Jeffrey K., 2006. *The Toyota Product Development System*, Productivity Press, New York, 2006, 363 pp.

7. Neufville, Richard de, Lee Yun S., Scholtes Stefan, 2008. *Flexibility in Hospital Infrastructure Design.*

8. Swensen S.J., M.D., M.M.M., Meyer S.D., M.D., Nelson E.C. , D.Sc.,et al., Cottage Industry to Postindustrial Care — The Revolutionin Health Care Delivery, *The New England Journal of Medicine.*

9. Rozich R.D., Howerd R.J., Justeson J.M. Jan, 2004. Standardization as a Mechanism to Improve Safety in Health Care, *Joint commission journal on quality and safety volume 30*, number 1.

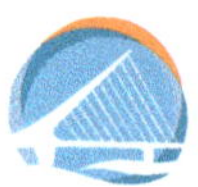

The Cause of Complications: Understanding the Relation Between Post-Operative Complications and the Systems and Processes of a Hospital by Means of an Influence Diagram

Rien L. Kooistra[1,2], Pieter G. Kamp [1,2], G. Maarten Bonnema[2]

r.l.kooistra@utwente.nl
[1]Health Care Technology Department, ZGT Hospitals, The Netherlands
[2] Laboratory of Design, Production and Management. Department of Engineering Technology, University of Twente, The Netherlands

Care for the patient is the core process of hospital care. Hospitals are becoming ever more complex and it is increasingly difficult to have a good overview of the hospital to ensure the quality of care. Among others, additional quality assurance and validation is required to remain in control of the situation. To acquire insight into the most important parameters in patient care, an influence diagram is made of the patient treatment process in the operating room. The outcome of this approach is an extensive diagram, giving an overview of the influences on post-operative complications in a hospital. Based on this, a concise abstraction is made, in which the occurrence of post-operative complications is summarized using a simple system diagram. The main challenges within the current system are identified, and will be used for further research. Preliminary solutions follow from the influence diagram: the essential parameters and the complex interrelations between these parameters are described.

Rien L. Kooistra *received his Master's degree in Mechanical Engineering, specializing in Systems Engineering, from the University of Twente in The Netherlands in 2012. Currently, he is pursuing a Professional Doctorate in Engineering in Hospital Engineering at the University of Twente and the ZGT Hospitals. This education focuses on the building-related systems in hospitals and application of Systems Engineering methods in this sector.*

Introduction

Hospitals are complex environments and are expected to become ever more complex. This is mainly due to technological progress and the increasing demands for greater quality and cost-efficiency. With this increasing complexity, it becomes harder to have an overview of the totality of the hospital systems and processes. The main objective has to be kept in mind: providing high quality care for the patient. Instead, attention is often focused on aspects such as technical possibilities or adherence to norms and rules set by external parties.

This paper aims to bring the focus back to the main objective. It gives insight into the way in which a hospital is set up to achieve this objective. This is done by means of an influence diagram. This diagram shows the parameters of influence

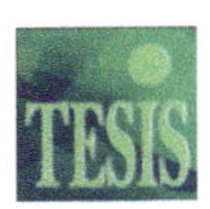

on one of the key indicators of quality of care: the incidence of post-operative complications after a hospital treatment. Several complications are recognized; post-operative wound infections (POWIs), electrical shock, mechanical damage, failure of medical treatment and succumbing of the patient due to treatment.

Research background

The diagrams are made in order to explore the effects that building-related hospital systems have on patient care. To date, little research has been done in this specific area. Therefore, it is useful to start off with a high-level description, both to explore the range of the discipline and to investigate the main difficulties faced by the discipline. This is echoed by (Blessing and Chakrabarti 2009), who name this first stage of the research process the 'Research Clarification Stage'. The goals of the research are identified during this stage. The outcome of this first stage is then used as the basis for the remainder of the project. One of the main activities followed by the authors is the creation of influence diagrams which they term 'reference and impact models'.

The outcomes of the research presented in this paper are used to initiate a research project into building-related hospital systems and the standardization of medically used hospital rooms (Kamp et al. 2014). Building-related hospital systems include systems such as the medical gas network and the electricity network, and may be seen as the infrastructure of the hospital. As such, they share a number of infrastructure properties such as being connected to a large number of other systems, supporting the production of goods and services and being critical to their users as rigorous changes to the system are not possible. This means that the building-related systems are connected to most other hospital systems, and often lead to complex interactions.

The research is carried out within the ZGT hospitals in Hengelo and Almelo, the Netherlands. Together, these two medium-sized hospitals form one of the largest hospital groups in the Netherlands, with a total of 3,200 employees and serving a population of around 300 000 people. In recent years, there has been increasing attention to the technology used in hospitals. The ZGT is a leading hospital in the field of medical equipment safety and is now focusing attention on the hospital building, including the installed medical systems. This is shown by a (Dutch) publication the title of which translates as 'The hospital is a single large machine' (Boeke et al. 2010) and by the establishment of an education programme aimed at understanding the building related systems in a hospital.

Method

The main tool used for our analysis of the hospital systems is the influence diagram, a tool proposed by Ross Shachter (Schachter 1986). An influence diagram contains nodes containing either a decision, a probabilistic variable (with unknown value), a general variable (with known value), or an objective. Nodes can be connected by means of links, signifying that they have influence on each other. This leads to insight into the essential elements in a system and their influence on each other. Figure 1 shows a simple example influence diagram and the types of nodes.

The influence diagram created contains highly uncertain information at a high level and is thus unsuitable for statistical analysis: patients cannot describe exactly how they feel, doctors cannot predict the exact influence of medicine or surgery, etcetera (Szolovits 1995). It is thus intended mainly to gain an overview of the factors involved, the main categories and, to a certain extent, the importance of all the factors. Therefore, the exact approach is, as also suggested by Schachter (Owens, Schachter, and Nease 1997) 'governed by convenience'. Several changes have been made to Shachter's original approach. Figure 2 gives an overview of item types used. A distinction is made between the items adjustable by different groups of hospital personnel. For example, the outdoor temperature cannot be controlled by anyone, the cleanness of the personnel's hand can be influenced by the medical personnel, and the OR (operating room) temperature setting can be influenced by both the technical and medical personnel. The diagram is created based on research and stakeholder input. It is kept in mind that the goal is not to be complete but rather to gain insight and overview. Step-wise improvement of the diagram is done using the approach defined by (Borches and Bonnema 2010), which iteratively repeats three steps: information extraction, abstraction, presentation.

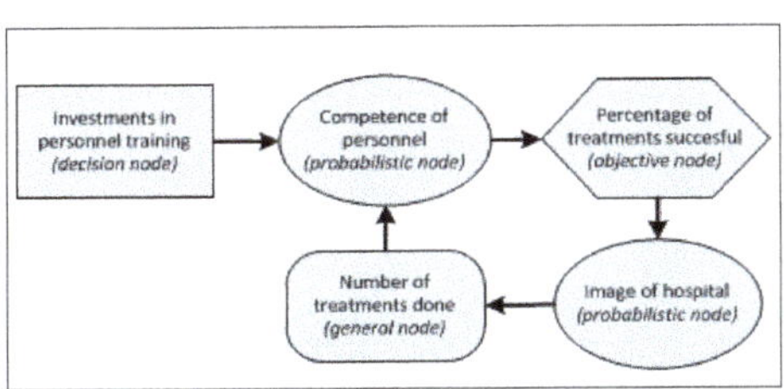

Figure 1. Example of a simple influence diagram with different node types (based on Schachter's approach).

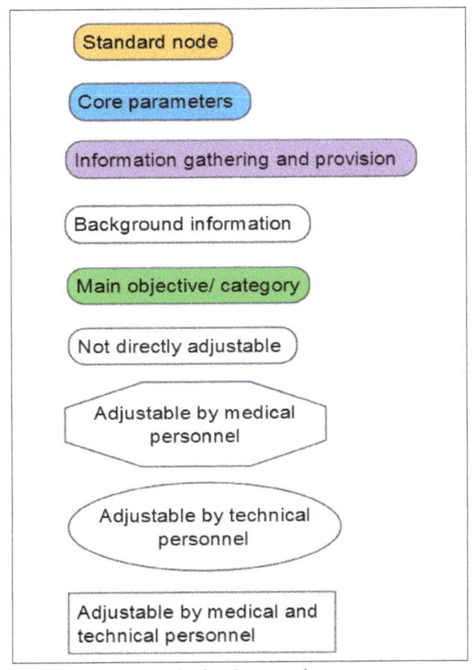

Figure 2. Legend of influence diagram items.

RESULTS

The resulting influence diagram is too large to be displayed in this paper. Therefore, an impression is displayed in Figure 3. The complete diagram can be downloaded from http://goo.gl/3M7RCQ. The diagram is best read by starting from the large objective node in the bottom right of the image, and moving outward to the influences on that node. As mentioned, a legend of item types is shown in Figure 2.

Influences on the core process – the percentage of post-operative complications – are categorized in four main groups: the state of the OR; the state of the personnel; the state of the patient and the type of procedure being followed. (Parush et al. 2011) confirm the core items as defined in the diagram, although this source groups the OR and personnel together as 'environment'

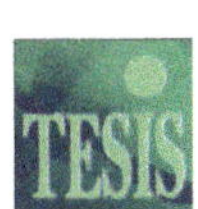

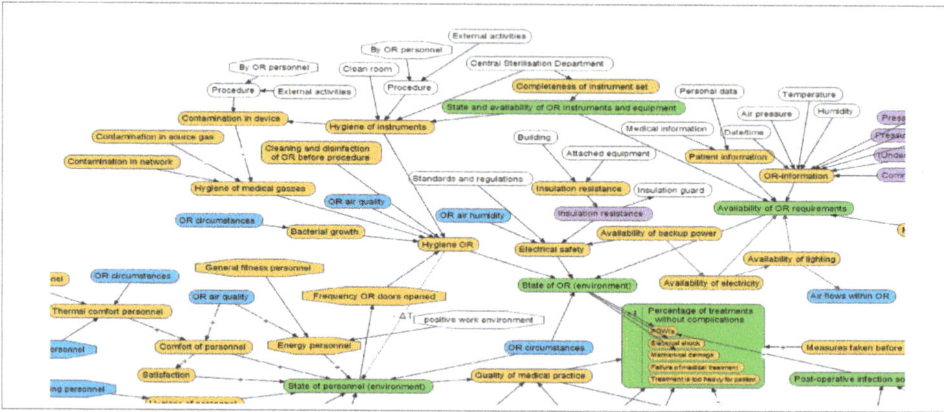

Figure 3. Impression of the created influence diagram.

and adds 'time' as a central item. This paper also recognizes time as one of the key parameters, as further described below.

Expansion of the influence diagram shows that several parameters keep recurring. These parameters influence the core process in many ways. The following key parameters have been identified: Duration of procedure (time); Clothing worn by personnel; OR circumstances; OR temperature; OR air humidity; OR air quality; Air flows within OR and Quality of air blown on patient.

Discussion

A single parameter may have influence on many different other parameters. For example, the temperature influences – among other factors– the comfort of both patient and personnel, air humidity and bacterial growth. This means that changing this node alters the objective node in several quite different ways. In other words: it has a complex influence on the objective node. Yet this range of effects also means that the parameters are likely to have a significant influence on the objective node.

Making an accurate estimation of this influence is difficult and requires extensive research. Another problem identified in the influence diagram is that the item measured is not always the parameter of interest. In ORs, the overpressure of the room relative to the outside pressure is measured, while this is not the required parameter.

The required parameter is knowledge about whether the required outward flow of air is intact, preventing micro-organisms and other pollutants from entering the room. This may lead to errors when indirectly related parameters are altered, since the exact effect on the objective parameters is not known. One example is that Dutch regulations, in a policy valid from 2001 till 2013 (Overheid 2001), state that an OR must have a fresh air ventilation rate of 20 times the volume of the room per hour. This was set in order to keep the level of nitrous oxide exhaled by the patient below 25% of the Maximal Accepted Concentration (MAC) and was based on the size of the OR. ORs have greatly increased in size, while the amount of nitrous oxide applied has reduced greatly in recent years in view of the perceived risks.

Thus, we consider the current approach to be out of proportion for the current ORs. In short, regulation has been surpassed by developments, but is still in place. A certain amount of air ventilation is required for other reasons, but no research has been undertaken into the optimum amount required.

Abstraction

In summary, the main priority in achieving the objective of minimizing the number of post-surgical complications is in maintaining the critical parameters at their optimums. Widely used cyclic models such as DMAIC (Define-Measure-Analyze-Improve-Control), LAMDA (Look-Ask-Model-Discuss-Act) and FOCUS-PDCA (Find-Optimize-Clarify-Uncover-Start-Plan-Do-Check-Act) all present process improvement approaches. The present paper, however, discusses how the current quality level is assured by analysing what influences the current quality. Quality assurance can thus be captured in a simple cycle, as shown in Figure 4. The figure shows the main points in bold font and some examples in normal font. A system will achieve its goal when these cycles are clear and all points are taken into account.

Conclusions

Examples have shown that, currently, there is not enough insight into control cycles within the process. Parameters have complex interactions and are often based on outdated objectives which are proven to work, but are not optimal in the current set-ups.

This paper attempts to give insight into the critical parameters that should be measured and governed by the control loop shown in Figure 4. The figure also raises a number of questions which are yet to be answered. An overview of questions raised is given. Italic font indicates questions (partially) answered by the influence diagram:

How to minimize the percentage of post-operative complications?
- What are the critical parameters?
- What are the optimum values of the critical parameters?
- What is the origin of values required by regulations?
- What measurable parameters need to be measured in order to accurately estimate the critical parameters' current values?

What parameters need to be controlled in order to accurately control the critical parameters?
- What changes to make to controllable parameters in order to achieve the required optima?
- What are the side effects of changing these parameters?
- What are the limiting factors in controlling the parameters?

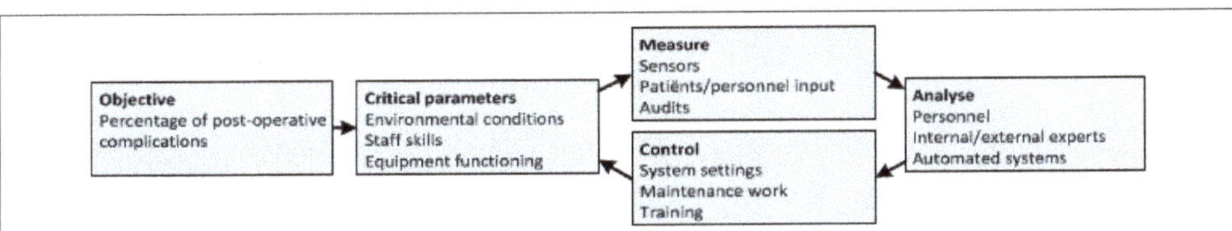

Figure 4. Generalization of the quality assurance cycles found in the influence diagram.

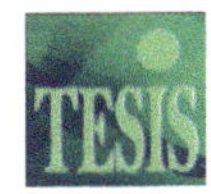

FUTURE WORK

The exploration into the systems in hospitals and the relation of these systems with the health care process described in this paper has achieved its main goal: creating an overview of the area of building-related hospital systems and their interrelations.

The insight provided by the influence diagrams is used as a starting point for further research into the relation between building-related systems of the hospital and the medical processes within the hospital. The influence diagram is used both as a means to analyse the processes within the hospital and to communicate with stakeholders regarding possible research topics. One such research topic, as mentioned before, which we are currently working on is the standardization of medical rooms (Kamp et al. 2014).

These research topics will involve clarification of the control cycles and investigation into the objectives governing these control cycles.

ACKNOWLEDGEMENTS

The authors would like to thank all who participated in brainstorm sessions regarding the contents of the influence diagram: Michaël Lansbergen, Petra Brummelhuis, Theo Weijmans, Jetze Posthuma, Irene ten Seldam and Erik Ankersmid. Furthermore, the creators of the tool VUE (http://vue.tufts.edu) are thanked for making the application freely available.

REFERENCES

Blessing, L.T.M. and A. Chakrabarti. 2009. DRM, a *Design Research Methodology*. Springer.

Boeke, A.W., M.D.I. Lansbergen, R.J. den Adel, and E.C.M. van der Wilden-van Lier. 2010. "Ziekenhuis is één groot apparaat." *Medisch Contact*, October 14, pp. 2122-2125.

Borches, P.D. and G.M. Bonnema. 2010. "*A3 Architecture Overviews - Focusing Architectural Knowledge to Support Evolution of Complex Systems.*" 20th Annual International INCOSE Symposium.

Kamp, P.G., R.L. Kooistra, H.A.H.G. Ankersmid, and G.M. Bonnema. 2014. *"Flexibility in Hospital Building and Application by Means of Standardized Medical Rooms."* Paper submitted for presentation at the IFHE 2014 conference, ZGT Hospitals department of Health Care Technology, University of Twente department of Engineering Technology, Hengelo/ Enschede.

Overheid. 2001. "*Wet- en regelgeving.*" Overheid.nl. Retrieved March 21, 2014.

Owens, D.K., R.D. Schachter, and R.F. Nease. 1997. *"Representation and Analysis of Medical Decision Problems with Influence Diagrams."* Medical Decision Making 17(3):241-262.

Parush, A., C. Campbell, A. Hunter, C. Ma, L. Calder, J. Worthington, C. Abbott, and J.R. Frank. 2011. *"Situational Awareness and Patient Safety."* Report, The Royal College of Physicians and Surgeons of Canada.

Schachter, R.D. 1986. *"Evaluating Influence Diagrams."* Operations Research 34(6):871-882.

Szolovits, P. 1995. *"Uncertainty and Decisions in Medical Informatics."* Methods of Information in Medicine 34:111-121.

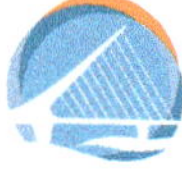

The Electrical Safety Concept for Medical Locations Acc. To National and International Standards – e.g. IEC364-7-710/ NFPA99 – Theory and Case Studies

Matthias Schwabe[1], Sergio Julian[2]

Matthias.Schwabe@bender.de, sergio.julian@bender-latinamerica.com
[1]Dipl. Ing., Association: WGKT / BENDER Group Germany
[2]Association: NCh4 – RETIE – CNE MINEM standard committees Bender Group Latin America

Electrical installations and equipment used in medical locations are subject to extraordinary demands. The life and health of a patient are at risk if only small electrical currents are flowing through his/her body or there is a break-down of life-sustaining apparatus and equipment used for diagnosis, monitoring or treatment. When safety and technical requirements are established, special considerations have to be given to the fact that patients may be connected to electro-medical equipment, their physical conditions may be restricted and that the application of electrical apparatus on or in the heart may be extremely dangerous, because of the high sensitivity of the heart muscle to electric currents.

Matthias Schwabe *University background: Dipl.-Ing. Diploma Engineer Electrical Energy and Automation Technology; University of Applied Sciences Giessen-Friedberg (Germany). Member of following associations: VDE (German Association for Electrical, Electronic &Information Technologies); ETG (Power Engineering Society); WGKT (German Scientific Society of Hospital Engineering). More than 15 years' experience in the field of electrical safety solutions for medical locations. Several papers on international conferences - guest speaker in various electrical institutes world – wide (e.g. Argentina, Brazil, China, India, Czech Republic, Malaysia, South Korea, Singapore, Viet Nam, the Philippines, USA, Poland, Holland, Austria, Spain, Norway etc). 2013 Matthias was announced as an active member in the IEC committee MT40: IEC60364-7 Electrical installations of buildings – Part 7-710: Requirements for special installations or locations – Medical locations.*

Sergio Julian *University background: Dip. Business Administration by Universitat Oberta de Catalunya (Spain); Lic. Economics by Universitat Oberta de Catalunya (Spain). Member of following associations: NCh4 (SEC Chilean standard committee); RETIE (Columbian standard committee); CNE MINEM (Peruvian standard committee). More than 20 years in the electrical field, among other developing OEM solutions as project leader in France, USA, Germany, UK, Hungary, Finland, Austria or Netherlands. Specialist in Energy Management Systems and marketing studies; in the other hand, he have participated as speaker in several forums -i.e. in Australia or Israel- related about politic systems and conflict resolution.*

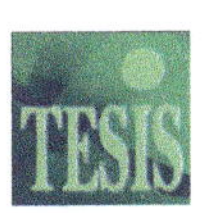

Introduction – The Electrical Safety Concept for Medical Locations

During an operation or medical examination the following technical conditions to the patient may have to be considered: the electrical resistance of the skin may be reduced through the insertion of catheters; body functions may be taken-over by apparatus, e.g. during surgery; natural reaction may be reduced through analgesia or switched off when anaesthetized. These risks have to be understood before objectives and measures for electrical safety may be established.

The complete picture of the dangers involved with the application of electrical equipment in high-tech medical locations, is made up by many sources: electrical and mechanical energy; high temperatures; fire; chemicals; micro organisms; defective or broken-down devices/equipment; incorrect handling of electrical equipment.

The aim of all electrical safety measures is the safety of patients, staff and installations. Safety can also be described in terms of risk minimization. The safety objective for patients, staff and installation may only be achieved, if the following requirements are simultaneously achieved: the site and the installation is safe; sevices and equipment are safe; procedures are defined and suitable training is provided for the handling of devices/equipment; regulations and instructions on hygiene are carried out.
To achieve these goals, a good sense of responsibility, competence and know-how, assignment as well as a good deal of willingness to cooperate by all involved, are essential.

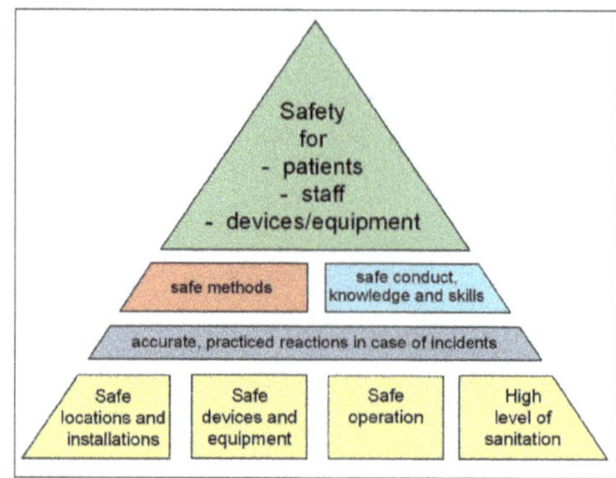

Figure 1. The safety concept in the hospital environment.

Electrical Devices/Equipment Used in Medical Locations

In view of the application of a multitude of electro-technical equipment in the medical environment, measures must be taken to prevent electrical accidents. There are two essential arguments for the installation of ungrounded power supply systems (medical IT systems) in hospitals:

- reliability of power supply;
- low leakage current to ground.

The electro-technical industries worldwide with their intricate knowledge about fault conditions in electrical installations see it as their responsibility to work with various national and international committees to establish safety standards. The application and monitoring of ungrounded power supply systems (medical IT systems) in hospitals are reflected in the different national standards.

The following are still valid basic statements according to IEC TC 62A:
- A patient may not be able to respond normally in a hazardous event (illness, unconsciousness, anaesthesia, or connect-

ed to electrical apparatus for therapeutic reasons).
- The natural electrical resistance of the skin normally provides an important protection against electrical current. With some treatments however this protection may be short-circuited, e.g. through the insertion of a catheter into the patient's body or by treating the skin when an electrode has to be placed on a patient's body. The human heart is more sensitive to electrical current than other parts of the body. Electrical current could inhibit the natural heart activity and could lead to heart-failure.
- Electro-medical equipment could be used to partly or permanently support or substitute vital bodily functions. A fault of the device/equipment or a power failure could be life-threatening.
- Interferences, e.g. from the power supply, could disturb the reproduction of action potentials, such as ECG or EEG.

The use of the ungrounded power supply system (medical IT system) may be desirable for the following reasons:
- Improves the reliability of power supply in areas where power failure may cause safety hazards for patient and user.
- Reduces the leakage currents of devices/ equipment to a low value thus reducing the touch voltage of the protective conductor through which the leakage current may flow. Lower ground leakage current levels substantially reduce the touch voltage of the protective conductor under fault conditions.
- Reduces the leakage currents of devices/ equipment to a low value, if approximately balanced to earth.

It is necessary to keep the impedance of the system to earth as high as possible. This is achieved by restricting:
- the physical dimensions of the medical isolating transformer;
- the system supplied by this transformer;
- the number of medical electrical devices/equipment connected to the system; and through;
- high internal impedance to earth of the insulation monitoring device connected to such a circuit.

Structure of an Ungrounded Power Supply System (Medical IT System)

The operation of the medical IT system with isolation monitoring and alarm forms the centre of the power supply. The base for the medical IT system is an ungrounded power source.
The essential advantage of a medical IT system is already evident in the case of a single fault condition. Only a small current IF flows, the value of which is determined through the system leakage capacitance C_e. This does not trigger a fuse, the supply voltage is maintained and the operation of the installation kept up.

The down-time safety is not the only argument for the use of an ungrounded power supply system or a medical IT system. It also reduces the leakage currents of the system to a low value, if the medical IT system is approximately balanced to ground.

Monitoring of ungrounded power supply systems (medical IT systems)

Increasing the availability of supply, a substantial aspect in the case of a first insulation fault, is guaranteed with the medical IT system. When operating an

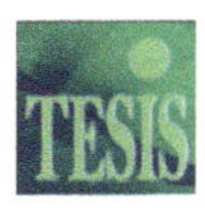

ungrounded power supply system (medical IT system) at single fault condition, attention has to be given to the fact that the original ungrounded system has turned into a system, comparable to a grounded system (TN system). An additional fault could then lead to triggering the short-circuit protection and hence to switching-off the entire system. To prevent this occurrence the insulation resistance is permanently monitored through a medical insulation monitoring device (IMD).

Electrical Safety in Medical Locations According to IEC 60364-7-710

IEC 60364-7-710:2002-11 the standard for medical locations was published in Nov 2002. In 2013 IEC/TC 64 MT 40 (International Electrical Committee) started a new draft for a new publishing in 2016.
Part 7: Particular requirements for special installations or locations, Section 710: Medical locations.

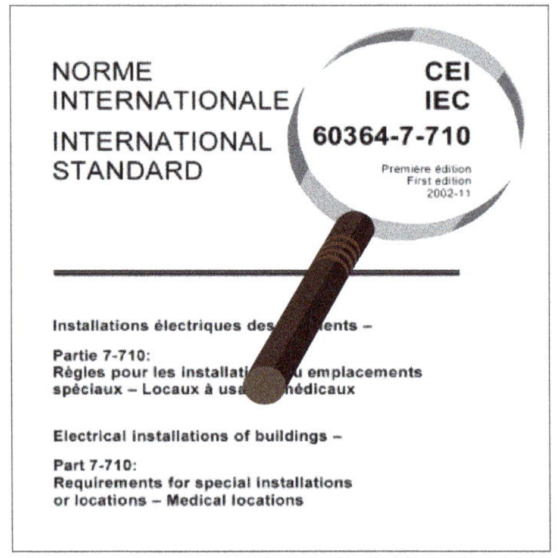

Figure 2. International Standard IEC 60364-7-710.

IEC 60364-7-710 classifies medical locations in three room groups:
- Group 0 medical location;
- Group 1 medical location;
- Group 2 medical location.

The Table 1 lists examples from IEC 60364-7-710:2002-11.

Clause 710.413.1.5 describes the medical ungrounded power supply system (medical IT system) as follows:

"In group 2 medical locations, the medical IT system shall be used for circuits supplying medical electrical equipment and systems intended for life-support or surgical applications and other electrical equipment located in the 'patient environment' excluding equipment listed in 710.413.1.3 For each group of rooms serving the same function, at least one separate medical IT system is necessary. The medical IT system is to be equipped with an insulation monitoring device in accordance with IEC 61557-8 with the following additional requirements:
- the a.c. internal impedance shall be at least 100 kOhm;
- the measuring voltage shall not be greater than 25V d.c.;
- the measuring current shall, even under fault conditions, not be greater than 1mA d.c.;
- the indication shall take place at the latest when the insulation resistance has decreased to 50kOhm. A measuring device/equipment shall be provided to test this facility;
- the indication shall take place, if the earth or wiring connection is lost.

For each medical IT system, an acoustic and visual alarm system incorporat-

Medical location	Group			Class	
	0	1	2	≤0,5 s	>0,5 s ≤15 s
1. Massage room	X	X			X
2. Bedrooms		X			
3. Delivery room		X		X [a]	X
4. ECG, EEG, EHG room		X			X
5. Endoscopic room		X [b]			X [b]
6. Examination or treatment room		X			X
7. Urology room		X [b]			X [b]
8. Radiological diagnostic and therapy room, other than mentioned under 21		X			X
9. Hydrotherapy room		X			X
10. Physiotherapy room		X			X
11. Anaesthetic room			X	X [a]	X
12. Operating theatre			X	X [a]	X
13. Operating preparation room		X	X	X [a]	X
14. Operating plaster room		X	X	X [a]	X
15. Operating recovery room		X	X	X [a]	X
16. Heart catheterization room			X	X [a]	X
17. Intensive care room			X	X [a]	X
18. Angiographic examination room			X	X [a]	X
19. Haemodialysis room		X			X
20. Magnetic resonance imaging (MRI) room		X			X
21. Nuclear medicine		X			X
22. Premature baby room			X	X [a]	X

[a] Luminaires and life-support medical electrical equipment which needs power supply within 0,5 s or less.
[b] Not being an operating theatre.

Table 1. Examples of medical locations according to their group.

ing the following components shall be arranged at a suitable place such that it can be permanently monitored (visual and audible signals) by the medical staff:

- a green signal lamp to indicate normal operation;
- a yellow signal lamp which lights when the minimum value set for the insulation resistance is reached. It shall not be possible for this light to be cancelled or disconnected;
- an audible alarm which sounds when the minimum value set for the insulations resistance is reached. The signal may be silenced;
- the yellow signal shall go out on removal of the fault and normal condition is restored.

Monitoring of Load and Temperature (Recommendation of IEC 60364-7-710)

To avoid overloading of the isolating transformer, monitoring of load and temperature is desirable, in order to protect the transformer and supply conductors between primary and secondary terminal and the distribution bus from overload or overheating. When the rated current or the temperature is over ranged an acoustic or optical alarm is released.

IFL (Insulation Fault Location System)

IEC 60364-4-41 Chapter 411.6.3.1

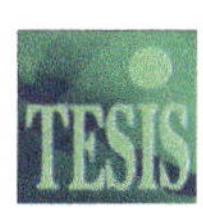

Note 1: recommends that a first fault hast to be eliminated within the shortest practicable delay. Modern monitoring systems will allow identifying the exact location of faulty electrical systems by on-line fault location => defect medical devices can be identified without switching off the supply system

Preventing Power Loss

Regardless of the implementation of a medical IT system and management of the total selectivity of the protection devices, a total loss of power in group 2 medical locations shall be prevented. This may be achieved either.

Provision of two independent supply lines:
- normal power supply;
- safety power supply (≤ 15s), e.g. Generator;
- special safety power supply (≤ 0,5s).

Provision of a ring-structure, capable to back up the mains supply, or local additional power supply unit, or an additional power supply unit for several rooms of group 2.

Electrical safety in medical locations according to NFPA99

Practical Case studies from Latin-American Hospitals

San Borja International Clinic in Lima, Peru; it's the second medical center facility in Peru installed with BENDER medical technology, it means IMD + EDS fault locators. It's a good and representative example of the real development and application of the standards, together with the technology in a continent as SA. Right now the system (technology) is working as expected, however the most interesting part is how the Clinic owners understood the technology, it was let's say a not easy process, therefore the real world in SA.

Conclusions

The patient is the focus of attention in the hospital. Even the slightest power failure can impair a successful diagnosis and therapy and therefore may be life-threatening to the patient. That is why ungrounded power supply systems (medical IT systems) with insulation monitoring are used, because this guarantees a comprehensive protection for patient, doctors and medical staff.

- Added safety at no additional cost
- No power interruption at first fault
- Early warning of faulty medical equipment
- Visual and audible indications of hazardous situations
- Inherent selective short circuit coordination
- Low leakage current to ground
- Reduced effects of common mode noise

The safety measures for testing medical devices/equipment regarding electrical parameters and faults complete the safety concept in the medical environment.

Modern indication and communication possibilities (web-based, SMS etc) will give medical and technical staff clear and detailed advises how to react in alarm situation.

Biosafety and Laboratory Facilities Design

Ana Teresa Rodríguez Quiala[1], Francisco Rodriguez Perez[2]

ana.quiala@infomed.sld.cu
[1]Dra. MSc. Dr., Havana, Cuba
[2]Architect, Consultant, Havana, Cuba

This article deals with the importance of minimizing all Types of Risks in the operation of clinical and microbiology laboratories.
Biosafety is the set of organizational scientific measures, human or technical, which include: a) those physical provisions designed to protect the workers of a facility, the surrounding community and the environment from the risks derived from the work with biological agents or the release of organisms into the environment, whether exotic and genetically modified or not, and also; b) those aimed at reducing the effects that may arise from contamination and quickly eliminate its possible harmful consequences in case of pollution, leakage or loss.

Ana Teresa Rodríguez Quiala. *Doctor of medicine. Specialist in Laboratory Clinical. Biosecurity Master. Member from de Community Cubans of Pathology clinical and Biosecurity. Teacher Assistant of Medicine Faculty Dr. ¨Salvador Allende¨ and Sanitation Faculty. It participation in exchange scientific in Areas clean, Seminar of Design, Cycle of life Analysis, Productions more cleans, Inauguration of Cathedra de Security and Risk in Cuba , II Congress International from Architecture and Engineer Hospitable Cuba 2013. Suitor a Science Doctorate now.*

Introduction

The organization of Biosafety in laboratories cannot be an individual, spontaneous or anarchic work. There must exist a Safety organization that evaluates all types of risks, and according to the recommendations made by experts, monitor and ensure compliance with the adequate safety measures to be adopted in each particular case. Two unavoidable aspects of Biosafety should be ensured in laboratories:
- Compliance with the current Technical and Safety Standards of each institution.
- Enforcement of a permanent Training policy for all staff on all the activities in which they are involved.

The key aspect to achieve risk reduction is the analysis thereof by competent personnel, on the spot where the tasks are performed, so that the evaluation results in a Methodology designed and expressed in practices and procedures that ensure safe working conditions.
The existence of Cuban Resolution 103 /02 as a standing rule for the establishment of Biosafety requirements and procedures of Biological Safety in institutions that make use of biological agents and products, organisms and fragments of these with genetic information, results a real tool in the daily work of laboratories, as it summarizes objectives and basic definitions, responsibilities of

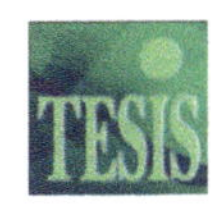

managers, requirements according to biosafety level, practices, procedures, equipment for biological safety, etc.
The Types of Risks analyzed in this study were: Biological; Chemical; Dependent on the design of the facility.

Biological: The probability of occurrence and magnitude of the consequences of an adverse event related to the use of biological agents that can affect humans, the community and the environment.
Biohazard Rating:
- Infectious: Infections and Infestations.
- Non Infectious: Allergies and Intoxications.

Chemical: This type of risk is one that generates the probability of damage, injury or death from exposure to hazardous chemicals. To relate chemical hazards with the damage they cause, it is advisable to apply the following classification.

Classification of chemicals according to predominant risk
1) Irritant: They cause local reversible conditions such as inflammation in exposed tissues.
2) Corrosive: Destroy the surfaces with which they come in contact.
3) Harmful: Substances which if inhaled, ingested or absorbed through the skin can produce noxious effects on health.
4) Toxic: Any material that can cause acute or chronic effects on the individual.
5) Highly toxic or Poisonous: Substances that can cause extremely serious or even lethal effects on human beings.
6) Extremely flammable: Substances that burn at a temperature below zero degrees Celsius and their boiling point is 35 degrees Celsius or less.
7) Flammable: Those that burn easily between temperatures of 21 °C or more and up to 55 degrees Celsius, hazardous to the environment.
8) Explosive: Substances very reactive against unstable products, that due to moisture absorption, spontaneous chemical changes or friction, burst and are sensitive to thermal or mechanical shock.
9) Oxidizing: Substances that provide oxygen, which in turn allows and encourages combustion. They produce highly exothermic reactions when in contact with other substances, particularly flammable or combustible.
10) Radioactive: They are divided into several categories according to the nature of radioactivity and the amount involved.

Dependent on the design of the facility

They are related with the external environment protection achieved by combining facility design and adequate operational practices, including: Contour Sealing, Solid Waste Treatment Systems, Waste Water Treatment Systems, Air Exhausts Treatment from Air Conditioning and Ventilation, Access controlled areas, Separate buildings or modules to isolate the laboratory, etc.

Groups of Risks	Biosafety Rating	Type of activity	Laboratory Classification
I	NBS 1	Teaching	Basic
II	NBS 2	Teaching, Diagnosis, Primary health care and Research	Containment
III	NBS 3	Diagnosis and Investigation	Containment
IV	NBS 4	Investigation	Of utmost containment

Table 1. Definition of Biosafety level for laboratories, depending on the biological agents handled.

Research Proposal

To investigate the percentages of Biological, Chemical and Facility Design Risks of the personnel occupationally exposed in the Clinical and Microbiology Laboratories of the "Dr. Salvador Allende Hospital".

Risk Analysis has different stages: I. Risk Identification; II. Risk Assessment; III. Risk Administration; IV. Risk Communication. The causes of Risks can be: Technical, Organizational, or Dependent on human behavior. For their analysis Risk Identification Techniques (RIT) are used.

Objectives: 1. Analysis and Risk Assessment in the Clinical and Microbiology Laboratories of the Hospital; 2. Description of the decreasing occurrence as a result of the analysis; 3. Design proposal for both Laboratories.

Material and Methods: This work was performed at the Clinical and Microbiology Laboratories at the "Dr. Salvador Allende Hospital" in the period between January and May, 2013, where an analysis and risk assessment procedure was performed.
Check-lists were prepared for each of the sections of the facility to verify compliance with the requirements of Biosafety, and subsequently the risk identification technique (What if .....?) was applied to weigh, from the standpoint of three different experts, the biological, chemical and facility design risks of the laboratories under investigation.

Results: In both cases, the results showed that although the three types of risks interlace to increase risk potential in the facilities that presently process the samples of each of the Hospital departments, the behavior of each type of risk expressed in percent was as follows:
1) Microbiology Laboratory: Biological Risks : 25 %; Chemical Risks: 8 %; Facility Design Risks: 67 %. In this laboratory the areas of greater risks were the Respiratory area in the first place and subsequently those assigned to Coprological and Parasitological tests.
2) Clinical Laboratory: Results in this section of the Hospital were as follows.

Biological Risk 35%: The analysis allowed us to propose the following order, starting with the areas of highest risk and moving down to those of the lowest risk: Major Risk areas in decreasing order: Scrub area; Disposal area; Manual Chemistry Area; Sample Extraction Area; Nephrology Area; Special Hematology Area; Basic Hematology and Automated Chemistry Area; Centrifugation Area; Reception Samples Classification Area.

Chemical Risks 5 %: Main areas with Chemicals Risks in decreasing order: Preparation and Storage of Chemicals Area; Manual Chemistry Area; Special Hematology Area; Nephrology and Basic Hematology Areas; Automated Chemistry Area; Scrub Area; Facility Design Risks: 60 %.

Given the results obtained in both laboratories, and because of the extremely deficient technical and engineering conditions of the existing facilities, with problems in their electrical and hydraulic services, ceilings, walls, bathrooms, etc. it was concluded that none of the above can be taken care of through minor renovations, and sustainable upgrading can only be achieved by complete repair of the property. Therefore, it was necessary to prepare and submit proposals at several

entities in charge of validating facilities dealing with biohazards, while undertaking the New Design of the facilities.
Once taken into account the former, the authorities of the Hospital decided to annex the two laboratories, since they have similar biosafety risk levels, and the patient samples often circulate simultaneously, since the studies are complementary. It was then decided to use one single pavilion of the Hospital to house both laboratories which, although working independently, have other similar characteristics. For instance, the hazardous waste that they produce cannot be sent to the sewer and will therefore be segregated and placed in a unified temporary room available for the entire hospital, close to the site where the two laboratories will be finally installed, ensuring a short transfer of the waste with minimum risk of spills, breakage or other accidents, before its final treatment outside the Hospital.

The design proposal of the laboratories to be remodeled took into account the existing regulations in CUBA. Clinical laboratories are biosafety level NBS II on a small scale, where different tests are being performed on different types of samples: serum, blood with anticoagulants, urine, body fluids, etc., whose analysis and risk assessment was used to determine the requirements according to each laboratory area. The exception was the Respiratory section in Microbiology laboratory, where tuberculosis bacillus is present and the biosafety risk level is NBS III because of the possibility of transmission by inhalation of this microorganism, as dictated by the competent Provincial Assessment Committee.

Conclusions

1. Risks categories were determined after proper analysis in both laboratories, and also the percentage of incidence of the three analyzed risk types.
2. In both laboratories the higher risk occurrence derived from those dependant on facility design issues, and then in decreasing order from biological and chemical sources.
3. The proposal thereafter elaborated resulted in a complete remodeling of a dedicated pavilion of the Hospital, to house both relocated laboratories, as their risk percentages due to facility design issues were nearly equally high: 67% at the Clinical Lab and 60% at the Microbiology Lab. The overall purpose of avoiding risks for workers, the community and the surrounding environment determined that such a comprehensive approach was unavoidable.

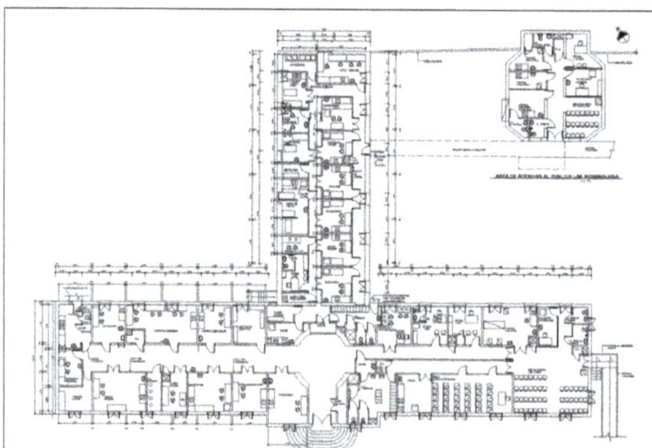

Figure 1. Design proposal for the relocation of Clinical and Microbiology Laboratories in Dr. Salvador Allende Hospital, Havana, Cuba.

Succession Planning and Workforce Development in Healthcare Engineering and Estate Management

John Thatcher

John.thatcher@eastwoodpark.co.uk
Cert Ed (FE), MA (Ed), CFCIPD, Hon MGI. Eastwood Park Limited

Healthcare engineering and estate management are highly specialised and technical functions that are delivered within Healthcare facilities by either in-house staff or outsourced specialist service providers. The workforce is aged and predominantly male, with recruitment and retention a real issue. This is partially due to the lack of awareness of the career opportunities and relevant technical skills held by young adults. This together with very limited specialised training and development provision, and a lack of progressive career frameworks being available, makes succession planning and workforce development in these areas a major issue for employers.

This paper will consider the implications of addressing this healthcare engineering and estates skills shortage by exploring strategies for Succession Planning and Workforce Development via: 1. changing the image of these work-roles to raise their profile and make them more attractive to young people of both genders; 2. developing and defining career pathways within healthcare engineering and estate management; 3. identifying and using existing qualifications and apprenticeship frameworks across all levels for these specialised areas and promoting them on a national basis; 4. Designing the specialised learning programmes and qualifications, from Traineeships to Advanced and Higher Apprenticeships to 'plug the gaps' in existing provision; 5. Forming clear relationships between qualifications, professional registrations and membership levels, Council status, competence compliance and the employers career and reward frameworks to ensure an integrated and coherent approach to staff retention and career progression.

John Thatcher *is the Chief Executive Officer of Eastwood Park Limited, a specialist training centre that focuses on Healthcare Engineering, Facilities Management and Support Services training and consultancy within the UK and Internationally. He has led Eastwood Park for over 20 years both from within the NHS and, since a management buy-out in 2003, as a private limited company. Amongst other things John has been instrumental in developing the Eastwood Park curriculum and customer base to the wide ranging portfolio of programmes and markets that they currently service.*

John is a qualified and experienced Engineer, Teacher and Director. Amongst his awards he has a Masters Degree in Education (MA (Ed)) and he is a Chartered Fellow of the Chartered Institute of Personnel and Development (CFCIPD). He was awarded Honorary Membership of City & Guilds of London Institute (Hon MGI) for his work in vocational qualification development and quality assurance.

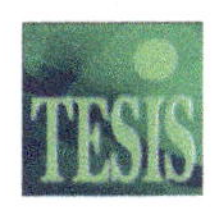

Development

Healthcare engineering and estate management are highly specialised and technical functions, delivered within healthcare facilities either by in-house resources or outsourced to specialist service providers. Worldwide the workforce is predominantly of mature age and male, with recruitment and retention proving a challenge globally; partially due to limited awareness of engineering and estates career opportunities, as well as a lack of relevant technical skills held by young adults within the health sector. Dr Peter Jarritt, President of IPEM states: "The role of technology in the provision of healthcare is set to increa se rapidly in all sectors from acute care to primary and social care. This will present a challenge to the engineering and technical workforce within this sector. It will require new skills as medical devices and computers become more integrated and the patient takes on more responsibility for their care..."[1]

This situation is also compounded by limited specialised training and progressive career development opportunities being available, making succession planning and workforce development an issue for both employers and employees alike.

This paper will seek to consider these and other issues by exploring strategies for succession planning and workforce development, within the following key areas: promoting healthcare engineering and estates management; attracting new talent; the complexity of designing career progression; developing existing staff; commissioning provision; new delivery models; meeting the challenge.

[1] *IPEM is the UK's Institute of Physics and Engineering in Medicine a professional organisation that represents physicists, engineers and technologists in healthcare.*

Promoting healthcare engineering and estates management as a career

Potential employees generally receive little information regarding career opportunities within the field of healthcare engineering and estates management. This coupled with a low uptake of maths and science subjects in secondary and tertiary education, particularly amongst females, is drastically limiting the pool of potential new talent. Perhaps as a consequence of this just 8.7% of British engineers are female, according to the trade association Engineering UK. This compared with 30% in Latvia and 40% in China. "The UK has fewer engineers than anywhere else in Europe... on the world stage it is worse." – says Sir Richard Olver, chairman of BAE systems[2].

Much more needs to be done around articulating healthcare engineering as a key career route and encouraging uptake of science related qualifications. Sarah Sillars, OBE, CEO of Semta said "We need to break out of the box and present the possibilities in an engaging and exciting manner. Young people are convinced that the subjects themselves are boring – even if they are good at them. Our job is to show the excitement and reward that a career in science and engineering can bring."[3]

Appropriate resources and recruitment campaigns need to be designed to promote jobs in this area and to clearly articulate the longer-term career opportunities. These need to reach the potential pool of talent using the most appropriate medium for the target group. The use of social media is key in engaging young people and increasingly

[2] *Quote extracted from Sunday Express July 14th 2013.*

[3] *Semta is the Sector Skills Council for Science, Engineering and Manufacturing Technologies within the UK.*

adults. However, to successfully promote healthcare engineering and estate management as a career the sector needs to ensure that suitable career paths with appropriate training are available.

ATTRACTING NEW TALENT

Attracting bright new talent to the sector is vital in developing engineers of the future and this can be achieved though the recruitment of apprentices and graduates.

Employing apprentices

Apprenticeships, which contain knowledge and competence-based qualifications, prepare new entrants for a specific trade. In some countries, government funding is available to support their education. Over the last 4 years apprenticeships have been extended from educational levels 2 and 3 to include higher apprenticeships at levels 4, 5 and 6 and level 7 (Master's Degree Level) apprenticeships are in development. Apprenticeships provide new entrants with a real alternative to more traditional academic routes to professional engineering roles and they are normally employed so they can earn and learn as they work.

However designing and delivering specialist apprenticeship frameworks is a challenge. The sector needs to support the development of suitable frameworks and not shoehorn healthcare apprentices into generic engineering programmes that do not develop the specialist skills and knowledge required.

Recruiting graduates

Another source of new talent is to recruit graduates into the healthcare and estates sector. Graduates will bring in-depth technical knowledge and important research skills but in some cases may lack the practical application that an apprentice will acquire during their training. To overcome this organisations are looking to supplement academic study with opportunity for hands-on training.

Qualification Levels			Other Country Qualification Levels		
England, Northern Ireland and Wales (QCF, CQFF)	Examples of types of English qualifications	Apprentice ships available in England	Scotland (SCQF)	Ireland (NQFQ IE)	Europe (EQF)
8	Doctoral Degree Vocational Qualifications e.g. QCF		12	10	8
7	Masters Post graduate Diplomas/Certificates Vocational Qualifications e.g. QCF		11	9	7
6	Bachelor Degrees Graduate Diplomas/Certificates Vocational Qualifications e.g. QCF		10/9	8/7	6
5/4	Foundation Degree Diplomas of Higher Education Higher National Diploma /Certificate (HND / HNC) Vocational Qualifications e.g. QCF		8/7	6	5
3	Vocational Qualifications e.g. QCF GCE AS and A level Advanced Diplomas (England)		6	5	4
2	Vocational Qualifications e.g. QCF GCSEs at grades A*-C, Higher Diplomas (England) Functional / Essential Skills		5	4	3
1	Vocational Qualifications e.g. QCF GCSEs at grades D-G, Foundation Diplomas (England) Functional / Essential Skills		4	3	2

Figure 1. Apprenticeships available in England.

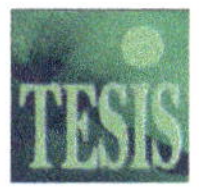

The complexity of designing career progression

Before exploring training programmes for existing staff it is worth reflecting on the need to align career progression with complex job roles, relevant qualifications, professional bodies and trade organisations.
There needs to be a clear focus on ensuring that new entrants and existing staff receive the appropriate training and qualifications required to meet the organisation's needs as well as their own. We need career pathways for internationally recognised roles such as Competent & Authorised Persons and Authorising Engineers. Within most countries these professional roles are normally linked to memberships of professional and regulatory bodies who have their own professional standards and membership criteria. These bodies may in turn relate to National Councils, such as the UK's Engineering Council which sets the professional standards and requirements for professional registrations leading to Engineering Technician, Incorporated Engineer and Chartered Engineer status. These statuses are recognised internationally by organisations such as the International Federation of Hospital Engineers (IFHE) which provides a global strategic forum for these disciplines.
In order to create and articulate career development linked to organisational, regulatory requirements and sector needs career frameworks need to be designed for each role.

Developing existing staff

Technical updating, familiarity with emerging technologies and developing a wider skill-base are all key areas that need to be addressed by organisations. Much of this training is likely to be undertaken by equipment manufacturers and estates services organisations as well as through Further and Higher Education development routes.
An example of 'blended' approach, which mixes Higher Education with a vocational route, is the UK's Foundation Degree in Medical Technologies where various healthcare engineering pathways are available. This programme enables full-time employees to also become full-time students by undertaking their studies in tandem with their job. They use a mix of work-based activities, on-line learning, weekend courses and assessment centres, held in a specialised healthcare engineering learning environment, to complete their studies. On achieving their Level 5 Foundation Degree, these students can then progress on to a BSc Honours top-up programme at the partner university.

Commissioning provision

Sourcing suitable training provision to meet the complexities already mentioned is not easy. Supply may be limited because of the investment training providers need to make in equipping facilities and developing high quality resources for relatively low numbers of trainees. However organisations have a number of options including:

- develop internal training opportunities to meet the needs;
- outsource the whole requirement to external training providers;
- use a blended learning approach working in partnership with an external accredited specialist educational provider to deliver some of the components with employers delivering others.

Whichever range of methods is used it is important to ensure that the training requested will meet the actual needs identified and that it is evaluated to confirm that it was effective.

Development Route	Qualifications	Role	Notes
Generic Management or Facilities Management as well as maintaining technical skills and knowledge where appropriate	Level 7-8 in strategic management and leadership, or equivalent Facilities Management Qualifications	Trust Medical Engineering Manager with deputies if appropriate	
As well as regular technical skills updating, could undertake foundation degree in medical technologies – leading to Master's degree + further additional development could be around people management – managing contracts, quality control, depending on role	Level 3 – 6 management qualifications Potentially Facilities Management Qualifications depending on role Level 5 Foundation Degree in Medical Technologies or Level 7 Masters Level 5 Foundation Degree in Medical Technologies or Level 7 Masters	Team Managers	Line manage all below staff including undertaking competence checks, appraisals, identifying training needs
		Specialist Medical Engineers in: • Anaesthetics/life support • Electronics • Infusion Devices Potentially involved in managing contracts	Also provide supervision/quality checks of the below
Regular skills technical updating provided by medical manufacturers	Bespoke training to meet needs of individuals and organisation	Fully trained medical engineers, but still subject to some additional supervision on high risk areas by the above	Appraisals are competency based and identify training needs
Level 3 Medical Engineering Apprenticeship using Engineering Manufacture (Craft and Technician – Engineering Maintenance pathway)	Level 3 NVQ Diploma (QCF) In Engineering Maintenance (servicing medical equipment pathway) + HNC in electrical electronics	4th Year Apprentices	Employed, released for training and on successful completion of qualifications and interview can progress to next level
		3rd Year Apprentices	
Level 2 Medical Engineering Apprenticeship using Performing Engineering Operations framework	BTEC national in electrical electronics	2nd Year Apprentices	
	Level 2 NVQ Diploma (QCF) in Performing Engineering Operations	1st Year Apprentices	

Figure 2. An example of a medical engineering development route from a UK hospital.

Case Study - Perceived training 'wanted' vs training actually 'needed'

Eastwood Park was commissioned by a hospital in Saudi Arabia, to provide training to enable their existing staff to achieve an American academic qualification. This training was commissioned to reduce non-compliance issues and ensure patient safety. An on-site competence analysis identified that what was 'wanted' would not provide what was 'needed'. After presenting their findings Eastwood Park proposed, and later delivered, the following phased development programme:

- reviewed and rewrote/updated local policies and procedures;
- designed a training programme based on the above that would also facilitate achieving the American academic qualification and an additional competence-based UK qualification;
- delivered the programme to the staff and supported them to achieve the desired performance outcomes and the two qualifications;
- as part of the organisation's succession planning, they trained and qualified department supervisors to support and assess their existing and new technicians.

This development programme gave them the skills-base and on-going structure to drastically minimise future threats and to support new staff coming into the department.

New delivery models

The sector also needs to beware of the developments in education that removes the barriers to providing staff training. This includes using technology to support mobile learning, social learning and e-learning.

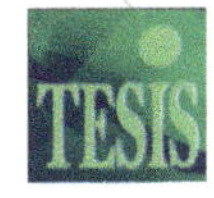

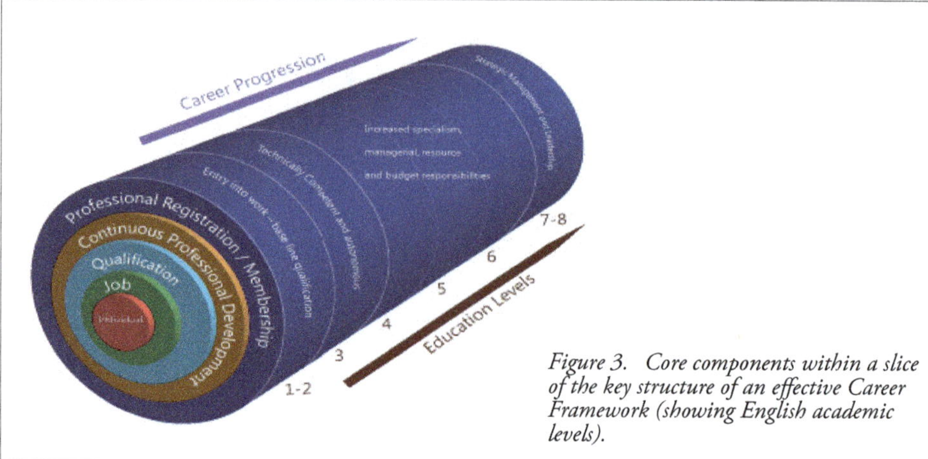

Figure 3. Core components within a slice of the key structure of an effective Career Framework (showing English academic levels).

Many universities and organisations are offering free MOOCs (Massive Open Online Courses). With the internationalisation of healthcare regulations it may be possible in the future for professionals from across the globe to come together to study.

In April 2013 a MOOC in Healthcare Innovation and Entrepreneurship attracted just over 36,000 students, of which nearly 14,000 have been active in the course so far. There are 1,800 students posting in to the discussion forum, into almost 750 threads so far.

Summary - Meeting the challenge

The sector needs to develop clear strategies to ensure we have a well equipped workforce that can support the advances in technology and the demand for services. The promotion and use of apprenticeships must play an important part in bringing new talent into the industry. The sector needs to ensure that apprenticeship frameworks are fit for purpose and harness best practice from across the globe.

Graduates are a vital source of exciting new talent but we do need to support their introduction into the workplace.

The training landscape is complex and designing suitable development programmes and career paths needs to done with internationalisation in mind. Finding and working with forward thinking providers must also be a priority. Practical training can be supported in the workplace by the use of low cost learning technology.

The challenges may be daunting but with a co-ordinated approach and by capturing best practice the sector can develop coherent, internationally recognised programmes that are vital to ensure we have an effective workforce for the future. At the core of this is the individual and their requirement to have appropriate training. This needs to relate to job roles and appropriate qualifications. A defined career path that progresses through the educational levels is required to provide continuous professional development. These pathways need to have multiple routes for those who specialise in highly technical roles or are to become the managers of the future. Finally all of these components must be aligned with professional registration and memberships at all levels that are internationally recognised.

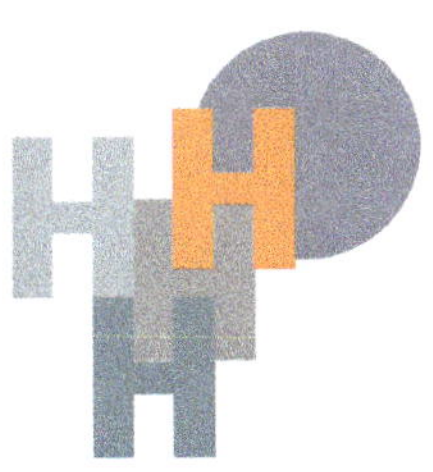

Design Focused on the Patient, Cultural Diversity

Session Introduction

The patient-centred design approach has come a long way and it is now possible to evaluate the success of the application of design principles related to the creation of the healing environment. The quality of the care settings has a significant influence on the wellbeing of patients, family members and the staff involved in the care processes.

In this regard the design solutions collected through evidence-based design research should be applied as far as possible in care environments. Designers of healthcare buildings should have the following common goals: design human-scale buildings; create environments that favour socializing and informal meetings; maximize views of the outside and the presence of natural light; use colour and light to encourage people to interact with the space; distinguish environments by using materials and furnishings capable of creating a non-institutional and homely atmosphere.

The task of healthcare designers implies a high level of complexity since the framework of needs and consequently the architectural choices to be made vary significantly according to the user profile and type of disease. Different design solutions may be adopted in environments for cancer patients or patients suffering from dementia. At the same time designers must establish a relationship with the hospital site and try to create a structure that can accommodate the constant changes imposed by technology and care in order to ensure equal access to the largest possible number of users.

The challenge for designers in the coming years will be to translate all these considerations into solutions fit for any country in the developing world, trying to adapt to the needs of different cultural models and limited resources.

Designing Hospitals in India: Challenges and Opportunities

Martin Fiset

martin-fiset@sympatico.ca
Architect, Montreal (Quebec), Canada

Hospital design in India offers a lot of opportunities for healthcare architects, engineers and other professionals. As the demand for healthcare facilities is forever growing, India has a huge gap to close to reach the WHO minimum of 3.5 beds per thousand. A multiplicity of factors, social, economic and cultural not to mention available building materials and current building practices not seen in the West impacts planning and design and challenges preconceived ideas and approaches. After a brief overview of the healthcare system both private and public in India, the speaker, based on his own experience, will present the impact these multiple factors have on planning and design of private hospitals in the country. These impacts will be contrasted with current design practices and standards in the US and Canada.

Martin Fiset *is an architect with over forty years of experience in all aspects of health care facilities planning and design. He has worked as a programming and planning consultant and project manager on numerous projects across Canada, the United States and abroad.*

His expertise has been sought for numerous health care facilities in Ontario, Alberta, Quebec, and New Brunswick, and, in the United States, in Washington, Baltimore, and Philadelphia. His foreign experience includes projects in India, Egypt, Germany, Argentina, The Bahamas, Algeria, Turks and Caicos Islands and Georgia. His Indian experience include programming, planning and design for four hospitals and he is currently involved in two new projects in that country.
He has been invited to lecture on hospital planning and functional space programming in Jaipur and Goa in India, in the USA in Washington (DC), Grand Rapids (MI), Denver (CO), and in Canada, in Montreal and Quebec City, as well as Paris, Buenos Aires (Argentina) and Valparaiso (Chile). Mr.Fiset established his own consulting firm in 1998, offering facilities programming and design services to the healthcare sector.

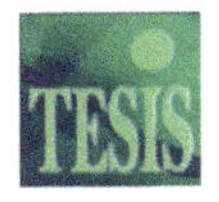

CONTEXT

Population

Life in India, with a population of 1.3 billion, is rife with many challenges: high income disparity, lack of infrastructure and high incidence of non-communicable diseases among others. In this context, delivery of quality affordable health care is one of the greatest challenges the country faces.
Whereas the private sector is well developed and is still growing at a quick pace – it accounts for 93% of hospitals, 64% of all beds and 80% to 85% of all doctors – the public sector is left far behind and practically nonexistent in rural areas.

There is a veritable boom in private hospital development. New hospitals are mushrooming mainly in large cities and entrepreneurs see the healthcare market as a lucrative venture. In metropolitan areas, hospital bed supply is almost at par with the global benchmark of 3.5 beds per 1000 people.

Care is available if you have the money to pay the bill. And the supply still cannot meet the demand as the rise of the middle class and the introductions of insurance make health care more accessible. The public sector on the other hand is terribly lagging behind.

Overall the bed supply in India is 7 bed per thousand. With the large concentration of beds in metropolitan areas, this leaves very few beds in rural areas.

Needs

There is obviously a huge gap between supply and demand in the public sector. To bridge the gap between what would be the WHO recommended level of 3.5 beds per thousand and to cope with population increase, India will have to add 3.1 million beds overall by 2018 according to some projections.

Expenditures

At the moment, India spends 4% of its GDP on healthcare. Its 11th development plan called for an increase to 6.5% of GDP by 2012, but this never materialized. During the recent election that brought to power the BJP and Narendra Modi as the new prime minister, the question of healthcare was never raised by any party, and neither was education. Health care is regarded by government as a loss not as an investment.

COMPARISON

Any comparison with countries that have a universal health care system would be unfair as the discrepancies are so wide. For example, Canada spends about 13% of its GDP on healthcare and provides access to health care to all its citizens.

A comparison with the US that spends 17% of its GDP would be more appropriate as it is the only industrialized country that's relies heavily on the private sector and does not have a universal healthcare system, an exception that the current president is trying to remedy.

Personal Experience in India

The presentation included detailed information about the following hospitals the speaker was involved in. Architects for these projects were ARCOP Architects Montreal and Delhi except for the Malabar Cancer Centre (Technicalya, Chennai) and the Aster DM Healthare Hospital (KHS, Dallas and Delhi):

- Malabar Cancer Centre, Thalasseri, Kerala;
- Medanta the Medicity, Gurgaon, Haryana;
- Jaypee Institute of Medical Sciences, Noida, Uttar Pradesh;
- GM Modi Hospital, Saket, Delhi;
- DM Healthcare Multi-specialty Hospital, Kochi, Kerala;
- Medanta GK Hospital, GKI, Delhi;
- Medanta Lucknow Hospital, Lucknow, Uttar Pradesh.

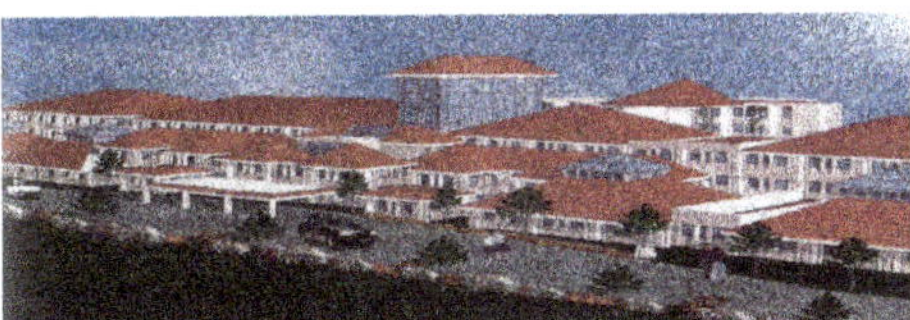

Figure 1. Malabar Cancer Centre.

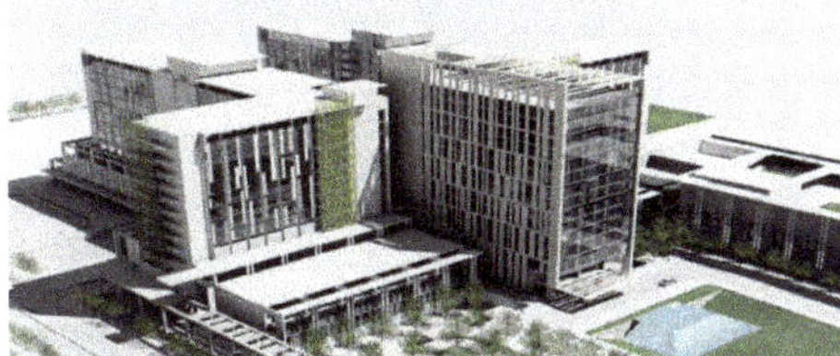

Figure 2. Medanta the Medicity.

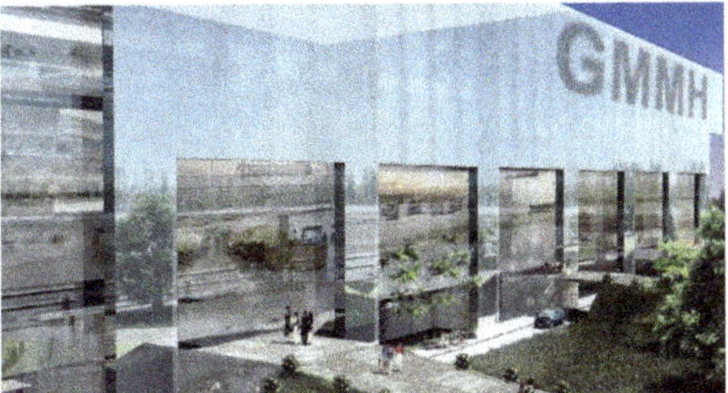

Figure 3. G M Modi Hospital.

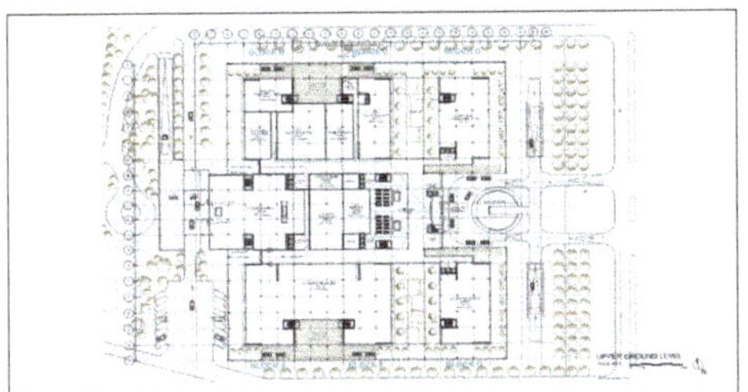

Figure 4. Jaypee Institute of Medical Sciences.

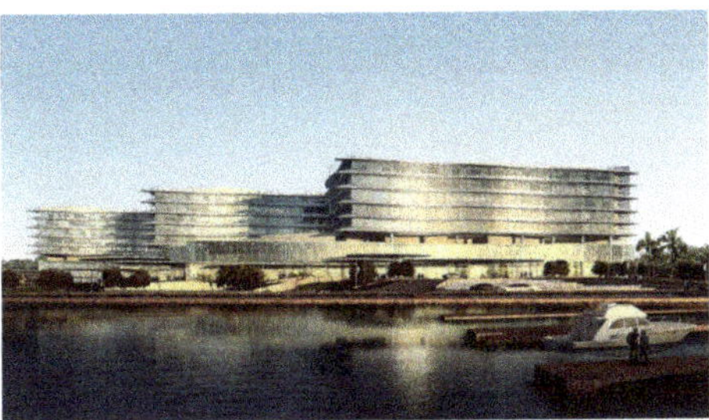

Figure 5. Aster DM Healthcare Hospital.

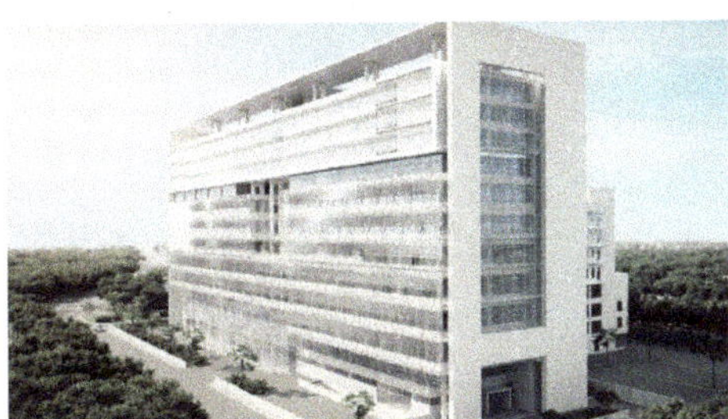

Figure 6. GK Medanta Hospital.

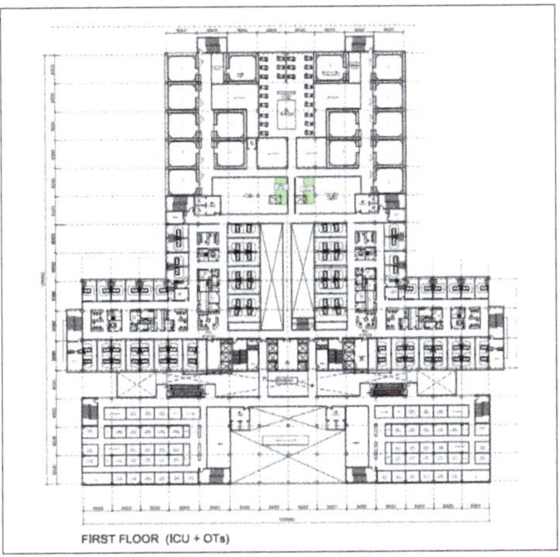

Figure 7. Medanta Lucknow Hospital.

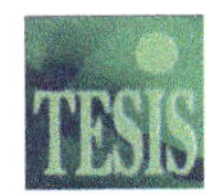

Factors to be considered

Several factors that a Western architect would not be familiar with and may clash with common approaches in North America and Europe have an important impact on planning and design. They include the following ones: Cultural; Socioeconomic; Environmental; Process; Medical practices; Building practices; Codes and regulations; Accreditation.

Cultural Factors

Family Unit

The family is at the center, the basic cell of Indian society. Three and even four generations of patriarchal lineage live together under the same roof. Members feel a deep loyalty to their family and it is in the family bosom that children's education takes place and cultural and social values are inculcated. This basic family unit extends to a wider kinship group also related by lineage.

When a member of this family unit is in the hospital, it is imperative that all members and even members of the kinship group come to visit the patient. Furthermore, an attendant is expected to be in the patients the room day and night for the duration of his or her stay. To accommodate this number of people, vast lobbies and large waiting areas have to be provided, number of elevators has to be increased and the patient room itself has to be larger to accommodate couches and chairs. At Medanta The Medicity to mention one, each patient at the time of admission is given two passes, one for a 24/7 attendant and one for visitors. Only one visitor at a time is allowed in the room, so to accommodate the whole extended family, one member will spend only 20 to 30 minutes in the room to give a chance to other members to see the patient. This means that over the two-hour visiting time, 4 to 6 relatives may come to see the patient.

For intensive care patients, the situation is different. No attendant is allowed to remain in the room and visitors can only spend five minutes at a time. One family member can however spend the night in the hospital. To accommodate these people, who can be quite numerous as the proportion of ICU beds to overall bed complement can be as high as 30% to 35%, night lounges furnished with comfortable reclining chairs and equipped with bathing facilities are provided.

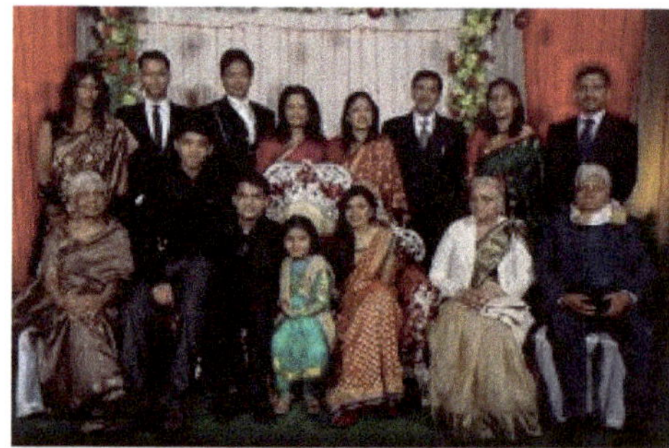

Figure 8. Family oriented.

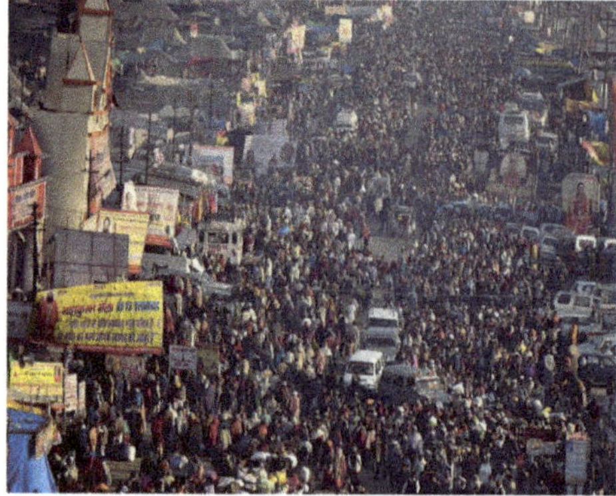

Figure 9. Demographics.

Caste

Status differences in Indian society are expressed in terms of purity and pollution whereas high status is associated with purity and low status with pollution, particularly if they are in contact or associated with bodily waste. Contact with or even view of these lower status people determine for example the placement of bathrooms in patient rooms to avoid patients seeing housekeepers coming to clean the bathroom or staff being in contact with lower status staff retrieving soiled material from soiled utilities. These lower status people have their own kitchen and dining room separate from other staff members and their own separate locker rooms. Within the higher status members, the medical and the higher echelon administrative staff have also their own dining room and so does the middle level staff. In some Surgical Suite layouts, it happens occasionally that clients would request a separate "dirty" corridor for the removal of soiled material so that the staff assigned to this function is isolated.

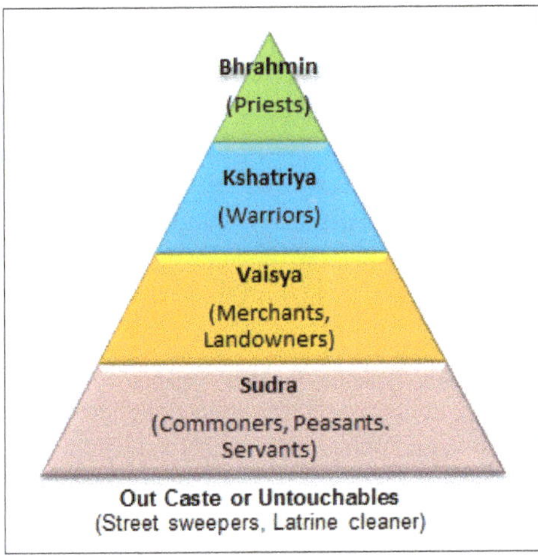

Figure 10. Castes.

Privacy

Privacy is of paramount importance in the hospital. On Inpatient Units, patient rooms' doors are kept shut and visibility of the patient from the corridor, contrary to North American practice, is shunned. This practice is obviated by the fact that there is an attendant in the room at all times. Some precautions have to be taken also in regard to segregation of the sexes.

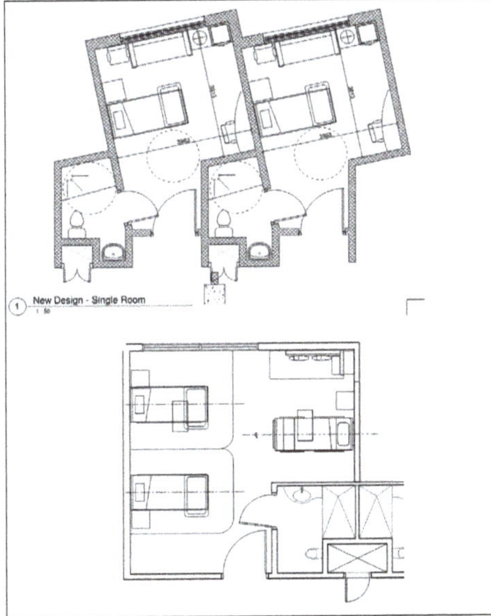

Figure 11. Inpatient accommodations.

Socioeconomic Factors

Socioeconomic status is also expressed in the hospital, particularly in inpatient accommodations. From the deluxe suite with salon for the family with kitchenette to multiple bedded wards for "charity" patients, accommodations run the whole gamut, which is a far cry from the all single same-handed rooms that has become common practice in North America.

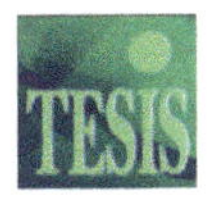

Environment

Northern India environment is far from being as temperate as one would believe. From near 0°C in winter to upward of 45°C in the summer with high humidity, it goes through wide variations that impact both architectural and engineering design. Surprisingly enough, it is only recently that energy conservation has been taken into consideration with the introduction of LEED-like guidelines. Walls are now insulated and double-glazed windows are installed. More recently, with the GK hospital presented earlier, double-skin walls with shading devices are introduced in India.

Water is a precious resource in Northern India and the aquifer is being depleted at an alarming rate according to environmentalist in part due to the paucity of rain during the monsoon. Hospitals are great consumers of water. To obviate this lack of resource, hospitals are required to have their own sewage treatment plant and use the output to water lawns and gardens. Furthermore, grey water from showers and sinks is treated and used to flush toilets.

Electrical power supply is also an issue. There is insufficient supply of power in general and interruptions are frequent. Hospitals therefore have to generate 100% emergency power.

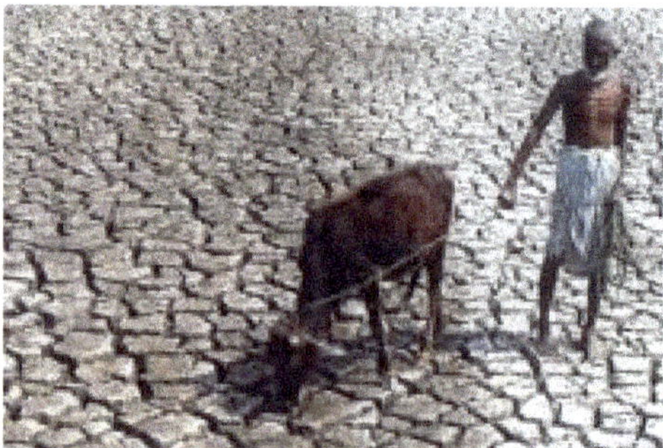

Figure 12. Environmental factor: water shortage.

Process

The unbelievable boom in hospital construction in the private sector caught in a way the industry unprepared. There is no formal planning process in place and very few rules and regulations so investors can more or less build what they want wherever they want. Market analyses are conducted and financial plans are developed in most cases but they are often perfunctory as there is practically no reliable epidemiology and demographic data. They consist in most cases of a survey of existing facilities in the area were a new facilities is planned to identify some service gaps. The attitude is often "let's build it and they will come" as there is such a shortage on the supply side.

In regard to planning and design, the brief received from the client is usually nothing more than a few pages outlining number and general distribution of beds, number of operating theaters, major equipment particularly for imaging and a brief list of clinics with a number of consultation chambers as exam/consultation rooms are called. The development of a comprehensive functional program with extensive users' input as we know it in Canada and other countries is not considered important and if it is done, the document receives scant attention. As investors are either physicians and surgeons or real estate developers, there is hardly ever any consultation with medical, technical and nursing staff members. It is quasi impossible to have an approved functional program before design starts: investors react to plans and other architectural drawings and may change their mind until the last minute even during construction. This lack of planning complicates the design

phase and imposes several iterations as programming is often done during design.
During layouts development, it is not unusual to come across what is referred to as the "chalta hai" attitude. Literally speaking, it means "it walks" but what it stands for is "it's ok, it's good enough, it will work", in other words, why go any further? why strive to do better? This attitude pervasive in many spheres of Indian society has been decried in media as leading to endemic mediocrity. Whereas the job of a medical planner through extensive consultations with users is to engage in the incessant pursuit of the perfectly functional layout striving to satisfy all requirements, the "chalta hai" attitude finds this pursuit counterproductive and a waste of time.

Medical practices

In India, stars are not only in Bollywood, they also exist in the medical field. Many hospitals are built around one or several physicians and surgeons, primarily surgeons, considered stars in their respective field, they are practically worshiped by their patients. Surgery is the meat and potatoes of private hospitals. A 200-bedd hospital will have 12 operating theaters. ICU beds are also an important programmatic element. As mentioned before, they represent 30% to 35% of an institution's bed complement whereas in Canada, for example, the proportionate would not exceed 15%. ICU beds are a good source of income but also this is where the more experienced nurses are concentrated. Hospitals have to train their own nurses as general nursing training in India is very basic and the profession is not highly regarded.

Not only is there a star system in the healthcare field, there is also what one could call "title inflation." There are no general hospitals or community or regional hospitals per se in India, they are multispecialty hospitals or super multispecialty hospitals and institutes of all kind. The main example is AIIMS, the national tertiary and quaternary care hospital in Delhi. AIIMS stands for All Indian Institute of Medical Sciences. Mimicking AIIMS, Medanta The Medicity was initially called the Indian Institute of Medical Sciences and Holistic Therapies, the hospital in Noida was called the Jaypee Institute of Medical Sciences. The name Medanta came when the hospital opened and later on as the term Medicity was used by other institutions, it was renamed Medanta the Medicity. Many hospitals are not organized around medical and surgical departments but around institutes with prominent names as chiefs. In this context, high buildings with imposing façades are preferred to more horizontal schemes. In any case, due to the scarcity and cost of land in most cities, high buildings are inevitable so the façades have to be treated with some panache to assert the institution's presence in the urban landscape. They are in a way a sort of billboard that complements other billboards around the city and full-page ads in newspapers promoting the unique expertise of each institution.
Chains of hospitals are important aspects of the industry. There are several chains in India and Apollo and Fortis are the major ones. In spite of the economic recession and the alarming dip in India's economic growth rate, they are still investing heavily in new facilities. This activity represents important opportunities for architects and engineers, local and foreign.

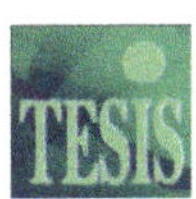

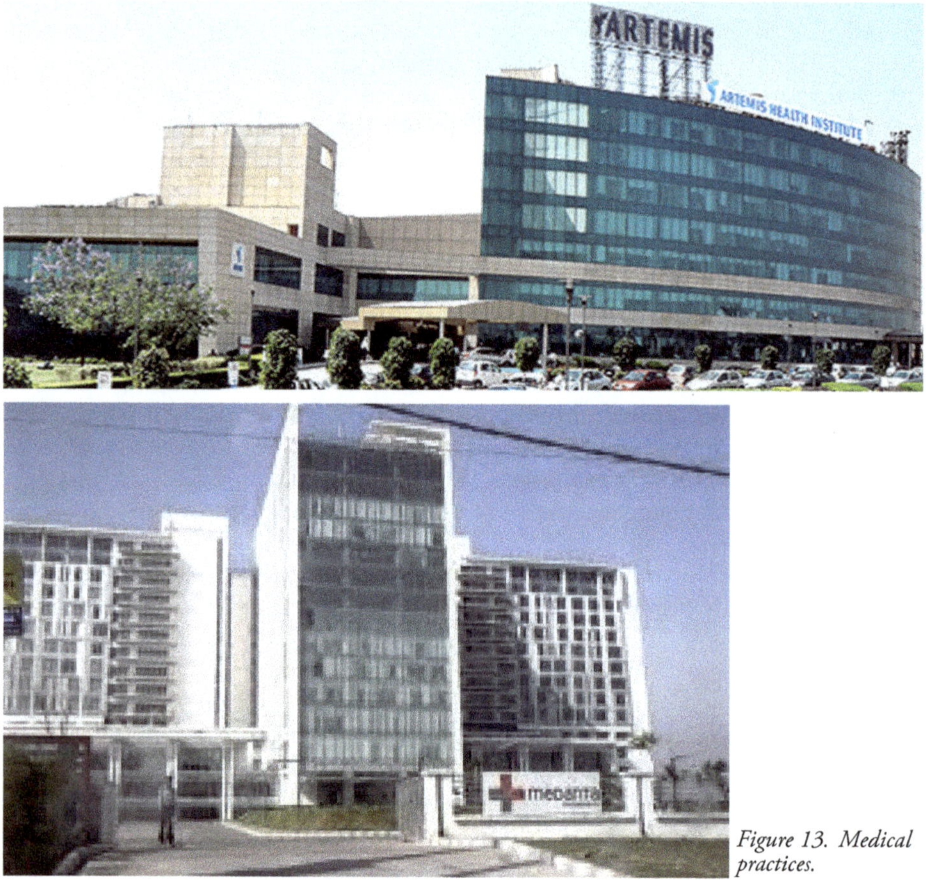

Figure 13. Medical practices.

Traditional medicines also play an important role in the Indian health care landscape. These different branches have been regrouped under a single umbrella that is called AYUSH, standing for Ayurveda, Yoga, Unani, Siddha and Homoepathy and they offer care essentially in facilities separate from allopathic institutions. Some public hospitals may offer one or another of these traditional medicines but they are few and far between.

Building Practices

Architecturally speaking, building materials and methods have not kept up with what we see in the West. Brick and sometimes aerated concrete blocks are still widely use, but drywall is making some headway. Polished floor slabs ready to receive finishes are not common: slabs have to be leveled first. Patient rooms in general do not have suspended ceiling as HVAC is provided by fan-coil units. En-

ergy conservation as mentioned earlier is starting to be considered in building envelope design.
Mechanical systems also follow traditional design methods. Provision of fan-coil units for ventilating and air conditioning patient rooms, no longer used in North America, is common practice. In general, HVAC systems are decentralized with AHUs dispersed within each floor area serving individual services. Each operating theater however has a dedicated AHU and receive 100% fresh air.

Plumbing is also of another age by North American standard. Plastic is seldom used for drainage and as it is assumed that plumbing will eventually leak, accessible shaft have to be provided behind every plumbing fixture and no piping can be concealed in walls. These shafts have to be continuous without elbows until pipes are transferred to other shafts at a service floor level. Service floors are therefore common between stacked Inpatient Units and Surgical Suite and other services to divert plumbing. This array of plumbing shafts complicates internal planning as one can well imagine. Power plants occupy a lot of space as they have to include water treatment, sewage treatment and 100% emergency power generators.

Fire protection codes are of another age in many aspects as they are more or less an accumulation of regulations that are not rationalized and are sometimes contradictory leading to conflicting interpretations. New laws are adopted as a knee-jerk reaction to some problem without any consideration for previous regulations. Building codes are also more of a compilation than a rationalized and well documented approach. They are contradictory as well with a whole series of exceptions and interpretations. Combined with municipal bylaws and regulations that vary widely from city to city, they form a complex and confusing intricate labyrinth in which even the most experienced practitioner can get lost. The cumbersome bureaucracy has a field day sorting out what is acceptable and not acceptable. Let's not forget that every law and regulation is an opportunity for corruption: as Tacitus, a second century AD Roman senator and historian said: "The more corrupt the state, the more numerous the laws."

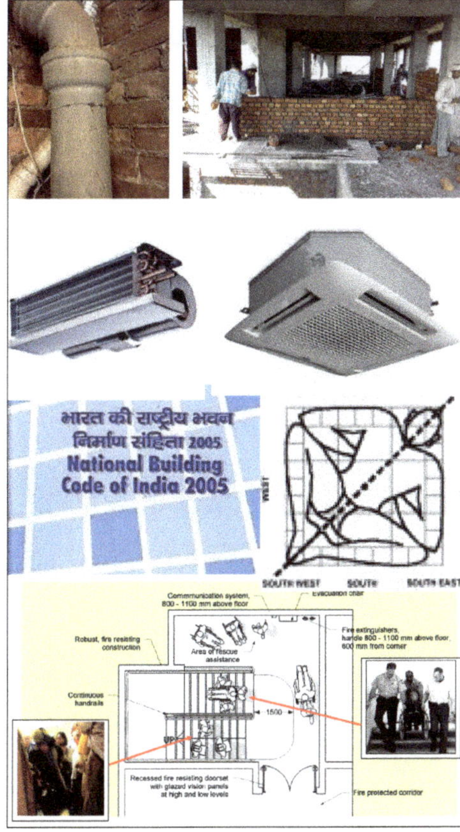

Figure 14. Building practices.

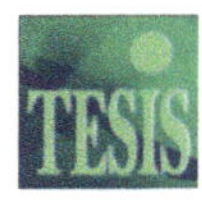

Accreditation

Accreditation of hospitals in India is a fairly recent phenomenon. The National Accreditation Board of Hospitals and Healthcare Providers (NABH) was created in 2006. It has its own set of standards primarily related to management and operations.

Accreditation from the US Joint Commission International (JCI), an offshoot of the Joint Commission on Accreditation of Healthcare Organizations (JCAHO) is sought by many private hospitals in India as it is perceived to be a prestigious seal of approval and opens the door to medical tourism. Medical tourism actually has had quite an impact on hospital design in India. Although JCI does not requires that design meets the FGI/AIA guidelines like JCAHO does in the US, to follow these guidelines is considered very important by investors in the private sector. Accredited hospitals are proud of their certification and advertise it widely.

Opportunities

Very little has been said so far about opportunities. The rapid growth of the private sector and the eventual revamping of the public one offer a lot of opportunities for local and foreign professionals. Several firms of architects and engineers have opened offices in India. In spite of some of the idiosyncrasies described above, foreign professionals in the health care field looking for new challenges can have the unique chance to participate in the design of outstanding facilities and contribute, however modestly, to the well-being of this country.

Architectures for Change

Mario Corea
info@mariocorea.com
Architect, España/Argentina

The interconnection between architecture and place: the 'place' is what defines the specific character of architecture. So we understand the place as the beginning of the whole process of design and a project is born out of the conditions offered by the place. The evolutionary hospital: the capacity to absorb physical, technological and medical changes – which is an ever-increasing demand today – means the possibility to transform the functional distribution or the technological equipment without the necessity to alter the structure, circulation or facades is a defining feature of the evolutionary hospital.
Projects to be presented:

- *Sant Joan de Reus University Hospital, Reus, Spain: this highly complex hospital integrates the functions of a general hospital with a subacute hospital as well as teaching activities.*
- *Mollet del Vallès General Hospital, Mollet del Vallès, Spain: although it is predominately a horizontal structure, because of the steep slope the building is resolved with volumes that step down over the site.*
- *Subacute Hospital of Mollet del Vallès, Spain: this is an example of how a hospital built in the 50s and 60s can be successfully recycled to meet current and future challenges that appear in the healthcare sector.*
- *Las Parejas Hospital, Las Parejas, Argentina: this hospital forms part of the new healthcare network in Santa Fe and was developed as a horizontal structure on one level.*
- *CEMAFE: Center for Specialized Outpatient Care, Santa Fe, Argentina: this facility will diagnosis and treat highly complex outpatient cases.*

Mario Corea *was born in 1939, in Rosario City, Santa Fe Province, Argentina. In 1962, he graduated from the School of Architec-ture, National University of El Litoral, Rosario City. In 1964, he earned a Master's Degree in Architecture and Urban Design by the Graduate School of Design Harvard University. Between 1962 and 1965, in Cambridge, Mario cooperated with architecture firm Sert, Jackson and Associates. The immediately following two years, he worked for architecture firms Desmond & Lord, and Paul Rudolph. In 1968, he began his academic career as a professor at the School of Architecture, Planning and Design Institute, National University of Rosario. In 1970, he earned a Diploma in Urban Studies from the London Architectural Association. Between 1976 and 2007, he was a professor at the Escola Técnica Superior d'Aquitectura del VallËs, Universitat PolitËcnica de Catalunya, Spain. In 2010, he was given Prize A+ for Lifetime Achievement, and he was appointed as Honorary Fellow by the American Institute od Architects. In 2011, the Mollet General Hospital was nominated for the Euroepan Prize for Contemporary Architecture Mies van der Rohe Award. Mario also earned the Architecture Prize for International Achievement, granted by the 13th Architecture Biennial Exhibition held in Buenos Aires.*

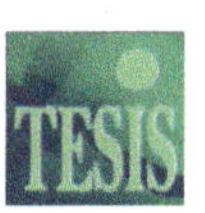

Before starting to develop the theme about hospitals of the 21st century, we want to bring up an issue of fundamental importance in our work as architects.

PERMANENT CONCEPTS OF ARCHITECTURE

The hospital before its specificity as a building for healthcare, is architecture. Therefore, the architectural considerations precede the specific design requirements of the hospital space. When we speak of architecture we are referring to a number of essential concepts that are universal and permanent regardless of the program.

The Interconnection between Architecture and Place

Louis Khan said that architecture does not exist, what exists is architectures and in this sense, architecture is recognized as a specific and unique process. The 'place' is what defines the specific character of architecture.

So we understand the place as the beginning of the whole process of architectural creation. A project is born out of the conditions offered by the place where it is to be developed. We understand the place as a complex and multidimensional reality where the geographical and topographical dimensions coexist with the economic, socio-cultural and historical dimensions. And we can see that the hospitals built in Barcelona, Spain; Santa Fe, Argentina; or Quevedo, Ecuador; have many common concepts in terms of the functional program development. But the issues arising from the location, climate and topography, as well as the building systems and cultural conditions contribute to the uniqueness and the specificity of the projects.

The Interconnection between Shape and Function

The second concept that we contemplate is the relationship between form and function. We have always reversed the famous principle of the Modern Movement: "Form follows function". This is because we think that form evolves into architecture. The function is always changing while the architecture remains permanent. Therefore, function must find its place in the form, which in reality could allow a variety of functions inside it.

The Interconnection between Architecture and Construction

The third concept that we consider important is that the constructive system needs to be defined from the beginning. To define a specific attitude towards the construction systems and materials used in each project is not a practical question of 'how to do it'. Rather it is an element of the conceptual evolution of architecture. And it implies a theoretical reflection about what kind of technology will be used, at what time, and in what place, in accordance with the ongoing development of each project.

THE EVOLUTIONARY HORIZONTAL HOSPITAL

The evolutionary hospital has a great capacity to absorb physical, technological and medical changes, which is an ever-increasing demand in contemporary healthcare.

The possibility to change the functional distribution or the technological equipment without the necessity to alter the support structure, the general circula-

tion or the facades is a defining feature of the evolutionary hospital.
The fundamental concepts of this type of hospital are based on a modular approach and on the use of a structural framework adapted to the different dimensions of the parts of the hospital.
In one of our latest hospitals in Reus, Spain the basic module is 7.60 m x 15.00 m with cantilevers of 1 m on each side.

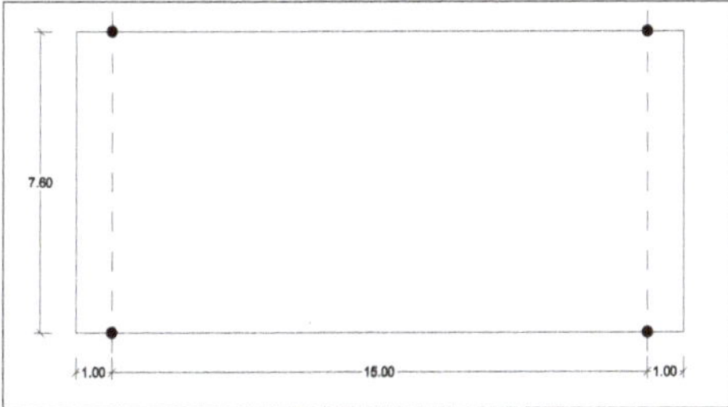

Figure 1. Module.

The module in Figure 1 allows the configuration of 7.60 m x 7.00 m for surgical areas, or for two consulting rooms, or two inpatient rooms on both sides of a corridor, etc.
This permits that the building works as a modular container capable of accepting all the functional demands of the contemporary hospital.
Another important element is the height between floors that varies between 4.00 m and 4.30 m with false ceilings usually of 1 m. A technical floor for installations is located between floors.

We must also consider the nature of the facades so that the distributional changes do not provoke conflicts with them. In this sense, in spite of the functional distribution, curtain walls and linear windows ensure good natural lighting.

Sant Joan de Reus University Hospital, Reus, Spain

This highly complex hospital integrates the functions of a general hospital with a subacute hospital as well as teaching activities.

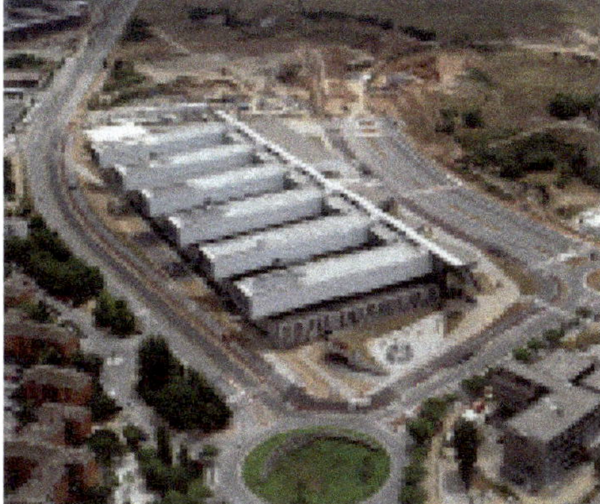

Figure 2. Sant Joan de Reus University Hospital, Reus.

Despite its large size of 107,000 m^2, the subdivision in pavilions where the main inpatient units are distributed on two floors, allows for its organization as a horizontal hospital. The spatial complex of four building units for the main hospital and two units for the subacute department is conceived as a horizontal system that is interconnected via mechanical escalators.

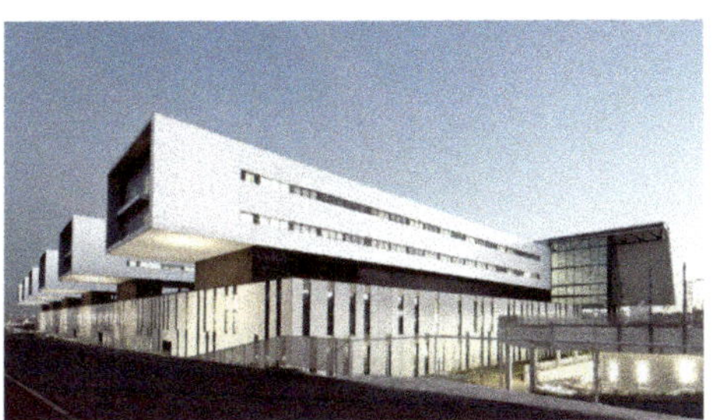

Figure 3. Street view.

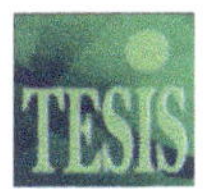

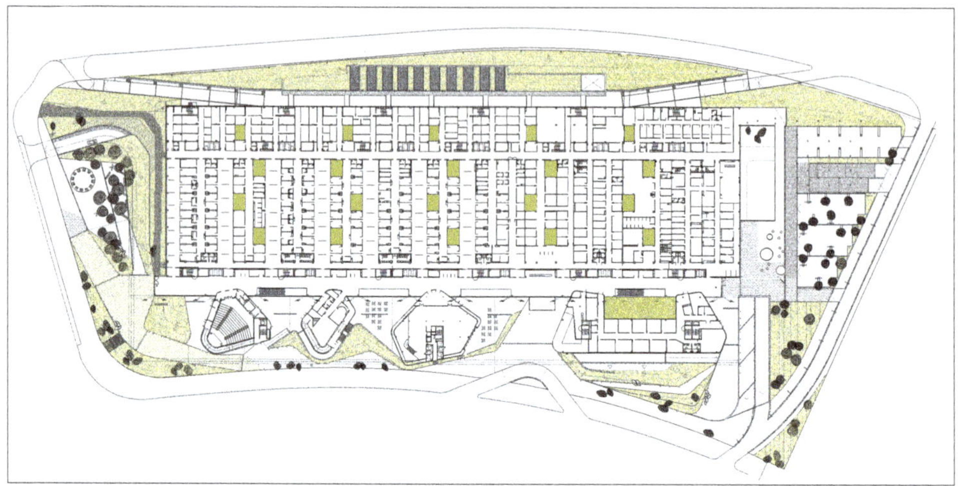

Figure 4. Ground floor plan, Sant Joan de Reus University Hospital. Reus.

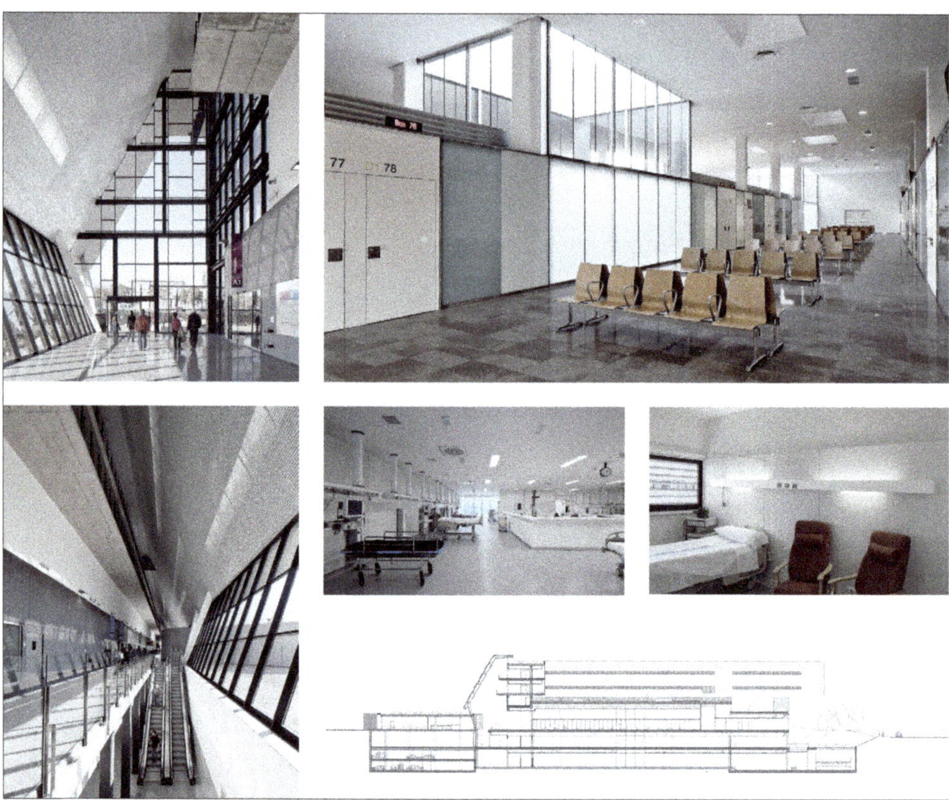

Figure 5. Interiors and section, Sant Joan de Reus University Hospital. Reus.

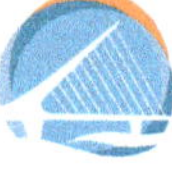

Mollet del Vallès General Hospital. Mollet del Vallès

The steep slope of the site places this project on the edge of the horizontal type as there are parts with four levels. At the same time the project design is a model for sustainability and energy efficiency. The use of geothermal power for cooling and heating was highlighted through the creation of 140 wells. Furthermore, rather than radiant floors, radiant ceilings were implemented in order to increase the insulation layer of roofs and facades. Finally, the main entrance is via a public square where an existing ancient oak tree has been preserved. The square becomes a key element in the project design that continues into the interior of the building, integrating a wide 'boulevard' of circulation, which connects the exterior with the intimacy of the interior space of the hospital.

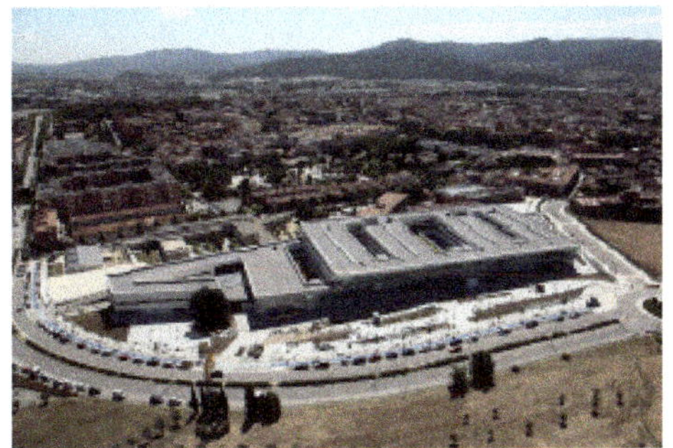

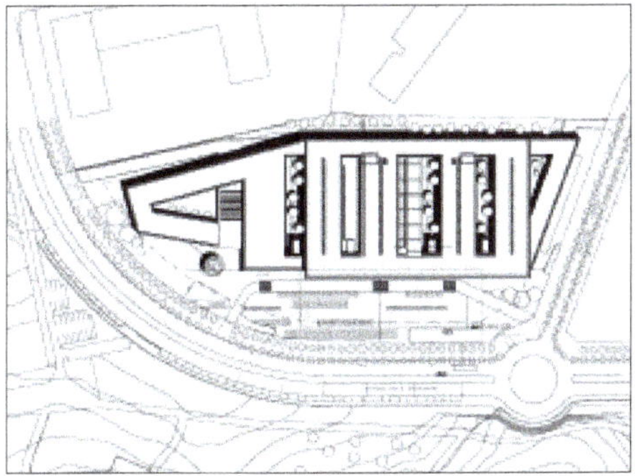

Figure 6. Photography and site plan Mollet del Vallès General Hospital.

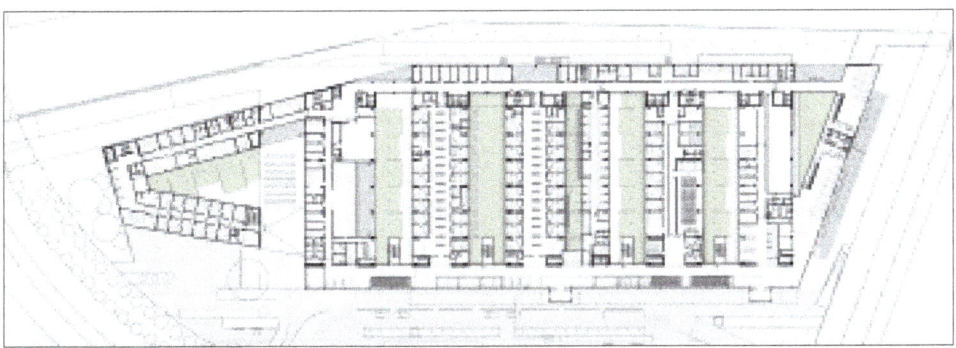

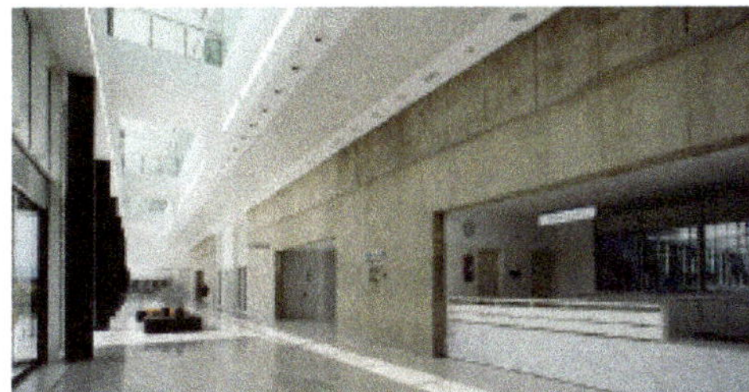

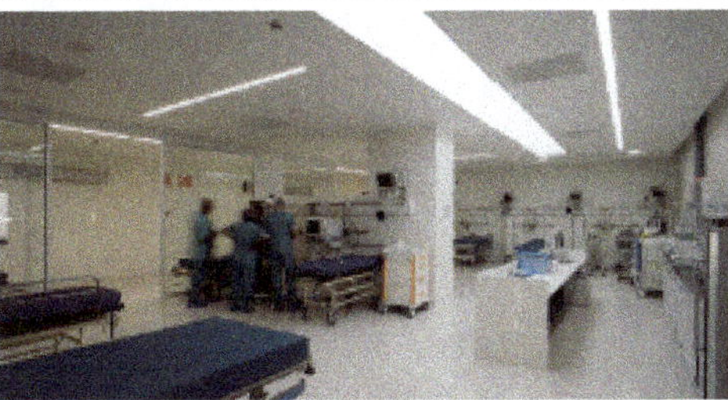

Figure 7. Ground floor plan and interiors views, Mollet del Vallès General Hospital.

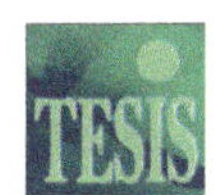

Subacute Hospital of Mollet del Vallès, Spain

The construction of the new general hospital on the edge of the city of Mollet resulted in the closing of the old hospital building in the city center. The decision was made to refurbish this existing hospital to accommodate a center for patients requiring rehabilitation or skilled medical care for a limited period. The Subacute Hospital of Mollet del Vallès is an example of how a hospital built in the 50s and 60s can be successfully recycled to meet current and future challenges that appear in the healthcare sector. The renovation project was based on simple and effective interventions that were practical as well functional, which resulted in a low-cost hospital with high energy efficiency, that undertakes an active role in the daily life of the neighborhood and the surroundings (Figure 8).

For the most part, the layout of the original hospital was conserved. The key design decision was focused on the open central area that had been previously used as a car park and service entrance. This space was enlarged and landscaped, transforming it into a garden patio for patients, visitors and staff. The transparent ground floor opens up to both this light-filled interior patio as well as the newly created public plaza across the street, which became part of the project during the design development.

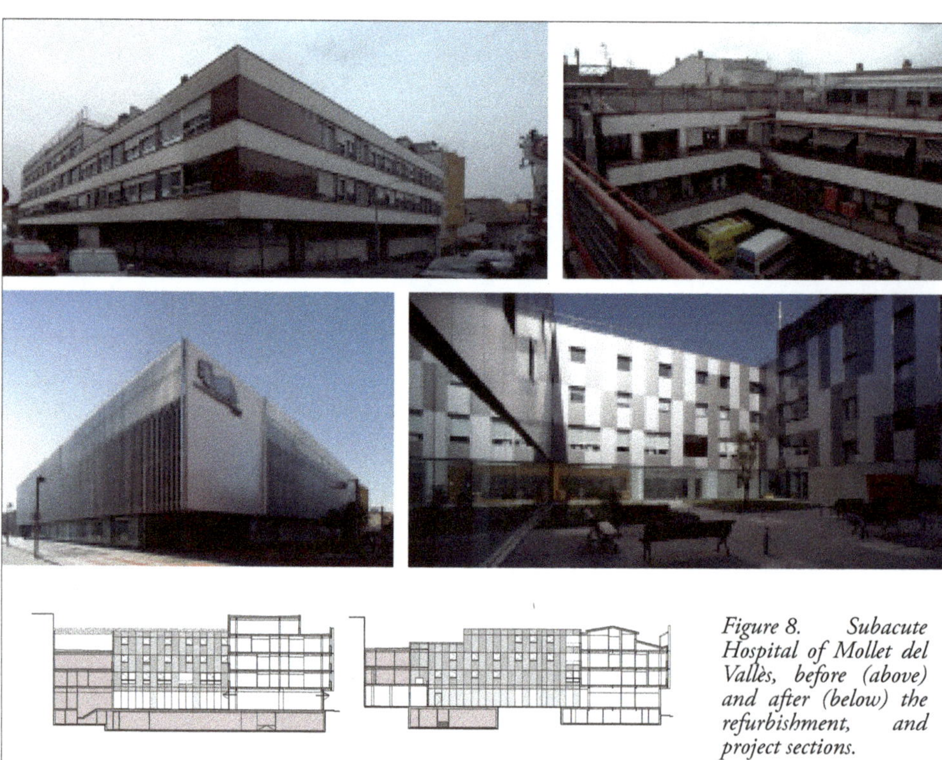

Figure 8. Subacute Hospital of Mollet del Vallès, before (above) and after (below) the refurbishment, and project sections.

Hospitals of Santa Fe

My experience in Catalunya is being developed simultaneously with my activity as Projects Director of the Office of Special Projects for the Ministry of Public Works in the province Santa Fe, Argentina (Figure 9).
Together with Silvana Codina, Francisco Quijano and a team of architects supervised by Jorgelina Paniagua and Evangelina Dania, we faced the task of building the new provincial healthcare services that integrates and refurbishes existing buildings. This network has been complemented by the construction of eight new hospitals and 80 healthcare centers of different complexity.

Las Parejas Hospital

Las Parejas Hospital forms part of the new healthcare network in Santa Fe. It is located in an urban area in Las Parejas, which is linked by a major highway to the city of Rosario, the nearest city where highly complex medical treatments are available (Figure 10).

The hospital was developed as a horizontal structure on one level, establishing a hierarchy of different zones according to function. Therefore, the technical, medical and public sectors are connected by circulation systems that form a sequence of accesses to the different areas of the building (Figures 10-12).

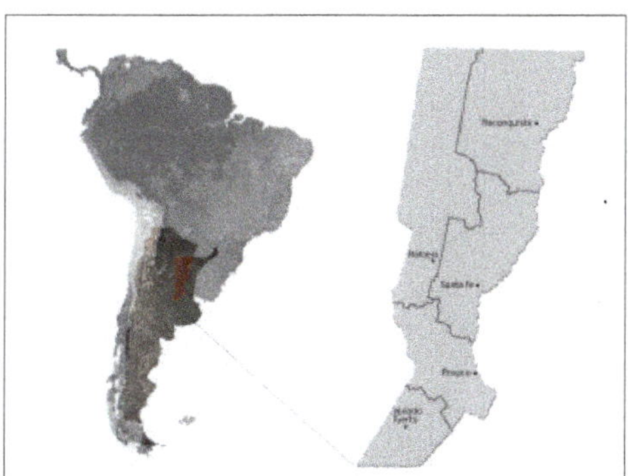

Figure 9. Argentina and Province of Santa Fe.

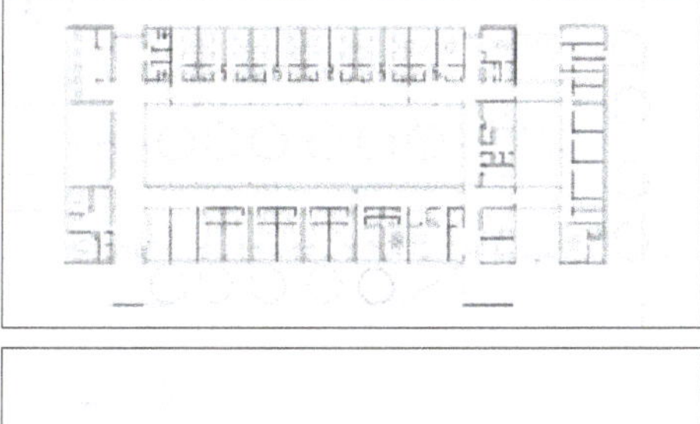

Figure 11. Ground floor plan and section, Las Parejas Hospital.

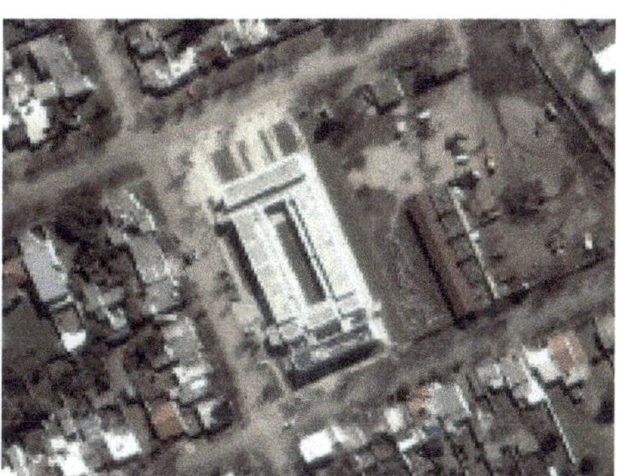

Figure 10. Las Parejas Hospital.

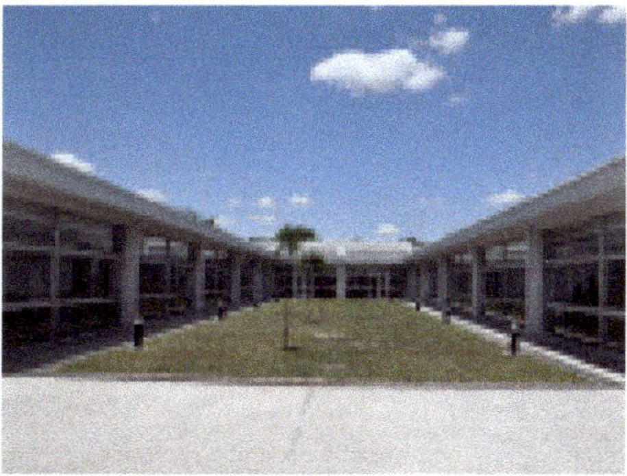

Figure 12. Hospital Las Parejas.

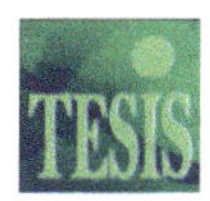

Natural light and ventilation in all functional areas as well as the spatial quality of the interior play a major role in the design, with the light being the main element of the construction of space.

The hospital is designed to provide diagnosis and treatment of diseases of low and medium complexity that require hospitalization and it has the capacity for rapid transfer of patients with complex health problems. The major medical departments are: clinical, pediatric, gynecology, surgery, dentistry, childbirth of low complexity, and the facility features 17 inpatient beds, as well as services such as x-rays, ultrasound and a laboratory (Figure 13).

CEMAFE: Center for Specialized Outpatient Care, Santa Fe, Argentina

The construction of the Center for Specialized Outpatient Care of Santa Fe aims to meet the demand for diagnosis and treatment of highly complex cases in an ambulatory way on the level of both the city and the region.

It will feature specialties from different disciplines (medical, biochemical, dental, surgical and outpatient oncology practices; central laboratory, etc.) and includes a dialysis service for chronic patients, which currently does not exist in the area of the city of Santa Fe. From the series of healthcare buildings that have been designed the CEMAFE stands out for the idea of a primary skeleton elevated above the functional levels, which allows the implementation of a construction of slabs that are literally hanging from an overhead structure.

Public, medical and technical areas are connected by circulations forming a sequence that imposes restrictions on the possibilities of access to different areas. In this way a higher clarity of users' trajectories is assured, interferences are avoided and hygienic control of the complex is provided.

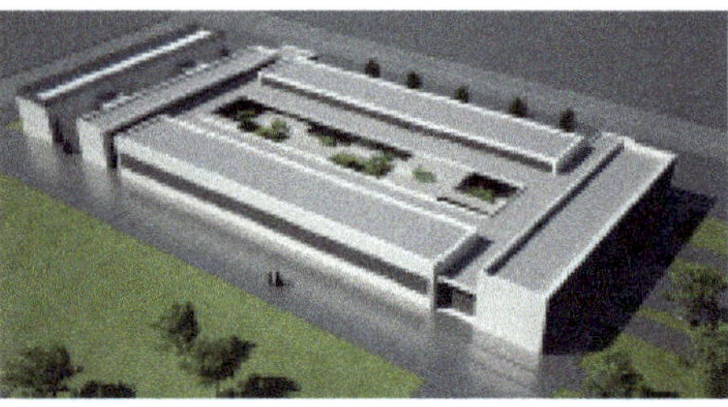

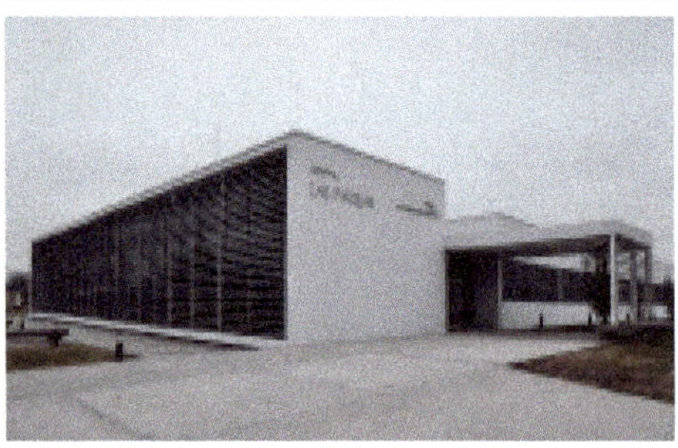

Figure 13. Hospital Las Parejas.

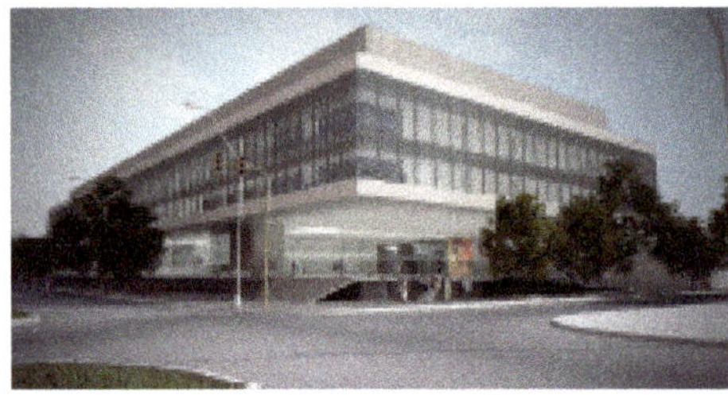

Figure 14. Center for specialized outpatient care, Santa Fe.

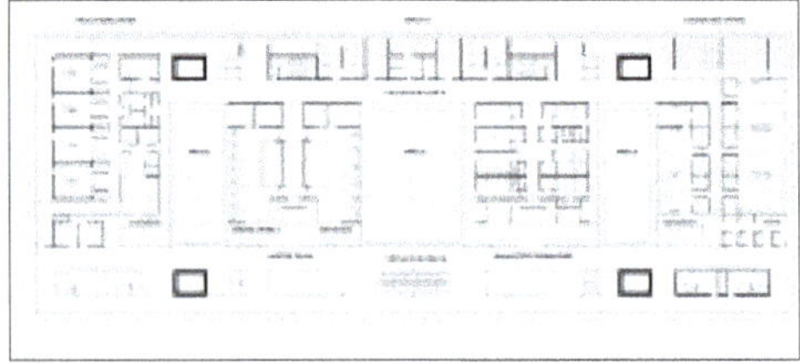

Figure 15. First floor plan.

Theory and Program of the "Intercultural Hospital" in Cuetzalan del Progreso, Puebla, Mexico

Eduardo Frutis-Gómez

edfrutis@hotmail.com
Architect, Universidad Nacional Autónoma de México

Various rights converge in the hospital: work, health, equity, fair treatment, information, and culture, among others. To guarantee the rights of its citizens, the state developed regulatory systems, which often have problems that are called loopholes and antinomy. These are resolved through temporary criteria, specification and hierarchy, or weighing the basic principles of the system itself. Some rights with high levels of subjectivity do not have specific standards that make them effective, becoming an important loophole in the system, an example being the rights related to culture and diversity. Given this, the architect has theoretical tools to resolve this type of problem, and, in turn, the state tends to create programs to compensate for such loopholes. The case of Cuetzalan General Hospital is an example of an architectural project that seeks to respond to a prototypical and standardizing model. In contrast, this model also comes from the Intercultural Hospital Program which seeks to promote and strengthen cultural diversity. The project acceptably complies with the standard model, but the same cannot be said regarding compliance with the program, a situation that could have been remedied through theoretical and architectural considerations.

Eduardo Frutis-Gómez. *Undergraduate degree in architecture with honors, Universidad Nacional Autónoma de México (2001). Masters degree in acrhitecture with honors, enphasis in law, Universidad Nacional Autónoma de México (2014).Presentations: Congress of the Mexican Society of Architects Specializing in Health (Méx. 2013), Latin American Congress of Hospital Architects and Engineers (Arg. 2013), Congress of Graduate Students UNAM (Méx. 2013). First level of diploma in Architecture for Health (SMAES-UNAM, Méx. 2013). Experience since 2006 in design, construction and supervision of hospitals of high and medium specialties, clinical laboratory units and remodeling of pharmaceutical laboratories.*

The Theoretical Tools of the Architect and the Regulatory Loopholes

According to the theory of habitability by Roberto Doberti, adequate appropriation of space can realize a means to exercise freedom and the application of justice, since architecture is the means to construct livability that allows for full development, personal, as well as family and social.

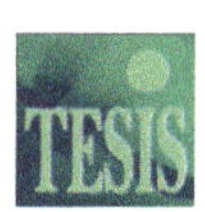

Within the theoretical and practical positionings one can find experiences with Universal Design Principles which are closely related to those established in the DUDH, as well as those proposed by José Antonio Juncà Ubierna, as shown in Tables 1-2.

Likewise, there are works of international organizations like the "WHO-QOL Measuring Quality of Life" of the WHO, where quality of life is defined as "the perception of an individual of their life situation, ranked in the context of their culture and value system, in relation to their objectives, expectations, standards and concerns." Within this document quality of life is comprised of six areas, which, in turn, are made up of various factors.

Cultural Diversity and the Regulations of Hospital Design

While the importance of cultural diversity has been shown in various documents from international organizations, when discussing their subjective aspects it has been difficult to establish the regulatory mechanisms which ensure compliance.

Key Factors of the Universal Project José Antonio Juncà U.	**Principles Related to the DUDH**	**Principles of Universal Design**
Accessibility	**Equality**	Equitable use Low physical effort
Comfort	**Dignity**	Simple and intuitive use
Density (overcrowding)	**Dignity**	
Division of space	**Dignity**	
Security	**Security**	Tolerance for error
Adaptability	**Equality, Dignity, Identity**	Flexibility in use
Communication	**Information, Equality**	
Signage		
Information		
Crossings	**Information, Independence**	Perceptible information
Equipment	**Security, Dignity, Equality**	Size and space for approach and use
Furnishings	**Security, Dignity, Equality**	
Temperature and air quality	**Dignity, Security, Health**	
Windows	**Dignity, Security, Health**	
Image	**Dignity, Identity, Culture**	
Finishes	**Dignity, Security, Independence**	
Control of the environment	**Dignity, Security, Health, Independence**	
Maintenance	**Dignity, Security, Health, Independence**	
Lighting		
Noise	**Dignity, Security, Health, Privacy**	

Table 1. Design principles proposed by José Antonio Juncà Ubierna.

Area	Factors
Physical health	Energy and fatigue Pain and discomfort Sleep and rest
Psychology	Image and personal appearance Negative feelings Positive feelings Self esteem Thinking, learning, memory and concentration
Level of independence	Mobility Activities of daily living Dependence on medication and medical assistance Job training
Social relations	Personal relations Social assistance Sexual activity
Environment	Economic resources Freedom, physical, medical and social security Accessibility and equality Family atmosphere Opportunities to acquire new information and skills Participation in and opportunities for leisure recreation Physical environment (pollution, noise, traffic, climate) Transportation
Spiritual, religious and personal well-being	Religion, spirituality and social wellbeing

Table 2. Design principles proposed by José Antonio Juncà Ubierna.

In Mexico, as in other multicultural countries, specific entities and programs have been created to guarantee that cultural rights are respected. For example, the national Ministry of Health has developed a Department of Traditional Medicine and Intercultural Development. Similarly, different states in the country have areas homologous to that direction, which, in addition to working in coordination with the Ministry of Health, have their own programs according to the needs of their population.

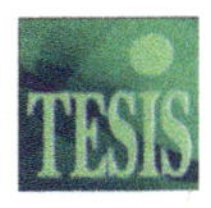

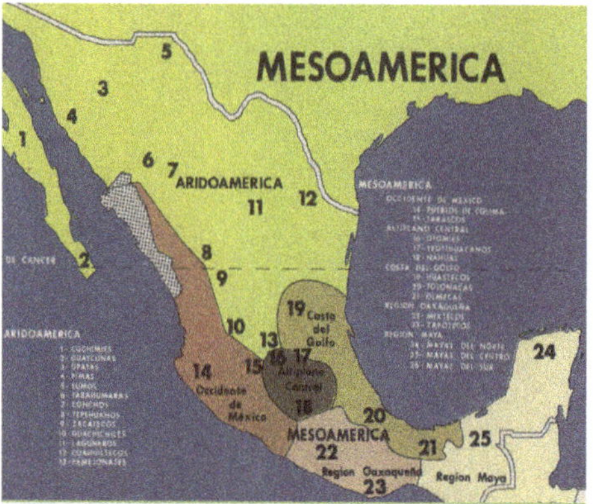

Figure 1. Cultural diversity in Mexico.

Mexico and the Intercultural Hospital

In Mexico there are communities that maintain languages, traditions and inherited territories from different cultural groups. For that reason the Ministry of Health in Mexico has developed different programs and projects which promote cultural diversity and equality, as well as the study of traditional medicine. Of those, "The Intercultural Hospital" stands out.

This program defines an Intercultural Hospital as "one in which elements are intentionally incorporated in architectural spaces and care procedures to strengthen the health conditions of the people and the environment, so that it is more efficient in the use of energy and resources, and to avoid and/or eliminate cultural barriers and to facilitate access to all users. In an integrative way, it also incorporates diverse elements for the care and strengthening of health from contributions offered by different medical models."

The proposal considers the following principles and criteria:

- participation of users and providers in the design and definition of spaces;
- healthy for the people (users and providers);
- healthy for the environment;
- economically and energetically sustainable;
- friendliness and cultural competence.

It integrates different cultural services including:

- translation module if the percentage of the indigenous population is significant;
- intercultural delivery care;
- intercultural enrichment of the hospital diet;
- services from other clinical and therapeutic models that are legally recognized in Mexico, as in the case of acupuncture, homeopathy and herbal medicine;
- services from traditional indigenous medicine;
- strengthening the health of the users, providers and local population through healthy diet, healthy exercise and good humor.

It includes a policy of recruitment and training of human resources, as well as an opening for the analysis, and, if necessary, an adaptation of the procedures and standards that have been applied.

This program is taken up by the Ministry of Health to develop the prototype called "Community Hospital," which is part of the Integrative Model of Health Holdings (MIDAS) of the Ministry of Health.

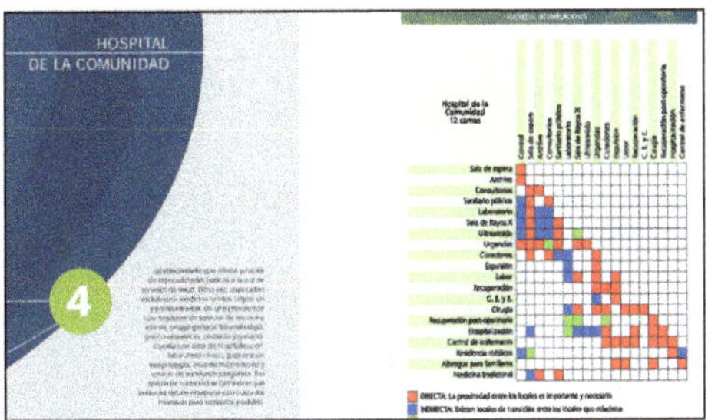

Figure 2. Integration of the intercultural hospital (MIDAS).

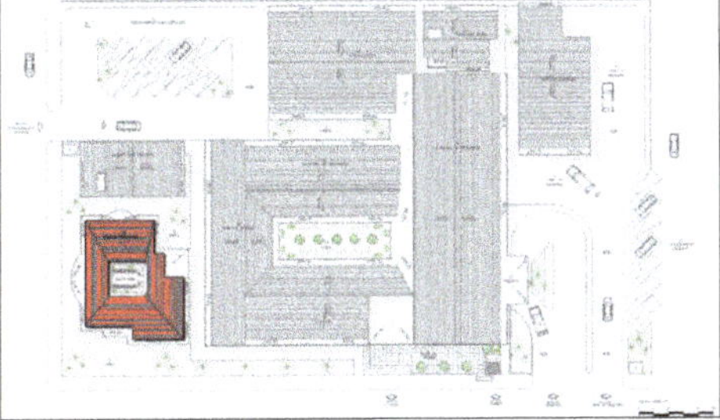

Figure 3. Rooftop facilities of the intercultural hospital prototype (MIDAS).

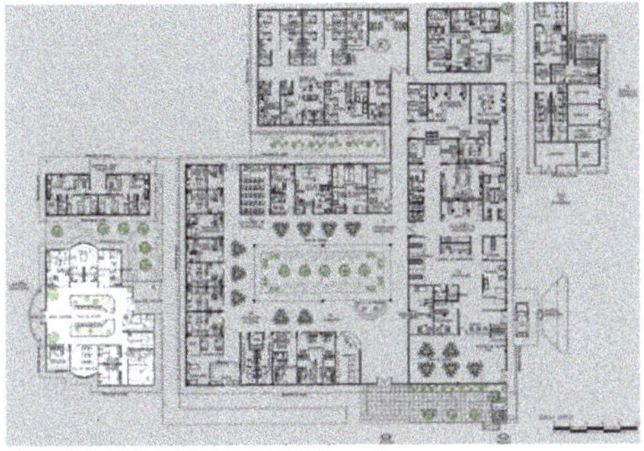

Figure 4. First floor of the intercultural hospital prototype (MIDAS).

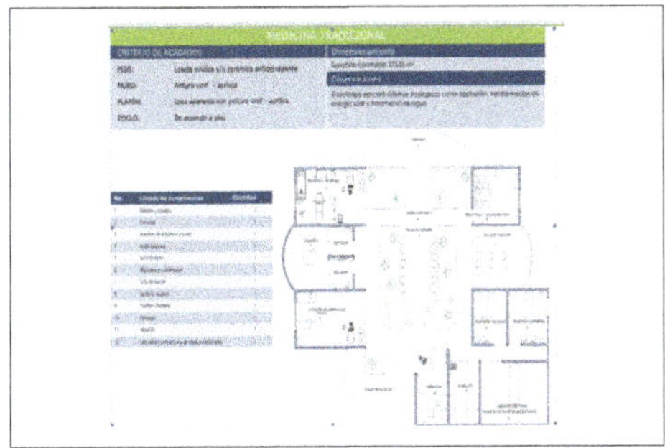

Figure 5. Traditional medicine unit prototype (MIDAS).

Case Study in Cuetzalan del Progreso, Puebla

Based on the MIDAS community hospital model and the intercultural hospital program, the project was developed to replace the General Hospital of Cuetzalan, in the Mexican state of Puebla.

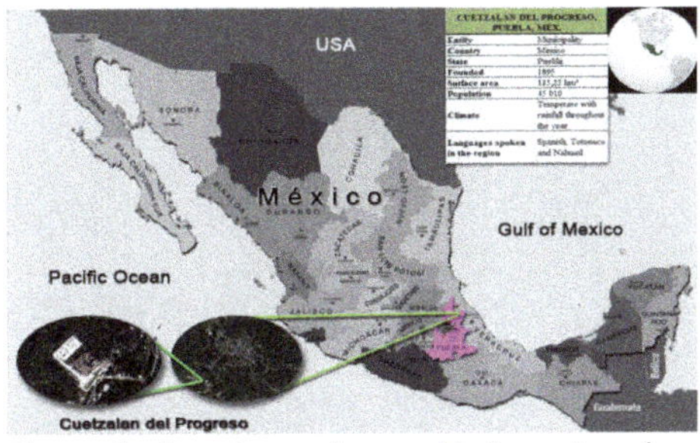

Figure 6. Location and general information about Cuetzalan del Progreso.

Cuetzalan del Progreso is listed as a "Magic Town." Through this classification in Mexico, the cultural value of diverse populations and their contribution to the national identity are recognized. Cuetzalan, with a principally Nahuatl influence, was awarded this designation for its architecture and traditions.

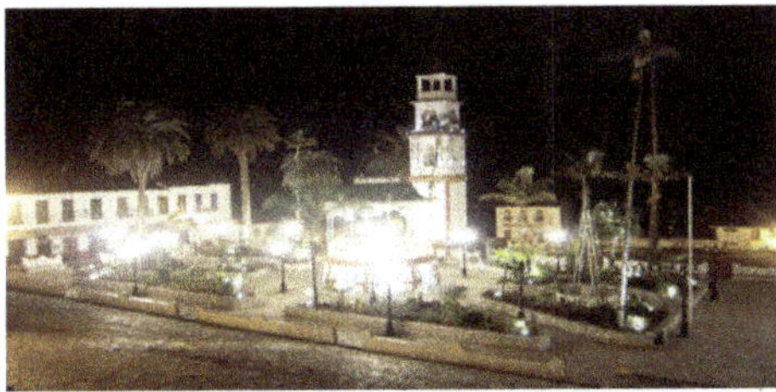

Figure 7. Central Plaza of Cuetzalan.

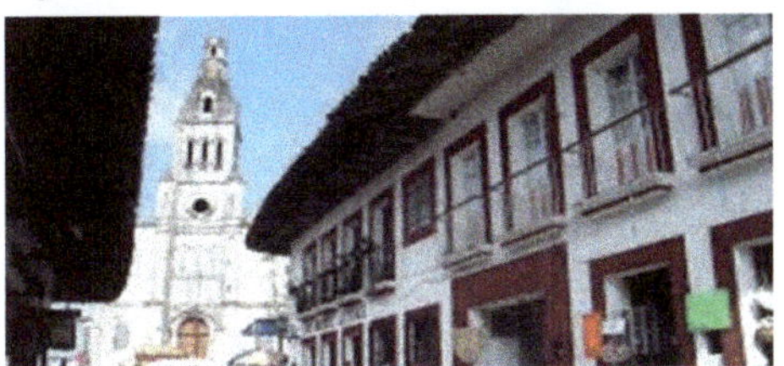

Figure 8. Center of Cuetzalan.

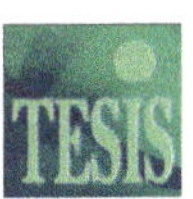

1958	The first rural hospital was inaugurated.
1978	The hospital was integrated into the National Indigenous Insitute, with traditional medicine services
1990	The unit was catalogued as a "Mixed Hospital"
2000	The hospital was taken over by the Ministry of Health of the State of Puebla.
2003	The hospital was called the "Integral Hospital with Traditional Medicine".
2008	Construction began on a new hospital on the outskirts of the town.

Table 3. Historical background of the unit.

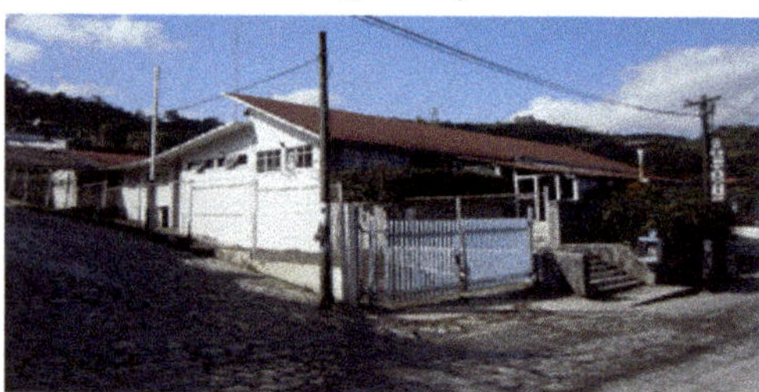
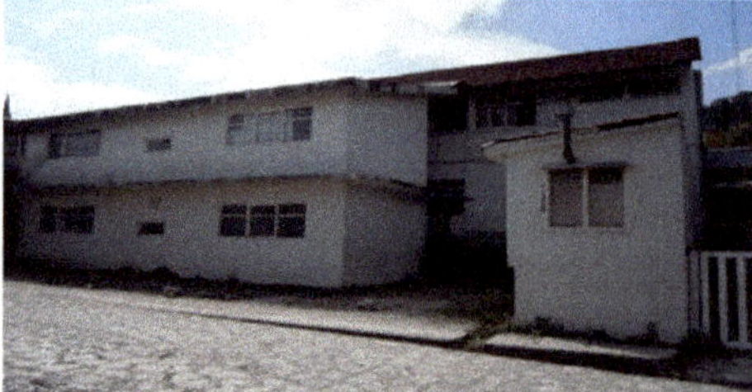

Figure 9. Former General Hospital of Cuetzalan del Progreso (1978-2011).

Originally, the new building, despite trying to follow the prototypical model of MIDAS, was conceived with an image that maintains a relationship with the architectural context of the place, and was inaugurated in January 2011. But, apparently for economic and administrative reasons, the building did not begin operation at that time, and was re-inaugurated in September of the same year. The official date, however, for beginning operation was June 16, 2011.

Population served	85, 732 Inhabitants	
Municipalities served	Cuetzalan, Zoquiapan, Nauzontla, Jonotla, Tuzamapan de Galeana, Ayotoxco.	
Date of construction	October 2008	
Start of Operations	June 16, 2011	
Services	Emergencies	
	General consultation	
	Dentistry	
	Pharmacy	
	Sample collection	
	Gynecology	
	Pediatrics	
	Trauma and orthopedics	
	Hospitalization	30 beds
	Outpatient consultation	12 locations
	Traditional medicine unit	

Table 4. Data from the General Hospital of Cuetzalan del Progreso.

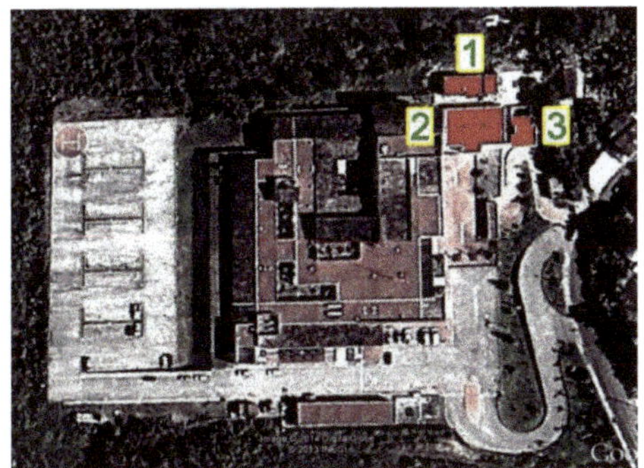

Figure 10. Aerial view of hospital: 1. temporary unit for traditional; 2. new medicine traditional medicine unit; 3. short term stay for women.

It is worth noting that between the first and second opening events, modifications were made to the facade, and sloping roofs with red clay tile, which are characteristic elements of the local architecture, were substituted for blue plastic flashing, thereby losing its primary and strongest link with the architectural context.

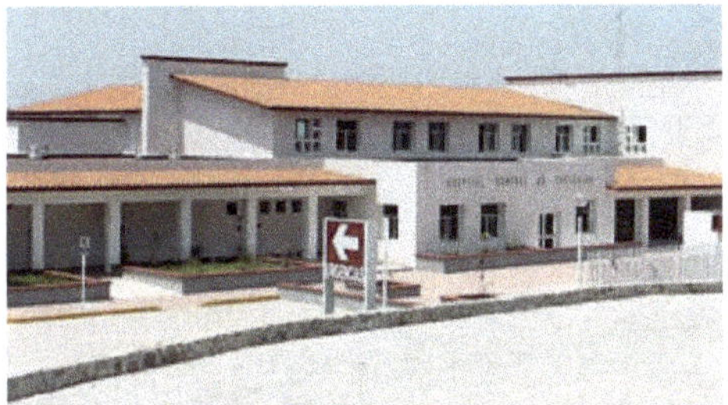
Figure 11. Inauguration January 2011.

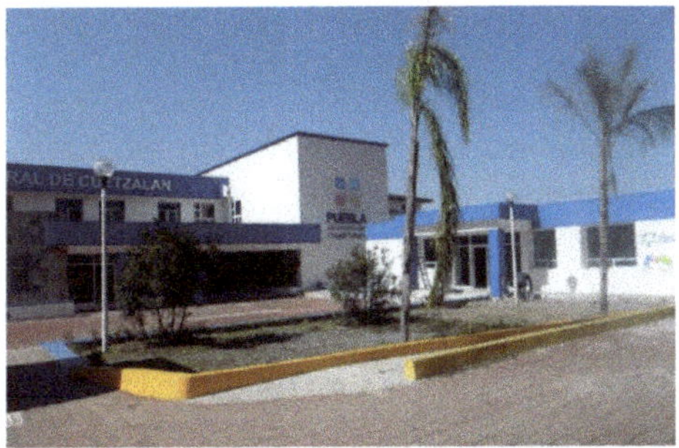
Figure 12. Implementation September 2011.

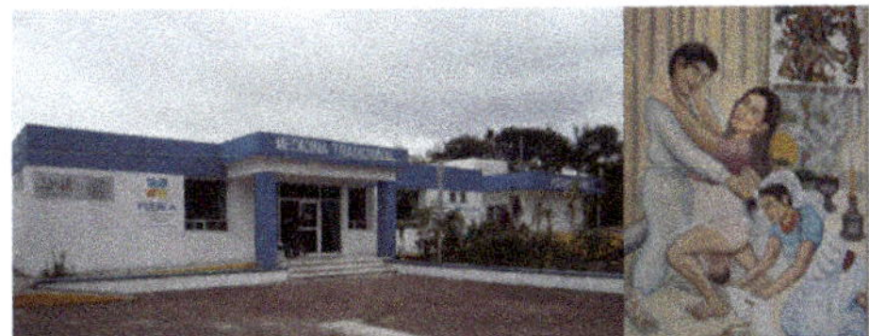
Figure 13. Traditional medicine unit and botanical garden and painting in the waiting room.

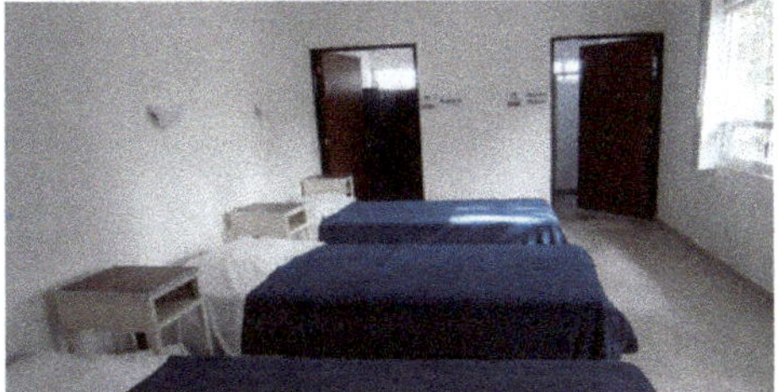
Figure 14. Dormitory for women in short term stay.

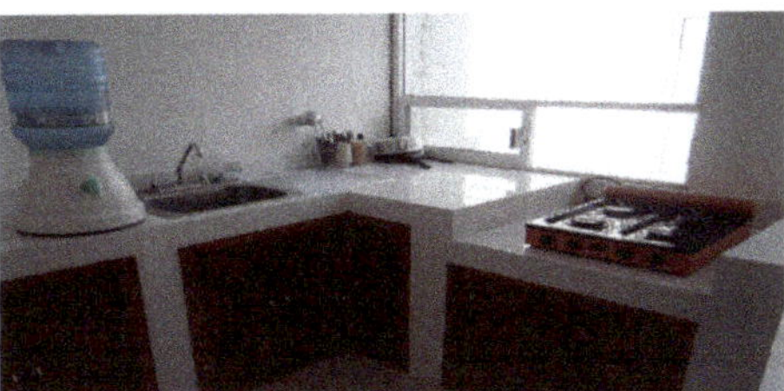
Figure 15. Kitchen for women in short term stay.

In addition, the traditional medicine unit has three clinics for midwives, bonesetters and healers, an area for vertical delivery, a waiting room and archives. Also, the clinics and the waiting room have altars that are used by the patients, as well as the traditional doctors to carry out healing rites. It also has an herbal pharmacy with a kitchenette and adequate equipment to prepare various potions and remedies.
Currently, work is being done to develop signage of the unit in the Nahuatl language.

During the first stage, the hospital had a small, temporary unit for traditional medicine, which included a temazcal that still operates. The rest of this small construction is currently used for storage.

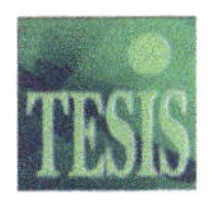

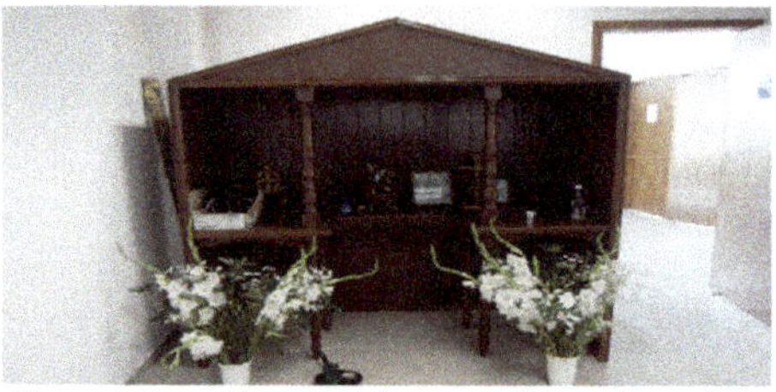

Figure 16. Altar inside a traditional medicine clinic.

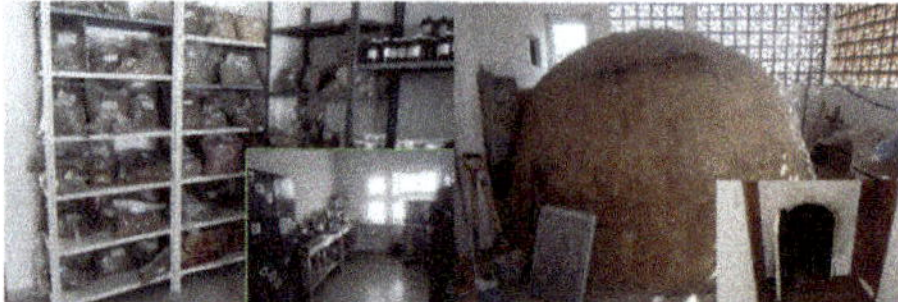

Figure 17. Traditional medicine pharmacy and kitchen and Temazcal.

This unit complies with various points and principles of the Intercultural Hospital and the MIDAS model, but there is a disconnect between the traditional medicine unit and the rest of the hospital.

In the former hospital the distance between the vertical delivery room and the operating room was a corridor of approximately 7 meters under cover, whereas in the new facility one has to pass through a parking lot, exterior corridors and the emergency room in order to arrive at the operating room. This rupture in the link between the traditional medicine unit and the hospital demonstrates a lack of architectural, cultural and social integration.

According to some of the traditional doctors, the unit complies with the basic characteristics necessary to do their work. However, they did not participate in the design process and there exist various points for improvement, such as the orientation and material of the altars, the lack of a stove in the clinic for preparing infusions or teas during consultation, as well as other details that weaken the importance of the role given to traditional medicine.

Conclusions

State programs, such as the Intercultural Hospital, are presented as a means to address the lack of adequate regulations and are of great value as a way to achieve just social development and to conserve an invaluable source of knowledge. Meanwhile, the specialized architect should be aware that the prototypical hospital models basically respond to budgetary and administrative needs with a general, standardizing approach to the type of population that is being served, and does not contemplate the specific needs of each group of users served by each unit.

It is necessary for the specialized architect to have a theoretical positioning for solving the regulatory problems posed by the most subjective elements of the work. These elements, such as the concepts of culture and tradition which are implicit in this type of architecture, lead one to transcend dogmatic fulfillment of regulations and programs in search of fulfilling the essential principles of livability and the law itself. In the case of Cuetzalan Hospital, if the project had responded more to the program of the Intercultural Hospital, or to some of the design principles such as those mentioned in the first part of this document, and if a greater deviation and flexibility had been allowed from the prototypical model, the response given to the traditional medicine unit would likely have been closer to the principles of equity, equality, cultural diversity and livability, essentially the reason for the existence of such units.

The Intercultural Hospital Program, theories of livability, diverse approaches to inclusive design, as well as other forces aimed at constructing more physically and emotionally livable spaces, will ensure full personal, family and social development which should be considered as fundamental to the search for a more just society.

Tropical Architecture for Cancer Treatment: A Radiotherapy and Chemoterapy Experience

Minor Martin Aguilar, Luis Alberto Monge Calvo

mamartin@ccss.sa.cr
Architects, Caja Costarricense del Seguro Social, Costa Rica

¨A great building must begin with the unmeasurable, must go through measurable means when it is being designed and in the end must be unmeasurable¨. Louis Kahn

The necessity of equality and accessibility in health for all patients in oncology services in all national hospitals and the capacity to offer Internal Social Security services instead of buying private treatment as a support plan to cover the excess of the demand, all this with a concept based in sustainability, bioclimatic solutions, humanized treatment is what brings us here. This was the trigger for the high authorities to commend this project to the recently created ¨Oncology Web Project¨ encharged of developing all the Cancer related infrastructure in Costa Rica´s Social Security, this building was design to host 2 linear accelerators, 1 Digital Tomography, 44 Chemotherapy adaptable chairs, 8 Consulting rooms and a Oncology pharmacy, with this the institution duplicates the number of radiotherapy treatments and better off the overall comfort of the patients attending Chemotherapy. Since the Hospital Mexico is the only one with two LINACS already, the strategy was to centralize the offer of radiotherapy because of the existence of the physical space and the human resource, never the less the Hospital Calderon Guardia and San Juan de Dios, which are the other two national hospitals, already have projects with this kind of technology in line just waiting to be develop. The overall cost of the project was of $18.000.000 being the Equipment Company (VARIAN) the responsible of the contract because of the cost of the equipment exceeds more than the 50% of the economic resources.

Minor Martin Aguilar. *Costa Rican Architect, graduated from VERITAS University. Currently finishing a Master's Degree in Tropical Architecture from the University of Costa Rica. Has worked for 6 years in the Social Security System of Costa Rica (CCSS), specifically in the Oncology Web Project as Chief Architect in the planning, designing and construction of the Health Infrastructure for Cancer Treatment. He is an Environmental Consultant for the National Technical Secretary of Environment (SETENA) and has been a practitioner in the Environmental Management Committee of the Special Projects Administration for the CCSS. Participated in the creation of the RESET national norm (Requirements for Sustainable Buildings in the Tropic) in the Institute of Tropical Architecture (IAT) and is a researcher on evaluation systems and design alternatives for Bio-climatic architecture in the Tropics.*

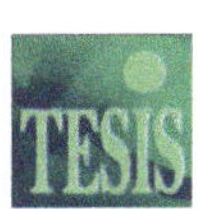

Design Process

An Investigation conducted in the outpatient services from Hospital Mexico before the Building design, help us collect a lot of useful information from the social, cultural and climate situations in the project area, this knowledge was pass on to the strategies used to propose an solve all the different variables of the design.

For the calculations made on the environmental and climate understanding of the project, some different procedures were used as asking for data from the Meteorological Institute of Costa Rica, as well as extracted from Meteonorm database and measurements on site with specialized equipment, so that we can have quite a good understanding and establish an accurate comfort zone needed for the patients, visitors and medical staff. At the same time we recognize some bad habits developed by the people that work in hospitals referring to energetic costumes, generally this are prompted because of a learned path and repetition, but architecture is a medium that can cure most of this paths with a good use of the resources that surround us, and inspiring people to have a different attitude towards its workspaces.

According to the different Comfort zones in all variables, Temperature, Ventilation, Natural lighting, humidity and sound, we establish a criteria that can be in an extended comfort zone and then the uncomfort barrier were most of the people will be displeased. And try to find its architectural causes so we don't replicate them in the new building, as

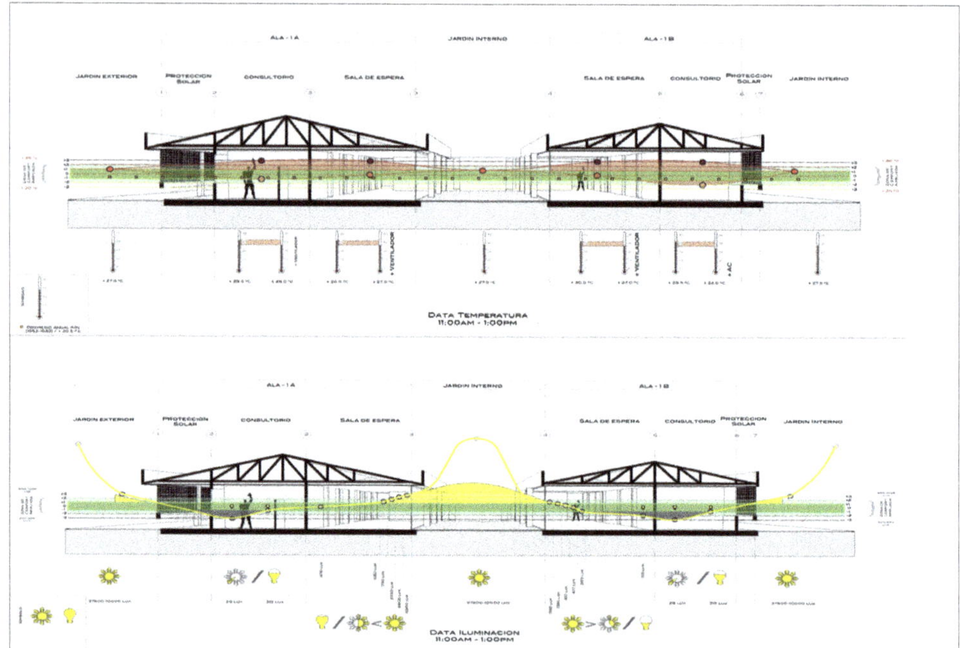

Figure 1. Temperature and illumination data.

its well-known, sometimes unplanned modifications to the original project ends up producing unwanted or unexpected effects to its overall functionality, from now on we call this phenomena: Building Pathologies.

It's a reality now days that sustainability must be a primal objective of all constructions, under this premise; hospitals have even an ethical obligation because they are bounded to promote health protecting the environment.

The form, orientation, the use of ventilation and natural lighting, the use of nontoxic reusable or recycled materials, the use of high efficiency equipment and lighting fixtures, recollection and reuse of water, amongst other solutions, must be imperative in health infrastructure.

Designing for Cancer Treatment

Nature

¨A contact with nature produces emotions that reduces the stress in the patient and distract or take him out of focus from its pathology, even reduces hospitalization time...¨ Ulrich 2006

Patient is the center of this design and it is represented in the beautiful tree we conserve from the existing site that is in the center of the geometrical composition to generate a positive distraction element to all visitors.

This tree is stationery, which means it loses all its leafs and flowers and has a dry dead look, then after that it flourishes again, in a majestic green and purple show, it has been called ¨The tree of life¨

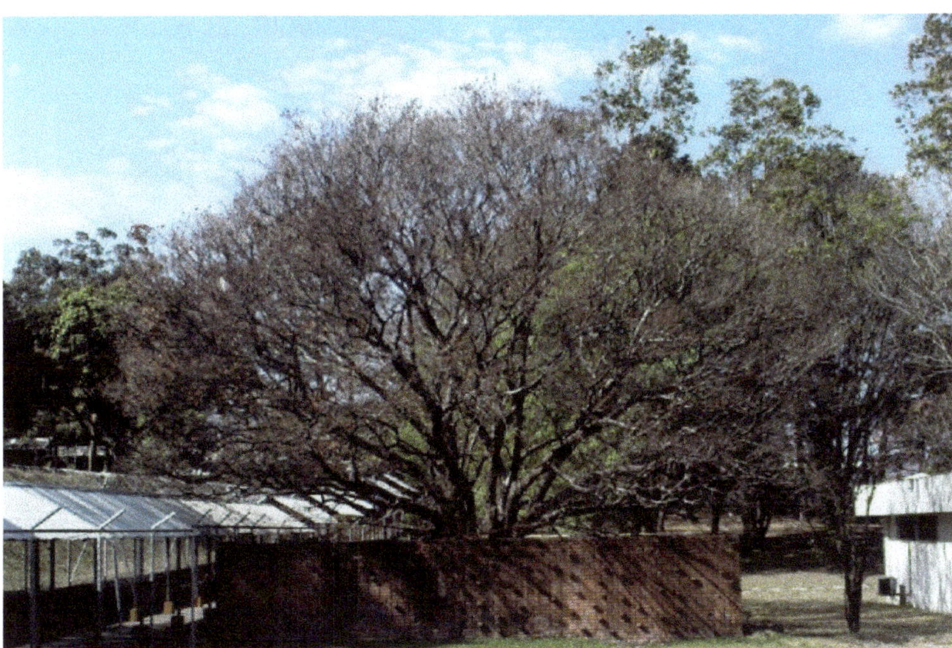

Figure 2. The existing "Tree of life".

because it is an analogy of the cycle of a cancer patient that endures its treatment cycle and goes on with his life, reborn.

This natural feature, not only have a visual effect on the project, but because of the prevailing wind passes through its shadow (measurements took in place shows there can be a difference between 3° to 5° Celsius from the outside to the base of the tree), and then enters the waiting room and public Radiotherapy facilities, it lowers spaces thermal charge and refreshes the interior of the building without the usage of air conditioning which our engineers calculate and estimate the cost of the extra equipment in near $ 500.000 and the savings in a year's electrical bill as $ 240.000.

Aside from the conservation of this tree, there were some other non-local species in the site that we had to cut down so that the project can be constructed, with the permits signed we proceed to have a forestall engineer to instruct us what kind of work we can do with each type of wood extracted from the trees, so that it will complement the architectural project and generate a reminder of what was part of the site before it exists. This type of savings reflect them self's in the pockets of every citizen since social security depends on the contribution of everyone, and represents money that can be used in other projects for the benefit of the country health system and the institution super habit.

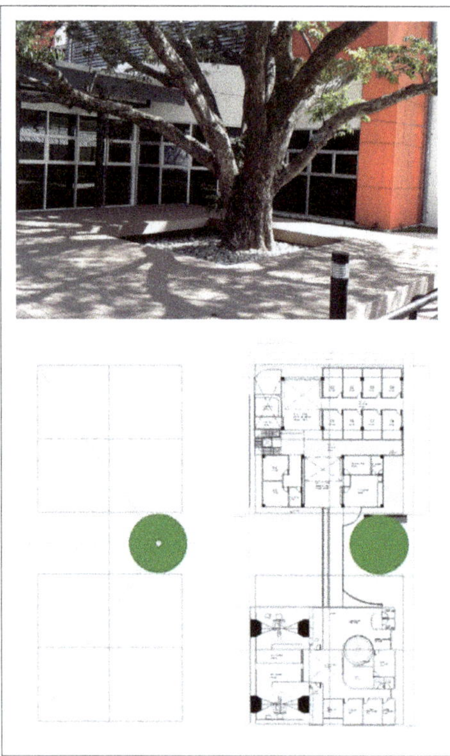

Figure 3. The existing tree is the center of the geometrical composition of the building complex.

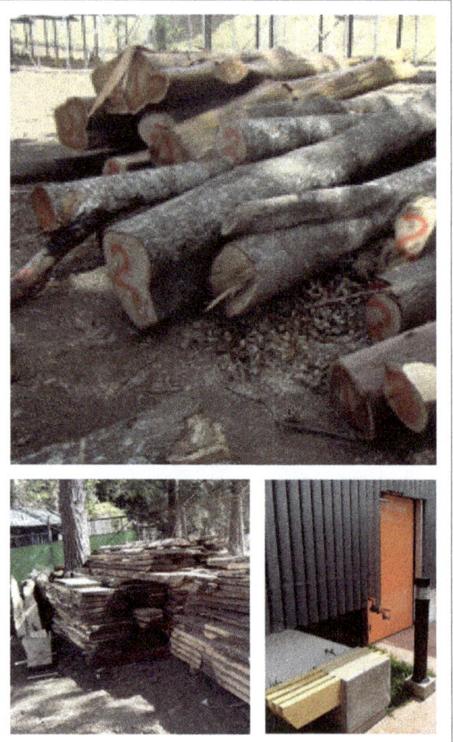

Figure 4. Type of wood extracted from the trees, so that it will complement the architectural project.

Colors

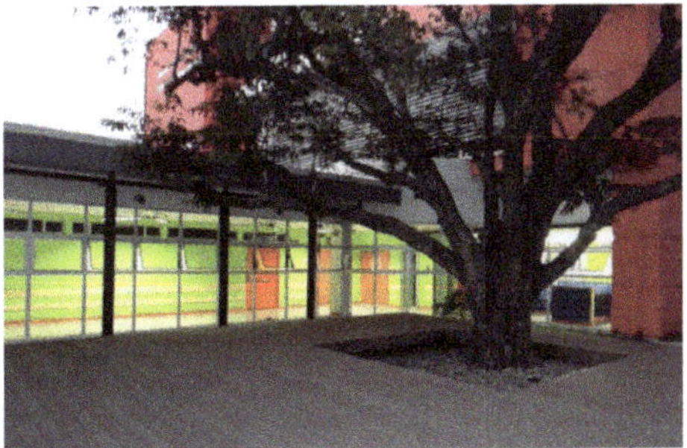

In order to affect all the senses of the human being through architecture and light, some sensitive color usage is necessary. The form of the building was complement by a study of Color therapy or cromotherapy which was conceptualize to activate the defense mechanisms of the organism, and create much happier and relax environments so they can interpose to a negative state of mind and offer a better life quality to the patient.

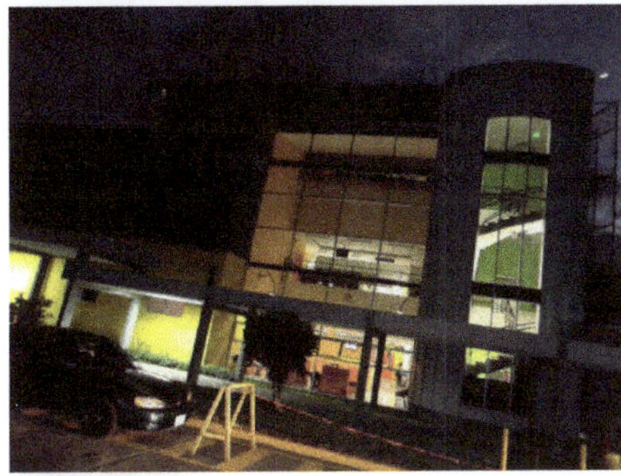

Yellow: Happiness, uplifts the spirit, comfort sensation, stimulates mental capacity and concentration

Red: Intensity, vitality, joy, will, passion, force, recommended to use in open spaces because it tires the eye, it simmers down with the contrast with the green of the tree.

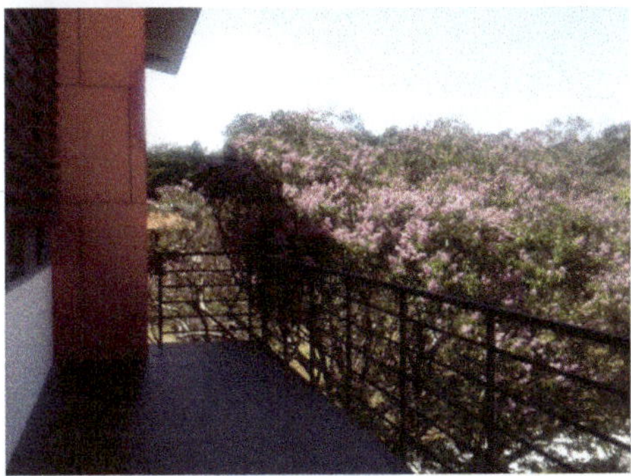

Orange: Regulates circulation and metabolism, stimulates the thyroidal gland, respiratory and hunger stimulant, promotes joy and happiness.

Green: Equilibrate energies, Increases sensibility and compassion, represents harmony, it has a relaxing effect on the nervous system.

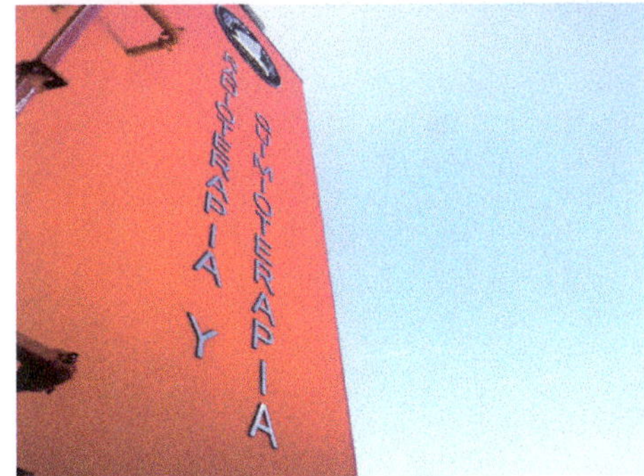

We use neutral colors for most of the interiors but try to experiment in strategic points with this color palette, quite different from the traditional colors used in health facilities, we hope to have changed the perception of the spaces and accomplish a certain degree of positive impact in the physiological state of mind of patients, visitors and medical staff.

Figure 5. Color palette adopted to changed the perception of the spaces.

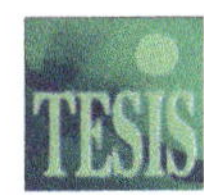

Comfort

Since sustainability is a conjunction of several components that has to do a lot with the consciousness of the owner or developer of the project, and our background is that of a governmental institution with budget limitations and standard specifications, our goal to have achievements as a sustainable architecture was based in the cheaper most basic way: Bioclimatic Strategies.

Ventilation

When it comes to achieve natural ventilation there are some golden rules we must respect and use to generate a positive thermal equilibrium:

1 - Search for the wind: one must know were the main winds (stronger and more frequent) come from so that you can capture or direction them into the building spaces. Air changes into Health facilities must be between 4.0 and 5.0 Changes / hour. In the project, prevailing winds come from northeast to southwest with an average velocity of 1.2 m/s must of the time depending of the height, there is some oblicuous flexibility of 40° from perpendicular wind that can maintain acceptable ventilation on the inside of the structure.

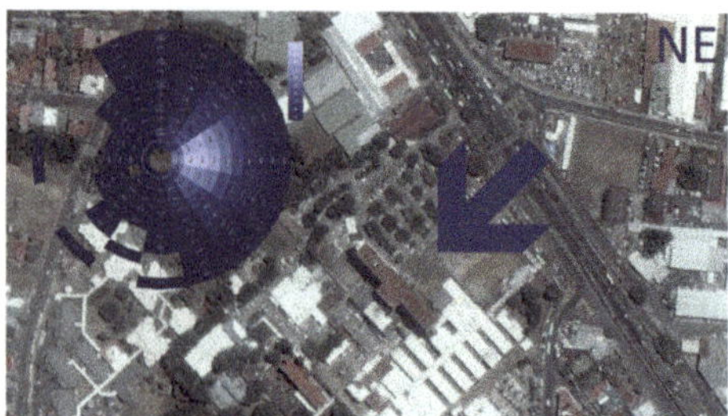

Figure 6. Search for the wind.

2 - Narrow volumes: the distance between 1 façade and the other must not be greater than 7 times the height of the spaces, this is so that the difference in pressures in each side is enough to generate the internal flow of air needed, so in volumes that are square like or to massive, it's almost impossible to have functioning natural ventilation.

This took us to the breaking up of the main volume and the creation of a Lobby of 30 m height in the middle, with the frontal volume being 1 story lower than the back one, we install metallic louvers so the prevailing winds can enter on the top of the building and renew the air volume on the inside.

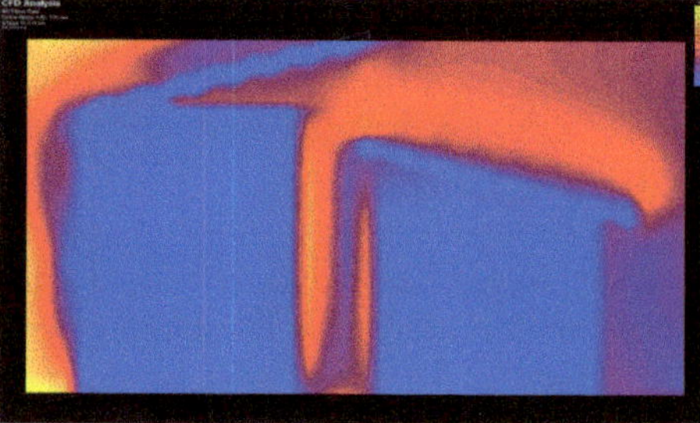

Figure 7. CFD Analysis, air flow race.

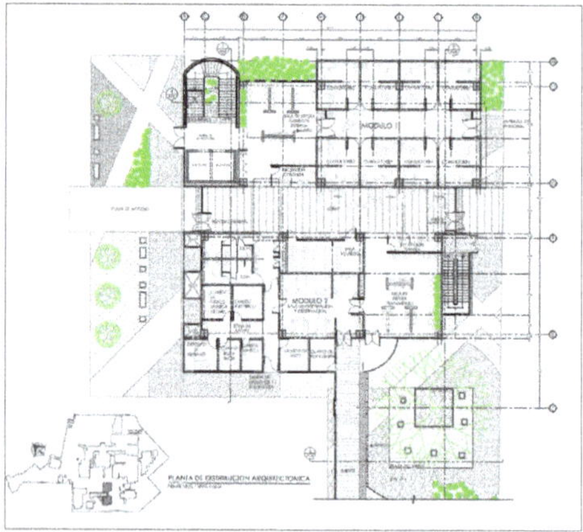

Figure 8. Two buildings and the lobby in between.

3 - Open up: in most Tropical countries the percentage of a glazing surface that allows the air to enter the building must be between 40% and 80% (Victor Olgyay) this is of critical importance so that the thermal gains and humidity leave the building, this strategy must have a control method, so that when the air outside is too hot or too cold that will produce uncomfort on the environment inside, one can isolate internal spaces.

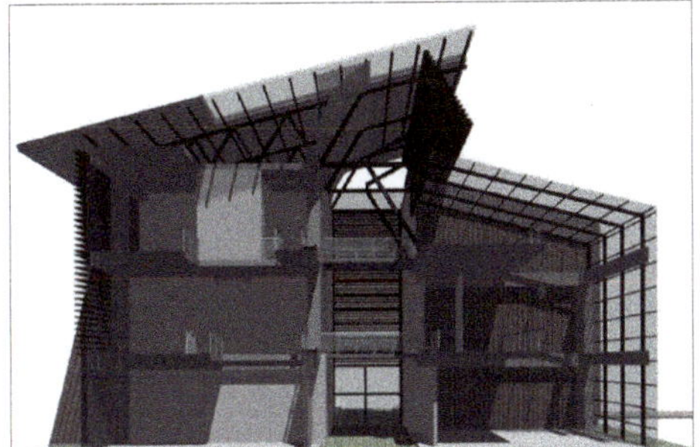

Figure 10. Building section.

4 - No obstacles: all of the strategies above will have no effect if the walls or divisions in the spaces reach top height, for this will represent an obstruction for the airflow, if there's no other option, then one must think in ventilating two different spaces, with different strategies.

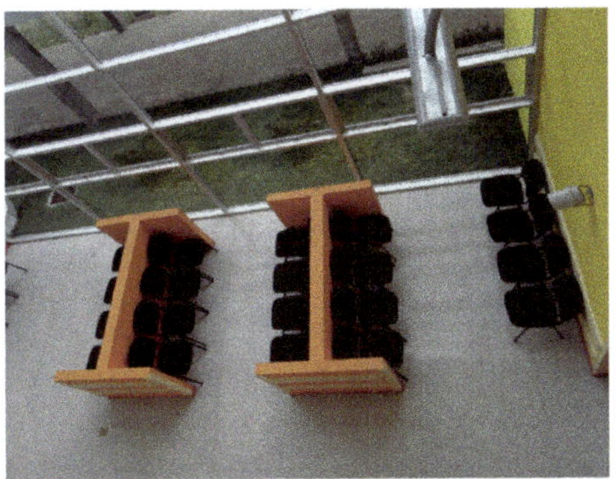

Figure 9. No obstacles.

5 - Hot air rises: another well-known strategy is to evacuate the hot vicious air on the top of the building; this is also called "stack effect" and bases itself in the physical principle that cold fresh air displaces hot vicious air and makes it rise and in the best case scenario take it out of the building. This is a very efficient way of closing the windows but continue to renew its air volume.

The Energy Performance of Buildings (or European directive 91) recognizes that health related buildings are particularly intensive energy consumers and expresses their worries about the growing air conditioning usage in the last years. They consider a priority to establish strategies to minimize dependence on mechanical ventilation.

Different studies prove that energy consumption based on fossil fuels has a direct impact in health, including premature death, chronic bronchitis, asthma complications, and visits to the emergency room related to contamination.

One directive that we realize and follow in the design process, was to use air conditioning only when the equipment in the room needed it for working properly and this was backup by the equipment supplier specifications or when there´s some legal requirement for a specific environmental condition in a room, aside from this two exceptions all the building functions with natural ventilation and we have prove it with measurements that internal temperature is within the established and desired comfort zone.

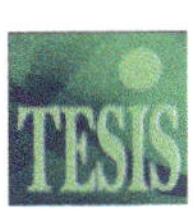

Illumination

Light is what makes forms and colors come to live before our eyes, it has been said that is the most important component of architecture, regarding natural lighting we had these considerations in our project:

1 - More light, less Rad: it is very important that in the localization and orientation of the building, solar geometry is taken in consideration as well as overall direct radiation charges, so that our design let pass the most of natural lighting without the radiation, that is the main cause of the increment in thermal gains for internal spaces.

2 - North overall: in our north hemisphere which Costa Rica has an inclination of 10° towards the Ecuador, the north light is the more desirable because of the low charge of radiation and the indirect appearance.

Light from the East is recommended to be uplifting for all people including patients, so in some parts of the morning it must be used as therapy.

On the other side, South and West lighting one must be protected at all times, mainly on the afternoons, this is the uncomfortable light and it is charged with lots of radiation that helps heat up spaces.

We protect our building with brise soleil and interstitial spaces like vertical circulation and electromechanical ducts that act as a shield so the rest of the building can stay cool in this critical hours.

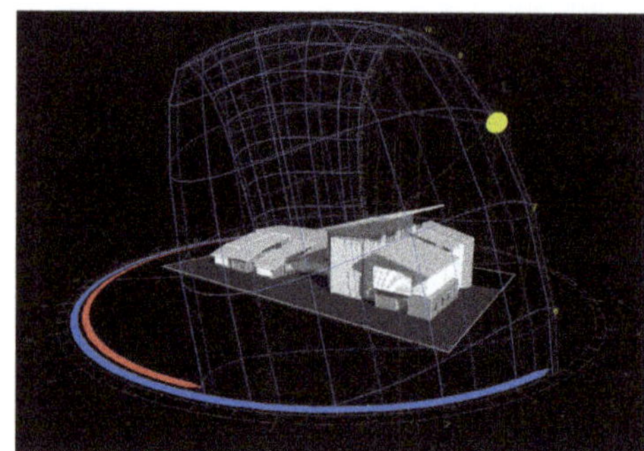

Figure 11. Building orientation.

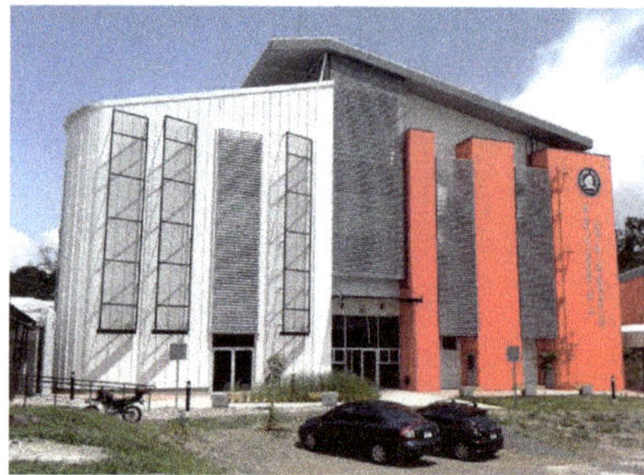

Figure 12. Building façade.

3 - More is better: when it comes to natural lighting, the correct amount of light to do the activities necessary for each space is better because it means you can use less artificial light to accomplish them, so we must have the standard criteria of daylight factor needed in each space depending on its usage, so we can measure external lighting and establish the percentage we must let come thru the skin of the building to accomplish this goals during day time, and hopefully create a beautiful spectacle in the meantime.

4 - Light is health: since a long time ago it is known that exposure to the morning sun is a therapeutic for most diseases, since it stimulates the immune system and help generate endorphins and other chemicals that give support to the body to generate defenses against viruses and bacteria as well as tolerate pain in a better way. Some studies shown that patients in a natural illuminated room need as much as 22 % less antibiotics and has a quicker recuperation in hospitalization times.

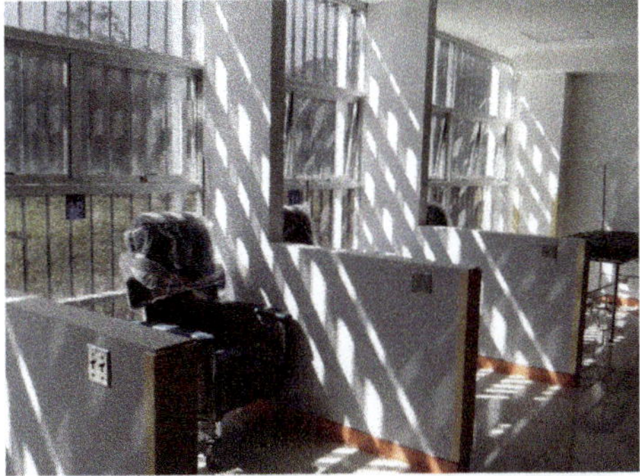

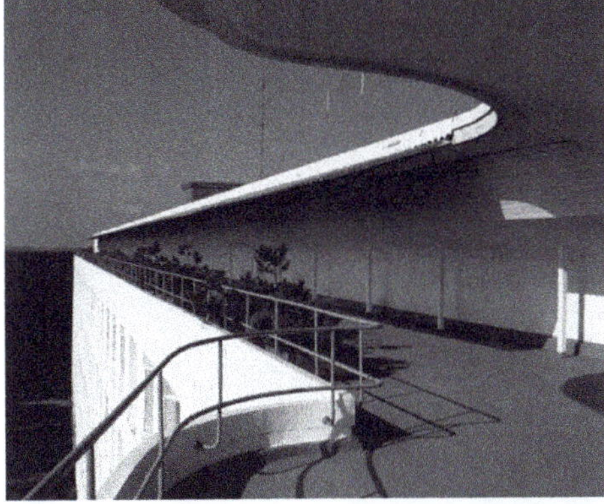

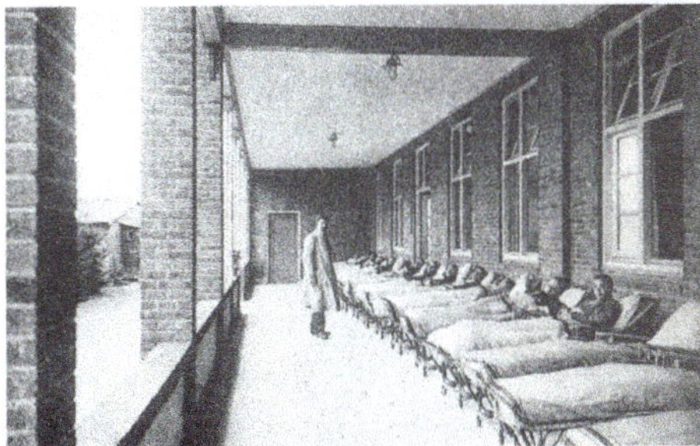

Figure 13. Natural illuminated environments.

Recently in Costa Rica, the Social Security System endorsed to instruct all of its staff that ¨Every new infrastructure project that it's made, must overcome all environmental jurisdiction, and guaranty that the product will be sustainable and friendly¨ in addition the institution promotes that ¨We must adopt architectural models for hospitals that are user friendly and environmentally correct, comfortable and highly functional.¨ This had been general communications in the last year, but we must now walk the walk.

Its unquestionable that all buildings in general, in its life cycle, construction, use and destruction, generate a vast number of environmental impacts in solid wastes, energy consumption and material extraction an usage, besides others. Good practices in construction can regenerate previously used sites, diminish water usage, used recycle materials, never the less this change must be design based which is the most difficult part because of the habits or standards that are being used now days and the resistance to change.

Equipment is a critical point in the energy savings in health infrastructure since its cost in regular conditions is near the 25 % of total budget, it has a great impact in the overall product. The fact that some of the equipment can be energy efficient can have saving in life cycle budgets up to 70% or 90%, so investigation in this field is required and capable professionals that can give the better solutions to each system is a great complement to passive strategies used in the design, and at a medium or long term can produce a positive cost & benefit numbers.

As a conclusion we are in a verge in history were technology has reach one of its peaks, but it continue to be the basic and essential things like reason, consciousness and good judgment which gives us the edge to propose intelligent, efficient and functional ways to solve our everyday problems, and make the health services a humanitarian way of making our world a better world for us and the rest of mankind.

Integral Centre for the Treatment of Elderly Adults Specialized in Alzheimer Disease, Citea

Eduardo Frank[1]
Erik Guth, Mariana Irigoyen, Luciano Monza[2]

efrank@estudioefrank.com.ar
[1]Architect, Estudio EFrank
[2] Architects ArquiSalud

In the last few years, Argentina is beginning the design and construction of specific effectors for the treatment of the Alzheimer disease, and one of them, the second to be inaugurated in the year 2015, is the CITEA.
In addition to the guarantee of the physical and psychic safety by means of concepts such as universal design, and maximizing the autonomy of the patients, the project intends to have non institutional characteristics, avoiding "hard architectures" typical for the buildings used for health-caring purposes. The program is articulated around an axis, a therapeutic "continuum", from the home up to the necessary institutionalization. The attention starts with the Domiciliary Attention administrated from the Centre, progressing with daytime activities, memory schools and tools to extend the patient's independence, etc. Afterwards, as the disease develops, the Centre offers a Daytime Hospital and three levels / hospitalization cells. Three hospitalization levels organized in an increasing way and according to the disease stage the patient is living.

***Eduardo Frank**, Architect Faculty of Architecture, Design and Urbanism, University of Buenos Aires. Specialist in Gerontology Architecture. Specialist in Planning of Physical Resources in Health. FADU, UBA. Collegiate Member of the Mexican Gerontology National Council. Since the year 1978 he carries out projects for Elderly Adults: Hogar Hirsch (Hirsch Home), Hogar Los Pinos (Los Pinos Home), Viviendas Vidalinda (Vidalinda Dwellings), Centro de Tratamiento del Mal de Alzheimer (Centre for the Treatment of Alzheimer), among others. Author of "Vejez, Arquitectura y Sociedad" ("Old Age, Architecture and Society"). Author of "Diseño y Calidad de Vida" ("Design and Life Quality") book "Discapacidad Intelectual y Envejecimiento" ("Intellectual Disability and Ageing") Editorial Universitaria de A Coruña, Spain, Dr. José C. Millán Calenti. Author of "Plan Maestro del Hábitat para la Tercera Edad" ("Master Plan of the Habitat for the Third Age"), "Temas Relacionados al Qué-Hacer Gerontológico" ("Issues Related to the Gerontology Duty") AGEBA.*

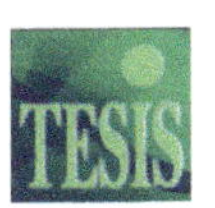

Summarizing, the target is implementing techniques contemplating the global approach of the patient and of the relatives and/ or formal or informal caregiver. The physical environment may have a significant role in maximizing the functional independence and the autonomy, and must be considered a partner or a tool for the care of the patient.

The role of the architectural environment must not be limited to the supply of the physical resources, it is not an isolated physical resource, but a part of a complex system that operates in organizational, social and therapeutic fields.
The three components framing the design model are the organizational, social and physical environments, which have the purpose of achieving the dignity and independence, both of the patients and of the team taking care of them.
The organizational component, in terms of policies, contemplates, by means of increasingly complex alternatives, and it accompanies the different phases of the disease, from the permanence at home through daytime homes, up to long-stay institutions. The social component, which is represented by the residents "neighbours", the family and the caregivers. Finally, the architectural component, which must add the attributes of the environment adequate for this pathology.
The project of the physical resources has been evaluated in due course by the interdisciplinary consulting team, in terms of the therapeutic, organizational goals and of the conceptual frame defined during the process by the consultants team and the professionals of the design.
The physical resource extends outside the specific building, first of all, to the patient's house. It will be prepared with the purpose of creating environments adapted to the needs of each patient according to the disease's evolution degree, in order to delay as much as possible the institutionalization, the patient and the family being accompanied by the professional team from the institution.

El Centre is located in the neighbourhood of Belgrano, in the City of Buenos Aires, at Vidal Street Nr. 2957 between Av. Congreso and Quesada Street, distant some metres from Av. Cabildo, with excellent public means of transport, on a plot of land of 1,105.10 m^2 (25.98 x 42.30). Total area of the project 3,000 m^2. The building has five levels, basement, ground floor and three storeys (Figure 1).

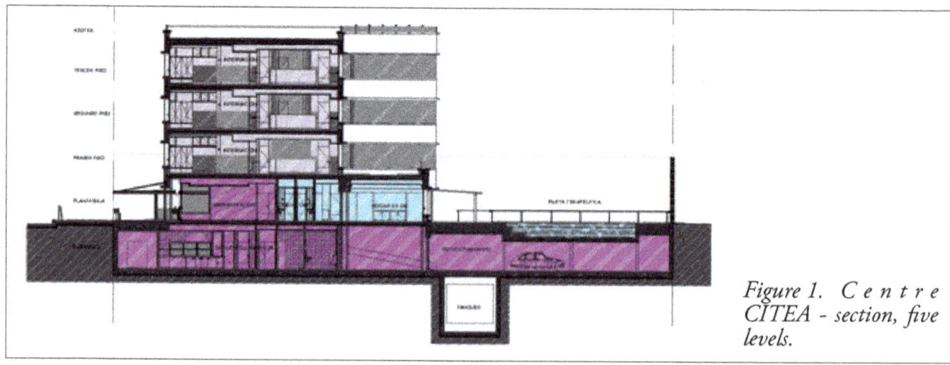

Figure 1. Centre CITEA - section, five levels.

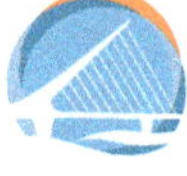

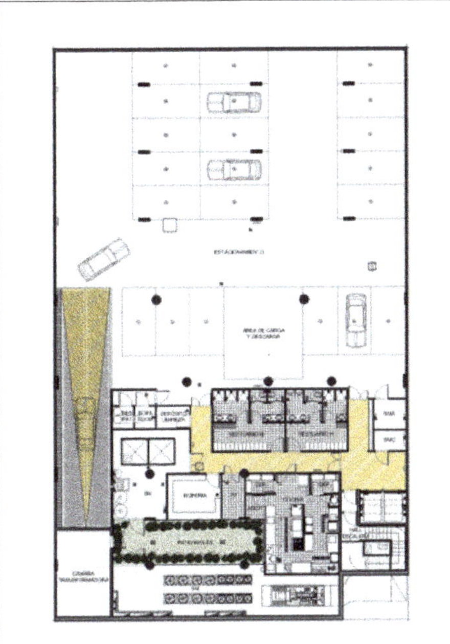

Figure 2. Centre CITEA, the basement.

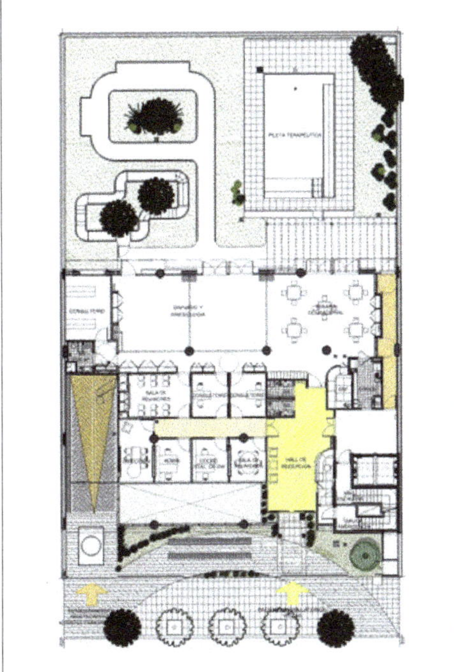

Figure 3. Centre CITEA, ground floor.

The Basement will lodge the kitchen, warehouses, lockers rooms, machine room and parking for twenty vehicles, as well as room for suppliers' loading and unloading operations (Figure 2).

The Ground Floor (Figure 3) has double access, one for the main hall (Figure 4) and the other one to the daytime centre. The Daytime Centre has a large multiple-function room that may be partitioned, to develop occupational therapy tasks, physical exercises / kinesiology, recreation activities, etc., as well as cabinets, doctor's offices, administrative sector and professional coordination area, infirmary, a workshop-classroom and sanitary installations (Figure 5). The same space will be used, outside the hours of the daytime centre, for training of domicile caregivers, meetings with families and promotion and awareness activities. There is also a therapeutic garden and expansion area of 470 m^2 with walking promenade and therapeutic pool.

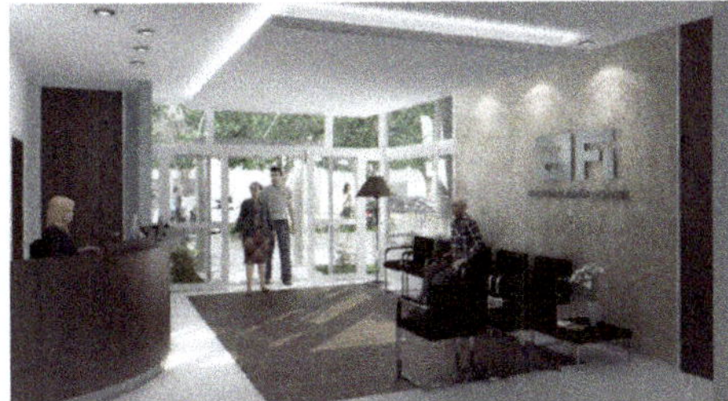

Figure 4. Centre CITEA - ground floor, main hall.

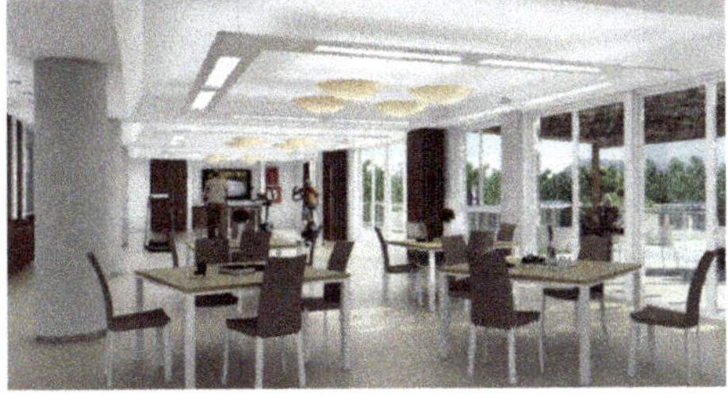

Figure 5. Large multiple-function of the Daytime Centre CITEA.

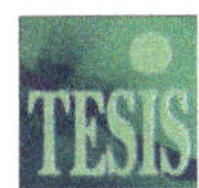

In the three upper storeys, there are three hospitalization "cells". Each of them consists of 10 rooms with private bathroom, with the possibility of lodging two beds each. All these rooms are directly connected, with no intermediate corridors, with a multiple-function room, and each level is completed with an infirmary office, place for used materials and meals office (Figure 6).

The inhabitants of each floor will carry out their daily activities in therapeutic communities according to the disease's evolution degree. The three levels will be occupied according to this criterion, the last one being destined for the most serious condition of the disease.

The building will be automated for the control and safety of the inhabitants, this fact not being evident for the patients: Each hospitalization level will be coordinated from a panoptic control in the infirmary office, and will be provided with a "phototherapy" system which will help with the regulation of the circadian rhythm of the patient, helping him or her to relax or to be active, as pertinent, thus helping to reduce medication.

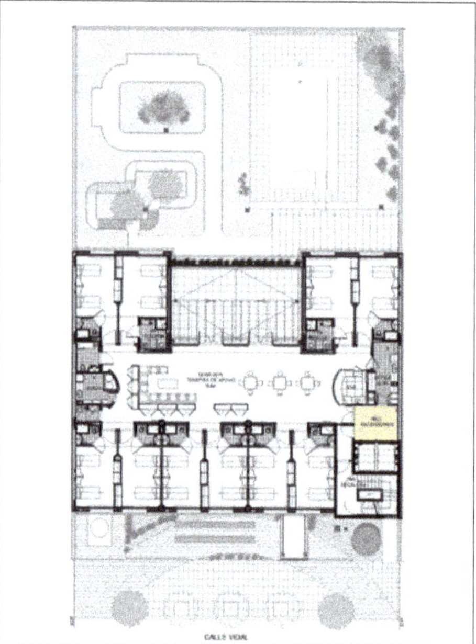

Figure 6. Centre CITEA, three upper storeys.

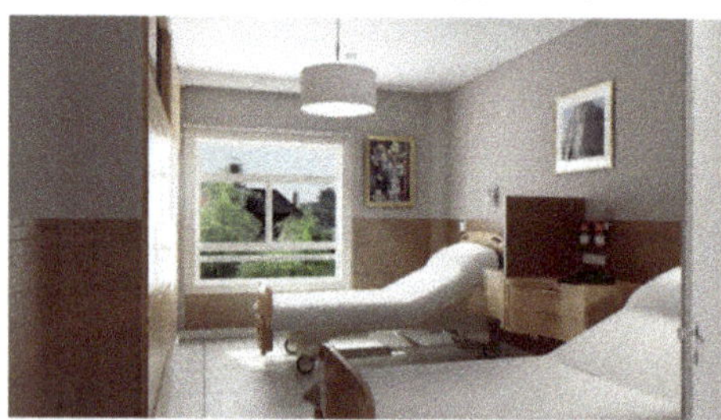

Figure 7. Centre CITEA, patient room.

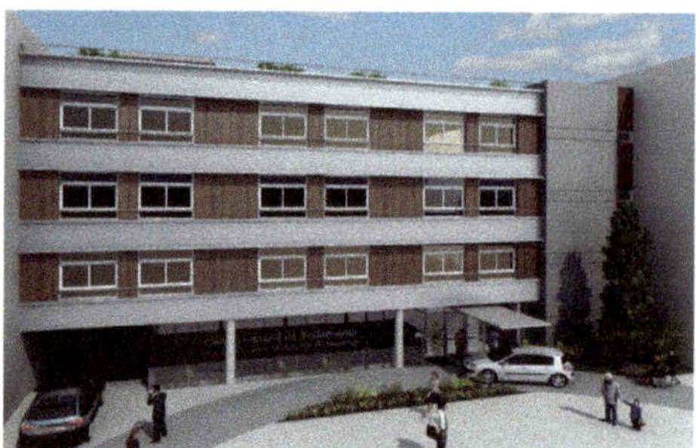

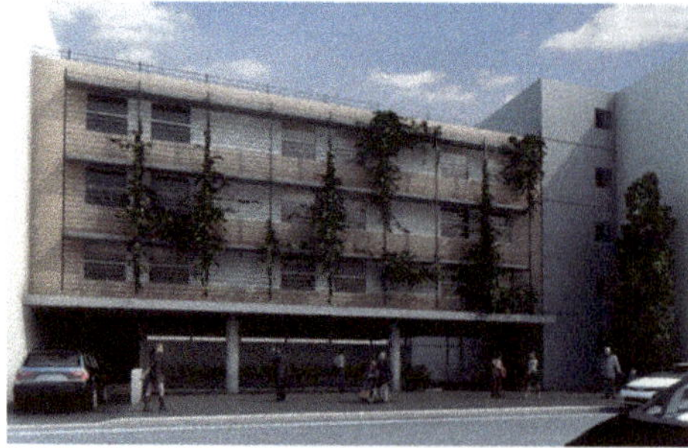

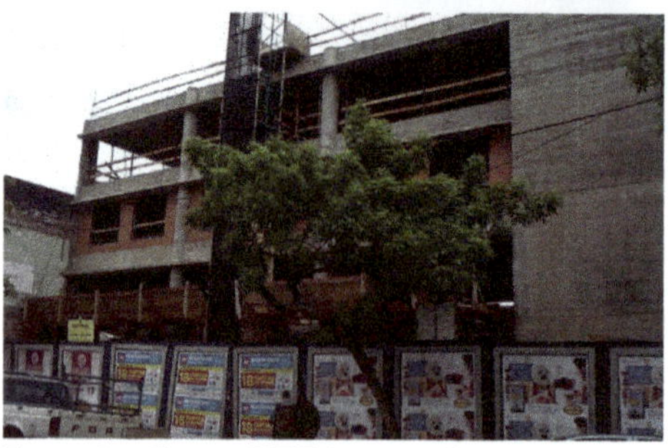

Figure 8. Centre CITEA, external views.

The Environment of Care for People with Dementia: Evidence-Based Design Solutions and Best Practices for Integrated Care Delivery in Times of Radical Change

Efthimia Pantzartzis, Andrew D. F. Price and Federica Pascale

e.pantzartzis@lboro.ac.uk
Loughborough University, United Kingdom

Populations in many countries are ageing at a rapid pace which is expected to rise over the coming years. People with dementia are predicted to increase by up to 100% by 2040 in developed countries, whereas in developing countries (i.e. Latin America, Africa, India, China, south Asian and western-Pacific regions) are estimated to grow even faster. Health and social care provision and infrastructure need to respond to the ageing population and its related conditions such as dementia. The healthcare built environment can impact on people living with dementia and the care pathway is highly relevant to quality of life, patients, residents, family, staff and carers. Evidence-based design solutions and best practice can help to improve the quality of life and deliver value for money during a period of rapid change where long-term solutions relating to the healthcare environment are required. Research and pilot studies can help to demonstrate the benefits of evidence-based design and best practice for integrated care delivery. This paper explores the current trend and future opportunities to deliver dementia friendly environments and integrated care through gathering of evidence, development of best practice guidance and integration of care delivery.

Efthimia Pantzartzis*, MArch, MSc Planning Buildings for Health - is a Research Associate at Loughborough University currently working on the Department of Health (DH) funded Dementia Capital Programme. A healthcare architect and consultant with expertise in acute and specialised hospital refurbishments and reorganisation of services, she has been working in the public sector on healthcare projects in Italy and on Engineering and Physical Sciences Research Council and DH funded projects on healthcare infrastructure value and critical infrastructure risk. She has worked at the European Topic Centre on Spatial Information and Analysis in Barcelona, in support to the European Environment Agency.*

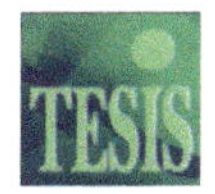

DEVELOPMENT

Aim

This paper aims to explore current trends with respect to dementia and the opportunities to deliver Evidence-Based Design (EBD) solutions and Best Practice (BP) for dementia friendly environments. This research mainly draws on a thematic literature review to set up the scene and determine the focus of the research literature focusing on demographic changes and their impact on the health and social care provision.

Scale and definition of the problem: ageing population and dementia

Populations in many countries are ageing at a rapid pace. The World Health Organisation (WHO) reported that by 2016 the number of people aged 65 or above would outnumber children aged five years and under. The increase in life expectancy and longevity combined with dropped fertility rates and reduced pandemics are expected to increase the number of people aged 65 or above from 524 million in 2010 to 1.5 billion in 2050 [1] (Figure 1). Worldwide the number of people aged 60 or above is expected to treble by 2100: ageing population trends in developing regions are expected to rise by 2.9% annually up to 2050, whereas in more developed countries the rate of increase is expected to be 1.0% per annum, but with a great transformation in the demographic profiles [2]. Ageing populations bring together a series of implications far beyond the social determinants for equity of care provision [3], among which are: non-communicable diseases; elderly related impairments; and long-term care. Dementia encompasses a range of conditions related to the impairment of brain functions, including language, memory, perception, personality and cognitive skills, which are progressive, degenerative and irreversible, and with currently no cure [4]; it presents a huge challenge to society [5]. Globally, it is estimated that 24.3 million people have dementia, which is expected to double every 20 years up to 81.1 million by 2040 [6]. This is predicted to increase by up to 100% in the developed countries, and much faster in developing countries, with an expected increase of: 235-393% in Latin America and Africa; and 314-336% in India, China, and their south Asian and western-Pacific regions [7]. In the United Kingdom (UK), 800,000 people live with dementia which is expected to increase to over 1 million by 2021 [8], with significant costs of health and care provision higher than the currently estimated £23 billion a year [9].

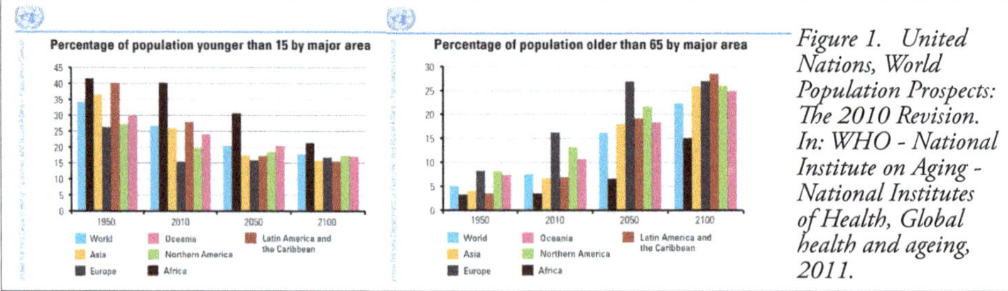

Figure 1. United Nations, World Population Prospects: The 2010 Revision. In: WHO - National Institute on Aging - National Institutes of Health, Global health and ageing, 2011.

Need

Health and social care services and infrastructures in many countries need to be significantly rethought if they are to appropriately respond to the needs of significantly ageing populations. Given the size of the challenge, future strategies need to consider highly innovative solutions and approaches capable of contribution to a significant step change, for example the increased use of:

- assistive technologies;
- integrated care pathways; and
- dementia and frailty-friendly environments.

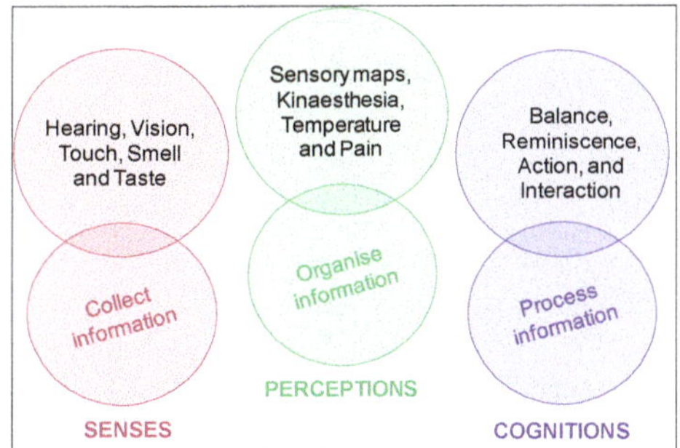

Figure 2. Dementia encompasses a range of conditions, which are progressive, degenerative, irreversible and with currently no cure.

Impact of the care environment

Contemporary research has established how the built environment impacts on the quality of care and on the wellbeing of people living with dementia [10-13]; design elements and layouts have been frequently associated with quality of care and behavioural outcomes [11, 13-16]. Reimer et al. have suggested that quality of life for adults with middle- to late-stage dementia is the same or better in purpose-built and staffed social care facilities than in traditional institutional settings [17]. Though, the quality and the understanding of existing evidence in relation to elderly population and people living with dementia is not always supported by research studies [18, 19]. According to Ulrich et al. and Calkins [19, 20] there is limited understanding and sometimes misunderstanding of issues specifically related to dementia and a lack of proven evidence on the implications of elements such as: design layouts; use of bedrails; views of and interaction with nature; use of abstract art; and observation of local information and images on the built environment for people with dementia.

The use of EBD and BP in relation to environments of care for people with dementia

Future guidance and long-term strategies are also urgently needed to deliver BP and EBD capable of supporting integrated health and social care delivery especially with regards to people living with dementia. Over the past 10 years, EBD has emerged as a scientific response to the questions about how the built environment impacts on patient, staff and resource outcomes. Its definition embraces the knowledge that can be transferred from evidence into best design options to improve service users' quality of life, well-being, healing and quality of care [19, 21-23]. Although previous research has demonstrated the benefits of EBD and performance and prescriptive standards have been developed to improve the quality of care provision, the use of evidence in practice has been limited mainly due to: a lack of time and cost resources to access rigorous evidence; and a common negative perception of evidence by the practitioners [24].

The term best practice is widely used; however, there are many definitions depending on the context. The concept of best practice in healthcare is related to the delivery of effectiveness efficiency in the healthcare systems [25]. It is the "best way to identify, collect, evaluate, disseminate and implement information [...], monitor the outcomes of the healthcare interventions for patients/ population groups and defined indications or conditions" [26]. The major complexities are identified on the transfer from evidence gathering to best practice delivery and a comprehensive structured approached is advocated at many levels [27]. Identifying the most appropriate framework, and specifically a "collective approach to information management", to improve effectiveness and efficiency in health and social care systems is fundamental [26], but skills, resources, patient-centric approach, and research and practice collaboration are required to make the model "evidence-based practice" work successfully [28].

Health and social care in the UK: pressures on the system and the built infrastructure

Furthermore to demographic change, there are other factors that contribute to escalate the pressures on the system and the built infrastructure. Notwithstanding the introduction of Private Finance Initiative (PFI) in 1997 to reduce the NHS England capital spending on new health and social care infrastructures, and of Foundation Trusts (FTs) in 2004 to allow financial and operational freedom at Trust level, inadequate buildings still exist [29, 30]. In the 2009-2010 17% of the standing NHS building infrastructure was reported as outdated and not fit for purpose [31]. The changes and adaptations required on the built environment impact on the care provision with risks to people, quality of service, costs of care. In the UK, health and social care are separated. The National Health Service (NHS) Reform in 2005 delegated budgets to the GPs and the right to supply the NHS to independent providers. In April 2013, the "NHS Health and Social Care Act 2012" came into force, recognising the rising demand and treatment costs together with the changing needs in scale and scope of service provision [32, 33]. The NHS England designated the Clinical Commissioning Groups (CCGs) to be in charge of commissioning services for Trusts, FTs, Primary Care and independent providers, while Public Health England was accountable for public health commissioning, through Local Authorities (LAs) and Social Care (SC) providers. Despite efforts to improve control on service commissioning to Primary Care providers and LAs, the management has been maintained within the NHS England, to some extent maintaining a lack of effective integration between health and social care service provision [34, 35].

EBD solutions, BP and strategies in the NHS and LAs: raising awareness and action

Today there is undisputable recognition of the need to: take due account of demographic change and its impact

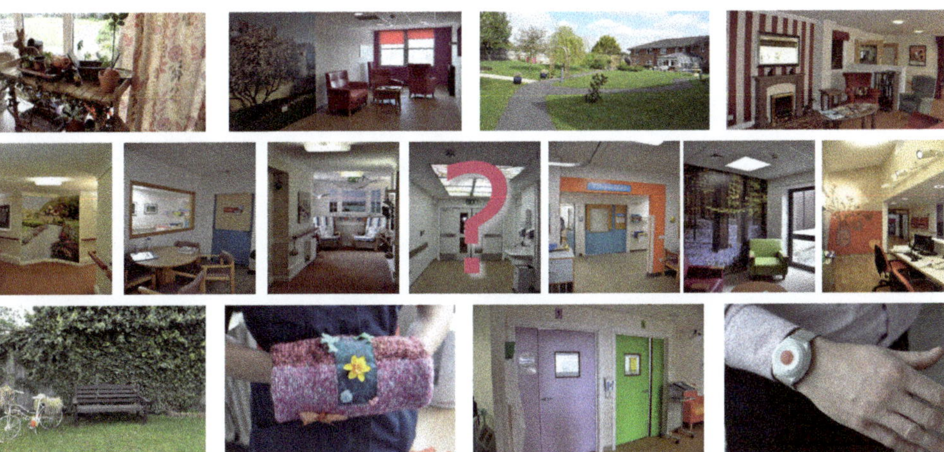

Figure 3. EBD solutions, BP strategies in the NHS and LAs.

on economic, environment and social issues , which is increasingly changing the design of the built environment [36]; and prove that dementia service delivery leads to an improved quality of care, hence health and social care productivity and efficiency is [37]. There is similarly a high level of understanding of the stakeholders and care providers, with dementia strategies developed at local level, which does not necessarily allow health and social services to liaise for an improved patient's journey across the care pathway.

Despite the increased awareness, issues have been captured on the commitment to provide integrated care following EBD and BP. Literature has demonstrated that: (1) there are important gaps in the design of the environment of care for people with dementia which to some extent accounts for lack of integrated care provision [38-42]; and (2) the focus is mainly on the development of management frameworks for integrated care pathways which does not necessarily take count of the environment of care or integration across different settings [43]. The NHS and LAs are challenged daily by: increased service and infrastructure capital and running costs; demand on A&E departments; acute service capacity; new service demands; extra-care provision; quality and safety issues; complex patients' journeys.

Moreover, the UK care provision for people living with dementia, including related funding and research, has not driven high quality design to integrate people with dementia, and more widely frail elderly population, to the entire local communities yet, if compared with the EU dementia care infrastructures [44]. Action is required to clearly, precisely and exhaustively apply EBD and BP knowledge and theories to design, build and operate environments for integrated care delivery.

Design towards decentralisation and integration of care: standards and guidance in the UK

In the UK, design standards and guidance - Design Guides (NHS Estates), Health Technical Memoranda (HTM),

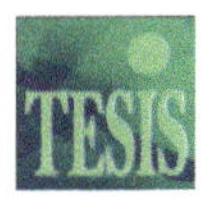

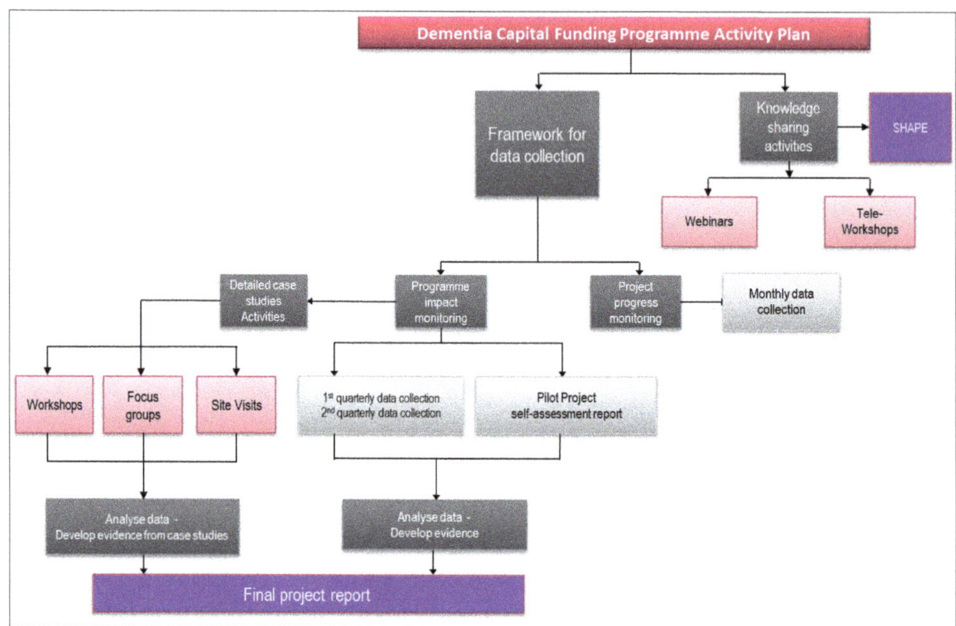

Figure 4. DH Dementia Capital Programme - Delivery plan.

Health Building Notes (HBNs), Health Facilities Notes, Health Guidance Notes, and Design Guidance - provide recommendations and guidance on purpose-built care facilities, specific elements of standards and operational issues. Nevertheless, there is no strategy in place to update this consistent corpus of knowledge with evidence from what works and what does not when the built environment is operated. Within this understanding, awareness and proactive national approach, the DH Dementia Capital Programme has approved £50 million funding of 116 pilot projects between NHS Trusts and LAs with the aim "to improve the care environment for people with dementia by means of conducting a series of NHS and SC National pilot projects" and to develop evidence and produce new Health and Care Building Note guidance derived from a clear identification of what evidence is required to demonstrate that people living with dementia benefit from purposefully created dementia-friendly care environments.

Although there is an actual recognition of the issues around the dementia condition and the "Challenge on Dementia" identifies key areas as: driving improvements in health and care; creating dementia-friendly communities that understand how to help; and promoting dementia related research [45], dementia stakeholders' semi-structured preliminary interviews pointed out as major constraints against an effective and efficient environment of care for people with dementia problems at different scales, including: raising costs of care provision; continuous staff training; discrepancy between and health and social care needs; lack of communication between health and social care providers.

Conclusions: the environment of care for people with dementia

Innovative approaches are needed to meet radical change, and as changes become more frequent the required approaches will have to meet rapid adaptation consistently over time. The rapid change in demographics impacts on the health and social care provision and infrastructure, and the environment of care is today not ready for people with dementia.

This research paper explored the current trend and future opportunities to deliver dementia friendly environments and enable dementia and frailty friendly communities, through EBD solutions and BP, through research and pilot studies, on the basis of a comprehensive literature review and of the DH Dementia Capital Programme, which is currently on-going and will report at the end of the year.

Nevertheless its announcement and set up has already had the power to determine a snow ball effect, in terms: of capital planning and funding strategy, learning enhancement, knowledge sharing, local expertise improvement, community engagement, business model, and others.

Capital economies, as the health and social care is, will increasingly be asked to promote service user wellbeing and quality of life, to cope with a changing built environment and a long-term strategy to enable the gathering of evidence, the development of best practice guidance and the integration of care delivery is advocated.

Acknowledgements

The research reported in this paper includes the outcomes of the stage 2 selection process of the DH National Capital Programme "Improving the environment of care for people with dementia" and of research projects funded by the Health and Care Infrastructure Research and Innovation Centre (HaCIRIC) and the Engineering and Physical Sciences Research Council (EPSRC). The authors wish to acknowledge the Department of Health England and IFF Research Ltd.

References

1. WHO - National Institute on Aging - National Institutes of Health, *Global health and ageing*, 2011, WHO.

2. UN - Department of Economic and Social Affairs - Population Division, *World Population Prospects: The 2012 Revision*, 2013, United Nations.

3. CSDH, *Closing the gap in a generation: health equity through action on the social determinants of health. Final Report of the Commission on Social Determinants of Health*, 2008, WHO: Geneva.

4. Access Economics Pty Limited, 2010, Alzheimer's Australia: Australia.

5. DH, *Living well with dementia: A National Dementia Strategy*, 2009, Department of Health: London.

6. Fleming, R. and N. Purandare, *Long-term care for people with dementia: environmental design guidelines*. International Psychogeriatrics, 2010. 22(7): p. 1084-1096.

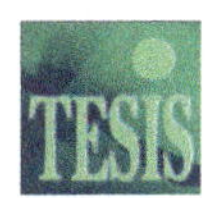

7. Ferri, C.P., et al., *Global prevalence of dementia: a Delphi consensus study*. The Lancet, 2005. 366(9503): p. 2112-2117.

8. Alzheimer's Society, *Dementia 2012: A national challenge*, 2012, Alzheimer's Society: London.

9. Matrix evidence, Spotlight on dementia care: *A Health Foundation improvement report*. 2011, the Health Foundation: London, UK.

10. Brod, M., A.L. Stewart, and L. Sands, *Conceptualization of quality of life in dementia, in Assessing Quality of Life in Alzheimer's Disease*. S.M. Albert and R.G. Logsdon, Editors. 2000, Springer: New York. p. 3-16.

11. Day, K., D. Carreon, and C. Stump, *The therapeutic design of environments for people with dementia: A review of the empirical research*. Gerontologist, 2000. 40(4): p. 397-416.

12. Lawton, M.P., *Assessing quality of life in Alzheimer disease research*. Alz Dis Assoc Disord. , 1997. 11(6): p. 91-99.

13. Kovach, C., et al., *Impacts of a therapeutic environment for dementia care*. American Journal of Alzheimer's Disease and Other Dementias, 1997. 12: p. 99-110.

14. Marshall, M., Brown M, and S. Stewart, *Tools for the future, in Making Design Dementia Friendly. Just Anoter Disability*, S. Stewart, A. Page, and C. Laurie, Editors. 1999, University of Stirling: Glasgow, UK.

15. Zeisel, J., et al., *Environmental correlates to behavioral health outcomes in Alzheimer's special care units*. Gerontologist, 2003. 43(5): p. 697-711.

16. Gitlin, L.N., J. Liebman, and L. Winter, *Are Environmental Interventions Effective in the Management of Alzheimer's Disease and Related Disorders?: A Synthesis of the Evidence*. Alzheimer's Care Today, 2003. 4(2): p. 85-107.

17. Reimer, M.A., et al., *Special care facility compared with traditional environments for dementia care: A longitudinal study of quality of life*. Journal of the American Geriatrics Society, 2004. 52(7): p. 1085-1092.

18. Rostenberg, B., M. Baum, and M. Shepley, *Sustainability and Evidence: The intersection of evidence-based design and sustainability*. 2009.

19. Ulrich, R., et al., *A review of the research literature on evidence-based healthcare design*. Health Environments Research and Design Journal, 2008(Spring): p. 61-125.

20. Calkins, M.P., *Evidence-based long term care design*. NeuroRehabilitation, 2009. 25(3): p. 145-154.

21. Ulrich, R.S., et al., *The role of the physical environment in the hospital of the 21st century: a once in a life time opportunity*. 2004.

22. Fleming, R., P.A. Crookes, and S. Sum, *A review of the empirical literature on the design of physical environments for people with dementia*. 2008, Dementia Collaborative Research Centres.

23. Malone, E., J.R. Mann-Dooks, and J.

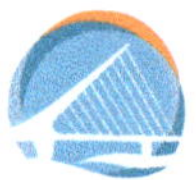

Strauss, Evidence-Based Design: Application in the MHS, 2007, HFPA Planning & Programming Division & TRICARE Management Activity PPMD.

24. Wanigarathna, N., A.D.F. Price, and S.A. Austin. *Improvement opportunities for evidence based design: an application of a critical realist's perspective in Proceedings 29th Annual ARCOM Conference.* 2013. Reading: Association of Researchers in Construction Management.

25. Employment & Social Affairs, *'Best practice': State of the art and perspectives in the EU for improving the effectiveness and efficiency of European health systems.* I.R.a.S.A. Eu Commission: Directorate-General for Employment, Editor 1999: Luxemburg.

26. Perleth, M., *What is `best practice' in health care? State of the art and perspectives in improving the effectiveness and efficiency of the European health care systems.* 2001: Elsevier.

27. Grol, R. and J. Grimshaw, *From best evidence to best practice: effective implementation of change in patients' care.* The Lancet, 2003. 362(9391): p. 1225-1230.

28. Rosswurm, M.A. and J.H. Larrabee, *A Model for Change to Evidence-Based Practice.* Image: the Journal of Nursing Scholarship, 1999. 31(4): p. 317-322.

29. Harker, R., *NHS funding and expenditure.* S.a.G. Statistics, Editor 2011, House of Commons Library. p. 16.

30. Harker, R., *NHS funding and expenditure.* S.a.G. Statistics, Editor 2012, House of Commons Library. p. 11.

31. Department of Health, E*states Return Infromation Collection (ERIC) 2009/10.* 2010, NHS Information Centre for Health and Social Care Leeds.

32. Department of Health, *NHS Autonomy and Accountability - Proposals for legislation.* 2007, The Stationery Office: Crown.

33. Department of Health, *Equity and excellence: Liberating the NHS.* 2010. The Stationery Office: Crown.

34. Robertson, H., *Integration of health and social care: A review of literature and models - Implications for Scotland.* 2011, Royal College of Nursing Scotland.

35. Priest, J., *The integration of health and social care.* 2012, Health Policy & Economic Research Unit.

36. Farrelly, L., D*esigning for the Third Age: Architecture Redefined for a Generation of "Active Agers" AD.* 1st ed. 2014: John Wiley & Sons Inc.

37. de Waal, H., et al., *Designing and Delivering Dementia Services.* 2013: Wiley-Blackwell.

38. Evans, G., *The built environment and mental health.* Journal of Urban Health, 2003. 80(4): p. 536-555.

39. Mitchell, L. and E. Burton, *Neighbourhoods for life: Designing dementia-friendly outdoor environments. Quality in Ageing and Older Adults*, 2006. 7(1): p. 26-33.

40. Alzheimer's Australia, *Dementia care and the Built Environment.* 2004, Alz-

heimer's Australia: Scullin, Australia.

41. Alzheimer's Society, *Support. Stay. Save. Care and support of people with dementia in their own homes*, 2011.

42. Verbeek, H., et al., *Dementia Care Redesigned: Effects of Small-Scale Living Facilities on Residents, Their Family Caregivers, and Staff.* Journal of the American Medical Directors Association, 2010. 11(9): p. 662-670.

43. Dubuc, N., et al., *Development of integrated care pathways: toward a care management system to meet the needs of frail and disabled community-dwelling older people.* 2013, 2013.

44. Astley, P., et al., *Active Aging: Comparative European case studies of facilities for people with dementia 2005-2008.* 2009, Medical Architecture Research Unit - LSBU.

45. DH, Prime Minister's Challenge on Dementia. *Delivering major improvements in dementia care and research by 2015: A report on progress.* 2012, Department of Health: London.

Designing Care on Human Scale.
The Latest Development in Netherlands

Reimar von Meding

KAW, Netherlands

KAW is the Dutch expert for the spacial, social and economic effects of demographic change. This is very much an international theme and we believe that international knowledge exchange helps us making big steps towards more sustainable, more social and more affordable solutions for people to live happily. We see our work as a contribution to strategic as well as practical matters. We work on investigation and strategy and continuously connect the results to our practical experience in architecture and urban planning. On the IFHE 2014, we will provide insight in the newest solutions in elderly cure and care from Dutch perspective. Also, we will show the latest developments that are still in design process. These will be completed and open for live visits at the IFHE World Congress 2016.

***Reimar von Meding** is chief architect at KAW. The architect of German origin decided to build a career in The Nether-lands, after studying architecture at the Technical University Delft. Under his leadership, KAW Rotterdam grew from 10 to 20 employees between 2004 and 2008. Still he spend most of his time at the drawing table. Reimar's motivation is designing for the 'forgotten targetgroup'. This group includes everyone who do not have the resources or the ability to choose his or her own living environment. Reimar belives that 'good living' is the basis for a better life. His specialty is the design of housing quality – and at low cost. He is also working on a better form of housing with care. In the article "Caring for the city, he shows how architecture residential care the quality of its entire environment can improve. He received several nominations and awards.*

Passive House Revolution

What is revolutionary about the 'Veilige Veste', is that this is the first large office block in the Netherlands to be renovated according to the Passive House standard. 'Passive House' is a standard for energy efficiency in a building, reducing its ecological footprint. It results in ultra-low energy buildings that require little energy for space heating or cooling. In this case, the fact that the former police stations' substructure was placed outside the building, meant an enormous energy abuser to be dealt with. The substructure created a thermal bridge that works exactly like a tunnel sucking in the cold outside air.

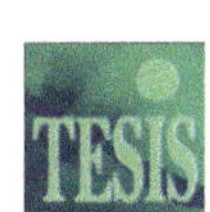

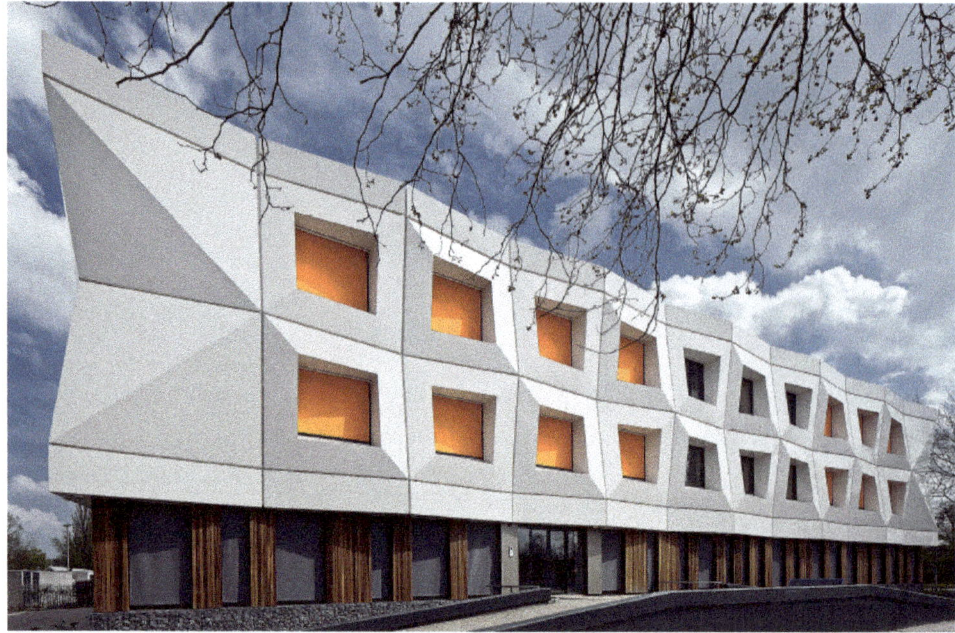

Figure 1. 'De Veilige Veste', used to be a police station and is now a safe house for victims of human trafficking.

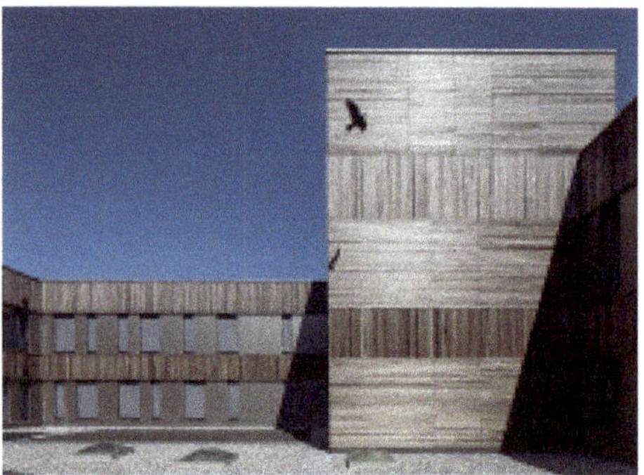

Figure 2. De Veilige Veste.

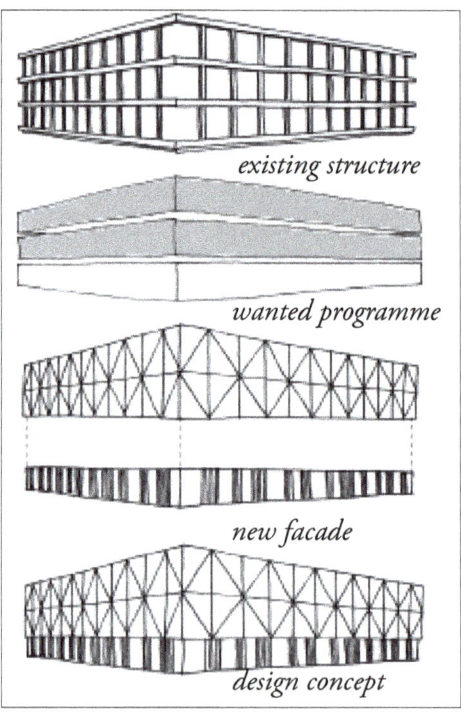

Figure 3. De Veilige Veste, project evolution.

By wrapping the building with the diamond-cut square panels, the substructure is now within the building and the whole building is covered by a thick layer of insulation. At some points, the façade is over 3 feet thicker now. Thanks to optimal insulation, draft proofing and the use of very little, highly energy-efficient equipment, the 'Veilige Veste' consumes exceptionally little power.

Dutch Design: brave, bold and safe!

In the Netherlands, design, energy reduction and the fight against human trafficking come together in one revolutionary project: the 'Veilige Veste'. Literally translated this means 'safe fortress', and that is exactly what it is. You cannot miss the bright white building, cut like a diamond, subtly gleaming in the sun. It is the new home for girls from all around the world that have been victims of human trafficking.

Bold, brave and safe is the concept for the new shelter for girls that have been victims of human trafficking. Not tucked away in anonymous houses in back alleys anymore, which is the way these girls are normally treated. No, these girls do not have to fear their perpetrators any more in their new home that is standing fierce in the midst of Frieslands' capital Leeuwarden. In their safe fortress they send out a clear message: we are no longer on the run, game over, giving their perpetrators the finger. 'Veilige Veste' provides security and protection, so the girls can build up their lives again.

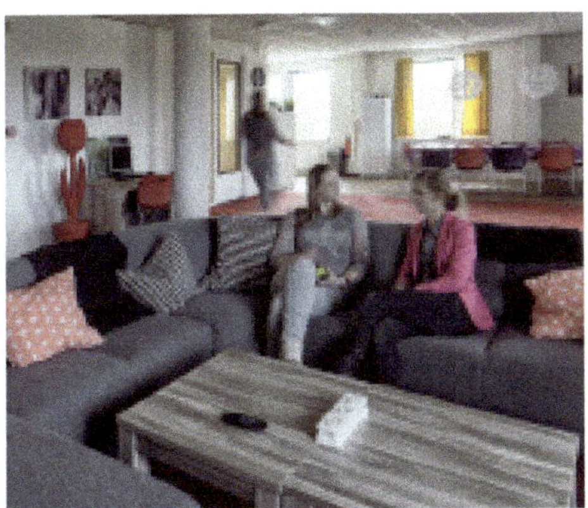

Figure 4. Veilige Veste'. Literally translated this means 'safe fortress'.

Village Elderly Housing
Care Housing Petterhusterstate, Stiens

Design of a new care residency for people with Alzheimer's or cognitive impairments. To minimize the influence on the environment, KAW designed a building that enhances the character of the landscape. The complex has a green roof framed by a striking border. Special is that one side of the roof is being lengthed over the facade, creating a unification of the landscape and the building. The wide landscape is honored by the spacious design of the apartments. The tranquil colors are consistent with the adjacent farmhouse, build in the early 20th century. The care center consist of four buildings, each containing six residential units. At the square you'll find a servicepoint, accessible for everyone that is in need of care.

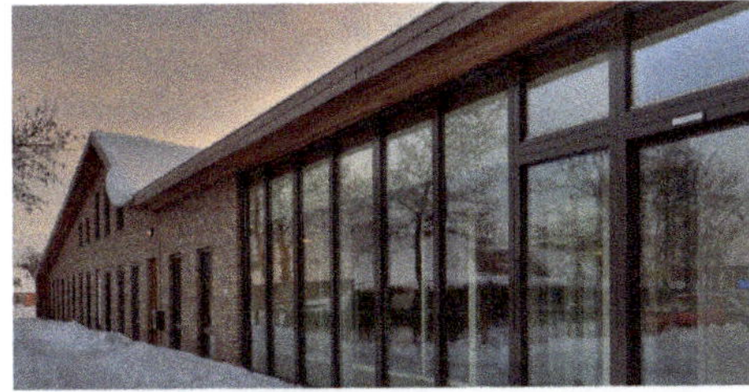

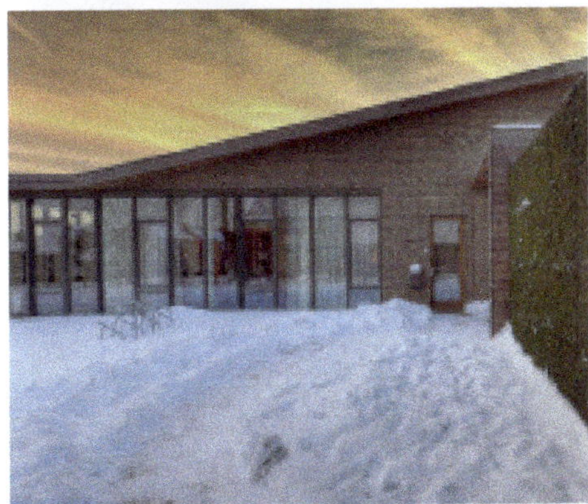

Figure 5. Care Housing Petterhusterstate provides elderly housing in small groups of 6-7 people.

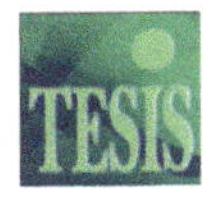

Healing Environment

Reimar von Meding about the project: "Occasionally you come across places so beautiful that you don't want to build anything there. But sometimes you have to. We found such a place in the middle of the village Stiens, a historic farm in Amsterdam School style, surrounded by grassland. We put an enormous effort in realising a residency here that both connects to its environment as to the village people. A healthy living environment starts with feeling at home. This is the main thought behind the Healing Environment theory. We put people and their mental, physical and social well-being first. This reflects in every aspect of this building, from the layout of the hallways to the colour of the toilet. Also the healing impact of nature and views cannot be underestimated.

Memory Walls

Design influences well-being of the elderly
The principal question for KAW was: How can the interior design support the life quality of its residents? Niches in the common living room provide access to the private rooms of the residents. So the people can more easily remember their room, each niche has a different colour and its own memorabilia to make it personal. Very important for elderly: keeping their dignity.

That means being able to retreat in your own private space if you wish to do so, and being able to do the things you want to do. In this care residency we eliminated all transport areas, like hallways or entrances. This resulted in a 25% increase of living space, adding to the comfort of the residents.

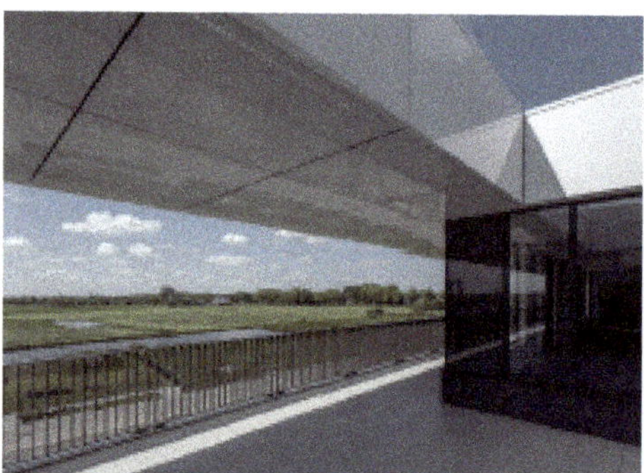

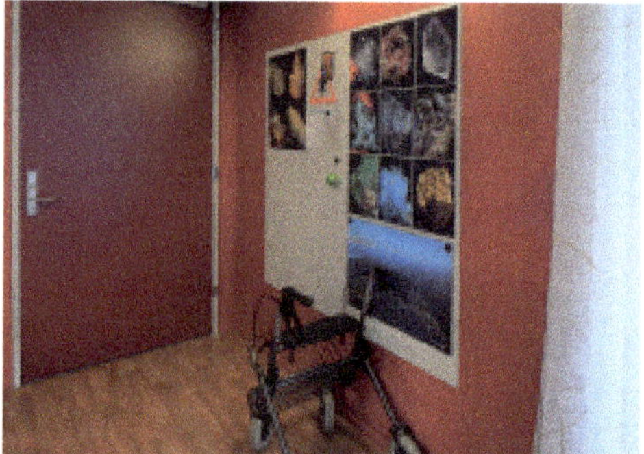

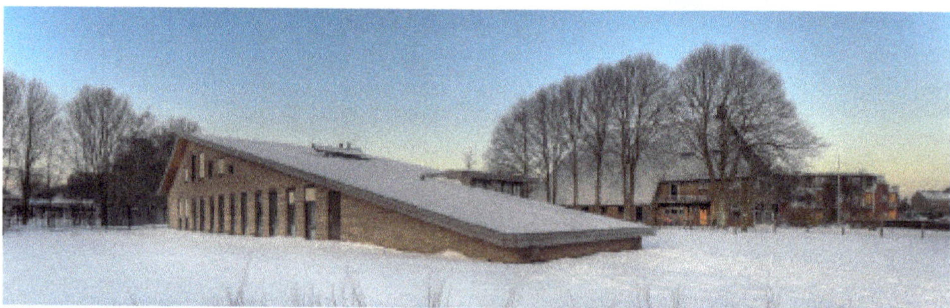

Figure 6. Care Housing Petterhusterstate, Stiens.

SENIOR INDONESIAN HOUSING NUSANTARA, ALMERE

A residence for senior citizens from Indonesian descent is developed at the edge of the commuter city of Almere. With a large amount of post-war immigrants now growing old, there is a sudden demand for housing for seniors with a shared background. The building concept is based on connecting building and landscape. The particular shape of the building allows it to blend in with the scenery. At the same time, the shape refers to the flowing lines of the Indonesian scenery.

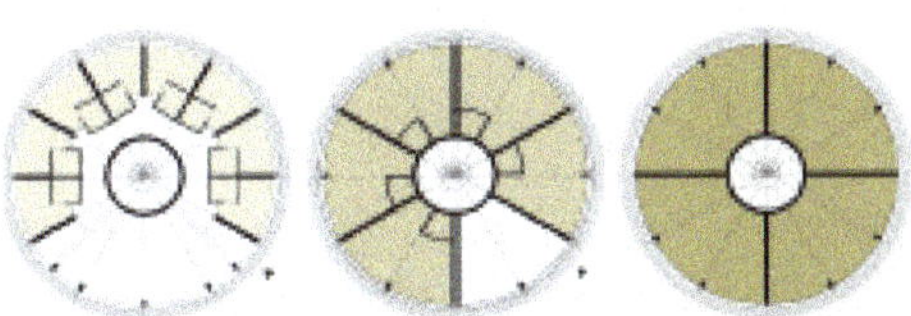

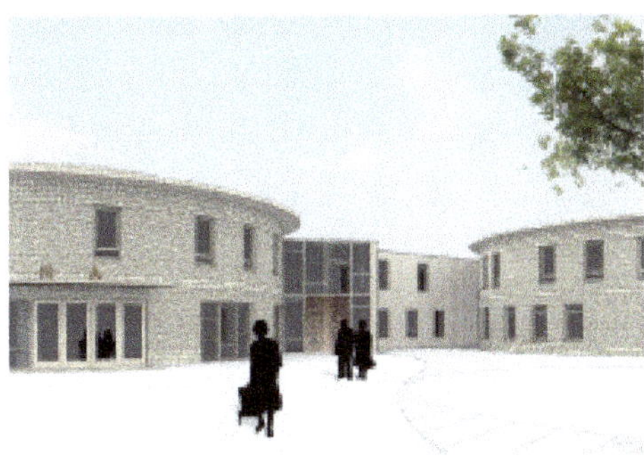

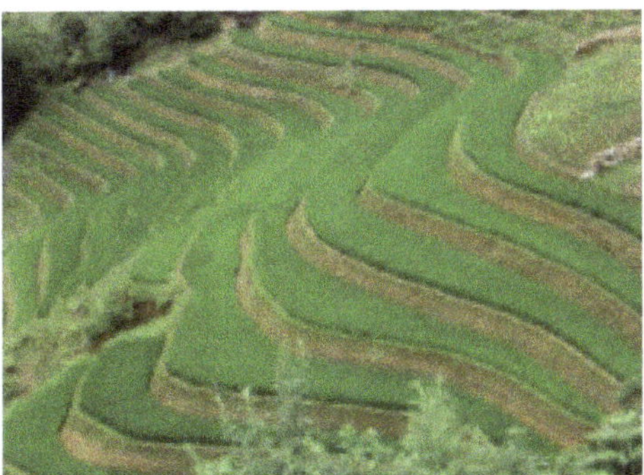

Figure 7. Senior Indonesian Housing Nusantara, Almere.

Feeling At Home

Reimar von Meding about the project: "KAW designs a care complex for people with an Indonesian background for the NPO Nusantara. In Indonesian, 'Nusantara' means 'between the islands'. That is exactly what marks the life stories of many of these people: as Dutch Indonesians they find themselves emotionally between the Netherlands and the old Dutch Indies. The living-with-care complex is also such an 'in-betweener'. It is located between city and landscape, between neighbourhood and large nature park. That makes it a building and a landscape at the same time. Although its shape reflects the Indonesian landscape, this is the result of practical Dutch thinking: the circle form beholds a larger content than any other form, resulting in a more affordable and energy-efficient building."

BACKGROUND THEORY

Residential Environment Strategy: The KAW Residential Environment Strategy allows us to typify residential and care areas in terms of spatial characteristics. It differentiates four residential environments that each are distinct in how people live together and the level of liveliness. Those environments differ in form and function of the public space, in type of access and in communal meeting areas. A Residential Care Environment Toolbox shows the most logical integration of care facilities.

Developing Assisted Living Areas in Rotterdam: For the development of assisted living areas in 'Delfshaven', an area with 70.000 inhabitants in Rotte rdam,

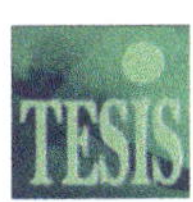

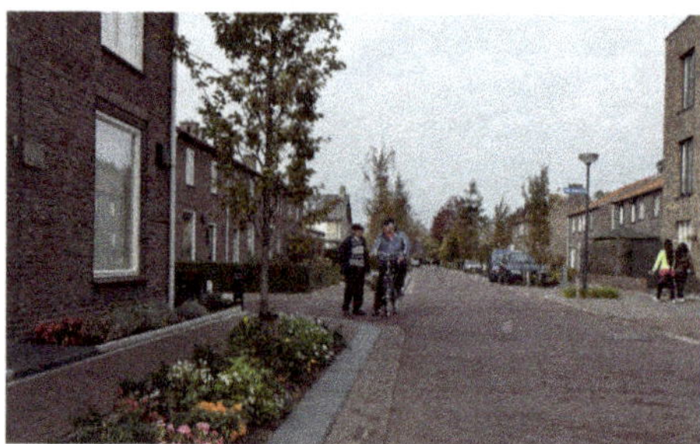

Figure 8. Age-proof neighbourhoods.

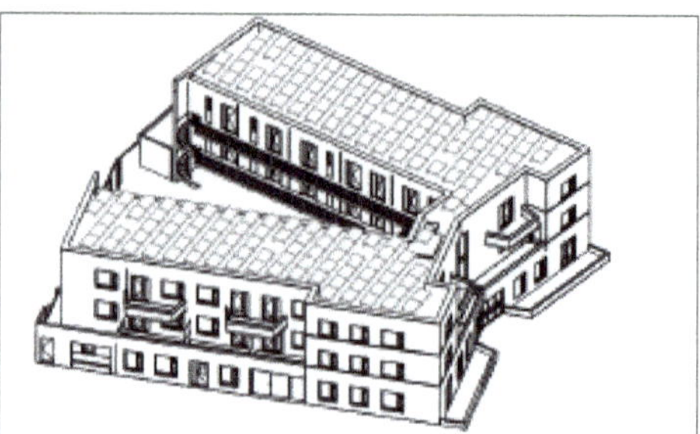

Figure 9. View of 'Vogeltjesbuurt' in Tilburg.

we used the Residential Environment Strategy. The Toolbox provides insight whether programmatic care ambitions can be easily realised or they come with large spatial challenges. The Toolbox joins social and physical aspects and proved useful in the understanding and collaboration between parties with a social background such as care institutions, and parties with a more physical background like housing corporations and the municipalities' urban development section.

A future-proof 'Vogeltjesbuurt' transformation
Renewal of the 'Vogeltjesbuurt' neighbourhood in Tilburg. The area is completely demolished and rebuilt as a future-proof residential area, that takes the elderly into account from an urban scale till the housing design. There was a large demand for large single-family homes and private elderly homes with garden. This has been translated in a broad series of housing typologies, with many suitable for the elderly. With an EPC of 0 the dwellings are very sustainable, adding to the neighbourhoods' affordability. Everything, even the floor plans, have been designed together with the residents. What they got was broad pavements, cosy residential streets, a spacious central square, enough parking spaces and even a communal 'neighbourhood living room' for community activities. Another feature developed on the residents' request, is a new square that forms the heart of the neighbourhood. Old and young come together here on the playground or on the jeux de boule zone.

Reimar von Meding about the project: "This is a neighbourhood with very tight social bonds, something the people value very highly. There are many families that stay here; two or more generations living close to each other. Now, with the Dutch care system ever more depending on volunteer care, such family ties are very important. So in our area transformation, we had to be very careful not to break down these social structures. Also, we designed the residential area in such a way, that people can grow old in their own neighbourhood. The urban planning was done in close cooperation with the residents of the neighbourhood. Through workshops, thematic meetings and questionnaires, the residents were able to set the standards for themes like public space, housing and parking. Look closely and you will find attention to elderly in every aspect of the plan: wheelchair friendly dwellings, very low and broad pavements and plenty of parking lots make the 'Vogeltjesbuurt' very accessible."

The Challenges of Architectural Human Scale in Hospital Environments: Brazilian Holy House of Mercy

Moema Loures

PUC-Rio - Pontifical Catholic University of Rio de Janeiro,
Imaginal Arquitetura, www.imaginal.com.br

We envision an argument that favours human senses in hospital ambiences. We are looking for potential in an atmosphere based on the human scale; the scale of social meetings; the scale that allows patients to be well orientated; the scale of sensory perceptions. We believe that a human-scaled space is the path to encapsulate beauty and simplicity.

Thus, we turn our gaze to the sensitivity of colour uses, light intensities, temperature variation, supporting orientation, way-finding system, and constant interaction of our bodies and movements within the environment in the architectural experience. We take into account the concept of a healing environment, improving sleep and reducing agitation and anxiety, as well as, increasing social relationships.

Moema Loures. *Architect and Urban Designer. Founder of Imaginal Architecture, a Brazilian office focused on healthcare architecture and design. Professor at the Architecture School PUC-Rio (Pontifical Catholic University of Rio de Janeiro). PhD in urban design at Federal University of Rio de Janeiro / École Nationale Supérieure d'Architecture Paris-Malaquais, France. Master at Federal University of Rio de Janeiro / University of Seville - Escuela Técnica Superior de Arquitectura, Spain.*

Our reference-case is the Holy House of Mercy Hospital in Juiz de Fora, Brazil, and the dialogue between architecture and ludic and its interfaces with art and design opposed to rigid institutional routines (Figure 1).

The Holy House is a philanthropic hospital founded in 1854. The main building was built in 1942, has 15 floors and represents the first vertical hospital in Latin America. It is a complex with 508 beds, a consultation and diagnostics centre, emergency services, operating theatres, intensive units, a nursing centre, knowledge, logistics and technical centres, an industrial kitchen and laundry. In the Complex there is a chapel and House, both dating back to the 19th century (Figure 2).

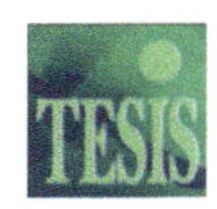

Over the past four years, the institution has been undergoing a period of big changes in its physical infrastructure. Important refurbishments were made to the consulting centre for the Public Healthcare System, the Hemodynamic and Endoscopy centre, the Centre of Sterile Supplies and the Coronary Intensive Care unit.

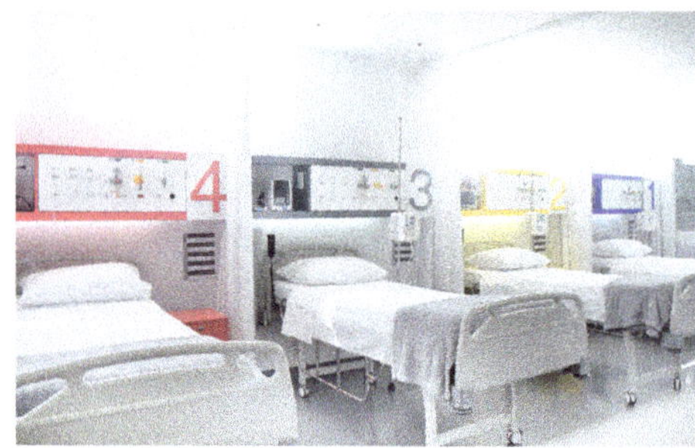

Beyond this, the refurbishment of the hospitality sector includes 55 new rooms. The Holy House of Mercy also incorporates in its complex a building that was refurbished to house the consulting centre for its private healthcare system (Figure 3).

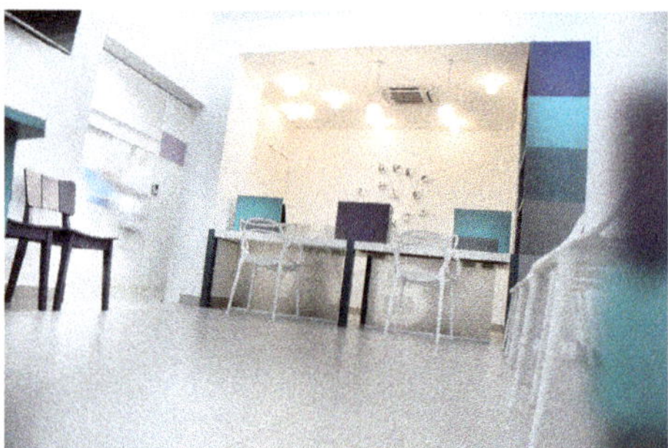

Figure 1. Endoscopy Centre. Stimulating a ludic atmosphere.

Having "the detail" as a keyword, for each work, we were learning how to approach the architecture on a human scale. The goal was always to awaken the playful in a rigorous and complex hospital environment. We start from small to reach a large scale.

Just as the great masters of Dutch architecture taught us in the past, the major design challenge is to master the urban, architecture or design scales. For us the most important thing to remember in a large-scale complex is to not lose the human scale (Figure 4).

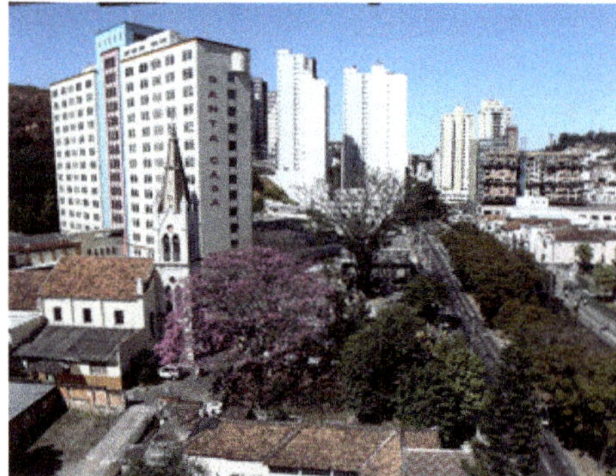

Technology and logistics are incorporated so that they function optimally but do not dominate the atmosphere of the interior space. The first impression of the refurnishing should be that it was easy to be done, and is simple and beautiful. In this project the patient has no idea about all the fills, gases and infrastructures that are needed to keep them alive (Figure 5-6).

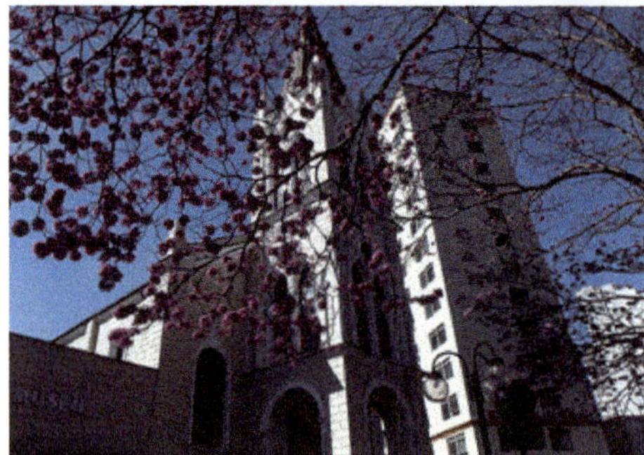

Figure 2. Juiz de Fora Holy House of Mercy.

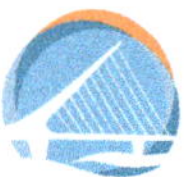

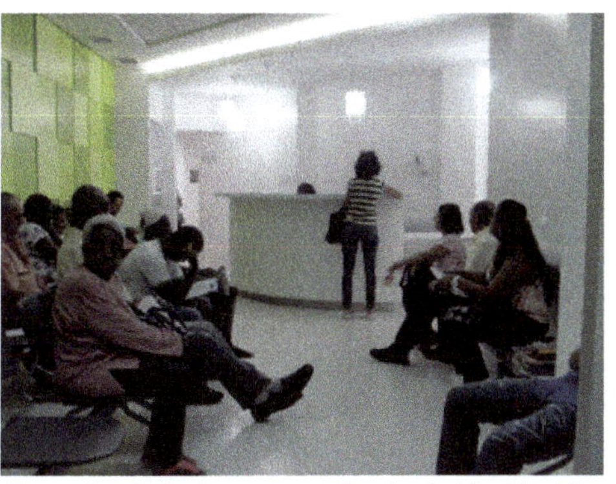
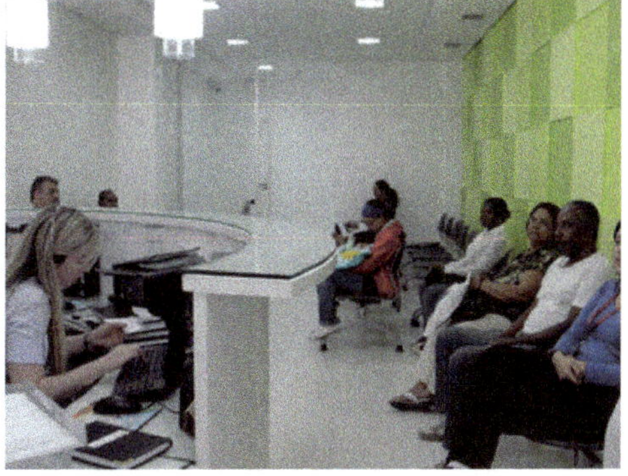

Figure 3. Consulting centre for the Public Healthcare System. The green panel supporting orientation and way-finding system.

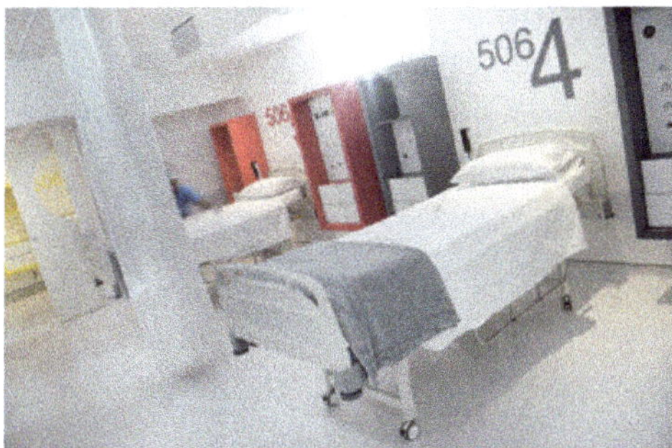

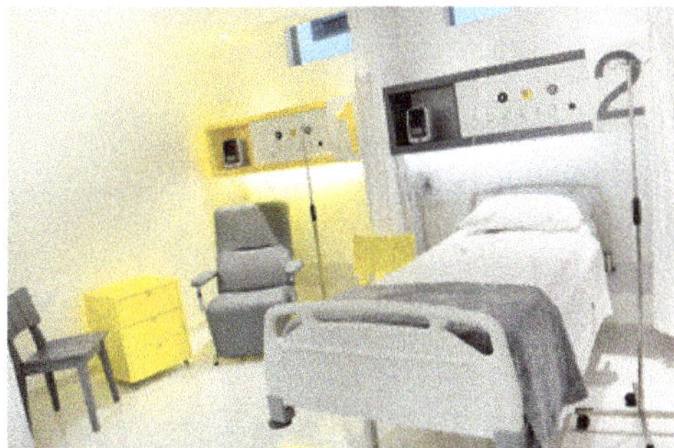

Figure 4. Coronary Intensive Care unit and Endoscopy Centre: designing the details.

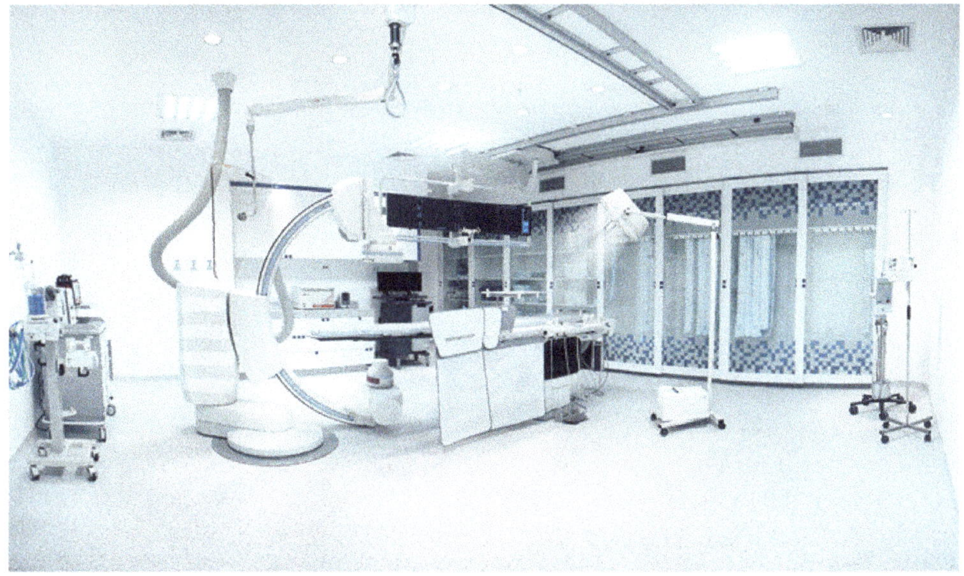

Figure 5. Hemodynamic unit. Interior space atmosphere inside a operate theatre.

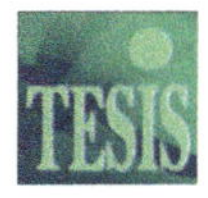

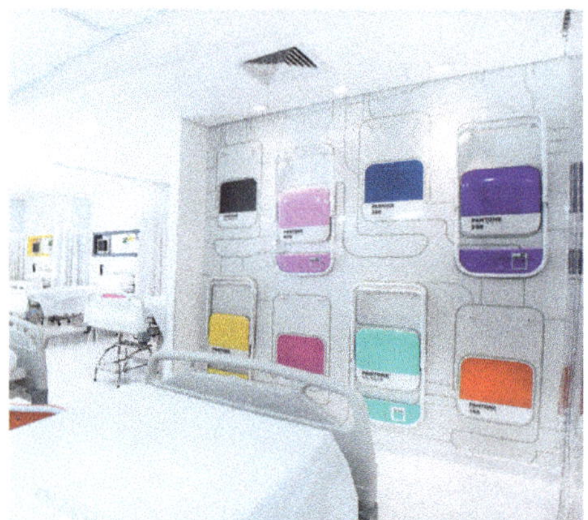

Figure 6. Hemodynamic unit. Resting centre and the chairs panel.

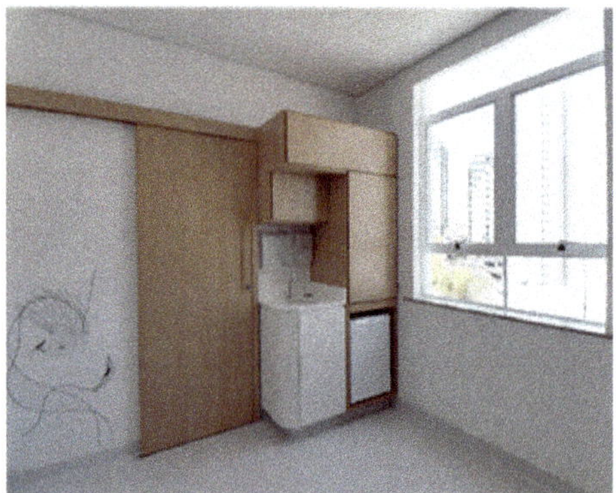

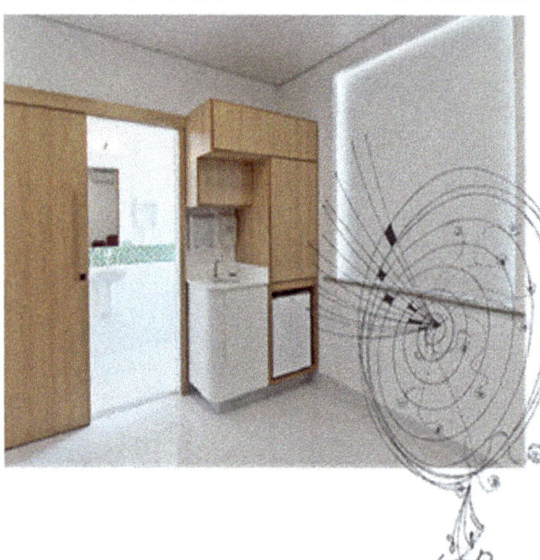

Figure 7. New rooms. Drawings behind the door.

The idea is to arouse curiosity of those who experience the architecture. The drawings, for example, are located in places where they are not evident, the patient will discover them. The forms are not clear, they instigate sensitive imagination (Figure 7).

Another example is the Hemodynamic project: the focus was on the notion of logical, chronological and topological time. Due to the objectivity of time on surgeries as well as the relativity of time in patient recovery, we decided to enhance this concept by creating different watches in which the exercise of seeing time becomes subjective, distracting the patient from focusing on their pain (Figure 8).

In each work we also take into account the context of the whole complex, trying to bring inside the natural light. Daylight is essential for the quality and functionality of a hospital and its adjoining inner areas. Architecture is especially the spatial experience that people undergo in buildings; the relationship with the outside for us is crucial. We are always interested in light, daylight, the light on things; it gives the feeling that there is something behind all understanding (Figure 9).

What made this possible was that the board of directors imposed no restrictions on the spatial orientation and was always supporting the architects' decision. The close relationship with nurses and doctors translating their needs in architectural terms was also essential to achieve our goals.

An integrated approach has resulted in

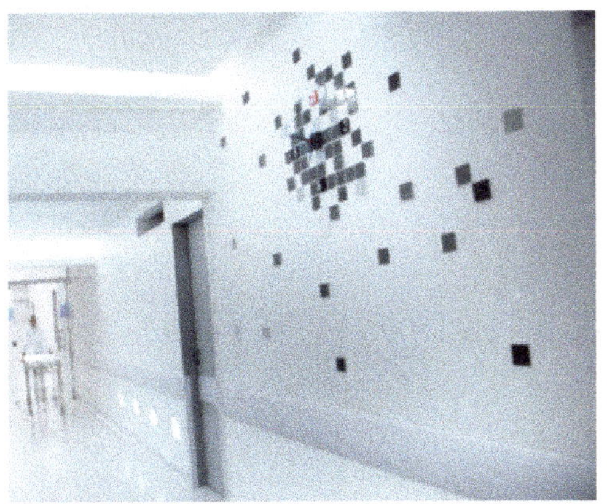

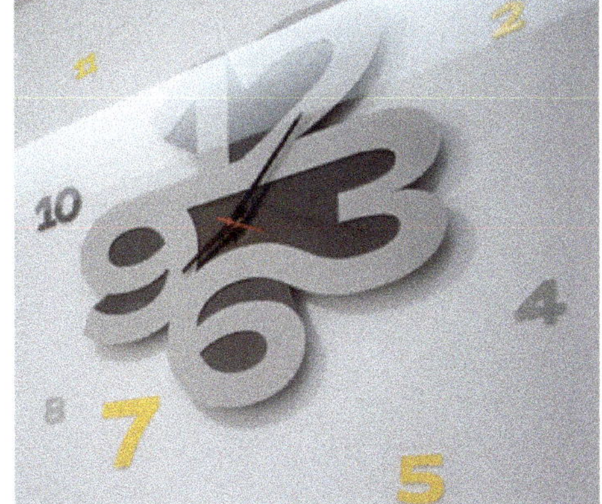

Figure 8. Hemodynamic watches. Distracting the patient and staff.

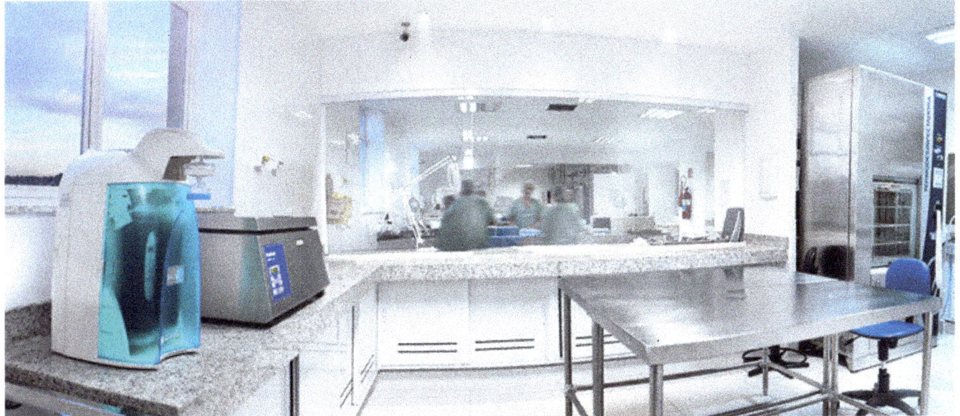

Figure 9. Central of Sterile Supplies. Looking for the health of the staff.

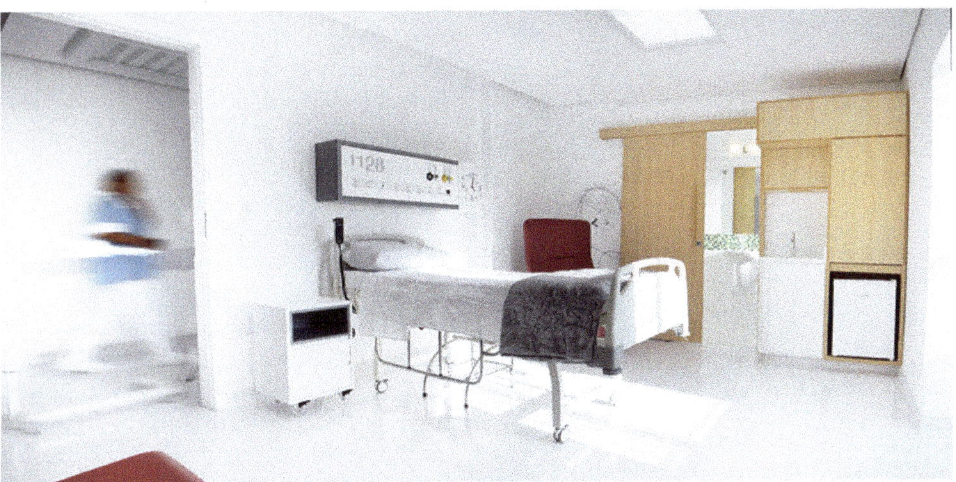

Figure 10. New rooms. Natural light all over.

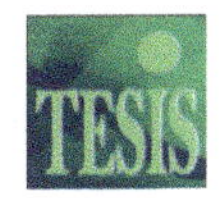

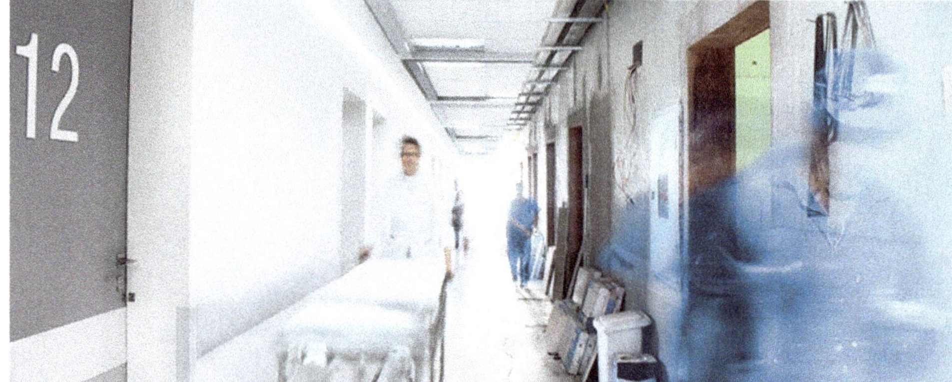

Figure 11. Corridors. Architecture and engineering side by side. Illustrative image.

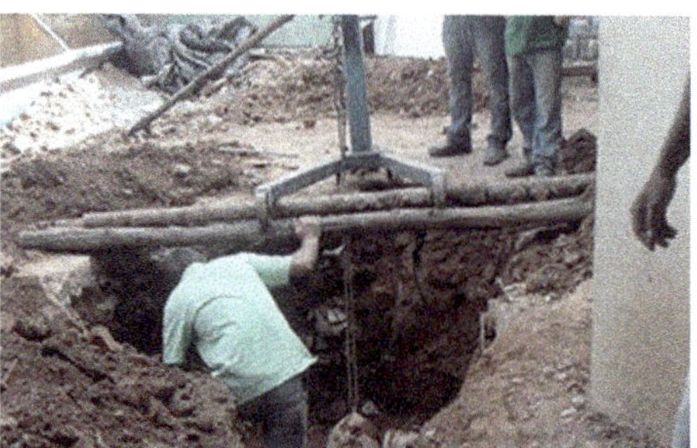

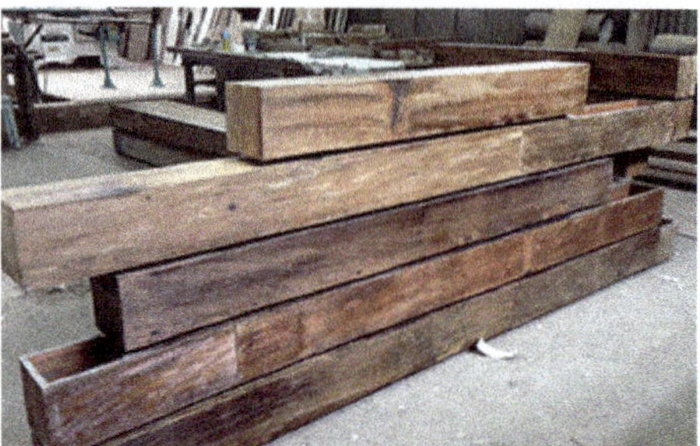

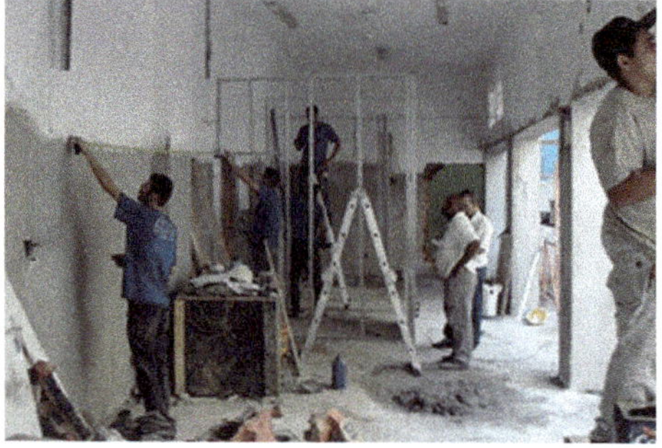

Figure 12. Immersing in the construction site.

our participation for the whole project process, since the first ideas and desires of doctors, nurses and boards right up until the units had started work. We have an architecture office inside the hospital and we work together with the engineers and the construction team. We are immersed in the construction site and in the hospital ambience.

This methodology of completed immersion in the hospital is giving us the opportunity to sense the character that surrounds it, we are able to feel the Hospital behind-the-scenes. Architecture not only to create functional and well designed spaces but also to provide possibilities to animate human instincts and habits by interacting with all of the human senses (Figure 11).

The most important aim of the architecture is the creation of an atmosphere inside and outside the building that helps the patient to recover as quickly as possible and to make the stay as pleasant as possible. We believe that the architecture can reduce the stress-levels of a hospital, medical errors and hospital infections.

Gradually, we approach the concept of living. By inhabiting space, individuals can sense the character that surrounds them. We argue that architecture and space are designed and built for people to use and experience. This feeling of presence, well-being, harmony and beauty is incorporated into the hospital ambience.

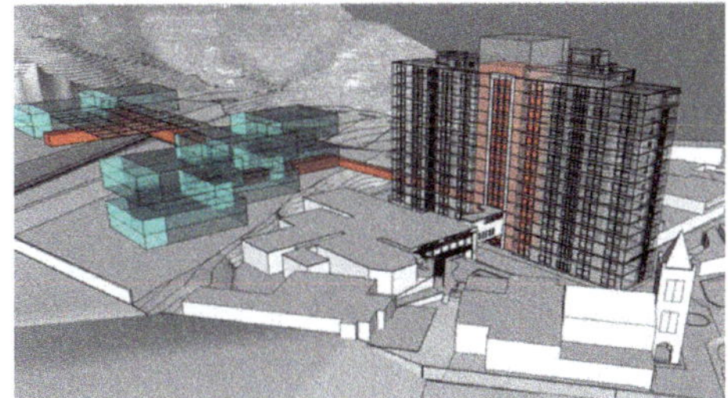

Figure 13. Diagram of Holy House of Mercy Hospital extension. The big boulevard in red.

This year we started the first ideas to build a Holy House of Mercy Hospital extension. Our main idea is to create a big boulevard that connects to the hospital. This space can give the visitors, staff and patients a clear sense of spatial direction (Figure 13).

At the same time, the boulevard is not just a circulation area but also a public space. A "between space" where you can stay to cast a quick glance outside, to talk with other patients or just to have a coffee. A space for socialising, meeting places for family and friends (Figure 14). The boulevard idea came together with a high level of daylight and a maximum support for the professionals and minimum inconvenience for the patients (Figure 15).

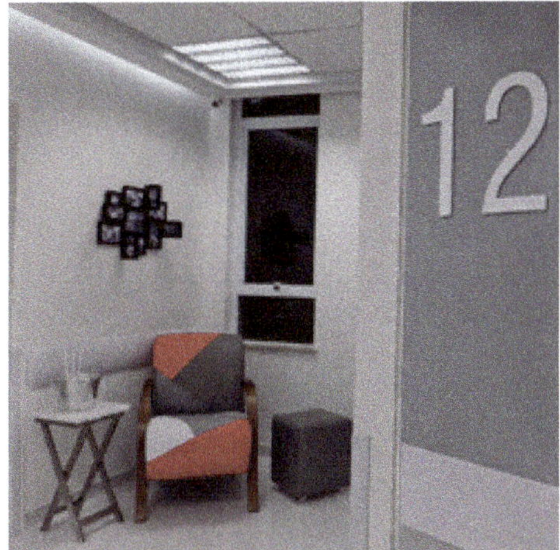

Figure 14. Juiz de Fora Holy House of Mercy Corridors. Place to take a break.

Some concepts came from an exchange trip we did to the Netherlands, vising more than 15 hospitals and some of the most important offices focusing on Hospital Architecture. What we had seen was well planned and designed buildings, with similar costs of Brazil's reality. Unfeasible is the use of certain prefabricated elements with high technology and industrial logistics of demountability and adaptability. This experience brings ideas and architectural solutions that can be leveraged in Brazil, altogether with respect for Brazilian's cultural diversity, traditions and landscape.

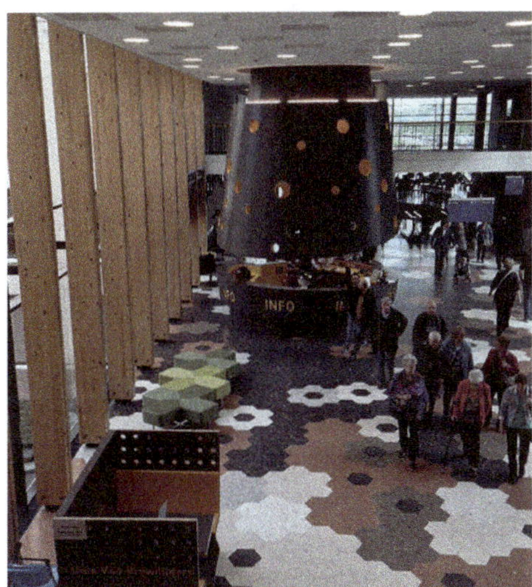

Figure 15. Den Bosh Hospital Boulevard.

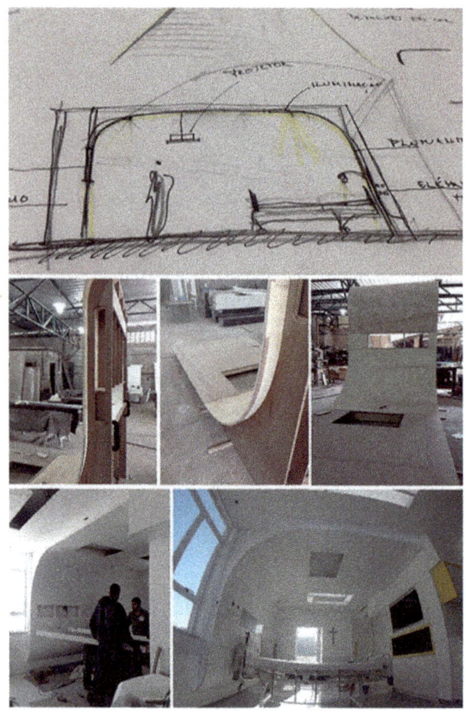

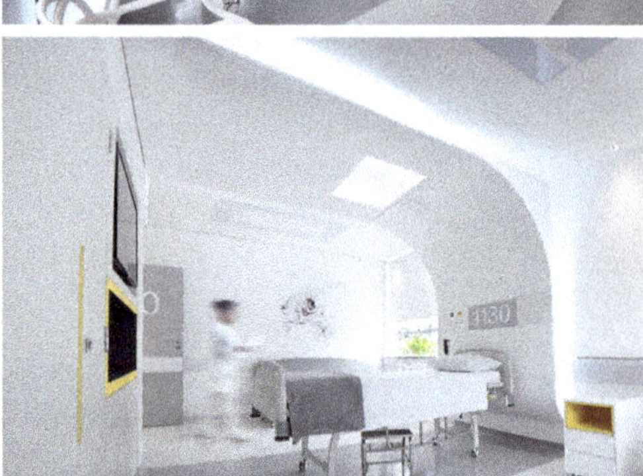

Figure 16. A concept room based on human scale.

Many questions about hospital architecture came to the forefront and were beginning to influence our projects: How the aging population impacts on hospital settings? How telemedicine impacts in reducing hospital beds? Why corridors are often narrow and monotonous and can give rise to common areas for patients and visitors to meet, as a living room? How natural light is utilised throughout the history of architecture and can drive design decisions inside a hospital?

We ask ourselves how we are shaping the infrastructure of the future, knowing that healthcare is changing very fast; a hospital that does not become outdated within a few years but where, in the future, new care concepts and technical developments can be added. At the same time, the only certainty we have is that the human scale will always be essential in architecture and in promoting the speedy recovery of the patient. Human scale will always be the challenge of architecture (Figure 16).

(…) what I am designing will be part of a place, part of its surroundings, used and loved, discovered and bequeathed, given away, abandoned, and perhaps even hated - in short, that it will be lived in, in the wildest sense." Peter Zumthor[1].

[1] *Peter Zumthor Works. Buildings and Projects 1979-1977.*

Wayshowing Systems and Productivity Enhancement in a Changing Environment? Consideration of Patient and Employee Diversity in Healthcare Organizations

Mario Alexander Pfannstiel

mario.pfannstiel@hs-neu-ulm.de
Faculty of Health Management
Neu-Ulm University of Applied Sciences

Due to complex streams of patients, visitors, and employees, hospitals are suitable environments for using signage and orientation systems. Streams of foot traffic are to be specifically steered in the correct directions in order to avoid any intransparent, confusing, or dangerous situations. Within this context, this presentation focuses on the influence of signage and orientation systems on the various user groups in the hospital. The diverse characteristics are presented as comprehension of complexity so that generally valid behaviors can be assumed and the actions of users in the system can be explained. Design possibilities are elaborated upon for improving the passage of users and for undertaking specific optimization measures within a hospital organization. Furthermore, recommendations are made for reducing cost and time and for increasing the quality of service and treatment. With a user-specific signage and orientation system, efforts to achieve organizational objectives should be prioritized and the necessary conditions established which contribute to the stability of a hospital.

Mario A. Pfannstiel*, MSc, MA, is a researcher and lecturer in the field of hospital and healthcare management at the Neu-Ulm University of Applied Sciences. He holds a diploma from the University of Applied Sciences Nordhausen in the field of social management with the major subject finance management, an MSc degree from the Dresden International University in patient management and an MA degree from the Technical University of Kaiserslautern and the University of Witten/ Herdecke in health care and social facilities management. He worked as executive assistant to the medical director in the Heart Centre Leipzig in Germany.*

Introduction to Wayshowing Systems

Wayshowing is a collection of maps, signs and other media that have been developed to aid peoples in hospitals in their journey. A successful wayshowing strategy ensures quality of service by carefully considering the individual needs of each type of user group, as well as the needs of the facility as a cohesive system. It requires a holistic approach, both geospatially and operationally.

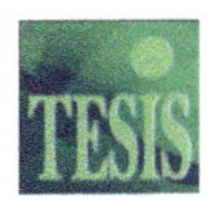

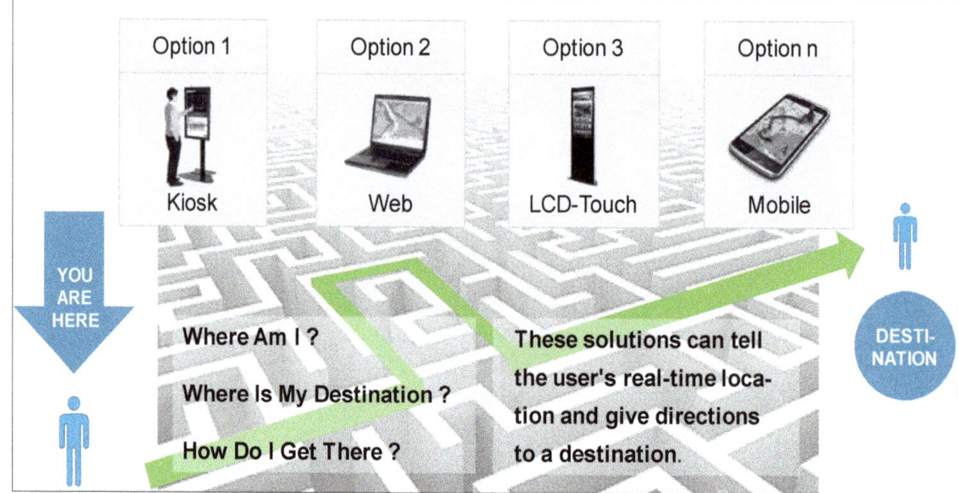

Figure 1. Definition and wayshowing solutions in hospitals. Source: Pfannstiel (2014), Dreamstime (2014).

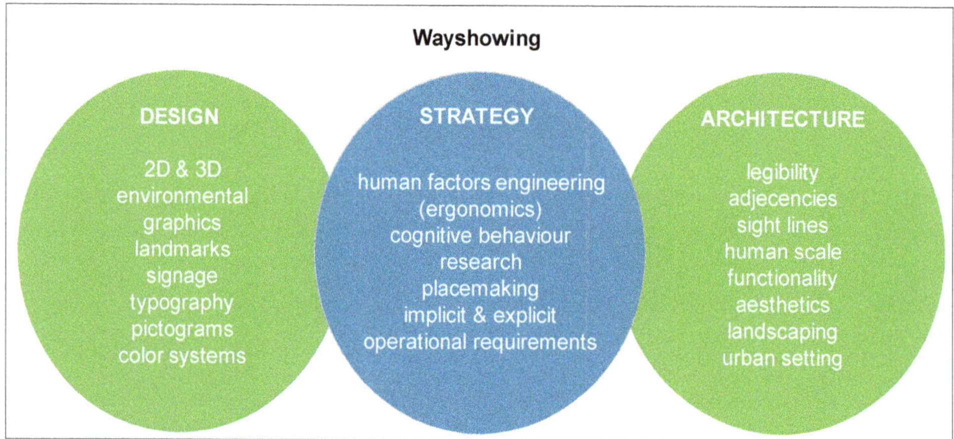

Figure 2. What is the right wayshowing strategy? Source: Blog Wayshowing (2014).

Principles of Effective Wayshowing Systems

Principles include:
- create an identity at each location, different from all others;
- use landmarks to provide orientation cues and memorable locations;
- create well-structured paths and create regions of differing visual character;
- don‘t give the user to many choices in navigation;
- provide signs at decision points to help wayfinding decisions;
- use sight lines to show what‘s ahead.

First time visitors frequently get lost, they go detours, they have larger distance trips and they are rarely on time at the destination.

Requirements for Holistic Wayshowing Systems

Wayshowing systems should:
- emanate a friendly and harmonious atmosphere;
- be safe, clearly and unambiguously structured;
- respond to the human perception;
- take into account the architectural features of the hospital;
be considered and designed for the different religious and ethnic backgrounds;
- address the cultural understanding and personal experiences and individual expections of peoples and groups.

What Role Will Perception Play?

An individual's understanding is always less than perfect.

This creates perceptual uncertainty, which means that our views of hazard risk and damage potential are at best partial and selective.

Every individual receives signals and stimuli from the environment around them, and uses these in building up an understanding of that environment and in deciding how best to respond and behave in relation to that environment.

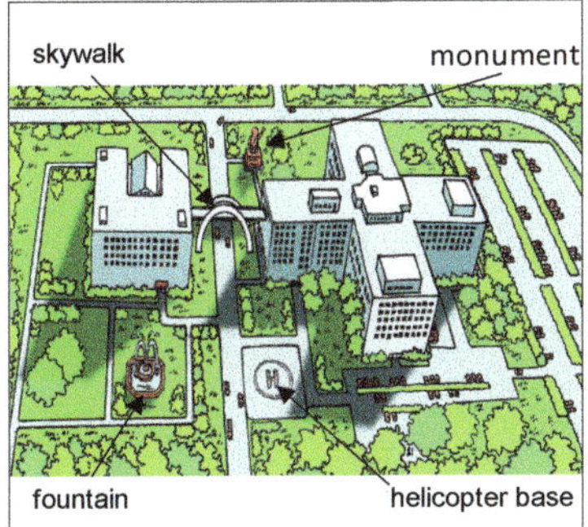

Figure 3. Scheme for applying the principles of effective wayshowing systems. Source: Pfannstiel (2014).

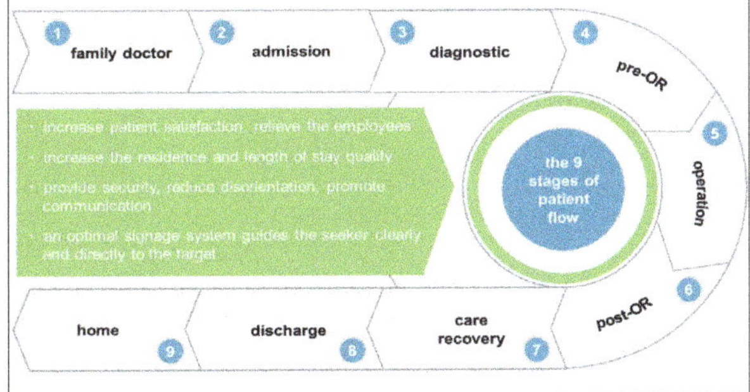

Figure 4. Advantages of holistic wayshowing systems. Source: Pfannstiel (2014).

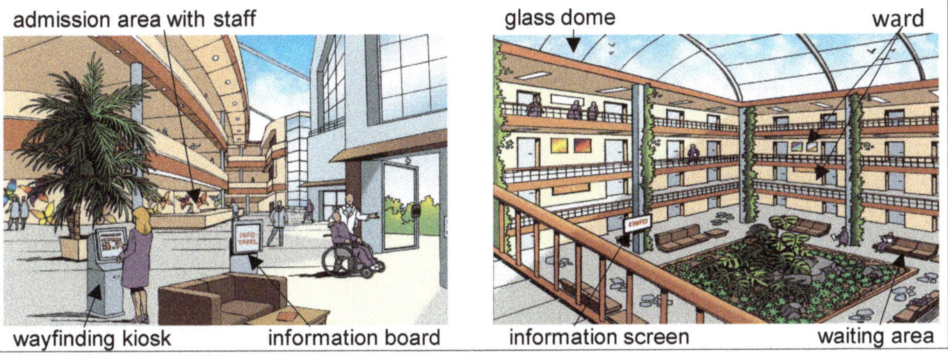

Figure 5. Requirements for holistic wayshowing systems. Source: Pfannstiel (2014).

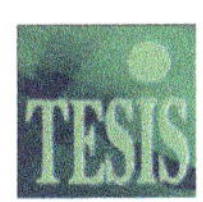

People Perception of the Hospital Environment

They hear strange noises, feel temperature differences and notice unknow smell. In conclusion the hospital environment affects well-being and motivation.

Questions about strategy-making:
- How will customers see us as exceptional?
- How can we create a valuable feel for our customers?
- What do we want our voice to say and sound like for our customers?
- What taste will we leave in customer‘s mouths?
- What smell will customers associate with us?

Colors

Why colors matter in hospitals: colors carry a message; colors can sway thinking, change actions, and cause reactions; color is one of the first things you notice; colors are responsible for different emotions; colors can irritate or soothe your eyes, raise your blood pressure or suppress your appetite; when used in the right ways, colors can even save on energy consumption; color sets a mood and it is a language; colors are a powerful form of communication.

Disadvantages of color guidance systems: two out of three people are unable to perceive color guidance systems in hospitals; color guidance systems usually generate higher costs; for people with color blindness and color vision defect there is no benefit; in low light conditions, there is the risk that colors are mixed; people remember different colors differently (depending on the culture).

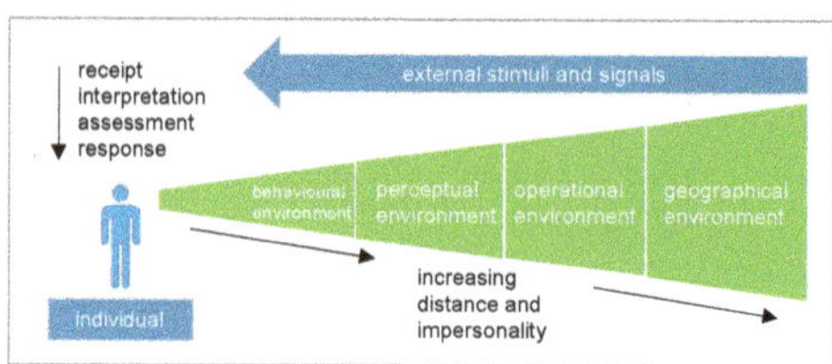

Figure 6. Perception role. Source: Park (2014).

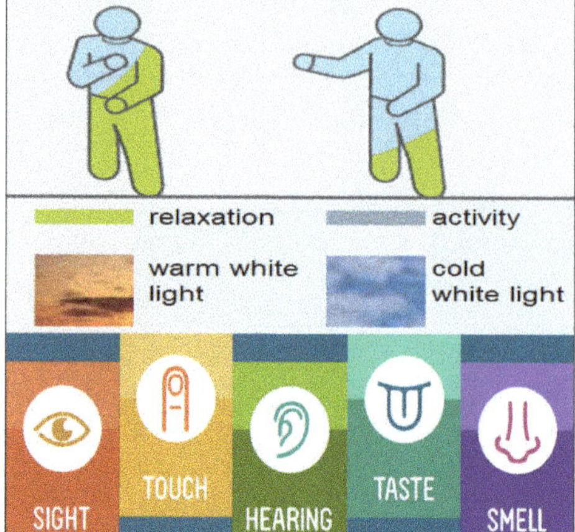

Figure 7. People perception of the hospital environment. Source: Siemens Healthcare (2014), Naphtali (2014).

OPTIMISM	CLARITY **WARMTH**	Yellow
FRIENDLY	CHEERFUL **CONFIDENCE**	Orange
EXCITEMENT	PASSIONATE **STIMULATING**	Red
CREATIVE	IMAGINITIVE **WISE**	Purple
TRUST	DEPENDABLE **STRENGTH**	Blue
PEACEFUL	GROWTH **HEALTH**	Green
PURE	INNOCENT **PRACTICAL**	White
BALANCE	NEUTRAL **CALM**	Grey
EARTHY	SIMPLE **DEPENDABLE**	Brown
EXCLUSIVE	PRESTIGIOUS **LUXE**	Black

Figure 8. Colors perception. Source: Pfannstiel (2014).

Design for Disabled People in Hospitals

Type of disability and medical condition: 63% physical disabilities; 10% mental or emotional disabilities; 9% cerebral disorders; 17% without reported type of disability. Source: Statistisches Bundesamt (2014).

Material Characteristics of Patient/ Employee Sidewalks

Advantages of carpets in hospitals: carpets absorb noise and thus increase the well-being; carpets can save energy costs by up to 30%; carpets with comfort back are price, environmentally, and health-conscious, moreever, they are easy to clean and maintain; carpets are dust binding and this is good e.g. if a person has a house dust mite allergy (the concentration of dust in the air can decrease up to 50%); one disadvantage: the transport of patients in beds over carbeting is a bit difficult.

Disadvantages of Multilingual Wayshowing Systems

Disadvantages: amount of information increases, costs increase by signs size; translation difficulties arise, literacy and language skills of patients/employees.

What should be considered: one language should be emphasised; multilingual handouts and cards provide the best support of symbol signs; two languages should be differentiated by contrast, lines and distance, but they should also have a visual connection at the same time.

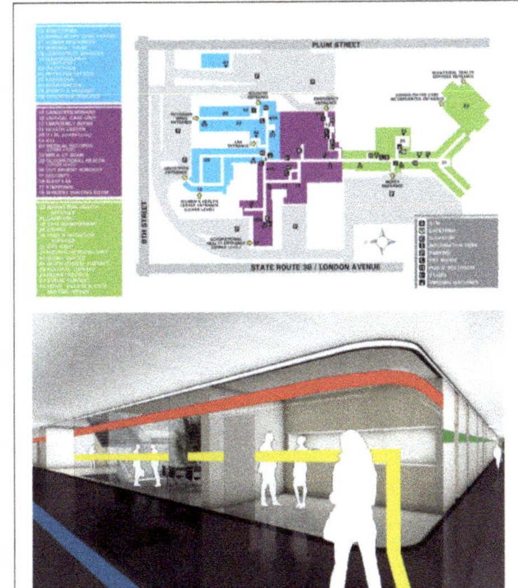

Figure 9. Disadvantages of color guidance systems. Source: Tiborplanet (2014), Hollback (2014).

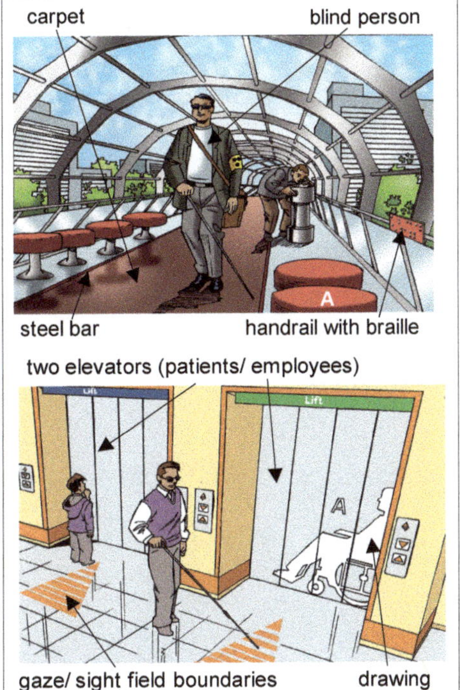

Figure 10. Design for disabled people in hospitals. Source: Pfannstiel (2014).

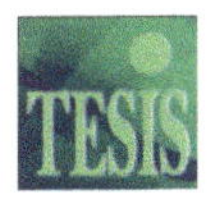

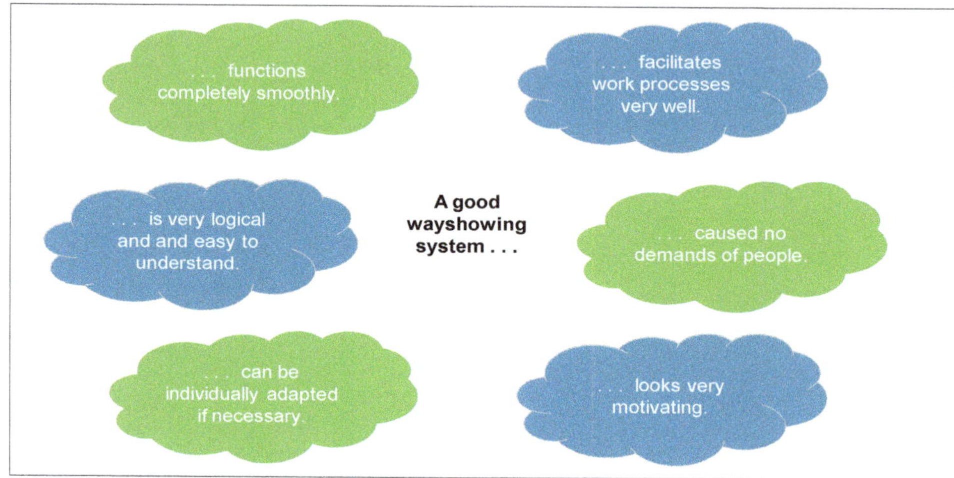

Figure 11. What are good wayshowing systems? Source: Pfannstiel (2014).

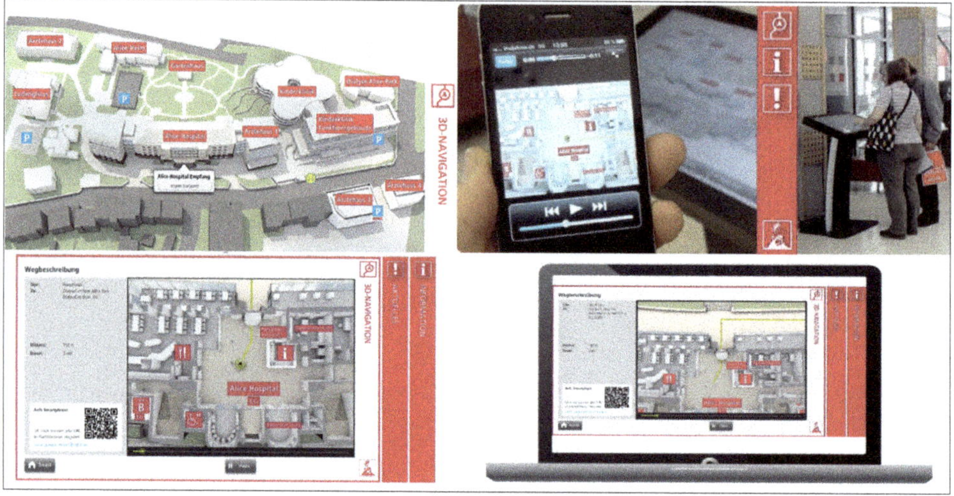

Figure 12. Example: Holistic Wayshowing System. Source: SIS (2014).

Example: Holistic Wayshowing System

The building navigation system «Guide 3D» implemented a new technology at the Alice-Hospital. Source: SIS (2014): the special feature of this solution is the option of having a start-destination connection in three-dimensional space or building displayed dynamically as an animated clip at your computer at home, at the info terminal on site or on your cell phone or smartphone. The contents are edited by the Alice hospital via a web interface and then immediately updated in the system. No additional costs arise for data main-tenance or content updates and all platforms are kept equally up to date.

Going to the Shopping Mall for Healthcare
The Case of Centro Médico Palmares

Paula Cepparo and Verónica Morist

cepparo.briggs@gmail.com
Cepparo.Briggs Arquitectura Integral & Pharus Asesores Económicos, Argentina

Since the early 80's separating the ambulatory services from the hospital environment has been one of the most important and consistent trends. This has generated new architectural as well as business typologies. One of these new typologies locates the ambulatory healthcare service within the retail store environment. In this presentation we aim to introduce a case study located in Mendoza, Argentina: Centro Médico Palmares. As professionals we have been able to work with the institution for the past 12 years following its footsteps and helping in its development and growth. We worked in an interdisciplinary team that included architects as well as economists, physicians and healthcare administrators. Today Centro Médico Palmares is the most important Outpatient Medical Center in the region having more than 700 patient visits per day. Our study also reveals that, locating the medical center in the shopping mall is not only beneficial for the institution, but also for the mall as well.

Paula Cepparo *– Achitect. Education: PhD Candidate (Universidad de Mendoza), LEED A.P., Master in Architecture (University of Arizona), Architect (University of Mendoza). Fellowships and Awards: Tradewell Fellowship (2001-WHR Architects – Houston, Texas), Graduate Student Fellowship Award (1998/2000 – University of Arizona – Tucson, Arizona), Interamerican Foundation Fellowship for field studies in LatinAmerica (1999 – Tucson, Arizona). Professional Experience in Medical Planning and Programming: Cepparo.briggs Arquitectura Integral (2006/today – Mendoza), Independent Practitioner (2004/2006 - Mendoza), Sr. Medical Planner at Morris Architects (2003/2004 – Houston, Texas), WHR Architects and Q Group Advisors Tradewell Fellow and Jr. Medical Planner (2001/2003 – Houston, Texas), Independent Practitioner (1996/1998 – Mendoza).*

Development

The benefits of separating the ambulatory services from the hospital facilities are countless. The first one refers to the sense of wellness of patients that are not sick. For these patients the hospital environment becomes scary and a real hazard, because there, healthy people has to interact with sick people.

Also, there are economic benefits in separating the ambulatory services from the hospital itself. Ambulatory services have less restrictive building codes and infrastructure than acute care hospitals so, in the end, they can live in a less ex-

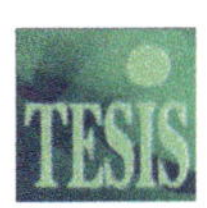

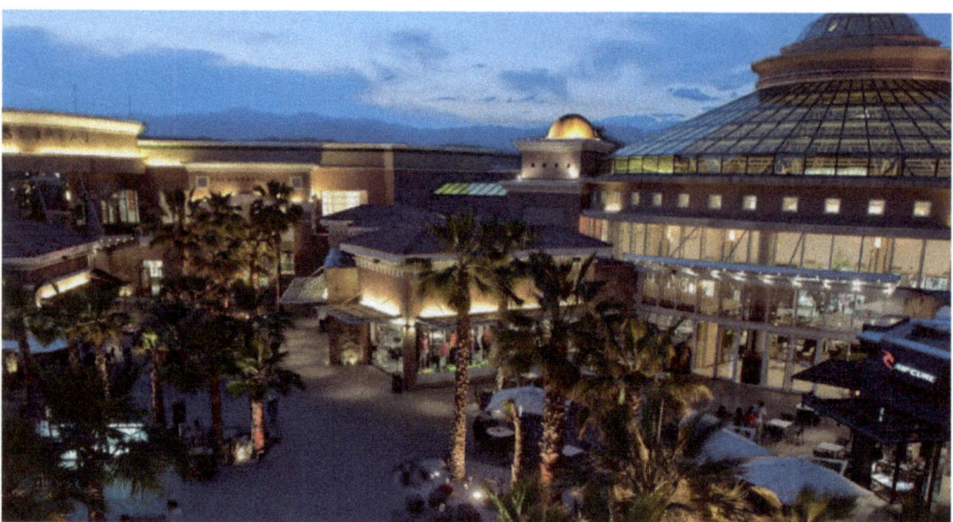

Figure 1. Palmares Open Mall, Mendoza - Argentina.

pensive building. The same happens in the operational end. The kind of personnel required for an ambulatory service is very different from the one required for a hospital. From the operational point of view, a hospital works 24 hours a day when an ambulatory service can work different hours and this has a huge impact in operational costs.
In the U.S. traditional typologies include Clinics, Medical Office Buildings, Ambulatory Surgery Centers as well as specialized centers like Cancer Centers, Trauma Centers, Rehab Centers, etc. Some of them are located within the site of a larger medical center like Memorial Hermann the Woodlands Medical Center or Memorial Hermann Memorial City Medical Center, both in Houston, Texas and others are located as freestanding centers like Kelsey Seabold Clinic (Houston, Texas).

New trends are directing ambulatory care facilities towards a new scenario directly related with retail facilities. Retail stores like Walgreens, Wal-Mart and Target are now offering what are called walk-in clinics. Leasing space in a retail store is cheaper than creating a stand-alone building and it has all of the benefits associated with the store location. These clinics treat a variety of no-life threatening diseases and help to keep people healthy, which, in the end means less healthcare costs overall. Unlike family doctors, they offer immediate healthcare in an easy to find location with plenty of parking space.
Currently other kinds of efforts are taking place. With the U.S. economy rundown, many spaces at shopping malls are free to lease and are being taken by healthcare facilities to develop ambulatory centers like Vanderbilt University Medical Center that occupies today what once was One Hundred Oaks Mall in Nashville, Tennessee.
In other cases, healthcare institutions are becoming tenants in a shopping mall such as Main Line Health Ambulatory facility located in Exton Square Mall,

in Exton, Philadelphia. These are new explorations and not all of them are successful. In 2012, the Mayo Clinic opened a space in the Mall of America called "Create Your Mayo Clinic Experience" to close it in 2013.
In South America we are ahead of the curve in this particular topic. In Chile it is common to have healthcare facilities incorporated into retail malls and it has been so for the past 15 years. In 1997 Parque Arauco Mall incorporated a Medical Center. One year later Plaza Vespucio Mall did the same. Today, most retail malls in Chile have a healthcare center as part of their programmatic requirements.

In 1999 my partner, Architect Viviana Briggs, was asked to design an Ambulatory Center within a shopping mall in Mendoza, Argentina. It was something really exiting and new. Because of the close relationship between Mendoza and Santiago in Chile, the group of physicians who hired her was able to visit the Parque Arauco Mall initiative and was inspired to do the same. They were offered 1000 meters of space in the first floor of the new addition of "Palmares Open Mall" in Godoy Cruz, Mendoza. Palmares Open Mall is located south of the city of Mendoza in one of the areas that grew the most on the past 15 years. It is surrounded by middle class and upper middle class neighborhoods.

Centro Médico Palmares opened its doors in 2001. Today it is the most important Outpatient Medical Center in the region having more than 700 patient visits per day. It includes services such as:

1) Physician consultation in several specialties such as general practitioner, pediatrics, otolaryngology, ophthalmology, nutrition, urology, orthopedics, gastroenterology, gynecology, obstetrics, pneumonology, etc.
2) Complete imaging center, including traditional X-Ray, mammography, echography, densitometry, dental X-ray, tomography and MRI.
3) Complete laboratory
4) And a vaccine and immunization service.

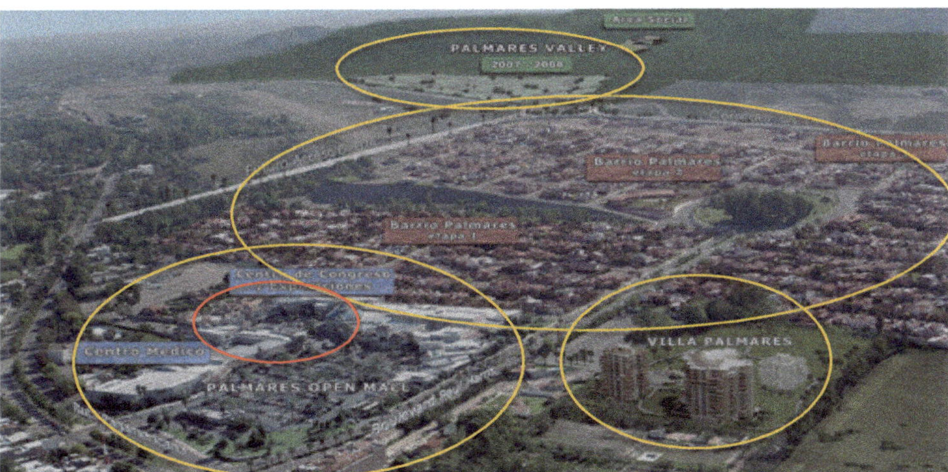

Figure 2. Centro Médico Palmares development.

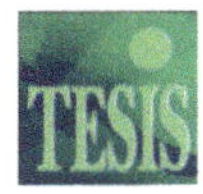

New centralized reception
40% increase in waiting area
New pediatric area
5 Exam rooms

Figure 3. Centro Médico Palmares 2014.

In the year 2008 we designed and build the Palmares Ambulatory Surgery Center with 3 OR´s and 8 recovery rooms. This is the case study we would like to present. Since Centro Médico Palmares has 12 years of experience and has been a very successful model we think it could help illuminate several issues regarding the development of ambulatory healthcare services within the retail environment.

In 2012 we were hired to work on a strategic plan for Centro Médico Palmares. We hold meetings with physicians and administrators using tools of graphic facilitation in order to develop a common vision that would help the institution grow.

During the first years of its existence, Centro Médico Palmares had no real competition because it was unique. However, when we were called to work on the strategic plan, this situation was about to change. Until then, Mendoza only had two shopping malls and only one of them had an outpatient healthcare facility, but new malls were arriving and the developers had seen the potential of having a medical center as an anchor store. Our analysis focused in these immediate threats and how to make Centro Médico Palmares more competitive not only from the medical point of view but from the architectural and business as well.

Many things had changed during its first 10 years of existence and in order to be able to grow it was important to align the new strategy with the physical space and operational changes. In order to achieve that alignment we had to work along with patients, personnel and healthcare providers as well as with sales representatives from the shopping mall.

In this presentation we showed our work process, the physical evolution of a healthcare service within a retail environment as well as the economic and patient data to support the decision making.

Today, the threats that were envisioned during our strategic plan are built and working, however, they hadn´t been as successful as once predicted. There are many reasons for that, but probably the main one is the lack of knowledge about how to approach a healthcare business within a retail environment. Centro Médico Palmares is still the leader in the region.

Concretion of a Palliative Care Facility from the Holistic Concept of Man. Casa de la Bondad

Alicia Pringles Belvideri

apringles@faud.unsj.edu.ar; arq.pringles@gmail.com
Dra. Arq., Instituto Regional de Planeamiento y Hábitat- Facultad de Arquitectura, Urbanismo y Diseño- Universidad Nacional de San Juan. Av. Ignacio de La Roza y Meglioli - Rivadavia - San Juan

A historical survey of the epistemological changes in medicine and architecture laid bare since ancient times, two sciences were closely related and humanize when they linked the man and his feelings, his physical and social environment; approach endorsed by anthropology, environmental psychology and neuroscience.

The origin of this research work showed that within the ideology of the architecture for the health of Argentina between 1980 and 2010, is this holistic approach to man and is consistent with the humanized medical thinking. Therefore, theories or project proposals, in addition to providing adequate development of medical procedures, are entered under the totalizing vision of man.

This paper presents the projective and materialization of the "House of Kindness" Casa de la Bondad San Juan, as a realization of a corpus of postulates or project proposals that views man as a holistic process. This institution is for palliative care of terminally ill cancer patients, and is an architectural type that predominates in the humanization of architecture and meet their psycho-social and environmental needs.

Alicia Pringles Belvideri. *Doctor of Architecture University FAUD-Mendoza. Architect FAUD-National University of San Juan. Academic Secretary of FAUD-National University of San Juan. Teachers (in the same house of higher learning) and researcher at the Institute of Regional Planning and Habitat -IRPHa-FAUD-UNSJ. Director and Co-Project Director for Research, Extension and Research Fellowships in UNSJ. Author of the book: PRINGLES Alicia. (2012). Architecture for Health and Medical Thought Humanized. Interpretation of architecture for health as holistic approach to man: Editorial Académica Spanish. Germany. ISBN: 978-3-659-04944-6. Member of Pringles and Bastianelli S.R.L.*

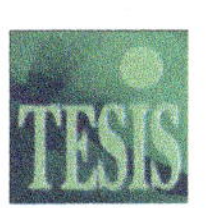

Introduction

> *"[...] The palliative care involve the comprehensive care of people in its total reality: biological, psychosocial and spiritual throughout all phases of oncologic disease: from prevention and diagnosis to treatment of symptoms , care of the end of life also comprising."* [1]

The "House of Kindness" or home hospice, provide comprehensive palliative care in terminal cancer patients, homeless without family support. It is a work that is part of the mission of Open Hands Foundation, Fundación Manos Abiertas, an organization of Christian inspiration born in 1992, and arises from the need to sustain this type of patients who are outside any therapeutic resource and where the national hospital structure is not prepared to address them, what motivates many patients to spend their last days in a state of loneliness and abandonment[2].

Therefore, the design of this architectural type was based on a research[3] made. The research, analyzed hospital architecture from its origins to the present in the transformation of the concept and types, and interpreted this evolution as the result of changes in the concepts and methods of action of the medicine.

The medicine of the twentieth century was marked by progress in science, instrumental developments, technology, specialization and the tendency to attend more to the disease than the patient. At the same time, the hospital architecture is addressed as one of the most sophisticated and complicated to solve housing concepts. The architects had to confront the complexity by distributing its use in mono-functional areas, conveniently solving their linkages. As perfect machines, hospitals and health centers became places of efficient operation but in return, became cold and alienating, they generated an uncomfortable stay, prolonged waits and prevented welfare, decreasing the efficacy of therapeutic actions.

In the late twentieth century, began to shift the focus of care and since, we understand the patient as sick man and tries to scientifically interpret how the disease is apprehended by medicine and the patients themselves. Likewise, anthropological research that helped identify the social imaginary about the causes of illness and healing were performed, and two representative models of medical thought were built: one focused on the disease or other streamlined and focused on the patient or humanized man (Laplantine, 1999).

With the interpretation of these models and the change in the concept of what the disease is and what should be the care of the sick man, the medical discipline initiated a conceptual translation that places the patient at the center of reflection and action. This humanization

[1] *Véase Instituto Nacional del Cáncer (2014). ¿Qué son los cuidados paliativos?. En: http://www.msal.gov.ar/inc/index.php/acerca-del-cancer/cuidados-paliativos. [Recuperado el 20-03-2014].*

[2] *Véase Manos Abiertas (2014). Cuidados Paliativos. Casa de la Bondad. En: http://manosabiertas.org.ar/Obra.aspx?id=11. [Recuperado el 20-03-2014].*

[3] *Pringles Alicia. (2012). Arquitectura para la Salud y Pensamiento Médico Humanizado. Interpretación de la arquitectura para la salud según el enfoque holístico del hombre: Editorial Académica Española. Alemania.*

of scientific concepts, is accompanied by hospital architecture and seeks to ensure that the passage through the hospital or care facility more bearable and pleasant stay in them.
The latter raises the need to generate a friendly environment that reduces the physical imprint of medical technology and promote the mood of patients. However, the proposed humanization often been approached from a superficial approach. Concepts related materials appear to meet a dual function cosmetic and hygiene, comfort and joy, etc. Therefore, it became necessary to find out where the truth lies in humanizing health buildings under the new medical thinking within the discipline of architects imaginary.

Hospital Architecture and Medical Anthropological Thought

From Classical Antiquity to the birth of the Modern Age, medicine and architecture regarded man as microcosm receptacle while the cosmos. That is, the nature of man contained a healing force and medical care with the environment around him and its architecture became consistent with that inner strength to eliminate the cause of the disease. Therefore, the physician, the atmosphere, the patient and family operated in coincidence with the curative action.
The man considered from the point of ontological, whole view. You could not understand the man in isolation from his body and the social length, between them a continuum linking the human condition stretched. Until the Middle Ages hospitals, where most monastic, gave assistance to the sick and infirm in the judgment of charity the Christian world.
In the modern age, with the rise of individualism and the mechanistic philosophy places man as a measure of the nature and rationalizes, body and soul, relegating sensory perceptions to the field of illusion. In architecture greater degrees of rationality are introduced to the detriment of mythological and religious legitimization, with minimal symbolic pretensions and greater efficiency and functionality. Thus began within the meanings of society, to miss the holistic man rooting for an individualistic view of the same.
The hyper-modern medicine of the twentieth century led to anatomical and physiological knowledge to the extreme degree of refinement. The anthropological model focused on the disease, comes to an isolation of disease and responds with an opposite measure: medication or surgery. The man is oblivious to his illness and abandoned passively medical knowledge (Laplantine, 1999:57-64). The instrumental relation of the body, brought on the complexity and automation of medical procedures and laboratory. Thus, the mid-twentieth century in Argentina, was characterized at the hospital and health center as an efficient technical-functional and evolving organism.
A mid-twentieth century a return to roots in holistic conception of man and the need to humanize medicine, its institutions and buildings are observed; anthropological medical model focused on disease-centered model is the sum sick man. In this second model, or tendency, every complaint or etiological interpretation of the causes of the disease, refers to a second reading comes from an oscillation between an external and an internal cause of the patient. In the latter

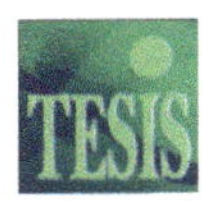

causality attends perceived importance to the individual not only as a participant but as a disease in its own generator in its current state.

From different theoretical views, one can infer that humanize means responding to man holistically. For example, satisfy your needs regarding your own person-body, soul and thoughts and their relationship with the social environment and the physical surrounding. The position of linkage between the physical and social environment man is also supported by other sciences such as anthropology, environmental psychology and neuroscience.

Also, from the basic postulates of the phenomenological tradition of existentialism, the architecture of the mid-twentieth century began to experience an aesthetic efficiency arising from the will of the subject by interacting with the world through the body. In this sense, the humanized space is created from the living man. But this living, is an intimate relationship in which something psychic or spiritual is introduced or amalgamated with some space.

Interpretation of the Discourse of Architects

Often, within the architectural guidelines are those latent rules but are operative as social meanings of architecture. They are presented as imaginary spatial and formal guidelines or are experienced as core indicators for the realization of projects. These imaginary serve several functions, including providing ammunition to design spaces. That is why, defines architecture as a symbolic mediation that translates through their languages and works of cultural significance (Sarquis, 2002).

Imaginary consist of representations of society that governs their conduct, ideals and values, and are configured in anthropological models from social practices and discourses. Therefore, opening the discipline and approach it from interaction with other knowledge, it can be inferred about the humanization of buildings on the medical thinking. In addition, the relationship established between the medical-anthropological models and projective positions that characterize a streamlined architecture for humanized or health may interpret the emergence of different hospital types in Argentina during the twentieth century.

The investigation sought to demonstrate that architectural patterns that guide the architecture for health in Argentina, from 1980 to 2010, meet the architectural requirements and are organized from the triple anthropological dimension of man, because they respond to the patient, their physical surroundings and their social environment. I mean that cultural meanings that arise from medical- anthropological models are reflected in the imaginary discipline of architecture and are present in the discourse of architects, when a projective position argues.

House of Kindness. Realization of a Project Process

The reinterpretation of this return to roots in holistic conception of man and the need to humanize medicine, its institutions and buildings emerged in the late twentieth century, devoting greater importance to the patient not only as a participant in their disease own generator but as it stands and is the result of multiple equilibria: between man and himself, between man and the surroundings, and between man and his social environment.

That is why it is possible to explain and predict an architecture for the human health when architectural patterns in three anthropological levels are ordered from this integrative approach of man, and answer is given:

- The patient as person, first man-anthropological dimension, and promotes: safe, intimate, comfortable and familiar environments, spaces for reflection and spiritual therapies that guide the imagination, and allow the patient to find its meaning with life and reduce levels of anxiety or stress (Figure 1).

- At the social environment of the patient, second man-anthropological dimension, and creates a comfortable environment for family and therapists, and spaces devoted to providing information to help the patient understand and adhere to treatment options (Figure 2).

- Finally, the environment surrounding the patient, third anthropological dimension of man, amalgamated with the general space or cosmos, and provides comfortable rooms with natural light and has views towards nature and images that provide positive distractions, with connections to gardens or natural environments that integrate the man with the environment and promote therapeutic treatments.

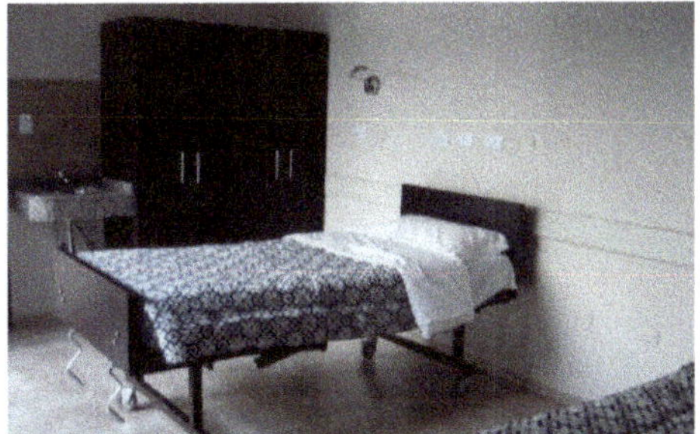

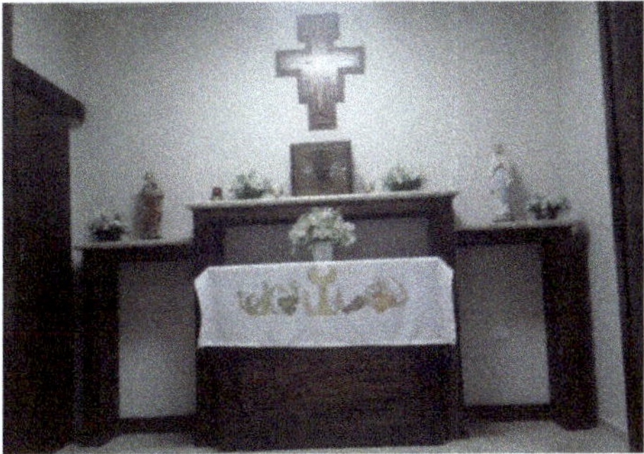

Figure 1. Patient environments.

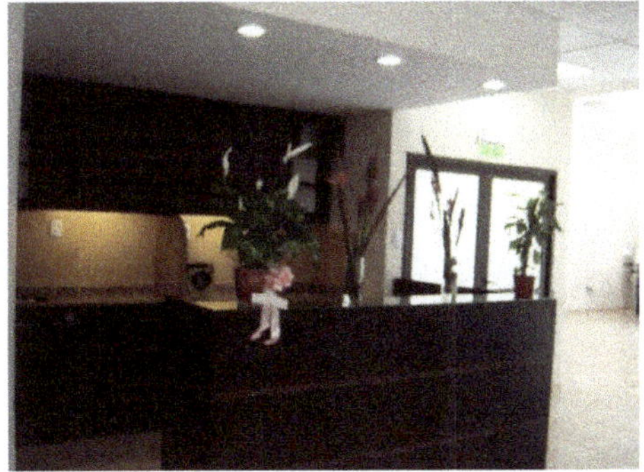

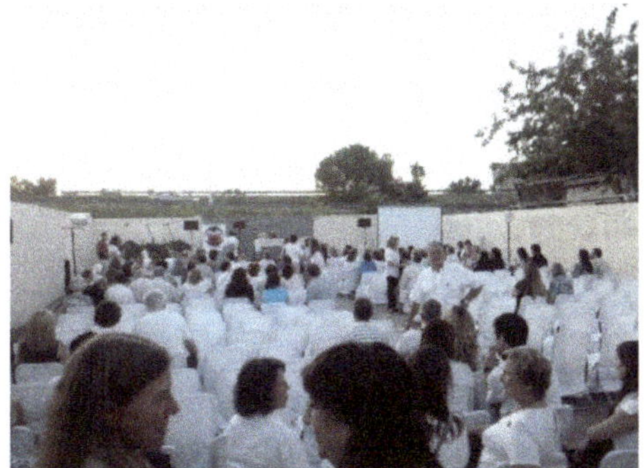

Figure 2. Social environments.

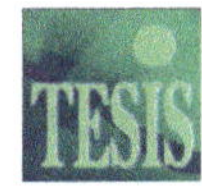

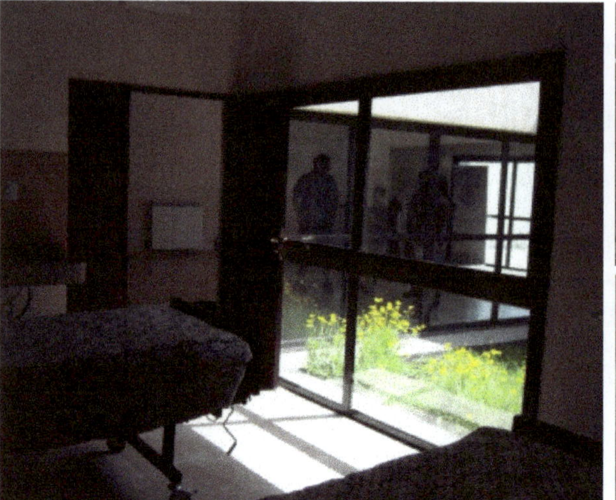

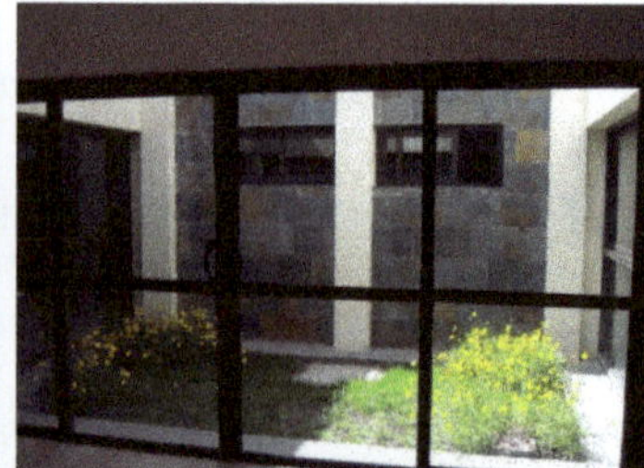

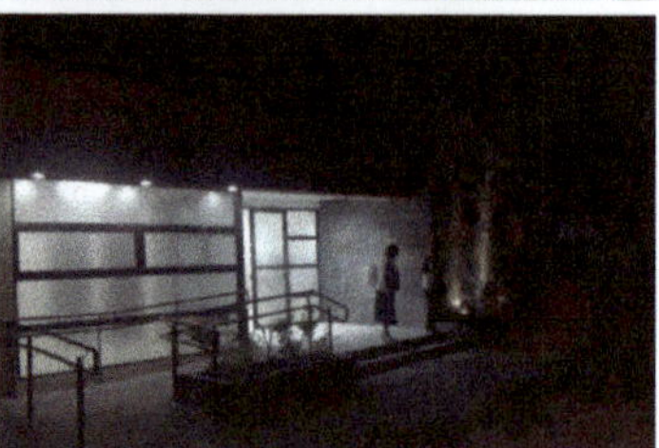

Figure 3. Environments surrounding the patient.

Conclusions

The House of Kindness, Casa de la Bondad, provides a support system that integrates patient physical care, such as psycho-social and spiritual. Also accompanying the family (if any) during the illness and bereavement period. It has permanent nursing care, medical care and other health professionals such as psychologists, care attendants, social workers, nutritionists and physical therapists, in addition to the work of volunteers trained in palliative care.

The Open Hands Foundation, a legal entity since 1994, has more than 30 works that involve volunteers and professionals who seek to alleviate the pain of suffering, offering their services in different areas: secretarial, kitchen, laundry, housekeeping, caregiving, health. It has four hospice houses built in the country.

The House of Kindness San Juan, incorporated since birth architectural guidelines ordered in a holistic anthropological view of man and thus are:
- responds to the whole man, your needs and desires, sensitive to their physical, social and cultural environment;
- humanizes the patient, considering it as a sick man in a social and cultural construction;
- reinforces the idea that patient care involves much more than clinical, pharmaceutical and technological capacity of the institution;
- exceeds the cosmetic interpretation is given to the architectural materiality of therapeutic environments;
- and finally, gives architects a holistic view of an architecture for the humanized health from a holistic approach of man, and aware of their existence, they can choose their paths do proyectual conscientiously being more lucid and free.

Learning from Aalto and Le Corbusier Paimio Hospital Venice Project Why are They Still Current Architecture?

María Elena Galesio, Silvina Pan, María Elizabeth Rial

silvinapan@gmail.com
HA-HI; Argentina

The construction system and the technical systems were tightly interlinked in Paimio Hospital. Along the centre line of the frame of the patient wing, at the side of each column, there is a system of horizontal and vertical ducts. All technical installations were placed in the duct shafts. Thus the repair and maintenance work could be carried out without having to enter the patient rooms. These innovative solutions were presented in the contemporary journals even before the sanatorium had actually been completed. The primary goal of the architectural competition for Paimio was to find new solutions for the placement and organization of the spaces. The design of the Paimio Sanatorium entailed a great challenge for Alvar Aalto because he set as his task to design and define a completely new building type, that is, a standard sanatorium. The new building type would include new tasks and new requirements. A new function justified the realization of a new form language. As Aalto said: "We can not create new form where there is no new content." It is clear that Le Corbusier was interested in the strategy of " Mat Building", may still not defined as such. What is a Mat Building? Mat is a flexible piece of tissue that is required to make thread and knots. Whether this system of nodes is repeated a pattern is generated. The pattern can change status by type of nodes or the number of threads. The most important aspect in the Venice Hospital is that it creates a fully planned organization and is also genuinely"no planned" with capacity to grow as a "Mat" although its formal organization solves a highly resolved and controlled growth system.

***Silvina Pan**, 1985 Architecture, Universidad de Buenos Aires, 1987 1991 Architecture for Health Buildings, U.B.A., 2000 Architecture for Medical Building Planning U.B.A., 2001 Bid for G.C.B.A. Public Hospital Master Plan in Buenos Aires, 2010 Specialization Facilities Management Austral University, 2010.2012 Master Planning and Design for Health Buildings, University of Catalunya.*

***Maria Elizabeth Rial**, 1984 Architecture, Universidad de Buenos Aires, 1987 1991 Architecture for Health Buildings, U.B.A., 2000 Architecture for Medical Building Planning U.B.A., 2001 Bid for G.C.B.A. Public Hospital Master Plan in Buenos Aires.*

***Maria Elena Galesio**, 1985 Architecture, Universidad de Buenos Aires, 1990 1993 Architecture for Health Buildings, U.B.A., 2000 Architecture for Medical Building Planning U.B.A., 2001 Bid for G.C.B.A. Public Hospital Master Plan in Buenos Aires, 2010 Specialization Facilities Management Austral University.*

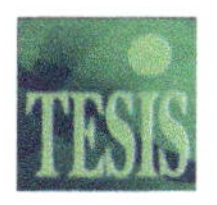

1930 - Aalto Paimio Hospital

An architectural competition for the design of the sanatorium was held in 1928, which was won by Aalto. Nowadays the building complex still operates as Hospital.

The hospital complex includes: the main sanatorium building, the chief physician's residence, the junior physicians' row house, the staff housing, the hospital morgue, the machine room and the garages, all completed in 1933.

The main building has been organized into five independent entities: the main entrance, the patients' rooms, the communal rooms, the operating theatre, and the kitchen/ maintenance. Each activity has its own wing, with each oriented in a direction most favorable to the activity in question (Figure 1).
This planning principle has produced a building which is naturally organized into parts, each with a different character and orientation, offering a dynamic whole with varying views outwards into the landscape (Figure 2).

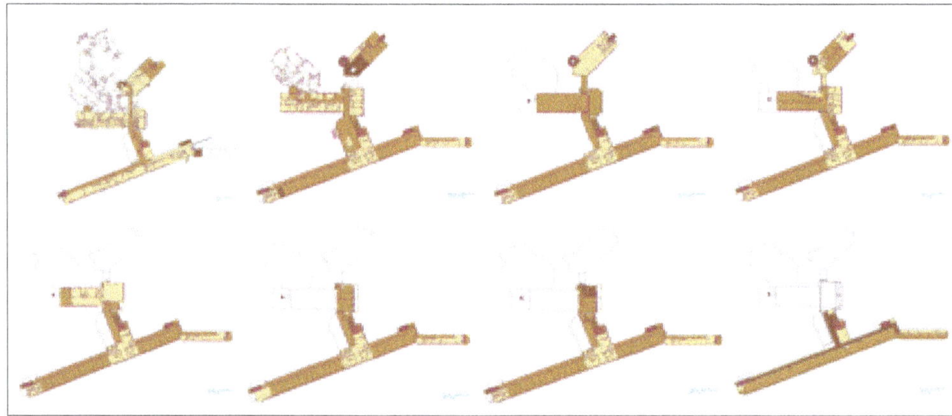

Figure 1. Aalto, plants of Paimio Hospital.

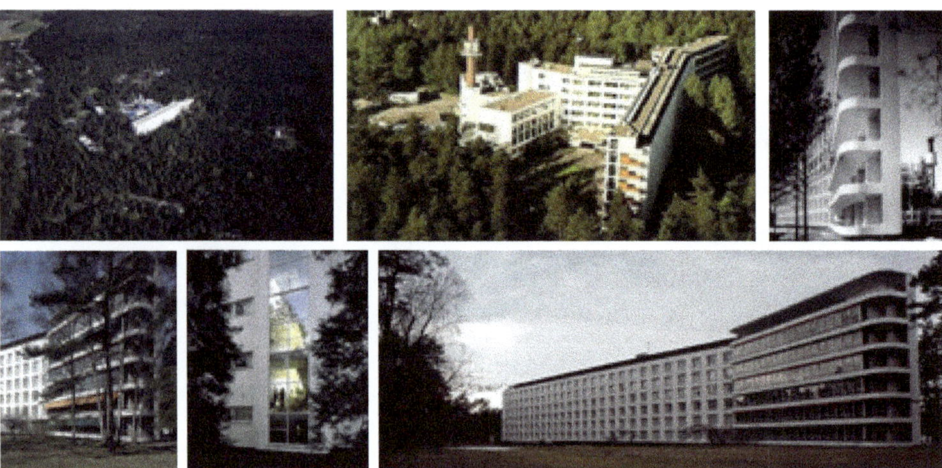

Figure 2. Aalto, views of Paimio Hospital.

1960 - Le Corbusier Venice Project

The Venice Hospital is one of the last projects of Le Corbusier before his death in 1965. Le Corbusier signs two projects for the Venice Hospital whose differences do not alter the design and implementation of the building. After his death, the project went on under the supervision de la Fuente to the early '70s, however, the project could not be completed because the authorities of Venice finally decided not to build the hospital.

The hospital is organized into three main levels. The first level is the level of the city where Le Corbusier organizes pedestrian access, water access, the vehicular access, the supplies access. At this level he also organizes: pharmacy, services, administrative offices, kitchen, laundry, chapel, morgue whose volume is expressed as an element suspended in the water (Figure 3).

The sectional strategy can be recognized in the form in which the plants are joined and articulated. Plants of the Hospital of Venice are a strategy where balconies create phenomenal doubles heights (Figure 4).

Although the Hospital of Venice is a functional structure that takes its formal idea from the context that is the entire city of Venice, the building has a disciplined geometric system that is much more than an outline or a geometric grid that organizes the project (Figure 5).

Figure 3. Le Corbusier, three main levels of the Venice Project.

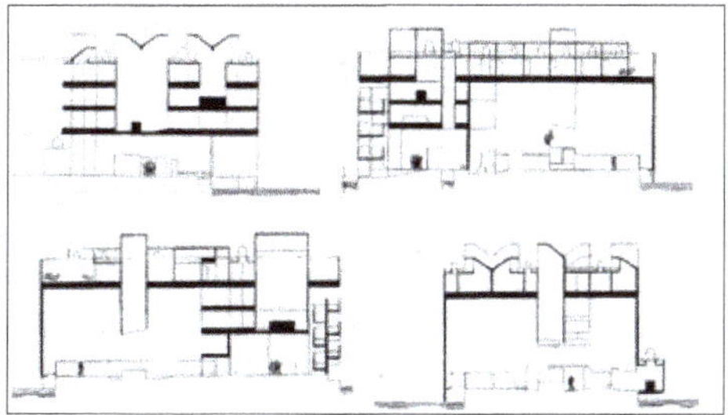

Figure 4. Le Corbusier, sectional strategy of the Venice Project.

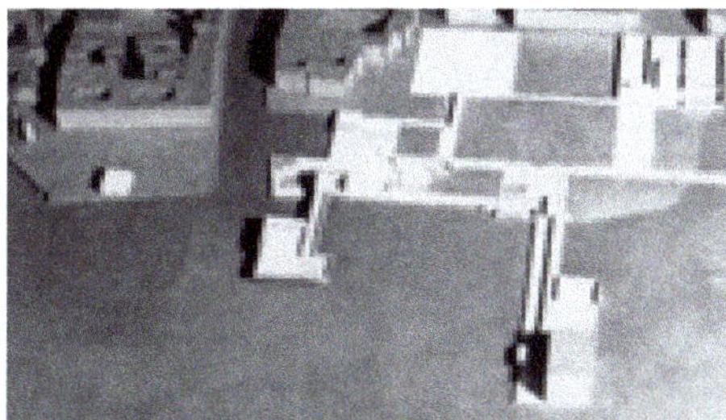

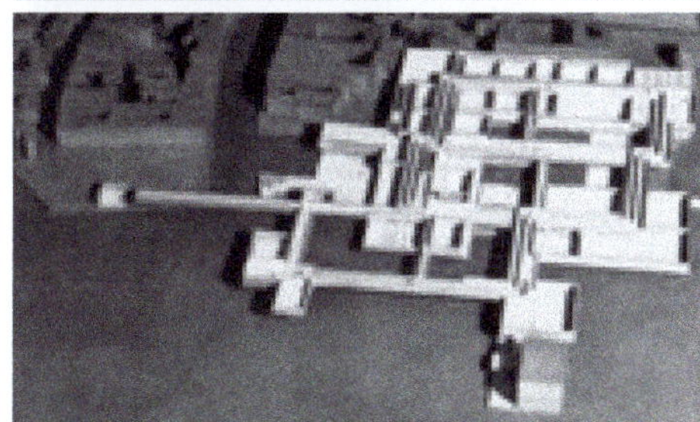

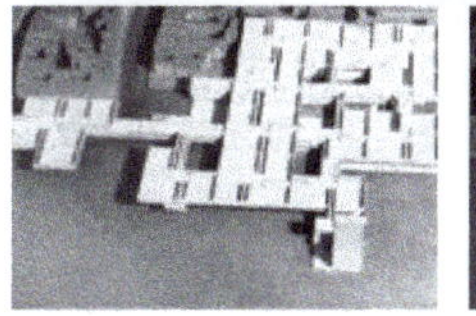

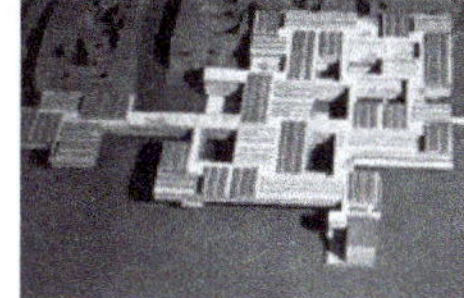

Figure 5. Le Corbusier, maquette of the Venice Project.

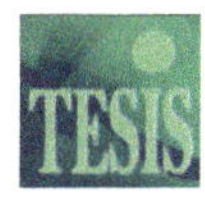

Why Are They Still Current Architecture?

Paimio Hospital – Functional and Technical Systems and Their Integration

The construction system and the technical systems were tightly interlinked in Paimio Hospital. Along the centre line of the frame of the patient wing, at the side of each column, is a system of horizontal and vertical ducts. All technical installations were placed in the duct shafts. Thus the repair and maintenance work could be carried out without having to enter the patient rooms. These innovative solutions were presented in the contemporary journals even before the sanatorium had actually been completed.
The primary goal of the architectural competition for Paimio was to find new solutions for the placement and organization of the spaces. The design of the Paimio Sanatorium entailed a great challenge for Alvar Aalto because he set as his task to design and define a completely new building type, that is, a standard sanatorium. The new building type would include new tasks and new requirements. A new function justified the realization of a new form language. As Aalto said: "We can not create new form where there is no new content".
In the Paimio Hospital two large subject matters are combined in a fecund way: the creation of a new type of sanatorium and the breakthrough of modernist architecture. The building responded in its time to the challenge of medical science like an instrument. It offered light, air and ventilation, thus implementing the ideology of Functionalism; namely, architecture in the service of society, and improving social disadvantages.

Venice Project - Flexible and Mat

It is clear that Le Corbusier was interested in the strategy of "Mat Building", may still not defined as such. What is a Mat Building? Mat is a flexible piece of tissue that is required to make thread and knots. Whether this system of nodes is repeated a pattern is generated. The pattern can change status by type of nodes or the number of threads.

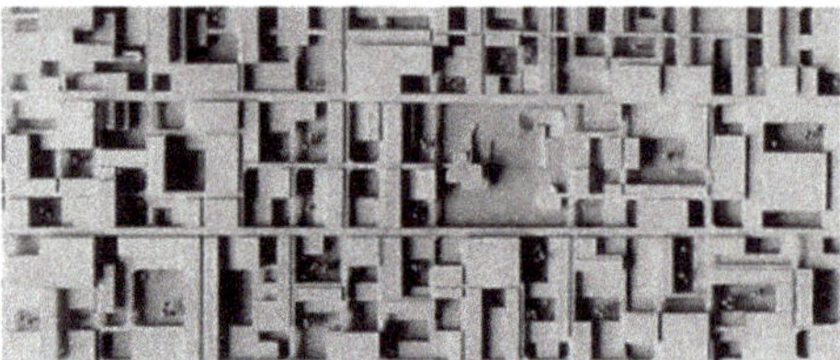

Figure 6. Le Corbusier, the strategy of "Mat Building" of the Venice project.

In the late 50s, Architects debate on innovative systems for urban structures concepts of integration , extension, flexibility and the "no horizontal monumentality" "Mat Building Concept" was intended to define a minimum and basic strategy around which the different functions can be added with alternating mesh and full.

It is a case in which a "Mat" building is both a building and a city. The internal organization is both structure and infrastructure, The project shows the classic principle according to which a building must be a small city, and a city is also a large building.

The most important aspect in the Venice Hospital is that it creates a fully planned organization and is also genuinely"no planned" with capacity to grow as a "Mat" although its formal organization solves a highly resolved and controlled growth system.

Effects of Traditions on Healthcare Service Delivery in Kenya

Salome Mwaura

salome2mwaura@yahoo.co.uk
Association of Medical Engineering of Kenya (Amek), Mbagathi District Hospital, Senior Medical Engineering Technologist

Kenya is one of the East African countries. It has a Population of 43 Million. There are 42 tribes and Kiswahili is the national language. The most common illnesses are HIV/Aids, TB, Malaria, pneumonia, cancer, high blood pressure, and diabetes. The ministry of health has 63,000 health care workers with only 2000 doctors. 51% of healthcare is provided by Public (Government) with two national teaching and referral hospitals, 10 level five hospitals, 42 level four hospital, health centres, dispensaries, 49% is provided by private/non governmental organisations. Each tribe in Kenya have their own traditions which are unique to a particular community. Some belief in witchcraft, religious sect which never go to hospitals for treatment, traditional medicine men and all sorts of things which make them not go to hospitals.
All this things have a lot of effect on our day to day operation in hospitals. Majority of these patients are brought to hospital on the verge of death and makes healthcare delivery very difficult. All these have had a lot of negative effects on healthcare delivery in the country. It has also contributed to high birth mortality rate of 42.18 deaths/1,000 live births (2013 survey).

***Salome Mwaura** is a senior medical Engineering technologist at Mbagathi District Hospital in Nairobi, Kenya. She has been working for the Ministry of health for the last 17 years where she has experiences in repair and maintenance of medical equipments.*
She has a Higher National Diploma in Medical engineering from Kenya Medical Training College in Nairobi and Diploma in Medical Engineering from Mombasa polytechnic. She joined AMEK in 2000. She is the treasurer of the association. Since joining AMEK, she has attended IFHE conferences in Argentina, Japan and Norway. She has also attended SAFHE/CEASA conference in South Africa.

Introduction

Despite newly free deliveries in Kenya, some mothers opt for traditional birth attendants. In Nairobi slums, the practice is very common as the mothers are told to avoid going to public hospitals because the services are poor, the nurses are very rude and that they are over crowded.
The government aimed to reduce Kenya's high maternal mortality rate by abol-

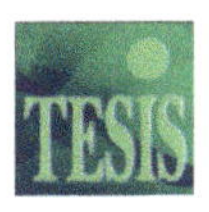

ishing delivery fees in public hospitals and discouraging mothers from using traditional birth attendants. Although many mothers are taking advantage of the newly free delivery services in public hospitals, some mothers say they still prefer traditional birth attendants, citing poor services in public health facilities. Traditional birth attendants say that they offer quality care which is equal to or better than hospital care. Some women have a lot of trust in traditional birth attendants and will always go to them. In addition, hospitals are difficult to access in rural areas, where traditional birth attendants typically work.

Witch craft is practiced by majority of tribes in Kenya. The most common form of witchcraft is often termed kamuti (kah-moo-teh), and is attributed to the Kamba people. It involves the use of charms, 'muti' and spells to achieve the client's ends. Therefore, most people believe that they are not sick but bewitched. In some communities, they believe that HIV/AIDS is witchcraft and not a disease. So in these communities, you find they are being wiped out by the disease since they don't want to go to hospitals.

Some religious sects don't believe in going to hospital so their followers are taken to church to be prayed for. In fact in the recent past there was an old man who was bitten by snake and went to church to be prayed for and it took the intervention of the area chief for him to be taken to hospital for medical attention. In traditional religions, diviners are believed to have the power to communicate with the spirit world, and they use their powers to cure people of diseases or evil spirits. Diviners are also called upon to help bring rain during times of drought. Sorcerers and witches are also believed to have supernatural powers, but unlike the diviners they use these powers to cause harm. It is the job of the diviners to counter their evil workings.

Of late, there are these traditional medicine men that are calling themselves "doctors" and have convinced a lot of Kenyans that their medicine work better and more effective than the hospital medicine. Due to the high cost of medication in the country, and these medicine men's medication is cheaper, most patients opt for them. About two years ago, there was one who was in Tanzania and was making a drug which he claimed that it was healing every disease. So those with terminal illnesses moved in masses to get the drug but unfortunately it did not work and most of them lost their lives and others got worse. Most of them put up advertisements everywhere on the streets and when their clients see the adverts, they go to where them for treatment (Figure 1).

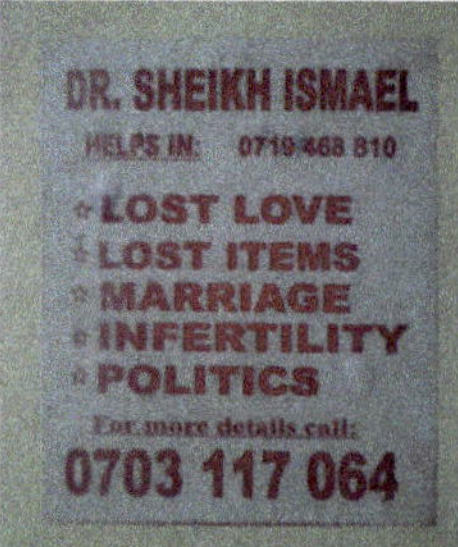

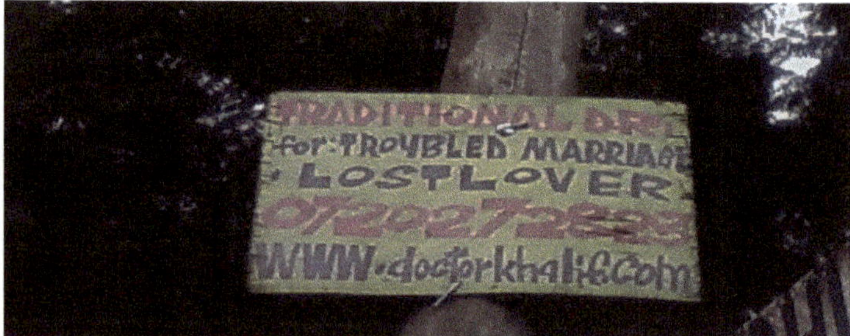

Figure 1. Some of the advertisements put on the streets by the traditional doctors.

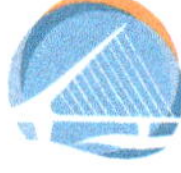

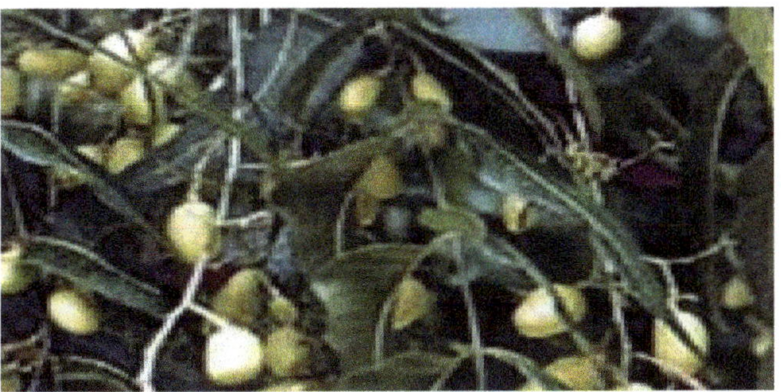
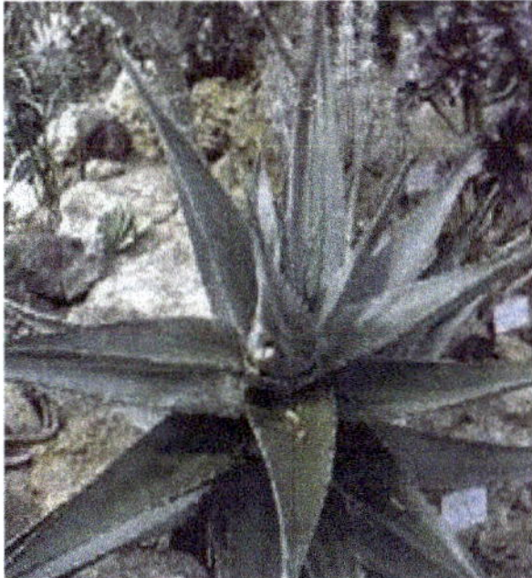

Figure 2. Commonly used herbs: the neem known in Swahili as Mwarobaini (left) and Aloe vera (right).

Herbalists are also on the rise and they use all sorts of weeds convincing people of their medicinal value and the patients go for them. They have even gone to an extent of wanting to be regulated and permitted to work without interference by the medical board in the country.

Traditions dictate that no one should go against them so many people follow them not because they would want to but in order to avoid any eventualities. For instance in Kikuyu traditions, they believed that if one is sick, he/she should slaughter a goat for the old men and sacrifice it to their God whom they believe lives in Mt. Kenya and he would in return heal the sick. This tradition is still held strongly by many of them and they keep offering sacrifices and the sick continue being sick. In some communities, they have disregard for women and group them as children. So if a man from such a community visits a health facility and finds that the healthcare provider is a female, he will refuse to be treated by her. Also, most traditional marriages are polygamous and this has led to an increase is the spread of HIV/AIDS. Wife inheritance also have led to the increase of the disease as those tribes which practice it continue doing it even after they identify what the deceased was suffering from. Healthcare workers are few for the growing number of Kenyans. With only 2000 doctors, then the workload is high and in effect the patients will continue looking for health services where they can be able to get them and more will opt to go for the traditional medicine men and herbalists.

The ministry of health has invested in training of counselors who talk to the patients and even go for outreaches to convince people to come to hospital when they fall sick. This is because when traditions take a tall order in the community, treatment becomes very difficult and in most cases, leads to death. During the outreaches, the health care worker at time are forced to even break into peoples homes to remove patients who are locked up and are suffering in the name of witchcraft.

The ministry has initiated very many campaigns in order to educate people on the need to visit a health facility when they are unwell. The county governments have also purchased many ambulances which will be able to transport patients to hospital when need arises. They have also tried to equip hospitals with necessary requirement so that patients are treated with ease.

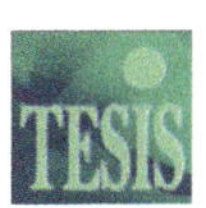

Conclusions

In conclusion, the government needs to put more effort in trying to reach the very remote areas where most of these practices are practiced and educate them on the need of seeking medical attention when they fall sick. There is need also for more health workers to be hired as the current number cannot be able to work and go for outreaches effectively. Infrastructure also needs to be improved to make the health facilities accessible to the patients.

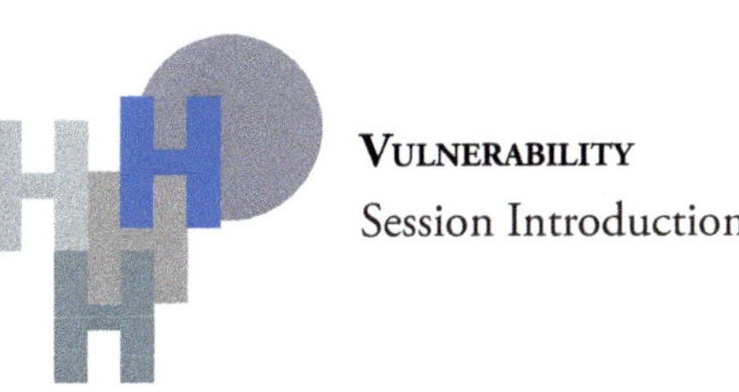

Vulnerability

Session Introduction

In a disaster situation a series of problems come to light affecting healthcare buildings and the territory in which the natural phenomenon occurs. Designing hospital environments to prevent damage caused by such events is an extremely complex problem that requires the collaboration of multidisciplinary teams made up of architects, engineers, medical staff, nurses and psychologists.

Healthcare environments should be designed so that any damage to the building in the event of a disaster is as limited as possible and the structure must be able to accommodate patients who are victims of adverse natural phenomena. For example, in the case of an earthquake, areas that are more structurally vulnerable such as as lobbies, cafeterias and waiting areas, require a set of specific measures. The configuration of the building and the materials chosen for its construction are very important, and the sustainability of the building is also assessed in terms of whether it can be recovered and reused in the event of damage.

Once a building is in the operational phase Facility Management (FM) tools play a vital role in the safety of users in buildings in the event of a disaster. To avoid care activities being interrupted by calamities it is necessary to provide plans capable of ensuring continuity in the delivery of energy.

In addition to considering the characteristics of the building under construction the plan must include safe places even outdoors where people can go if the severity of the event does not allow them to remain inside the building in safety, and from this point of view managing the event also involves planning the urban area adjacent to the building.

In a disaster situation relief must be brought to the victims of the calamity, and this requires planning. It foreshadows the need to bring medical devices to the site where the adverse event occurred, and it is necessary for first aid teams to have a complete overview of the structures in the area so the wounded can be brought to the closest facilities in a timely manner. Proper risk management includes an evaluation of where the primary care stations are located and provides rescue equipment systems, non-site-specific-architecture able to reach the wounded at the place of the disaster.

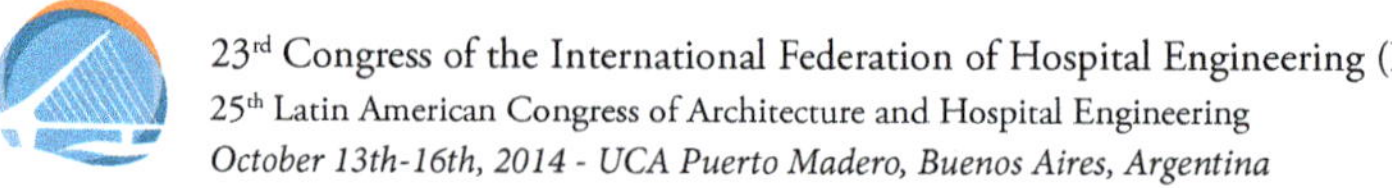

Disaster Mitigation through FM (Facility Management) and Hospital BCP (Business Continuity Plan)

Nagasawa Yasushi

donpayasusin@gmail.com
Past President, IFHE (International Federation of Hospital Engineering)
Vice President of Kogakuin University, Dean & Professor in School of Architecture,
Professor Emeritus, University of Tokyo
Vice-President, HEAJ (Healthcare Engineering Association of Japan)

Facility management (FM) of healthcare buildings will become increasingly important in healthcare facilities planning including hospitals and other health related facilities, both in developed and developing nations. When it comes to the issues of the most expensive part of all the life of a hospital in terms of life cycle cost (LCC), 80 % of LCC is devoted to operating stage cost, while 19 % is consumed to construction stage cost. It means that more consideration should be put on the planning of operation after accomplishing buildings. The problems of natural and man-made disasters (earthquake, landslide, avalanche, flood, cyclone, etc.) requires interdisciplinary cooperation between architects, engineers and medical faculties (health care staff, crisis management clue, etc.) as well as psychologists in some cases to be solved. Architectural solutions for the protection against the above hazards: e.g. Shelters in Bangladesh, etc. are in need. Research on disaster management has produced a shift of focus from the structural strength of materials to the elasticity in human living. The purpose is to enhance sustainability (synonymous with recoverability after disasters including provision of disaster medical services and maintenance of healthcare for those suffered), and management in both ordinary and disaster situations is relevant. For example, it is important to provide pathways and squares for people to walk and stay in a city in the event that most buildings are destroyed. The reservation of such vacant spaces in urban areas is more meaningful if they can be used to full advantage in non-disaster situations and understanding gained from disaster experience needs to have more impact on future planning.

Nagasawa Yasushi. *Immediate Past President of IFHE (International Federation of Hospital Engineering (2010-2012), He organized the 21st IFHE Congress in Tokyo in 2010, and appointed as President of IFHE. Professor Emeritus, University of Tokyo (2007-) Immediate Past-President of JIHA (Japan Institute of Healthcare Architecture (2006-2010), Vice President of HEAJ (Healthcare Engineering Association of Japan (2001-), Vice-President of JAHMC (Japanese Association of Healthcare Service Management Consultants (2003-2012). He was graduated from the UT (University of Tokyo) in 1968. Designing various buildings and carrying out research works in the Ministry of Health, Japan, then obtained Diploma in the UK as a British Council Scholar in 1978 and Doctor of Engineering (PhD) from the UT in 1987. Moved to the UT in 1989 as Associate Professor, then in 1993 full Professorship in Graduate School of Engineering, UT until 2007 followed by current position as Vice-President of Kogakuin University, Dean & Professor, in School of Architecture.*

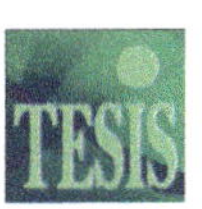

A hospital is built to cater for maintaining health of local people and treating diseases. However, diseases and injuries can occur in any incidence at any place, and health facilities should be able to serve for such sudden emergency occurrences. In the case of earthquakes, large fires and accidents, tidal waves, landslides, wars as well as spread of epidemics, and chronic shortages of health facilities in remote areas, building permanent hospitals is not realistic but carrying mobile facilities is more effective and efficient (Figure 1).

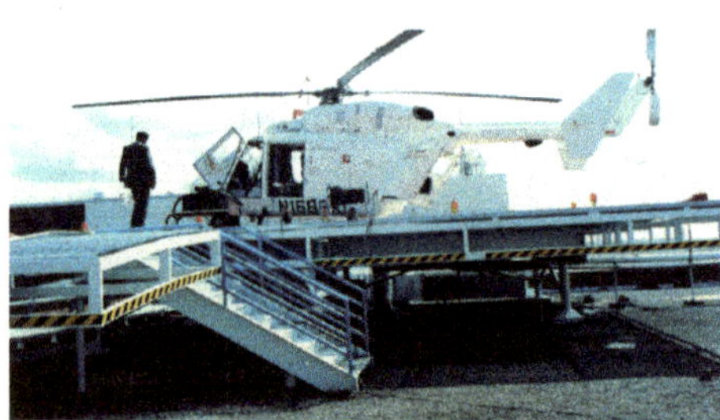

Figure 1. Ambulance system with fire brigades.

Such circumstances can be found throughout the world, both in developing and developed parts of the earth. Future hospital will be non site-specific architecture, to have a thought on mobile structure, not just as a machine of providing health services but having beauty in it.

Barrier-free planning for handicapped people (physically and mentally handicapped, elderly, sight/hearing/speaking handicapped). Health care, training, development of relief devices, etc. are needed and require interdisciplinary cooperation. Safety and Security are basically 2 different concepts. Security will not be satisfied even in sufficiently safe conditions, unless the users themselves consider being safe. On the other hand, non-safe conditions can also become a secured condition, as long as the users regard it as such. However it is not a preferable situation. It is very important, in the healthcare environment in the year 2050 that both safe and secured situations be attained.

As an integral part of fostering both better relationships in communities and health maintenance, we need greater self-reliance and opportunities to exercise individual will. This becomes more critical in the case of those, e.g. elderly or handicapped, who must often rely on others to accomplish daily activities. The built environment should not restrict but rather encourage everyone to participate as fully as each would like.

The blossoming of personal communication technologies allow us more readily to meet and have great potential to contribute to forming stronger community ties at the same time as individual independence. Realization of their full potential will depend on how we cope with the shift in their nature from direct to indirect, and whether applications remain humane. In this sense, 'Universal Design' concepts should be fully utilized. The morale and cultural issues will influence the healthcare system. We can identify in the Western world at least the medical culture in USA, Middle Europe, Nordic Welfare, Russian and Japanese are all different. Powerful Chinese medicine will be integrated with western medicine, a process which may take some 50 years. Cultures have their own diagnostic methods with related industry. However, the globalization process is fast and even more so in the future. The new generations will be educated more homogeneously, yet we will still see in 2050 several identical medical cultures.

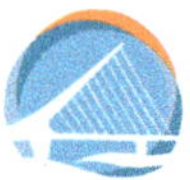

A Comparative Study on the Disaster Recovery of Hospital in Tokyo Japan. Focusing on Lifeline in BCP Manuals

Shigeta Takuro[1], Kobayashi Yuta[1], Nagasawa Yasushi[1], Saruwatari Fumiko[2], Nanba Nobuyuki[3], Matsumoto Jun[3]

kobayu110@gmail.com, donyayasusin@gmail.com, sarufumix@gmail.com, kangaroo@tokyo-gas.co.jp, matsu-jun@tokyo-gas.co.jp
[1]School of Architecture, Kogakuin University. Japan
[2]Yamashita Sekkei, INC
[3]Tokyo Gas Co.,Ltd. Public Sector Sales Section. Medical and Welfare Unit Japan

Past experiences in the case of functional damage of hospitals during and after attacks by devastating earthquake show that several main lifelines, e.g. supply of electrical power, city gas, portal water, sewage, etc. greatly affected their business continuity of hospitals. Particularly, electrical power supply is turned out to be great contribution to keep medical function. It is therefore that implementation of multiplexing energy source for supply electric power will play an important role.

The paper aims at considering Blackout start (BOS) cogeneration system as one of the crucial tools to sustain multiplexing energy source for supply electric power. The questionnaire-interview surveys were carried out to Tokyo Metropolitan Disaster Base Hospitals, asking their current situation on lifeline systems mainly based on their Business Continuity Plan (BCP) Manuals.

Shigeta Takuro. *Born in 1993. Graduated from Tokyo Metropolitan Kurume Nishi High School. Enrollment of Kogakuin University in 2011. Studying on disaster mitigation of hospitals as a senior student in Kogakuin University. Tokyo Japan.*

Kobayashi Yuta. *Born in 1993. Graduated from Tokyo Metropolitan Roca High School. Enrollment of Kogakuin University in 2011. Volunteer Service for Kids Camp. Studying on disaster mitigation of hospitals as a senior student in Kogakuin University. Tokyo Japan.*

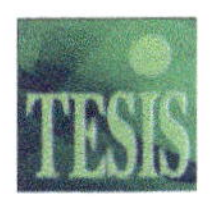

We asked for cooperation with 70 hospitals.
However, only 11 hospitals cooperated.
We suspect that many Disaster Base Hospitals have still not completed a BCP manual.

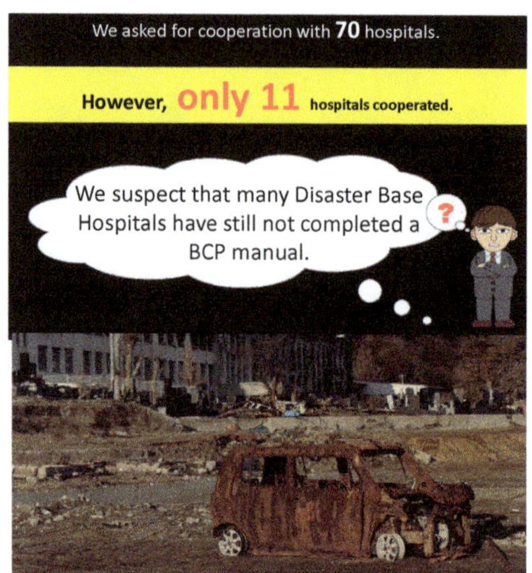

Figure 1. The importance of BCP has been recognized after the Great East Japan Earthquake.

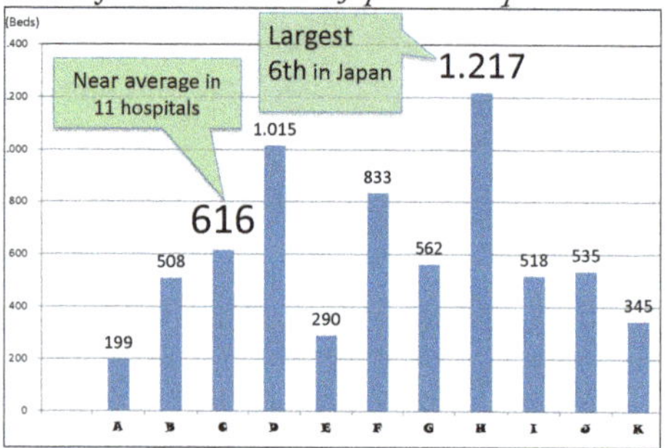

Figure 2. Number of Hospital Beds in 11 Disaster Base Hospitals. From 200 beds to 1,200 beds.

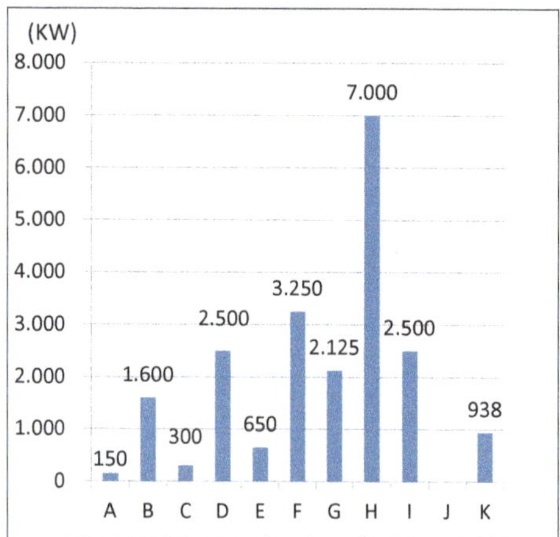

Figure 3. Capacity of Emergency Generators in 11 Disaster Base HospitalsFrom 150KW to 7,000KW.

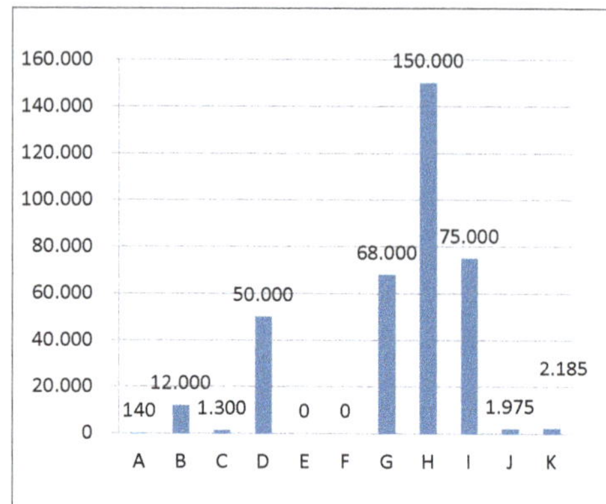

Figure 4. Quantity of Fuel for Emergency Generators. Up to 150,000ℓ.

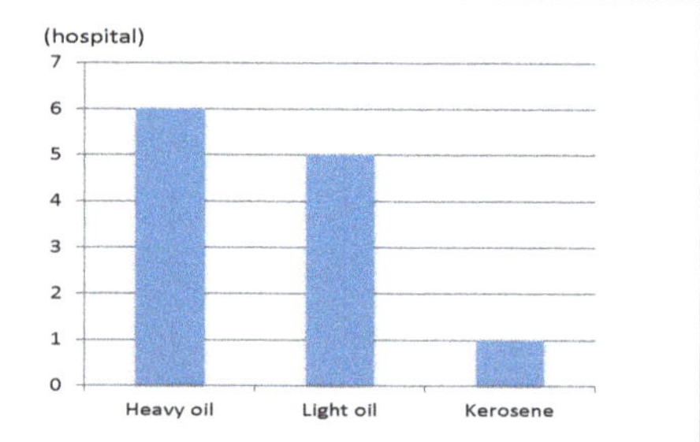

Figure 5. Number of Emergency Generators Classified by Fuel Source.

A comparative study of each hospital manuals showed that the impression of countermeasures have a lack of flexibility, although countermeasures of each focus item of the lifeline system show clearly identified. In particular, it is highlighted that BOS specified cogeneration system combined to standby generator is capable of providing electrical power as long as city gas is supplied during and after disasters. In addition, consideration should be made that installation of Gas BOS system for hospital operation is not only from the stand point of BCP, but also daily operation and business in order to attain effective and efficient energy saving tools to support hospital management.

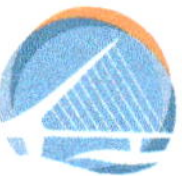

Study on First-aid Stations of Disaster Medical Services in Hospital District

Egawa Kana

kanaegawa@mail.dendai.ac.jp
Assistant Prof. School of Information Environment, Department of Information Environment, Tokyo Denki Univ., Dr. Eng.

There are many local governments in Japan planning setting up first-aid stations for disaster medical services to carry out triage a number of causalities suffering from devastating disasters and transport critical cases to designated District Disaster Base Hospitals. The study aims at finding out crucial items to consider hospital plan/design in relation to appropriate location of first-aid stations in the hospital districts.

The survey was conducted on current situation of regional disaster mitigation plan, especially on the way to set up first-aid stations in each 23 ward in the Metropolis of Tokyo in March 2013. As the result, first-aid stations are located in various places such as in health and welfare center, primary and secondary schools, clinics and hospitals. In addition, the number of first-aid stations per unit population are found to be different from one ward to another.

Egawa Kana. *Born in 1976. Graduated from Kogakuin University in 2000. Completed Post Graduate Master Course In Tokyo Denki University in 2002. Designing various buildings as qualified architect at K. ITO Architects and Engineers Inc. from 2002 to 2008. Obtained Doctor of Engineering (PhD) from Kogakuin University in 2012. Since 2012, working for Tokyo Denki University as Assistant Professor, School of Information Environment, Department of Information Environment.*

Background

Devastating earthquake disasters will occur on Japanese archipelago in near future. Consequently, a number of casualties will need medical care. Effective triage for casualties is needed before visiting district hospitals in order to cut down ineffective treatment in hospitals. Four grade of triage color are: immediate (red), treatment is needed immediately; delayed (yellow), treatment, even if somewhat delayed, no danger to life; minor (green) minor injuries, ambulatory; dead (black), already dead or no possibility of resuscitation.

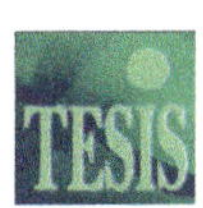

First-Aid Medical Station(FAMS)	To provide medical treatment to Yellow and Green triaged peaple
Emergency Medical Aid Station(EMAS)	To provide first aid medical servises
Medical Support Base(MSB)	To provide medical support to peaples at home and at FAMS

Figure 1. Tokyo Metropolitan Government defines 3 kinds of medical stations. Source: Tokyo Metropolitan Government, modification of Tokyo regional disaster prevention plan, 2014.8.

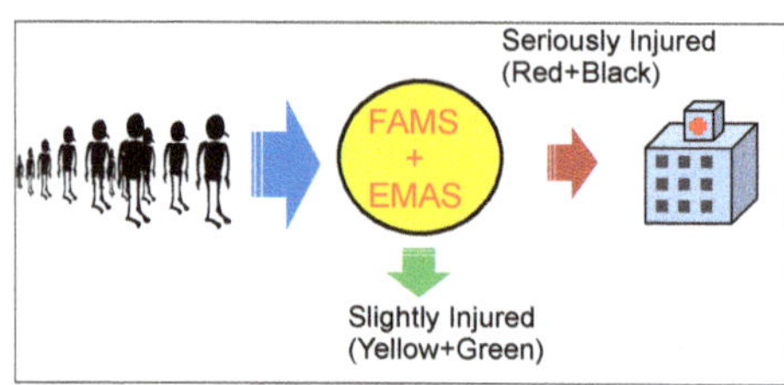

Figure 2. Study objectives: To find out appropriate planning tools of First Aid Medical Station (FAMS) and Emergency Medical Aid Station(EMAS).

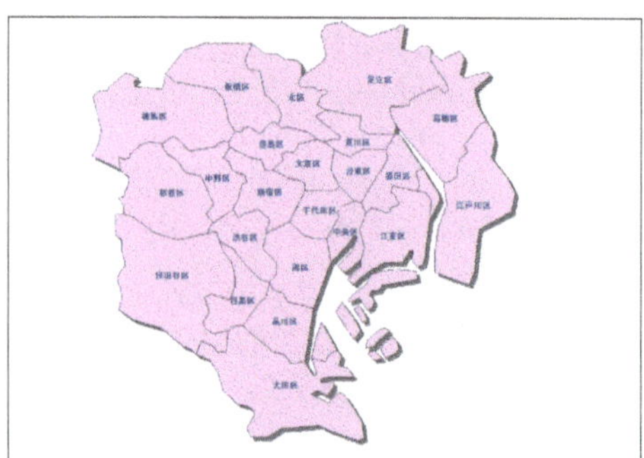

Figure 3. Investigation to find out the way to set up FAMS in mitigation plan of 23 districts in Tokyo Metropolis. Source: Tokyo Metropolitan Government Bureau of Taxation.

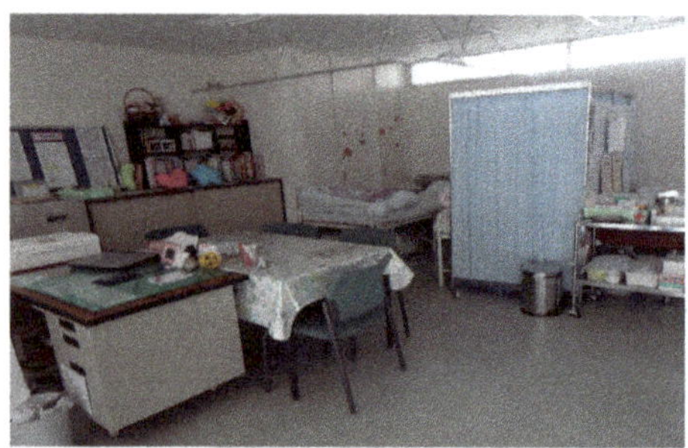

Figure 4. Location of FAMS in Junior High Schools.

DISCUSSION 1

Most schools allocate FAMS in and around the health room. Floor space of the health room is limited. It is necessary to consider providing enough space to carry out triage around the health rooms.

DISCUSSION 2

About 30% of district hospitals allocate EMAS in hospital site. Locating near hospital OPD entrance is considered. Building tents to provide appropriate places is considered.

DISCUSSION 3

Triage activities were found at its peak on the second day after the earthquake. Back up activities should be planned even in the situation of life line disruption. Effective flow of people and goods should be planned as well.

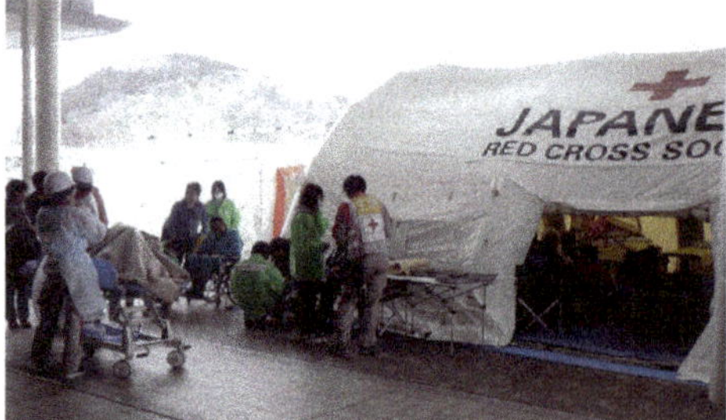

Figure 5. Example of discussion 2.

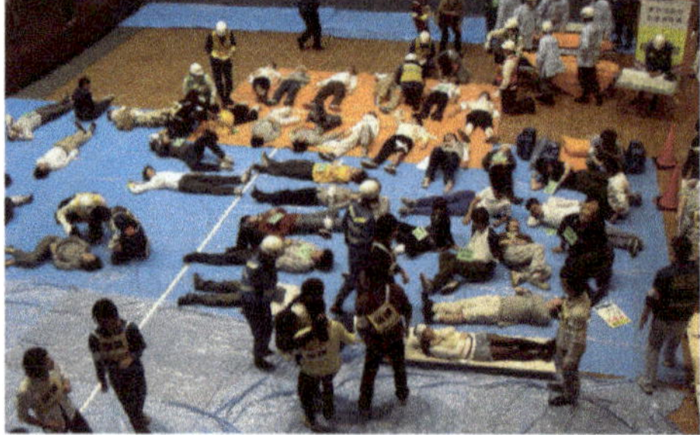

Figure 6. Example of discussion 3.

Tools of Business Continuity Plan for Hospitals suffered from Recent Devastating Disasters in Japan

Kosaka Osamu[1], Taguchi Shigehiro[2]

kousaka.osamu@takenaka.co.jp, shigehiro.taguchi@mj-sekkei.com
[1]Japan Facility Management Association/Healthcare & Educational Facilities Dept., Takenaka Corp. Japan
[2]Japan Facility Management Association/Environment Design Dept., Mitsubishi Jisho Sekkei Inc. Japan

Japan has been suffered from devastating earthquake for many years in the past. Especially a couple of recent big earthquakes attacking to Kobe area (Hanshin Awaji Earthquake) in January 17, 1995 and attacking to North East Coast of Japanese archipelago (Great East Japan Earthquake) in March 11, 2011 influenced a great deal to recognize the importance of disaster mitigation of suffered areas. The paper aims at outlining these two earthquakes in terms of continuing hospital function during and after disasters and proposing effective tools of Business Continuity Plan (BCP) for hospitals. Inter-alia, after the Great East Japan Earthquake, increasing attentions has been paid to Hospital BCP, and recognized as one of the most important subjects for hospital management. As the result, utilizing Facility Management (FM) tools to examine medical activities of actual hospitals experienced disasters, check points for hospitals resistant ability to disasters can be proposed and to measure these FM tools during ordinary times is the key to ensuring medical functional continuity for the surrounding hospital districts.

Osamu Kosaka. *Born 1950 in Kyoto prefecture, Japan; joined Takenaka Co., Ltd. in 1973, Japan Facility Management Association. in 2001, and is currently Chief of the Healthcare Facility Management Research Group. Extensive supervisory design experience in creating medical facilities such as clinics and hospitals, campus facilities such as universities and institutes. Occasioned by the advent of the Great East Japan Earthquake, has been engaged since 2011 in research on facility management tools for business continuity planning for hospitals. Certified Facility Manager Japan. Architect. Member of Architectural Institute of Japan.*

Shigehiro Taguchi. *Born 1960 in Shizuoka prefecture, Japan; joined Mitsubishi Estate Co., Ltd. in 1990, Mitsubishi Jisho Sekkei Inc. in 2001, and is currently head of the Healthcare Facility Design Office, Residential & Living Environmental Design Department. Extensive supervisory design experience in creating medical facilities such as clinics and hospitals, care facilities for the elderly such as special care homes and health care facilities, and care-provided accommodation for the elderly such as pay-for homes. Joined the JFMA Healthcare FM Study Group in 2006. Occasioned by the advent of the Great East Japan Earthquake, has been engaged since 2011 in research on facility management tools for business continuity planning for hospitals.*

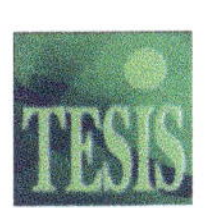

Surveys on Disaster Mitigation and Business Continuity situation in 50 Hospitals suffered from Great East Japan Earthquake in 2011

Kosaka Osamu[1], Taguchi Shigehiro[2]

kousaka.osamu@takenaka.co.jp, shigehiro.taguchi@mj-sekkei.com
[1]Japan Facility Management Association/Healthcare & Educational Facilities Dept., Takenaka Corp. Japan
[2]Japan Facility Management Association/Environment Design Dept., Mitsubishi Jisho Sekkei Inc. Japan

After the Great East Japan Earthquake, Business Continuity Plan (BCP) for hospitals has been increasingly attracting attentions, and it becomes one of the most important subjects for hospital management. The purpose of the paper is to propose tools of Facility Management (FM) in order to support Hospital Business Continuity Plan (BCP) at the time of natural disasters. According to surveys carried out on disaster mitigation and Business Continuity situation in 50 Hospitals suffered from Great East Japan Earthquake in 2011, the FM tools could be describing hospital activities during the disaster, including not only conditions of the hardware, such as structure / infrastructure of buildings, but also including conditions of patients, provisions of medical equipment, catering services, health care staff, materials. In addition these physical and human resources could be describing in chronological order. As one of the conclusions, facts and figures founded in the back of the reports on 50 hospitals suffered from the East Japan great earthquake, the importance of the FM tools is highlighted.

Osamu Kosaka. *Born 1950 in Kyoto prefecture, Japan; joined Takenaka Co., Ltd. in 1973, Japan Facility Management Association. in 2001, and is currently Chief of the Healthcare Facility Management Research Group. Extensive supervisory design experience in creating medical facilities such as clinics and hospitals, campus facilities such as universities and institutes. Occasioned by the advent of the Great East Japan Earthquake, has been engaged since 2011 in research on facility management tools for business continuity planning for hospitals. Certified Facility Manager Japan. Architect. Member of Architectural Institute of Japan.*

Shigehiro Taguchi. *Born 1960 in Shizuoka prefecture, Japan; joined Mitsubishi Estate Co., Ltd. in 1990, Mitsubishi Jisho Sekkei Inc. in 2001, and is currently head of the Healthcare Facility Design Office, Residential & Living Environmental Design Department. Extensive supervisory design experience in creating medical facilities such as clinics and hospitals, care facilities for the elderly such as special care homes and health care facilities, and care-provided accommodation for the elderly such as pay-for homes. Joined the JFMA Healthcare FM Study Group in 2006. Occasioned by the advent of the Great East Japan Earthquake, has been engaged since 2011 in research on facility management tools for business continuity planning for hospitals.*

Effects of "Free Plan" Modern Architectural Configuration in Seismic Performance of Hospitals

Teresa Guevara-Perez

tereguevara@gmail.com
Departamento de Arquitectura, Facultad de Arquitectura y Diseño, Universidad de los Andes, Bogotá, Asociación Colombiana de Arquitectura e Ingeniería Hospitalaria, Colombia

The modern architectural configuration known as free plan or open floor, is a commonly design tool used by architects in hospital projects. This configuration exists, when one of the stories of a frame structure, is mostly free of walls, while in the rest of the floors, stiff walls are present. It provides design advantages to the architect when designing hospitals, since it is mostly used for accommodating spaces that require free of walls layouts in the building: large entrance halls, cafeterias, large maintenance service areas, physical therapy gym, or car parking lots.
Earthquake engineering around the world have recognized, however, that this architectural configuration leads to the formation of soft story and weak story seismic irregularities, that if not treated in a special way could produce severe structural damage and even the collapse of hospitals when an earthquake occurs.
Currently the majority of seismic codes in the world include special requirements and penalties for the seismic analysis of buildings with these irregular configurations, especially in hospitals.
An emblematic example of the effects of the 1971 San Fernando, California, Earthquake on the modern Olive View Hospital that was severely damaged, and some conclusions and recommendations, are presented.

Teresa Guevara-Perez. *Architect, Universidad de los Andes, Venezuela; AAGradDip in Industrialized Construction Management, London. Master of Architecture and Ph.D. in Architecture, specialized in Buildings Seismic Design, UCBerkeley. 1972-1989, Researcher in Industrialized Housing Technology and Architectural Seismic Design, Instituto Nacional de la Vivienda, Caracas.*
1990-1992, Head of the Research Department in Consejo Nacional de la Vivienda, Caracas. Since 1992, Independent consultant, and Visiting Professor in diverse universities. 1994-2003, PAHO/WHO Temporary Advisor.
Recent books: "Terremotos en El Salvador 2001," PAHO/WHO, Washington: 2001; "Arquitectura Moderna en zonas sísmicas," Editorial Gustavo Gili, Barcelona: 2009; "Configuraciones urbanas contemporaneas en zonas sismicas", Ediciones Sidetur/ FAU-UCV, Caracas: 2012.

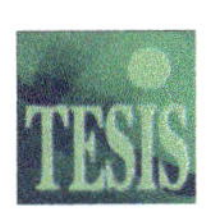

Introduction

The origin of free plan or open floor configuration, so common in the design of modern hospitals is mainly derived from three of the "five points for a new architecture" published by architect Le Corbusier (LC) in 1926 that defines the tenets of modern architecture: pilotis (open first floor); free plan; and free façade.
The application of these principles was possible by the development of modern construction techniques and materials, specially by the use of reinforced concrete frame structures (RCFS) that consisted of solid slabs that transfer the gravity loads to very slender columns and finally to the footings, leaving behind the rigid structural wall system, that prevailed until early 20th Century and generated dark and damp interior spaces.
Von Moos (page 159) mentions: "Light, air, openness were the qualities emphasized by this new building type and lung sanatoriums came to see as prototypes of the new way of life: the most recent studies in the field of medicine concerning hospitals coincide with the intention inherent in the whole field of architecture; the doctor, too, requires a maximum dissolution of the walls in glass, the freest possible access of light".

Soft Story and the Weak Story Irregularities

These seismic irregularities are derived from the open floor architectural configuration. The soft story irregularity, refers to the existence of a building floor that presents a significantly lower stiffness than the others, hence it is also called: flexible story. It is commonly generate unconscientiously due to the elimination or reduction in number of rigid non-structural walls in one of the floors of a building, or for not considering on the structural design and analysis, the restriction to free deformation that enforces on the rest of the floors the attachment of rigid elements to structural components that were not originally taken into consideration. Because of the effects produced by non-structural components on the seismic performance of the building, the term non-intentionally-structural has been assigned to these components since the end of the 1980's (Guevara, 1989). Table 12.3-2 in the ASCE/SEI 7-10 document, (p. 83) defines soft story as irregularity type 1. If the soft story effect is not foreseen on the structural design, irreversible damage will generally be present on both the structural and nonstructural components of that floor. This may cause the local collapse, and in some cases even the total collapse of the building.
In a regular building, the earthquake shear forces Vn increase towards the first story (Figure 1). The total displacement (ΔT) induced by an earthquake tend to distribute homogeneously in each floor throughout the height of the building. Deformation in each floor (Δn) would be similar (Figure 2a). When a more flexible portion of the lower part of the building supports a rigid and more massive portion, the bulk of the energy will be absorbed by the lower significantly more flexible story while the small remainder of energy will be distributed amongst the upper more rigid stories, producing larger relative displacement between the lower and the upper slab of the soft story (interstory drift) on the most flexible floor and therefore, the columns of this floor will be subjected to larger deformations (Figure 2a-2b).

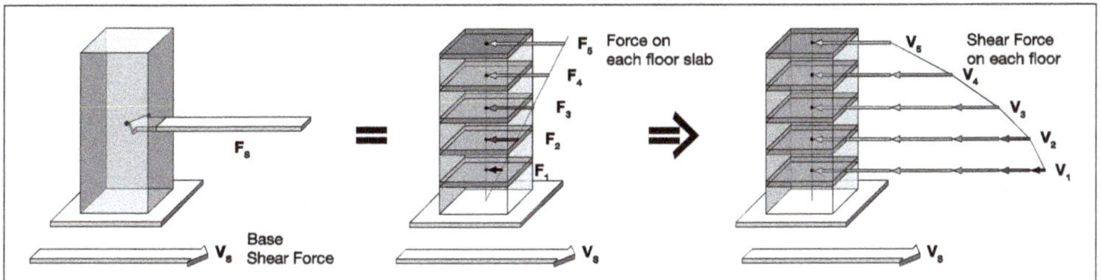

Figure 1. Lateral forces and shear forces generated in buildings due to ground motion.

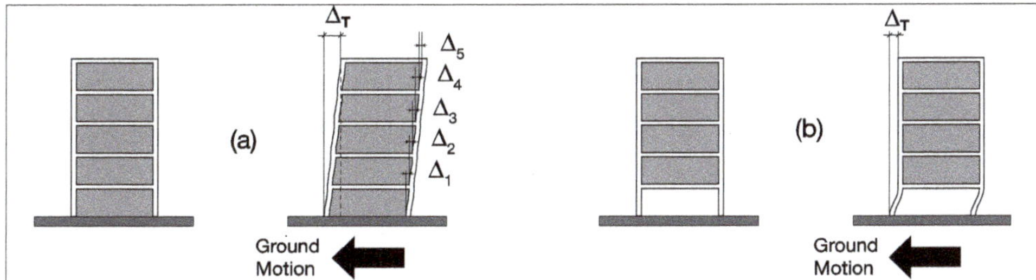

Figure 2. Distribution of total displacement generated by an earthquake in: (a) a regular building; and (b) a building with soft story irregularity.

The lowest more flexible portion, in the path of force transmission, may create a critical situation during an earthquake; the stiffness discontinuity between the first and the second stories might cause significant structural damage, or even the total collapse of the building. One of the most common examples observed is the first story of modern residential buildings used as car parking. The structural elements are homogenously distributed throughout the building, but the apartments are located on the upper floors with many masonry walls, while the lowest floor is left totally or partially free of partitions for parking vehicles and for social areas that require wide spaces. In the case of double height first soft stories, columns are very flexible not only due to the total or partial absence of walls but as result of their significantly greater height in relation with those from the upper floors. This configuration is one of the characteristic models of modern design for hospitals, in which the main lobby or entrance hall of the hospital, and other large distribution spaces for general public have great importance, and they require free of walls layouts. This configuration may also exist at intermediate floors.

The weak story irregularity refers to the existence of a building floor presenting a lower lateral structural resistance than the immediate superior floor or the rest of the floors of the building. The building's weakest part would suffer severe damages due to its inability to withstand the different types of loads (lateral, vertical and moments) produced by the ground motion. Current seismic regulations at the beginning of the 21st Century in most seismic countries, following the parameters initially established in the 1988 Uniform Building Code (UBC-88), and, recent versions of the National

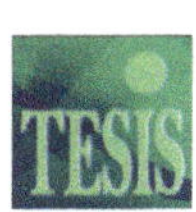

Earthquake Hazards Reduction Program (NEHRP) and the International Building Code (IBC), have included numeric values to the assessment of weak story. As an example, table 12.3-2: Vertical Structural Irregularities in the ASCE/SEI 7-10 document, (p. 83) of the American Society of Civil Engineers (ASCE) and the Structural Engineering Institute (SEI), illustrates this irregularity.

Weak story can be generated by: (1) elimination or weakening of seismic resistant components at the first floor; (2) mixed systems: frames and structural walls, with wall interruption at the second floor or at intermediate floors (Figure 3). This irregularity can be present also at the first floor or at intermediate floors. There are numerous examples of many buildings presenting a combination of these types of irregularities, soft and weak story, making them particularly seismically vulnerable.

Emblematic Example

The main building of the Sylmar Olive View hospital (OVH) in the 1971 San Fernando, California Earthquake is an emblematic example of failure due to the effect of both, soft and weak story.

The OVH consisted of four bodies joined around a courtyard, as shown at the structural layouts in Figure 4. Each body had six floors and a penthouse.

Bertero (1978, p. 114) describes: "The structural system has significant discontinuities. While the upper four stories consisted of shear walls combined with moment-resisting space frames, the lower two stories had only a moment-resisting space frame system. The floor system consisted primarily of a flat slab-column system with drop panels at the columns.

Tied and spirally reinforced concrete columns were used. The shape and reinforcement of these columns differed from story to story." Bertero (1997) explains that the large interstory drift in the main Treatment and Care Unit, which induced significant non-structural and structural damage and which led to the demolishing of the building, was a consequence of the formation of soft and weak story at the lower story levels because on the lower floors there were columns only, while there were reinforced concrete walls above the second floor level (Figure 5).

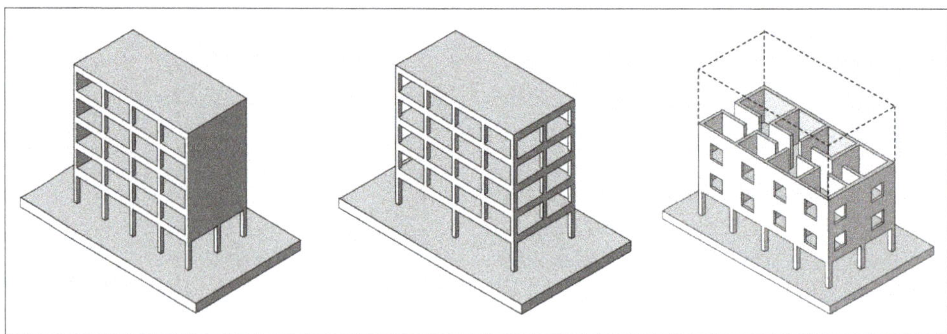

Figure 3. Examples of weak first story irregularity.

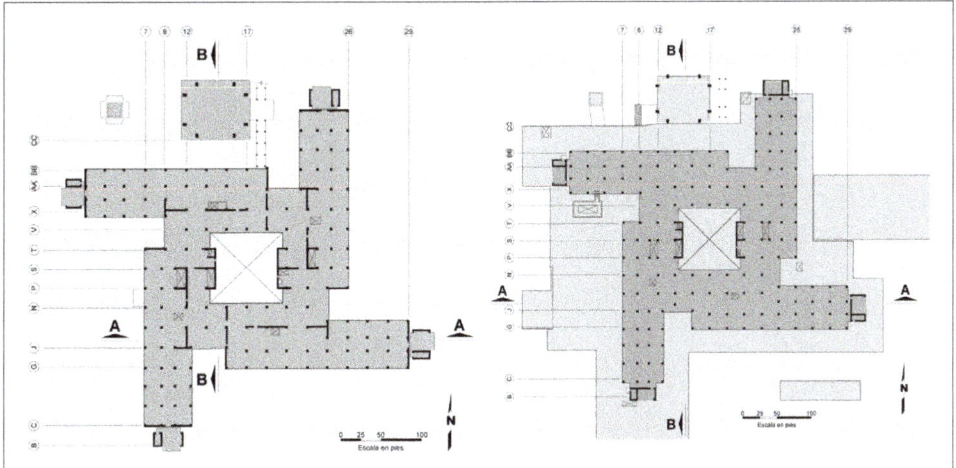

Figure 4. Structural layouts: left, typical floor plan from the second floor level up; right, floor plan of the lower floor levels.

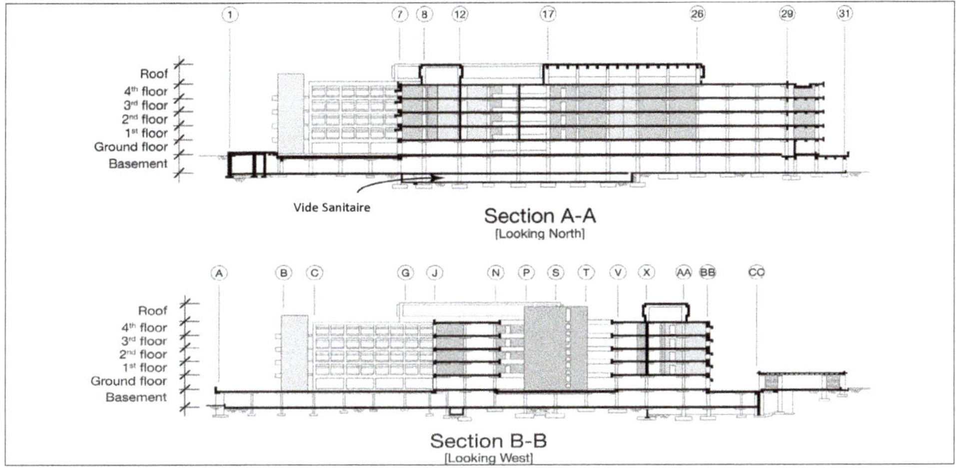

Figure 5. Structural sections illustrating discontinuity of loadbearing walls in the lower stories.

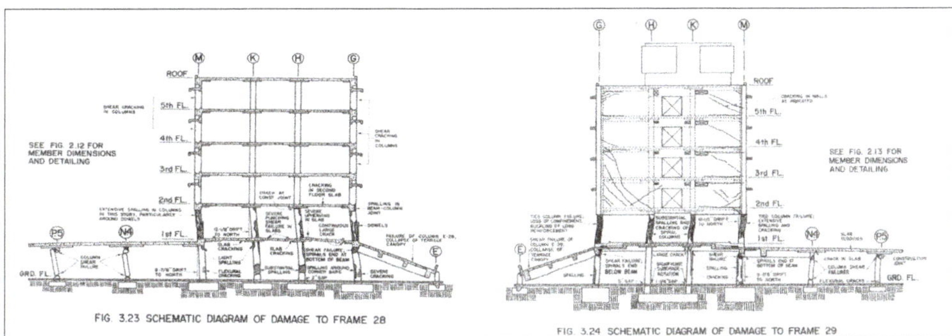

Figure 6. Schematic diagrams of damage to frames 28 and 29 (Mahin et al. Page 26).

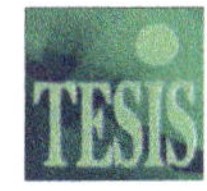

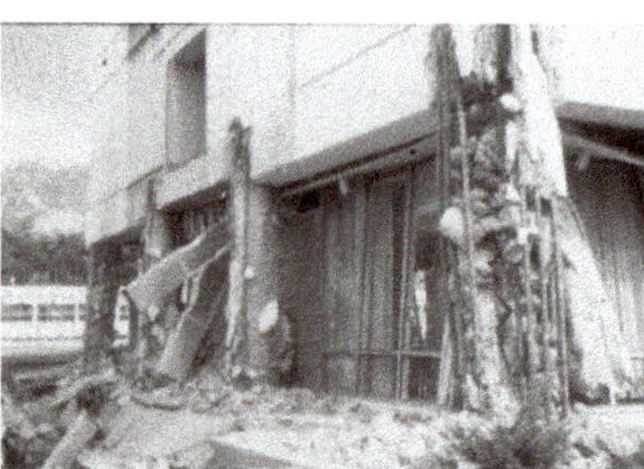
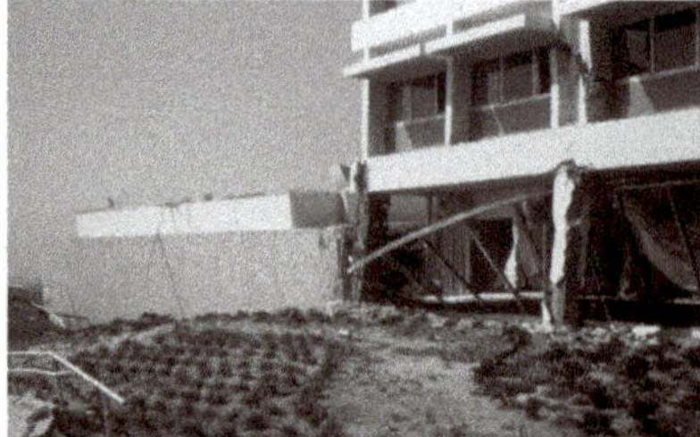
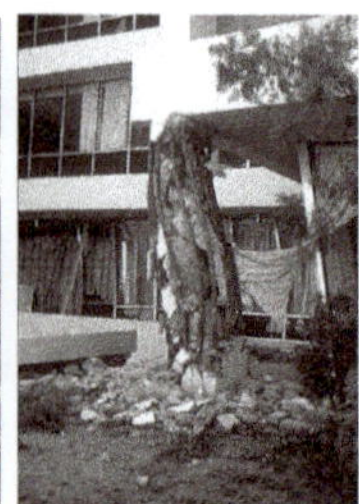

Figure 7. Deformations in the first story level.

Final Remarks

The open floor configuration is an architectural design feature that will not be easily eliminated from the design criteria of architects. It gives to the designer a series of functional and aesthetic advantages that are encouraged in schools of architecture.

Arnold and Reitherman (1982, p. 120) recommend:

> When shear walls form the main lateral resistant elements of the building, they may be required to carry very high loads. If these walls do not line up in plan from one floor to the next, the forces created by these loads cannot flow directly down through the walls from roof to foundation, and the consequent indirect load path can result in serious overstressing at the points of discontinuity. Often this discontinuous-shear-wall condition represents a special, but common, case of the weak first story problem. The programmatic requirements for an open first floor result in the elimination of the shear wall at that level, and its replacement by a frame. It must be emphasized that the discontinuous shear wall is a fundamental design contradiction: The purpose of a shear wall is to collect diaphragm loads at each floor and transmit them as directly and efficiently as possible to the foundation. To interrupt this load path is a fundamental error. To interrupt it at its base is a cardinal sin. Thus the discontinuous shear wall which stops at the second floor represents a "worst case" of the weak floor condition.

Since 1988 most seismic codes worldwide have included penalties for the use of these irregularities which results in the increase of the design lateral force or shear at the base. Since the beginning of the 21st Century new "extreme" categories were incorporated for controlling and even forbidding the use of these two types of configuration.

Lessons include in international post-earthquake reconnaissance reports, regarding the influence of open floor in buildings' seismic performance, barely reach architectural practice, or decisions takers that continue encouraging the use of this configurations in urban zoning regulations (UZR). Most seismic codes are written in analytical terms for engineers who are specialists in seismic design and difficult to be understood by architects and decision takers. For understanding the influence of architectural configurations on building seismic performance, conceptual knowledge on

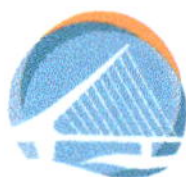

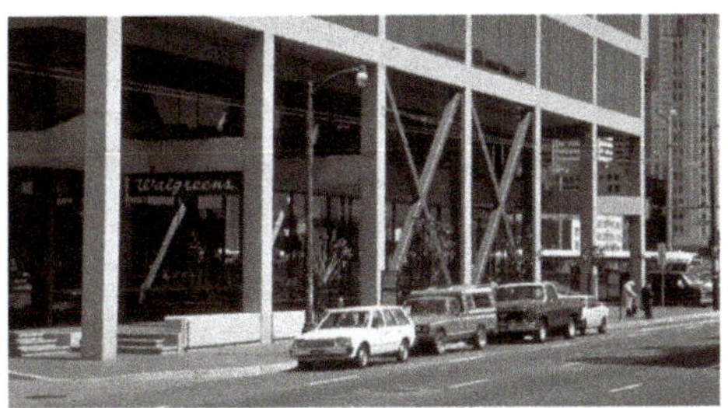
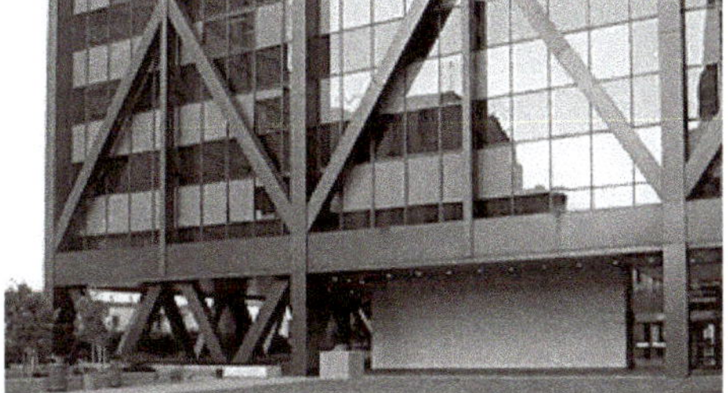

Figure 8. V. V. Bertero (left); former Alcoa Bldg (right).

the effects of mass, stiffness and resistant distribution in buildings is necessary. Earthquakes lessons have taught that it is not sufficient for reducing seismic vulnerability of buildings to apply structural engineering building codes.

The problem has to be untangled with a holistic approach where engineers of different disciplines, architects, local authorities and medical community that take decisions in the design of hospitals, participate, not only in reducing vulnerability of existing hospitals but avoiding the construction of future seismic risk.

As a final remark, it is necessary to: (a) Strengthening communication and collaboration between earthquake engineering disciplines; architecture disciplines; and decision takers; (b) Establishing a common vocabulary in earthquake-resistant terminology across disciplines; (c) Active participation of architects in the development of regulations that affect the earthquake-resilience of hospitals; (d) Development and implementation of a cross-disciplinary approach in the design of hospitals; (e) Teaching cross-discipline courses in undergraduate and graduate schools of architecture and engineering, including in the program topics related to the influence of architectural configurations on seismic performance of hospitals.

RECOMMENDATIONS

If in the design of new hospital buildings in seismic zones the widespread use of the open first floor is unavoidable, the recommendation is to take measures to avoid soft and weak story formation at any cost. Therefore, it is necessary to include prescriptions or restriction for designers that allow them to reduce the vulnerability of hospitals in seismic hazardous zones, as it is being done already in California. Authorities in Alameda, Berkeley, Fremont (http://enginious-structures.com/pages/softstory.html) are already including in the UZR, some restrictions and in some areas prohibiting the use of these configurations. At present, there are many analytical studies available on this regard in the structural engineering field, worldwide. Guevara and Paparoni, (1996), gave some solutions; some of them: (1) Design based on the use of diagonal members in the soft first stories are feasible. All the foregoing assertions can be considered as reliable under the condition of having very weak walls in the uppers stories, that is, that they will not increase the rigidity of the structural elements. (2) One influence which in many instances tends to be ignored is the large increase of the member forces in the first stories of buildings due to torsional effects. Besides the dy-

namic influences, the simple fact that most of the first stories of buildings are designed as if they had built-in columns and theoretically rigid foundations gives rise to very high concentrations of design forces there. In the case of seismic torsion, we have the additional effect of warping, due to the particular nature of most of the framing schemes in current use. When we add to that, sudden changes in rigidities caused by the disappearance of relatively rigid claddings over the soft story level, then large force concentrations appear which can be attributed to torsional effects. It is necessary to avoid abrupt changes.
In 2010 Mayor Gavin Newsom of San Francisco, California, proposed seismic mandates for retroffiting buildings with soft story configurations in the city. (See http://sfdbi.org/san-franciscos-soft-story-buildings-lie-vulnerable-quake and ATC-52-32 Report in http://www.sfgsa.org/modules/showdocument.aspx?documentid=9759). Figure 8 illustrates some examples of methods that have been used in the San Francisco Bay Area to retrofitting buildings with first soft story.

References

Arnold, CH. y R. Reitherman (1982), *Building Configuration and Seismic Design*, John Wiley & Sons, Inc., New York.

American Society of Civil Engineers (ASCE). (2010). *Minimum design loads for buildings and other structures: ASCE Standard ASCE/SEI 7-10. Reston*, Virginia.

Bertero, V.V. (1997), en "Distribution of mass, stiffness & strength", W. G. Godden, Editor. Structural engineering slide library. Set J: Earthquake engineering, V. V. Bertero. National Information Service for Earthquake Engineering, University of California, Berkeley.

Bertero, V.V. (1978). *Distribution of Mass*, Stiffness & Strength. Anal. Acad. Ci. Ex. Fis. Nat., Vol. 31, 1979. Buenos Aires.

Bertero, Vitelmo, (1997) *Distribution of Mass,* Stiffness & Strength, Structural Engineering Slide Library, W. G. Godden Editor. Set J: Earthquake Engineering, V. V. Bertero. NISEE On-line, U.C. Berkeley.

Building Seismic Safety Council (BSSC). (2015) *NEHRP Recommended Seismic Provisions for New Buildings and Other Structures presents commentary to ASCE/SEI 7-05*. Washington, D.C.

Guevara-Perez, T. (2012), *Configuraciones urbanas contemporáneas en zonas sísmicas*, Fondo Editorial Sidetur and Ediciones FAU-UCV, Caracas.

Guevara-Perez, T. (2009). *Arquitectura moderna en zonas sísmicas*, Editorial Gustavo Gili, Barcelona, Spain.

Guevara, L. T. and M. Paparoni. (1996). *Soft First Stories Treatment in the Municipal Ordinances of a Hazardous Sector of Caracas, Venezuela*. Paper No. 1065. Proceedings 11WCEE. Elsevier Science Ltd.

Mahin, Stephen, et al. (1976) *Response of the Olive View Hospital main building during the San Fernando earthquake, Report No. EERC 76/22*, October 1976, Berkeley, California, Earthquake Engineering Research Center, College of Engineering, University of California.

Von Moos, S. (1979). *Le Corbusier: Elements of a Synthesis.* Cambridge, MA: MIT Press.

Project Hope: A Case Study

Walter Vernon

adeboisfroge@mazzetti.com
Mazzetti, United States

In November of 2013, Typhoon Haiyan struck the Philippines, destroying large swathes of the country. Numerous international NGOs responded in the months that followed. Project Hope, a US NGO that has been providing disaster relief services for years was one of the first on the ground. Project Hope set up services at two different locations on two islands, providing various kinds of medical services and capacity re-building. One focus of the Project Hope volunteers has been the reconstruction of the Filipino healthcare facilities, including the entire health infrastructure of the island of Poro. One of the key design elements of the Project Hope Approach is disaster resilience – to better equip the facilities with the ability to both withstand and operate effectively operate after the next such severe weather incident.

The systems include on-site DC solar generation systems, certain DC-powered medical equipment, and on-site water treatment systems. The systems are designed to provide essential primary care services, and larger, more conventional AC-generation PV systems for larger clinics and hospitals. The scheme involves unique financing methodologies, including the sale of carbon offsets and power purchase agreements. This session will detail the design and financing details for the systems.

Walt Vernon *is the CEO for Mazzetti, a national consulting and engineering firm headquartered in San Francisco. He has been working with healthcare clients to plan, design, and operate healthcare facilities globally for more than 25 years. Walt Chairs the NFPA99 Electrical Systems Technical Committee and is the former Electrical Engineer for the California Hospital Building Safety Board. As one of three co-coordinators for the Green Guide for Healthcare, the nation's first Green Healthcare rating system, and co-authored the IEEE/ANSI White Book, the international standard for Electrical Systems in Healthcare Facilities. Walt co-chairs the ASHRAE 189.3 committee, which is currently writing a model national green building code for healthcare facilities. Walt chairs the Research and Development Committee for the Facilities Guideline Institute, the body that writes the Guidelines for Healthcare Construction, which is the model licensing code for most states in the country.*

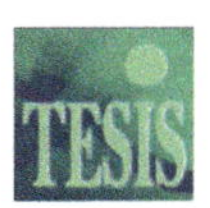

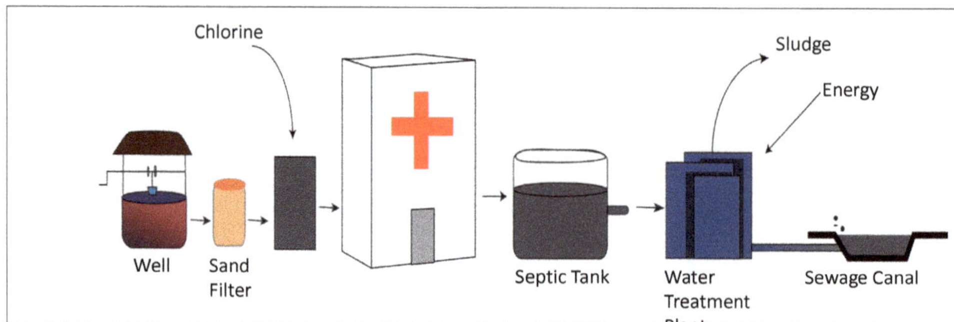

Figure 1. Conventional approach.

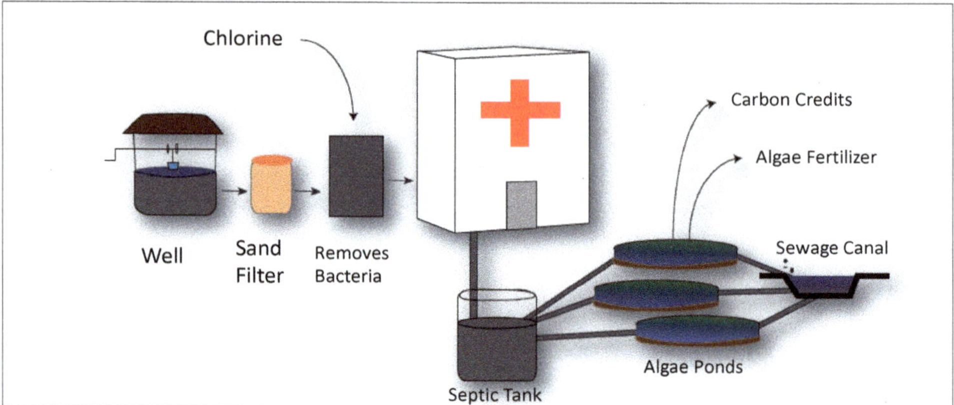

Figure 2. Engineers without borders solution.

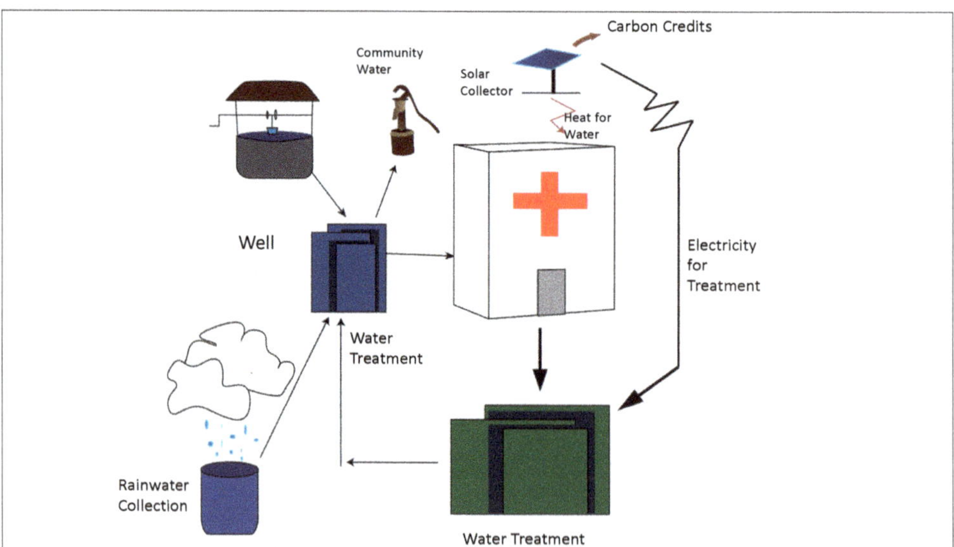

Figure 3. Walt's idea.

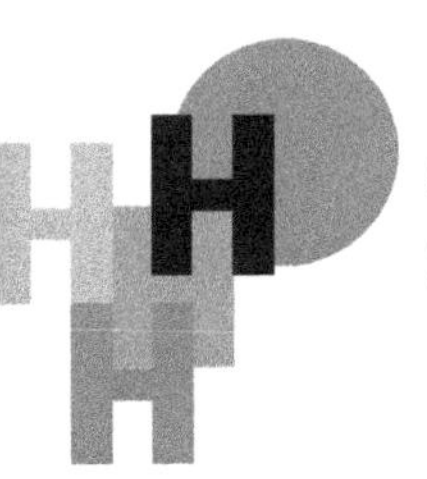

Status of Health Services and Systems

Session Introduction

The efficiency and development of the healthcare system is an indicator of the welfare of a country. On the other hand, the recent economic crisis has resulted in the need to reduce construction costs and the use of healthcare facilities.
In this scenario, the choices that affect health and welfare policies have a direct impact on healthcare architectures, determining plans to redevelop existing buildings or plans to construct new state-of-the-art buildings.
Similarly, the presence of public or private investments determines the choice of different types of procurement and execution of the works, and this can have a strong impact on the spatial and qualitative connotation of healthcare environments. Furthermore, this assistance, organized according to the intensity of care, determines differing types of healthcare buildings according to different levels of care.
The design choices can lead to significant reductions in the operating costs of a hospital, especially using technologies to reduce energy consumption and carefully organizing the functional spaces.
The technological changes of recent years have affected care practices and procedures resulting in alterations to care environments. It is still of primary importance to design the space in line with user needs, and create environments in which the wellbeing of patients, relatives, physicians and nurses is taken into account.
Buildings should be designed to take advantage of the possibilities offered by the terrain, orienting buildings so as to favour the infiltration of natural light. The application of prefabricated elements should be assessed on the basis of how the structures adapt to the needs of the local populations, and the actual accessibility of prefabricated modules in different areas of the construction site should be considered. Any intervention considered should first undergo a careful needs analysis taking into account both the characteristics of the place and the requirements of the population.

Preliminary Studies and Design of 20 Healthcare Service Provider (IPS). Facilities Located in Several Departments throughout Colombia

Sergio Gonzalez, Natalia Laurens

sergosigma@gmail.com
20 + Member Interdisciplinary Team, Consortium Sigma GP – SERGO

The 2010 - 2011 La Niña phenomena caused damages to the public healthcare infrastructure, impairing the water and sewage and epidemiologic conditions of the population in Colombia. As a result, 20 of the 223 healthcare facilities affected by the phenomenon contacted us to substantiate the existence of damages, analyze the risks of or threats to the new plots of land to be developed, evaluate the legal issues of the plots of land chosen, and draft the architectural and technical designs of the new facilities within a six-month term. This paper presents some examples of the projects, from the survey of the location of the affected facility, to the design of a new facility in a new plot of land chosen by the Healthcare Provider, including all the information that builders will need to carry out the work. This work was carried out by an interdisciplinary team of architects, engineers and attorneys, under the supervision of the United Nations (UNOPS) and the Antioquia Government (Comprehensive Management). The contracting agency is the "Fondo Adaptacion", a governmental entity established to carry out the building, rebuilding, recovery and economic and social reactivation of the areas affected by the 2010 - 2011 La Niña phenomenon.

Sergio Luis Gonzalez. *Born in 1949, Bogotá, Colombia. CEO, SERGO Ltda, Architects. Architecture Degree, Universidad Nacional de Colombia, 1974. PhD, Universidad de Navarra, Pamplona, Spain, 1980. Has authored articles on the Theory of Architecture. Beginning in 1974, Dr. Gonzalez has been faculty member: Universidad Nacional de Colombia, Universidad de Navarra (Spain), Universidad de Los Andes, Universidad Autonoma de la Costa, Universidad de la Costa, CUC. Beginning in 1987, Dr. Gonzalez has devoted his time to architectural projects for healthcare facilities. Member of the Sociedad Colombiana de Arquitectos, SCA and the Sociedad Colombiana de Arquitectura e Ingenieria Hospitalaria, ACAIH, among others.*

Natalia Laurens*, a Civil Engineer specialized in Project Evaluation from the Universidad de los Andes in Bogotá, participated in the team responsible for structuring the Metro project for Bogotá in 1998 and 1999. She was also in charge of implementing the infrastructure for the TransMilenio System for more than 4 years. Likewise, she was Director of Project Studies and Design at the Urban Development Institute of Bogotá (IDU, according to its acronym in Spanish) for over 3 years, where she contracted and executed more than 120 urban infrastructure projects, among which the following are worth highlighting: TransMilenio Phase III, the Western Longitudinal Avenue, the expansion of the Autopista Norte, and 75 projects related to roads, bridges, intersections and public space, financed through property appreciation taxes. She has also served as advisor in transportation and infrastructure projects in various Colombian and Latin American cities.*

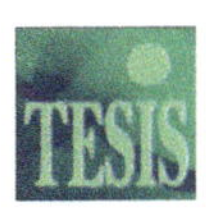

IMPLEMENTATION: 2010 – 2011 LA NIÑA PHENOMENA

The Phenomenon had a direct effect over 60% of Colombia, leaving more than 2.4 million victims. The heaviest rainfall took place between the months of December 2010 and March 2011, causing floods and landslides, leading to the declaration of economic, social and ecologic emergency.

THE "FONDO ADAPTACION"

The Colombian Government established the Fund in 2010 as part of the Ministry of Finance "for the recovery, building and rebuilding of the areas affected by the La Niña phenomenon". The Fund is in charge of the building and rebuilding projects and of the furnishings and equipment required by the public healthcare facilities of the country.

As mentioned above of the 223 facilities affected, SIGMA GP – SERGO was commissioned to assess the damages caused by the 2010 - 2011 La Niña phenomenon, analyze the risks or threats of the new plots of land to be developed, study the legal issues of the plots of land chosen, and draft the architectural and technical designs of 20 facilities located in five different departments as follows: two in Antioquia, seven in Choco, two in Cordoba, four in Norte de Santander, and five in Sucre, all within a six-month term. Supervision is in charge of the International Organization UNOPS.

The team (more than 20 professionals) that was put together by the consortium included an engineer - as administrative director -, an architect - as technical director -, two architects - as coordinators -, two engineers - as coordinators -, and work teams comprised of engineers specialized in risks, bioclimatic and biomedical architects, hydrologic engineers, forestry engineers, topographers, soil engineers, structural engineers, hydraulic engineers, water and sewage engineers, fire extinguishing systems engineers, electrical engineers, telecommunication engineers, fire control systems engineers, mechanical engineers specialized in air conditioning and ventilation systems, engineers specialized in natural gas, medicinal gas and compressed air pipe networks, financial administrators and attorneys specialized in real estate law.

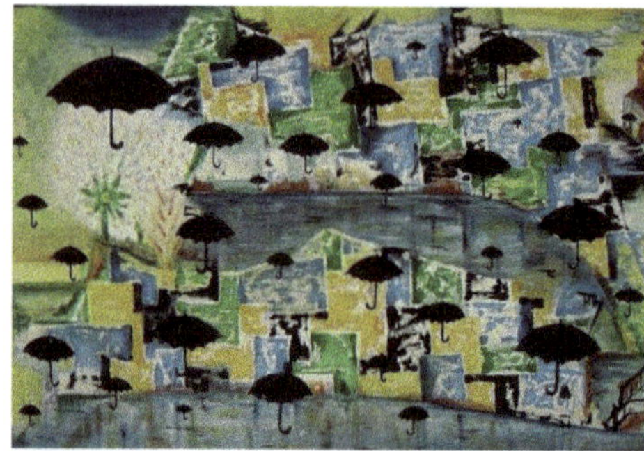

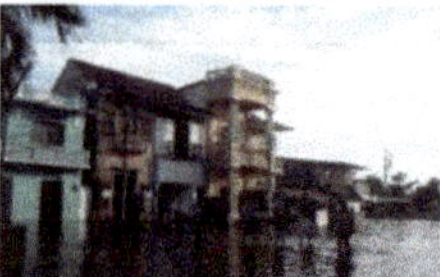

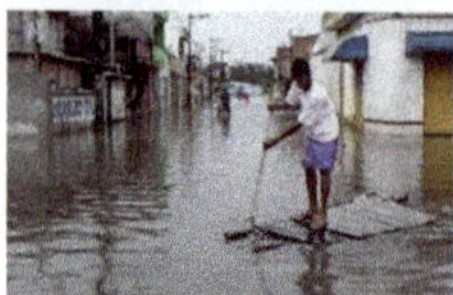

Figure 1. Town of Sucre, Sucre (top, left), any settlement affected (below, left). Landscape, Jose Abelardo Narvaez, oil, 2012 (right).

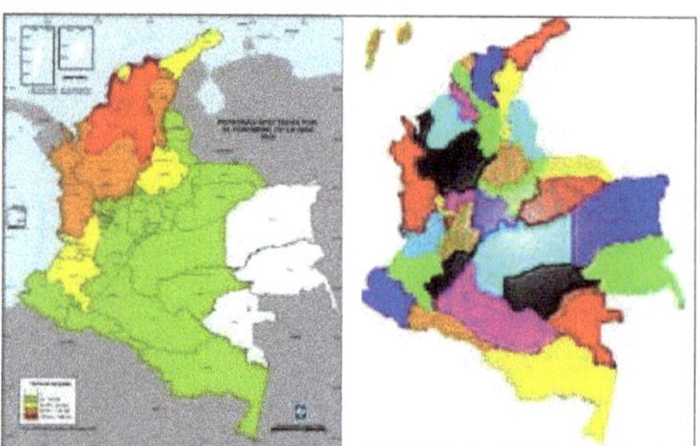

Figure 2. Colombian areas affected by the La Niña phenomenon. Of the 32 Departments, 11 were affected.

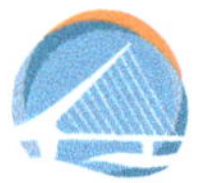

Validation of the damages

To be able to initiate the audit of the facilities of an IPS (provider health care institution), a field inspection must be conducted to substantiate whether or not the facilities were affected by the 2010 - 2011 rainy season. Supporting documentation of the municipal, regional and national entities corroborating the damages suffered has to be submitted. Once the inspection is made and the documentation is obtained, our expert drafts an opinion about the damages with his recommendations concerning the rebuilding or relocation of the affected facilities. By way of example, the following pictures show the area and the facilities of the Puerto Santander, Norte de Santander, IPS. In conclusion, the report states: "Our recommendation is that the facilities be relocated to a plot of land at least 1 meter higher than the current location of the IPS, with proper access and risk levels to provide the service".

Threat and/or Risk

Once the recommendations are given, which most likely will include the relocation of the facilities, the local government has to suggest a new plot of land of the size required to be able to build the new facilities.
Our architects make sure that the plot of land meets the local legal requirements (use of the soil and zoning regulations) and the size requirements, since the facilities cannot occupy more than 60% of the area of the lot.

With the involvement of engineers specialized in risk, our consulting services include an assessment of the level of risk involved in the event of a natural threat that may place the new facilities at risk. The following pictures show the facilities of the Centro de Salud Coveñas, located in the Morrosquillo Gulf, Sucre department, on the Atlantic coast.

DESCRIPTION	EXISTS	CONDITION		
		GOOD	NOT SO GOOD	BAD
RISKS				
Flood	X	X		
Landslide				
Collapsing				
Torrential				
Lateral undermining of river				
ACCESS				
Overland routes	X	X		
Sidewalks	X	X		
CONSTRUCTION				
Floors	X	X		
Walls	X	X		
Roof	X	X		
Other				
TECHNICAL INSTALLATION (PUBLIC SERVICES)				
Water supply network	X		X	
Sewer system	X		X	
Electrical network	X		X	
Natural gas network				
Telecommunications				
FUNCTIONALITY				
Consulting rooms	X		X	
Laboratory	X			X
Emergencies	X		X	
Obstetrics and Gynecology	X			X
Hospital beds	X			X
ACTA				

Figure 3. Puerto Santander and summary of the assessment of damages suffered by the facilities.

MEDICAL-ARCHITECTURAL PROGRAM (PAM)

The Health Department provides the size parameters of the facilities according to the epidemiologic requirements of the region and the guidelines of the National Hospital Network, which establishes the needs of each healthcare facility so that healthcare providers may provide adequate services within the Colombian territory.

In drafting the Medical-Architectural Program, we include supporting areas in addition to the parameters provided by the Health Department. The PAM must be approved by the Subdireccion de Prestacion de Servicios de Salud and the Subdireccion de Infraestructura en Salud, in order to meet the requirements of the architectural designs, which must be reviewed and approved by the Health Department.

Titling

The IPS has to hold the title to the plot of land where the facilities are going to be built. To that end, our team has attorneys specialized in Real Estate Law who study each property, their titles and any other property matters, to make sure that the properties meet all the legal requirements; as well as to make sure that any land purchases are made in compliance with the law.

Topographic Survey

Once the plot of land has met all the aforementioned requirements, a team of topographers travels to the location to analyze the property.

Basic Plan

An interdisciplinary team of architects, urban specialists and bio-climatic experts drafts a preliminary plan based on the functional requirements approved by the Health Department and the characteristics of the plot of land.
The following is an example of the basic plan of the Centro de Salud, located in the town of Nueva Colonia, Turbo municipality, Antioquia department, near the Uraba Gulf:

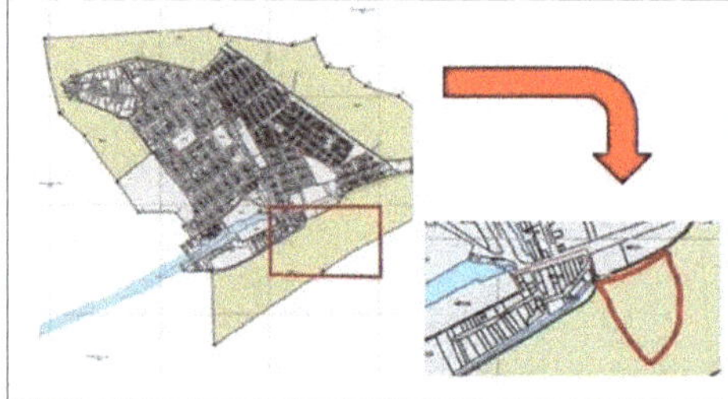

Figure 4. Nueva Colonia localization.

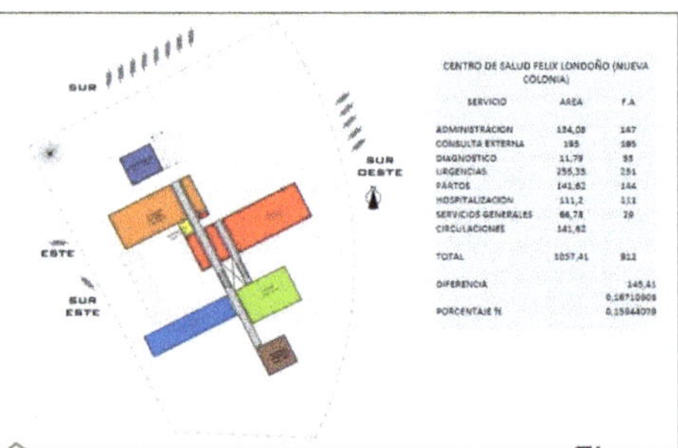

Figure 5. Nueva Colonia basic scheme.

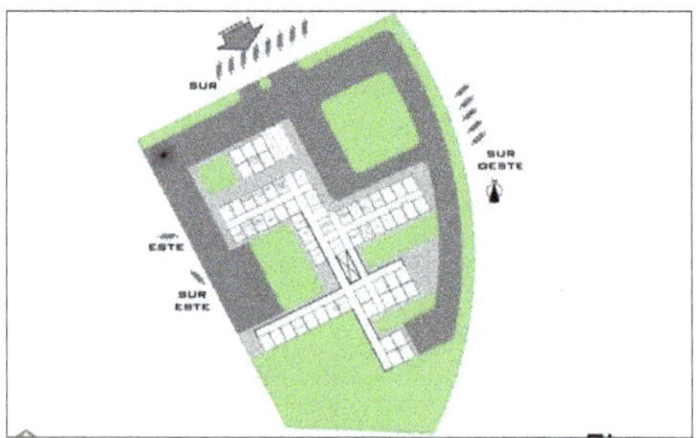

Figure 6. Nueva Colonia zoning.

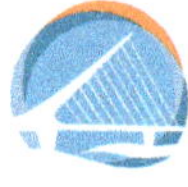

Soil Survey

The soil engineer gives the basic plan in order to perform the required digging, in compliance with the earthquake-resistant regulation NSR-10, which regulates all the procedures to carry out the structural designs in accordance with the specific characteristics of the structure and the area where the structure will be built.

Architectural Designs and Technical Studies

The architectural project is drafted after all the information is obtained. Throughout the different phases, the different technical designs seek innovation, energy savings, ease of handling of materials, etc. Concerning the characteristics of the architectural designs, main topic of this presentation, we have developed a modular design that can be adapted to the regional characteristics of the area, the plot of land, materials to be used in the region, transportation of materials when the location is difficult to get to.

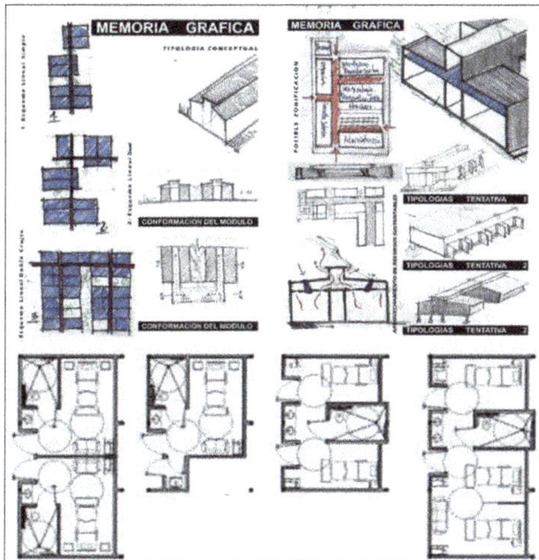

Figure 7. Modular system.

In determining the construction systems to be implemented, light pre-fabrication systems were ruled out due to the following reasons:

1. Future changes or modifications required to install new equipment that the healthcare provider may want to acquire cannot be made.
2. Uncertainty as to the duration of the construction systems and materials used to make the prefabricated systems, as opposed to properly chosen traditional methods that ensure long life of the buildings if properly maintained.
3. The adaptability of the building to the cultural environment where it will be located, since IPS users need to feel comfortable in it. The building needs to improve the quality of life, without introducing elements foreign to the cultural environment.
4. High construction costs, because prefabricated systems for this type of buildings are not well developed in Colombia, which requires the use of systems developed in other countries. In addition, maintaining the buildings becomes a difficult since replacement items are not readily available locally; with the resulting uncertainty as to how well will the chosen prefabrication system hold over time.

The studies and designs ensure that the technical regulations in effect for the healthcare sector are complied with, regulation NSR10 of 2010 for structural systems and fire protection requirements, environmental and water and sewage regulations and other applicable regulations for the drafting of the designs and studies subject matter of this preliminary study.

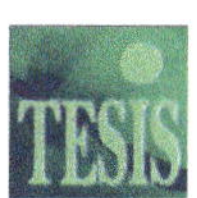

We are presenting some designs with their characteristics, using a modulation method that can be adapted to different planning requirements and different topographic characteristics, including, looking to obtain bioclimatic effects to generate proper temperatures without having to use too much mechanical ventilation. Most IPS are located in warmer climates, where temperatures average 32°C and the humidity is high, especially in the Department of Choco, on the Pacific coast, which is mostly an area of rain forest and where it rains throughout the year.

The following designs show the facilities of the Centro de Salud Currulao, located in the Urabá Gulf, Antioquia department, on the Atlantic coast:

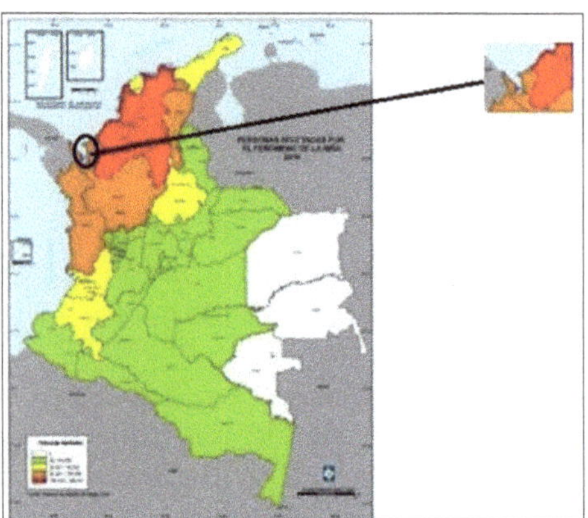

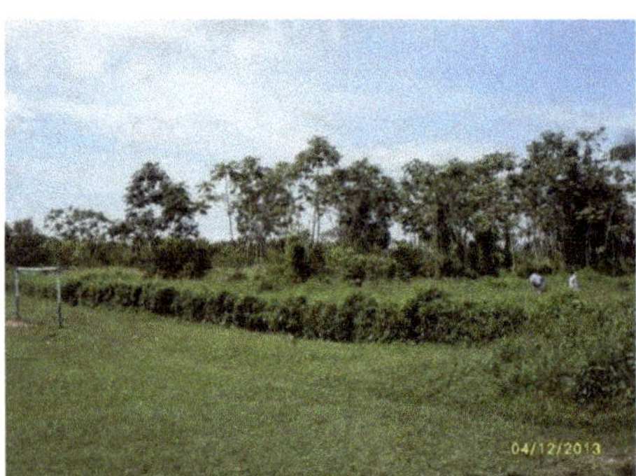

Figure 8. Centro de Salud Currulao, area and localization.

SUR
ESTE
SUR ESTE
ACCESO 1
ACCESO 2
CENTRO DE DON BOSCO (CURRULAO)
SERVICIO AREA F.A
ADMINISTRACION 143,48 147
CONSULTA EXTERNA 195 221
DIAGNOSTICO 18,4 59
URGENCIAS 230,29 231
PARTOS 150,8 144
HOSPITALIZACION 111,25 131
SERVICIOS GENERALES 61,8 29
CIRCULACIONES 214,4
TOTAL 1125,18 940
DIFERENCIA 185,18
PORCENTAJE % 0,197

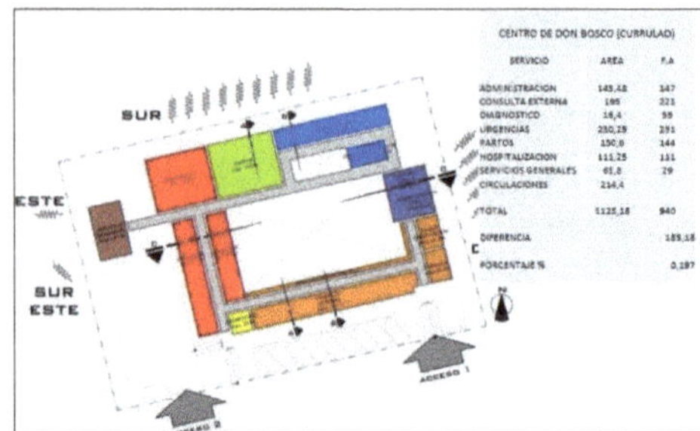

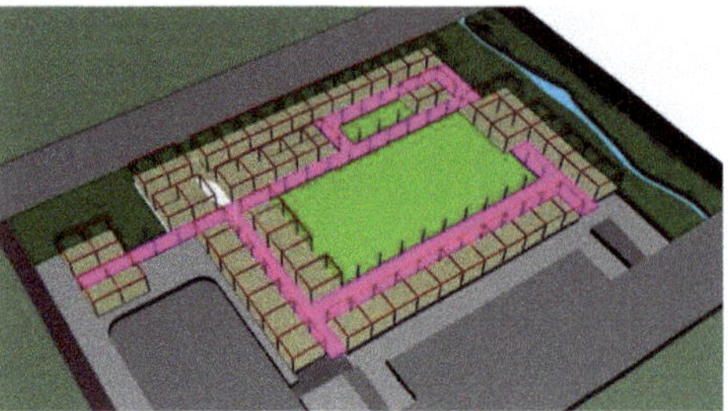

Figure 9. Centro de Salud Currulao basic scheme and structure.

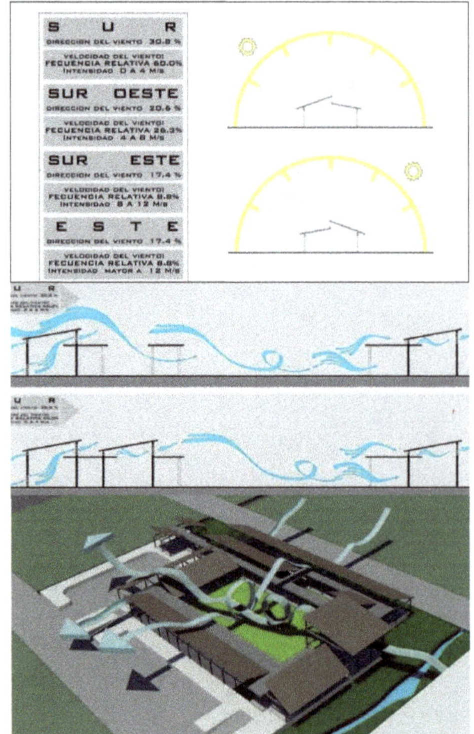

Figure 10. Sun and winds.

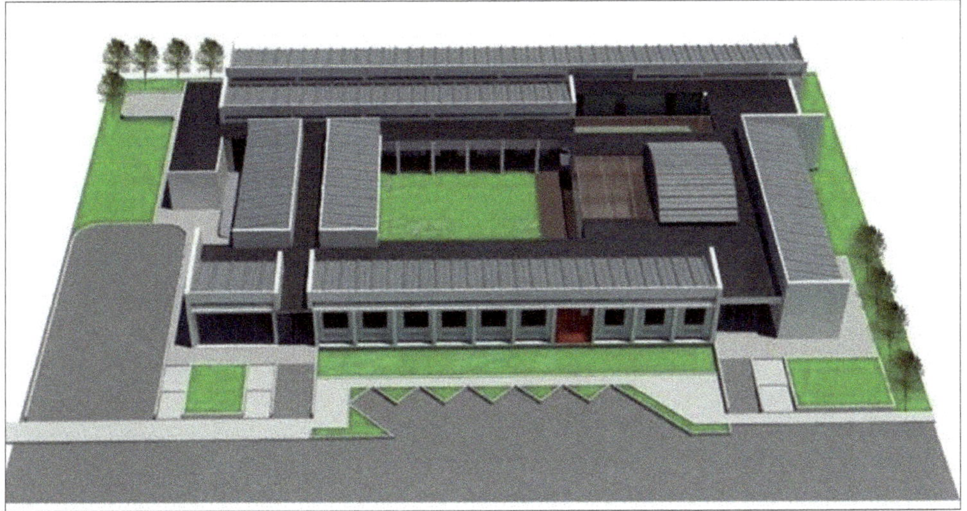

Figure 11. Rendering aerial view.

Specifications, Amounts of Work, Construction Costs and Licenses

Our consultancy services end by submitting all the requirements so that a builder may complete the work in the shortest amount of time, with a high quality and low cost construction system. We include designs that have been properly approved by the Health Department, construction licenses and any permits are required to be able to begin the construction work.

The average cost is US$1.250 per square meter, without including furnishings and with some basic urban works.

Characteristics of our Contract

We have felt it important to include the contracting method because it gives us some flexibility in the execution of each one of the works. The works are paid based on deliverables:

1. Report on the validation of the damages suffered by each IPS as a result of the 2010 - 2011 La Niña phenomenon: 2%;
2. Report on the risk and/or threat study performed for each one of the lots: 2%;
3. Report as to the titling status of each one of the lots: 2%;
4. Topographical surveys of each one of the lots: 4%;
5. Soil surveys of each one of the lots: 4%;
6. Medical Architectural Program of each facility, approved by the Health Department: 5%;
7. Drafting of the architectural design of each facility, approved by the Health Department: 30%;
8. Drafting of the structural design of each facility to include: blueprints, construction details, technical specifications, amounts and budget with their respective per-unit price analysis: 10%;
9. Drafting of the electrical and tel-

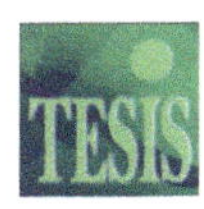

ecommunications design of each facility: 10%;

10. Drafting of the hydraulic, water and sewage and natural gas design of each facility (the latter, when applicable): 10%;

11. Drafting of the medicinal gases design of each facility (when applicable): 3%;

12. Drafting of the air conditioning and mechanical ventilation design of each facility (when applicable): 3%;

13. Submitting applications for construction permits and any other permits required for the construction of each facility before the applicable authorities:%;

All of the above ads up to 90%; the balance of 10% will be paid at the time the contract liquidation minutes are signed. In addition, a fixed monthly amount will be payable for each report submitted with the activities carried out during the month.

Reimbursable expenses are also acknowledged, including:

1. Expenses incurred because of risk and/or threat studies, soil surveys and other unanticipated surveys.
2. Travel and lodging expenses of the consulting team.
3. Local travel expenses (whether by air, land or water), i.e., cost of traveling outside of the limits of the towns where the lots are located.
4. Regional premium for the technical, operating or support personnel when such personnel have to travel away from home to perform activities requiring more than 30 days.

Current Trends in the Healthcare System and Facilities in Venezuela

Sonia Cedrés de Bello

bello.sonia@gmail.com
Instituto de Desarrollo Experimental de la Construcción. Facultad de Arquitectura y Urbanismo
Universidad Central de Venezuela

In 1999, a new government came into power in Venezuela. This new government, labeled "Socialism of the XXI Century" introduced many changes to the Health Care System and in doing so, created a parallel system to the existing one. These changes impacted healthcare delivery, facilities, administration, medical personnel and staff. Additionally, medical facilities architecture, project management and construction were also affected. The government dedicated extensive time and resources to implement this new system, including remodeling and modernizing existing facilities, but the program has proven unsuccessful. The construction process has left public hospitals with limited operational capabilities and as a result, private hospitals have seen a surge in demand. To meet this demand private hospitals have had to invest in capital projects to expand capacity. This research paper is an analysis of the impact of the changes to the healthcare system on the architecture, construction and programming of healthcare facilities in Venezuela.

Sonia Cedrés de Bello. *Architect (UCV, 1973), Master of Architecture (University of Washington, 1978) and Doctor in Architecture (UCV, 2006). Professor and researcher at Facultad de Arquitectura y Urbanismo at the Universidad Central de Venezuela (UCV) since 1982. Visiting Professor and lecturer at: Universita La Sapienza, Roma (1991-92), University of Tokio (1996), Texas A&M (2002) and Universidad Católica de Chile (2008). Over 40 years of experience in different areas of healthcare facilities planning and design, founding member of the Asociación Venezolana de Arquitectura e Ingenieria Medico Sanitaria (AVAIMS), official member of the International Union of Architects Public Health Group, and member of EXAIS. Author of books and specialized articles. Speaker at national and international conferences and seminars. Healthcare facilities design and programming consultant.*

The Health System and the Health Facilities

In Venezuela, a country with 28 million inhabitants, the healthcare system is provided by two large sectors: public and private. Each sector has its own facilities, but with the same rules and regulations for design and construction established by the Ministry of Health (now titled the Ministry of the Popular Power for Health, Ministerio del Poder Popular para la Salud MPPS). Health care in public hospitals is free of charge as

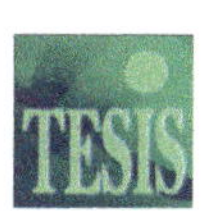

established by the Constitution, and private care is financed by insurance companies and the patients. The MPPS estimates that 80% of the population utilizes the public sector and 20% the private.

There are several public institutions that deliver health care, the main ones are: MPPS, the Institute for Social Security (IVSS), and the military health service (SSFA). Since their founding, the IVSS and SSFA provided services strictly to members and family, but in the last decade they have opened to the public. While they are open to the public, they are still dependent on social security and the military for funding. For years, a new law for a National System of Health has been pending approval. This law would unify healthcare services through an integrated and decentralized network of defined services with clear competencies at the national, state and municipal level.

Since 1983, the public health care facilities have been classified by the Ministry of Health as Ambulatories (urban and rural) and Hospitals (type I: 20-60 beds, type II: 60-150 beds, type III: 150-300 beds, type IV: >300 beds). This classification determines the level of complexity, level of medical care and population coverage.

The public hospitals now in operation are 20 to 50 years old and during this time been remodeled and modernized. They are currently in the process of installing new technologies.

Dependency	Nº Hospitals
MPPS	217
Social Security	33
Military Hospitals	13
Petroleum Company PDVSA	3
Total	**266**

Table 1. Amount of public hospitals and dependence. Venezuela 2009. Source: MPPS. Misión Barrio Adentro III 2009.

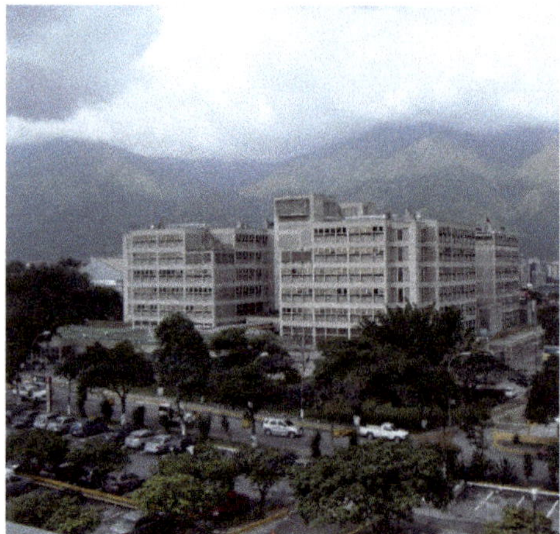

Figure 1. Hospital Domingo Luciani. Type IV, (IVSS), build in 1984.

In addition to the public health system there is a private system made up of more modern, specialized hospitals, ambulatory services and day hospitals. These facilities are smaller and have less capacity than public facilities. Among the 457 existing private hospitals (profit and nonprofit) only 35 have capacity larger than 60 beds.

In the last 30 years Venezuela's population has doubled while the government has only built 5 public hospitals increasing capacity by only 1%. Public hospitals have a maximum capacity of 42,000 beds, currently only 16,000 function properly. The private sector, as of 2013, had 7,300 beds representing 50% of the actual public functional beds.

At this time the number of operative facilities does not meet demand and cannot provide the level of services required. This is due to a deficit in infrastructure, inefficient and obsolete architectonic capacity, poor distribution, limited availability of physical, human and technological resources, unprofessional institutional management and lack of criteria and best practices that support the construction of hospitals by pathologies instead of general hospitals The most critical areas to specialize by are: emergency departments, surgical suites, maternity and delivery rooms, and intensive care (Oletta, 2013).

MISSION BARRIO ADENTRO

Beginning in 2003 a new model of heath care was established: Mission Barrio Adentro (BA). This model was inspired by the Cuban model and a co-operation agreement was signed with Cuba which created a system parallel to the existing one[1]. This Mission is adscript to MPPS with its own doctors, staff, programs, procedures, budget, and facilities. This fact needed a new typology, classification, and operatively of the services delivered.

Facilities	Quantity
Consultorios Populares	6.708
Popular Clinics	12
CDI	499
CAT	21
SRI	545

Table 2. New facilities build under the Program Barrio Adentro I and II. Source: Dirección General de Hospitales. Misión Barrio Adentro. 2008.

[1] *Different researches (Rodriguez, et. al, 20, p.; Diaz Polanco, 2008, p. 31-2), lets confirm a strong tendency to cubanization of the public health in Venezuela, since Barrio Adentro has been inspired from the first stages in the Cuban health system and the formation of the communitarian integral doctor under the premises of the communitarian integral medicine.*

This Plan has been implemented in 4 stages: Barrio Adentro I, started in 2003 with the construction of popular consultation (consultorios populares) to provide primary care services. These offices are 100 m^2, and have the objective to cover 1.200 inhabitants or 250 families each one. They include a residence for the doctors, 24 hours attention, and are located in barrios with high population density, located on the outskirts of large cities.

Barrio Adentro II, started in 2005; provides services for the second level of health care, the facilities are named Center for Integral Diagnosis (Centros de diagnostico Integral CDI), Rooms for integral rehabilitation (Salas de rehabilitacion integral SRI) and Center for high technology (Centro de alta tecnologia CAT). Some function in new buildings and others in remodeled existing buildings. All of them in an outpatient (ambulatory) basis. The CDI provides emergency attention with appropriated areas of: intensive care, some have surgery suites, X ray, ultrasound, endoscopy, clinic laboratory and clinic ophthalmology. The program includes a basic area of 700 m^2. The CAT offers services of clinic laboratory and imaging including tomography, magnetic resonance, X ray, mammography, endoscopy, and ultrasound in a basic area of 500-700 m^2. Some of them have few beds for a short term observation (10- 20 beds).

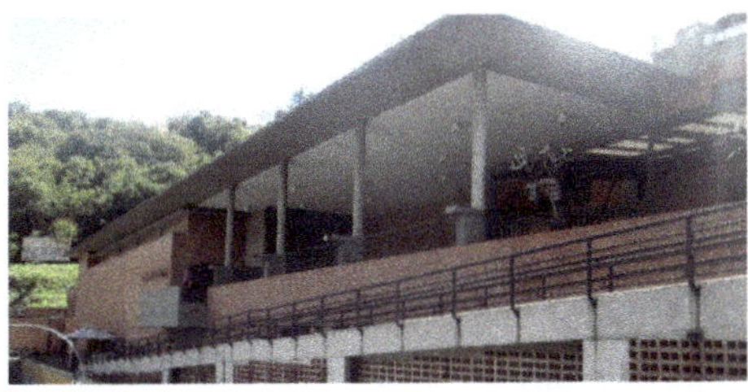

Figure 2. Center for Diagnosis of High Technology (CAT) 2009.

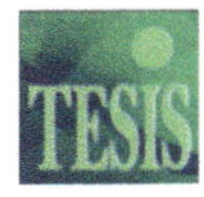

Barrio Adentro III, started in 2006. This program oversees the renovation of the existing hospitals including implementing new technology and building additions to meet the new requirements. The priority areas to be updated are: surgery suites, emergency departments, intensive care units (adults, pediatrics, neonatal) imaging and dialysis units. Areas for cardiology, radiotherapy and oncology are also included.

Barrio Adentro IV, started in 2007 plans for the construction of 15 new specialized hospitals, the first 6, with 200 beds and 14.000 m2 are under construction using a prefabricated Turkish technology. Phase III of Barrio Adentro, consisting of modernizing hospital structures and equipment, has been realized through partnerships with other countries including: Argentina to supply equipment for oncology, radiotherapy, neonatology, and obstetric for all the hospitals and to manage the construction of the facilities, installation for the equipment. China to install medical equipment and Cuba to manage the purchase of equipment and additional installation. All of these partnerships are financed with petroleum.

The inefficiencies of the parallel system Barrio Adentro, to provide primary care have made that the influx of patients to the conventional system (ambulatories and hospitals) continue.

In May 2011, a high number of construction left unfinished in the existing hospitals, due to poor management, budget shortfalls besides the mistake of the simultaneous intervention of many hospitals with different construction companies without coordination between them, brought the reduction of the capacity of response of the public hospitals network, limiting the operational capabilities.

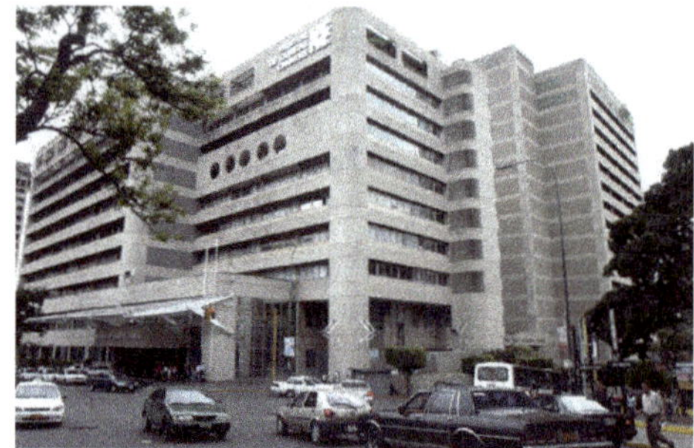

Figure 3. Clínicas Caracas. Private hospital.

Meanwhile, an important segment of the population cannot meet their healthcare needs in the public system and are turning to the private sector. It is estimated that the private sector is now servicing 30% - 38% of all medical consultations, and 50% of the emergencies. This is putting immense strain on the private sector driving construction projects in an attempt to meet demand. This is made more difficult due to economic restrictions that restrict free enterprise and reduce production and investment. In addition, competition has declined and inflation is the highest of the world.

References

Diaz Polanco, J. Barrio Adentro (2008), *Continente afuera*. Ediciones CENDES, Universidad Central de Venezuela.

Rodriguez Y, y otros. Misión Barrio Adentro: balance y perspectivas. *Revista Nuevo Mundo*. Universidad Simón Bolívar. Caracas. Año IV, No. 10; p. 139-182.

Oletta, J.F. (2013), *Balance de Salud del año 2012 en Venezuela*. Alerta Epidemiológica No 246. Red de Sociedades Científicas Medicas Venezolanas. Disponible en: www.rscmv.org.ve

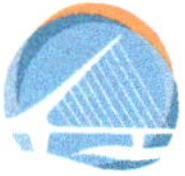

Public Health Care in the Province of Santa Fe, Argentina
Scenarios in Consolidation

Silvana Codina, Jorgelina Paniagua

silvanacodina@hotmail.com
Architecture Department - Ministry of Public Works - Government of Santa Fe

The province of Santa Fe is consolidating transformation scenarios in health care, based on a model defined in 2008 which has resulted in buildings that introduce innovative architectural concepts.
Three strategies are being materialized:

- *A homogeneous distribution of facilities across the provincial territory, intended to establish territorial balance and proper access.*
- *Health care facilities operate in a network, in three different levels of care, in diverse building models.*
- *Comprehensive architectural concept based on typological systems of design, aimed at planning the different interventions to project and management execution periods.*

The notion of typological systems of design surpasses the idea of prototype known until now; it was dormant in paradigmatic projects built in Argentina in previous decades (i.e. Amancio Williams' three hospitals in the province of Corrientes). This strategy enables open architectural systems, adaptable and configurable to different programs, scales, plots and orientations, always taking into account the physical conditions imposed by each and every location.
Multidisciplinary work has proven to create fertile soil for experimentation, leading to technological solutions, combining architecture, engineering and building techniques that feature a certain degree of innovation.

Silvana Codina. *Architect (National University of Rosario) and Expert on Physical Resources Planning in Health Care (National University of Buenos Aires). Former Director of Hospital Architecture, Rosario Municipal Secretary of Public Health. 2007-2011, Special Adviser, Government of Santa Fe. Current Secretary of Architecture, Ministry of Public Works. Has planned and created the design concept of over 365,000 sq. m, most of which have been actually built and some are under construction; 200,000 sq. m. correspond to health care facilities. Author of several books, articles and publications. Associate professor at FADU-UNL and guest professor in different universities. 2011, 12th Architecture Biennale, Public Management Award.*

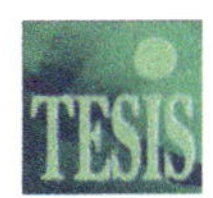

Development

Santa Fe population, a little more than 3 million, is characterized by its immense cultural diversity and wealth of natural resources. Most of the province consists of green flatlands but it presents unique features at the four points of the compass. There is significant heterogeneity in every dimension of human settlements (social distribution, economic base, environmental characteristics).
The clear understanding of such diversity implied establishing a participatory process to organize the 132,638 sq. km in five regions. The process represents a scale of proximity that acknowledges regional identities and values open dialog between the community and the environment, manifesting an intermediate scale of belonging for 51 municipalities and 312 communes.

Provincial administrations in office since 2007 have had this perception of the territory, enabling public policies aimed at decentralization. With respect to health care policies, the intention has always being bringing services closer to the people, from diagnostic to the implementation of specific solutions, resorting to the principles of universal, equal and efficient health care and looking forward to overcome long standing imbalances and territorial deficits.

Architecture plays an essential role because it accepts the challenge of meeting collective demands and hopes, and responds by deploying different ways of adapting the physical, geotechnical, regulatory, cadastral, constructive and technological elements of the urban environment.

R1
RECONQUISTA NODE
37 TOWNS AND VILLAGES
R2
RAFAELA NODE
97 TOWNS AND VILLAGES
R3
SANTA FE NODE
98 TOWNS AND VILLAGES
R4
ROSARIO NODE
96 TOWNS AND VILLAGES
R5
VENADO TUERTO NODE
56 TOWNS AND VILLAGES

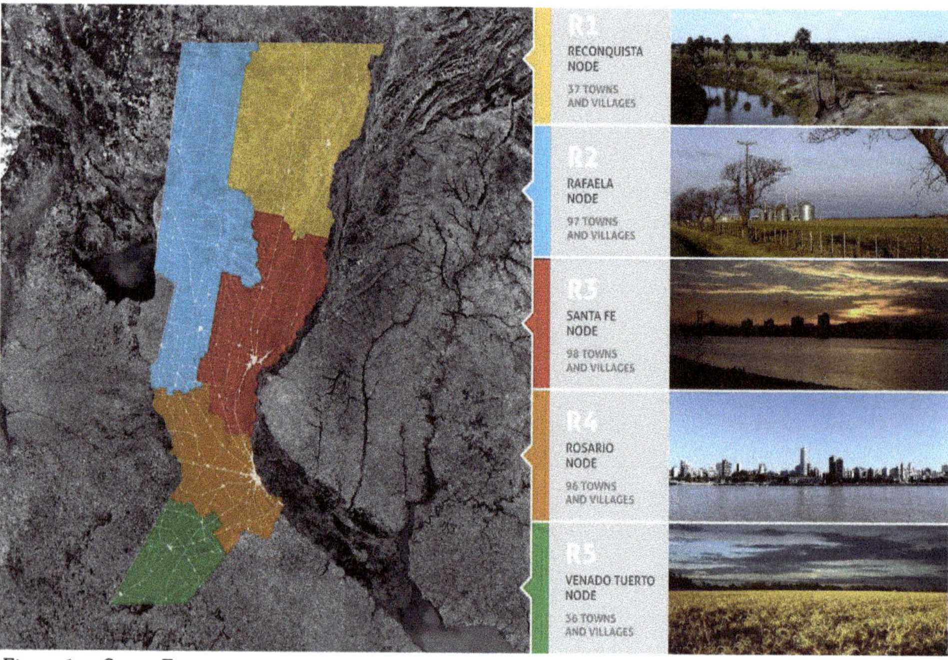

Figure 1. Santa Fe.

MATERIAL INTERVENTIONS INCLUDE THREE DIFFERENT ACTIONS

First, a homogeneous distribution of facilities across the provincial territory, intended to establish territorial balance and proper access. This is not just providing equal opportunities to exercise citizens' rights; it also understands that health care facilities should be located strategically in order to be accessible to all.
Currently, the provincial strategy revives the precedent established seventy years ago by the architect of modernity Wladimiro Acosta, then advisor of the Public Health Care Department. Under the 1938-1942 Health Care Plan, only partially executed, 58 rural health care stations, an asylum in Oliveros, a mental hospital in Santa Fe and a leper colony in Recreo were built.

Second, a system that operates in three levels of care in diverse building models: health care centers, mid-complexity hospitals, outpatient centers and high complexity regional hospitals that follow a progressive care scheme and work in line with specialized hospitals. All located strategically following epidemiological data and based on the efficiency and sustainability of public finance and on sound criteria for the rational use of resources.

Third, the development of a comprehensive architectural concept based on typological systems of design. Architecture has no limits; it constantly touches other disciplines, synthesizing the relationship in a design. This synthesis results in a culture that transforms reality. Buildings already designed and built are open, permeable, transparent they occupy the space without affecting the landscape.

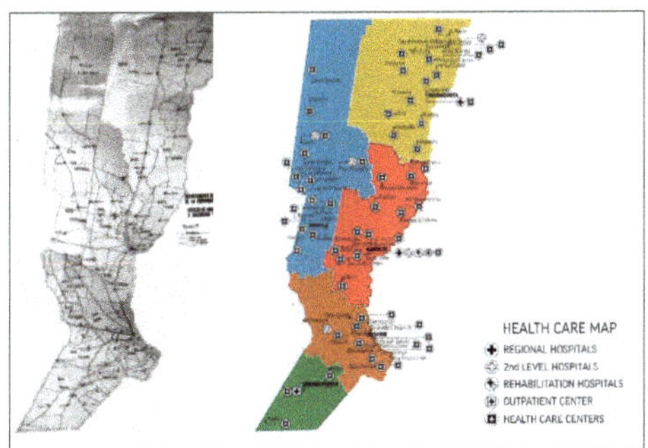

Figure 2. 1938-1942 Health Care Plan (left) and Public Works in Health Care since 2008 (right).

Typological systems of design reinforce this concept of public architecture. They give shape to this institutional image, the representation of a State that has accepted the responsibility to provide health care to its citizens in buildings easily recognizable in their many locations and shapes.
The idea of place, of location, is thought as a vital component in the genesis of each building. Buildings share basic concepts but present their peculiarities, due to the number of people served, the climate, the location and the services actually provided.

Health care facilities' design is mainly horizontal, inspired in the topographic features of the plot and intended to favor the natural access to services, to facilitate circulation of people and materials by avoiding vertical circulation and the waiting times proper to mechanical systems, especially for the disabled.

Design appeals not only to an architectural language but also to a common technological solution to problems presented by infrastructures, equipments and finishing. Furthermore, solutions need to be adapted to the territorial di-

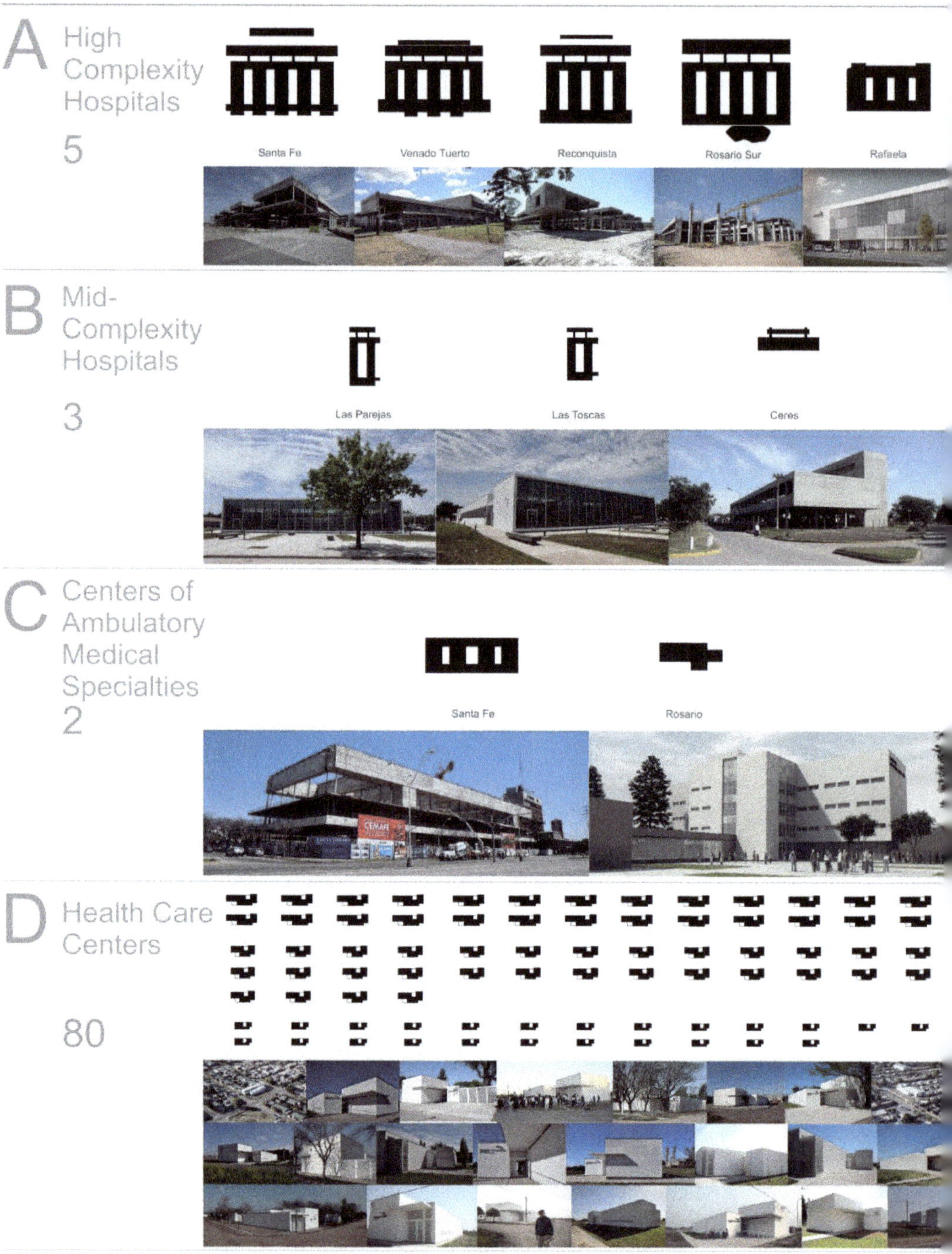

A High Complexity Hospitals 5

Santa Fe | Venado Tuerto | Reconquista | Rosario Sur | Rafaela

B Mid-Complexity Hospitals 3

Las Parejas | Las Toscas | Ceres

C Centers of Ambulatory Medical Specialties 2

Santa Fe | Rosario

D Health Care Centers 80

Figure 3. Healthcare buildings typologies related to assistence levels.

versity and to the chosen location. The idea is to enhance building quality, interior comfort and to create adequate and flexible spaces for outstanding medical performance.

The notion of a project-based system is superior to the idea of a prototype because it allows open, systematic, adaptable and configurable projects that can be adapted to different programs, scales, territories and orientations. We mean a single project but with different specific solutions, materialized based on the location, the circulation of people and materials and the size of functional modules controlled by project guidelines that link and define how to face the challenges at hand. The whole is in the part and the part refers to the whole, which relates directly to the location.
Metaphorically speaking, the typological system of design can be compared to a chess game. The chessboard is the supporting modular grid. The pieces are designed following a common module. The strategic distribution follows functional criteria and the physical constraints of the plot. The game, that is, the project played every time, is unique, unrepeatable and singular. As are the location and the specific users of this built public space.

The systematic planning of the different stages, from territorial planning until the facility comes into operation is supported by a professional, multidisciplinary team that is constantly consolidating the Special Projects Unit. This Unit gathers young professionals, mostly architects and engineers that are fully identified with the criteria above. Their mission is to interpret the needs and requirements of infrastructure and equipments derived from each ministry and to interact with teams of experts.

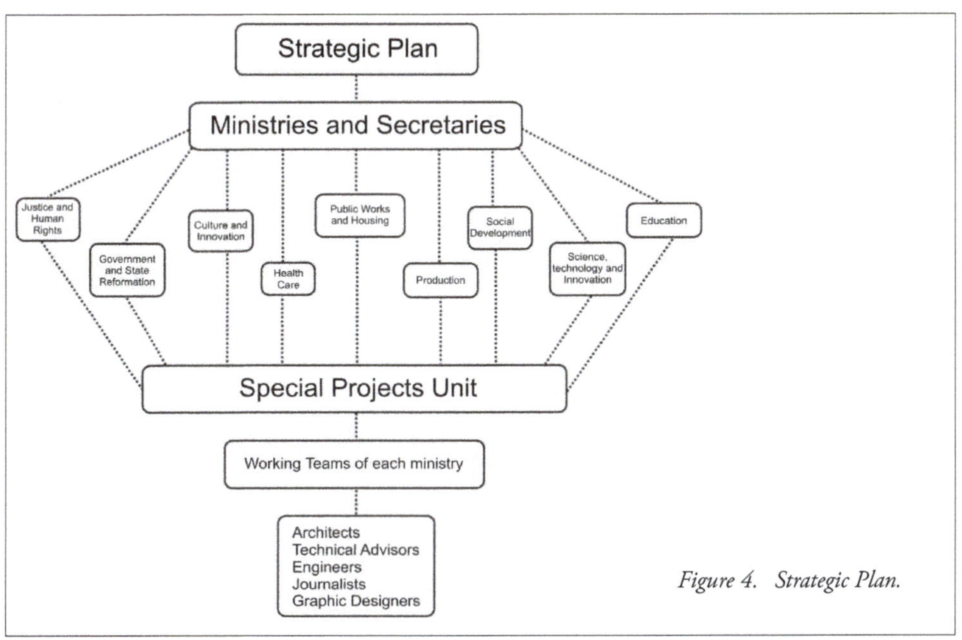

Figure 4. Strategic Plan.

Professionals are organized by themes: health care, culture, education, justice, etc. However, transversality instances are promoted because they express the willingness to optimize and perfect the design, based on the implementation and evaluation of construction solutions. On occasions, there are clear manifestations of innovation.

If we think of traditional methods, we can state that multidisciplinary work has introduced new construction concepts that have resulted in a quality leap. Completing the execution of the works has demanded a fair combination of technical expertise in architecture, engineering and construction, melted with the willingness to explore new horizons in design.

Structural, technical and technological approaches derived from experimentation are the natural way of transferring knowledge to new projects, irrespective of their size or scale, in order to foster a significant impact on the functional, formal, spatial and symbolic qualities of architecture.

Why Management and Technology Will Change the Hospital Design

Luis González Sterling

Asociación Española de Ingeniería Hospitalaria (AEIH), Spain

In the last few years, not only the agents that intervene in the process of producing the health facilities but also their roles are changing radically. Specially concerning architects and engineers, for whom their client is moving from the public to the private sector.
I am referring to the increase, all over the world, of hospitals promoted through using Private Finance through Public Concessions by applying systems of Outsourcing, like APP, PPP, PPF. A few years ago when the PPP started in the UK there was a saying that said: "The Prince has become Cinderella" in reference to the government who had made decisions on hospital design and was leaving a big part of these decisions to housekeeping and building maintenance: changes in how the hospital are promoted and who runs the design, construction and services management; other changes in the management's software that change the needs of spaces in accesses, waiting areas and space for procedures; changes in the requirements and planning of space, due to technology and new medical procedures; changes in the topological relation between the flows and the areas, will lead to new lift and vertical communication requirements as well as the need of a new scheme; changes in the communications facilities available that will develop the procedures and long distance healing that will change the concept of the hospital itself; changes in the outsourcing of services that will lead to a unification of resources and provide long distance medical services; changes in the models and software to process the information, and the increasing possibilities of sharing this information. All of this implies necessarily the need for a new design model.
The conclusions of my study will show the new tendencies and the most probable changes that will be needed, and how these changes will affect the design and the model of the future hospitals. This study will demonstrate the theory based on evidence and the resulting positive and negative consequences.

***Luis González** is a qualified architect with over 40 years' experience working for the Spanish National Health Service (Insalud) since 1978, and is a frequent guest speaker at healthcare international conferences. He has developed great number of major healthcare buildings both in Spain and abroad, and has extensive experience as a senior consultant and healthcare architecture expert. Luis is co-founder and CEO of Argola Arquitectos, a firm established in 1990 specializing in healthcare architec-ture. Argola has International experience in Europe. South America, Africa and the Middle East.*

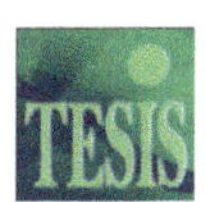

The Spanish Experience

Spanish Context in the Last 10 Years

After 14 years of continuous growth came a very tough crisis in 2008. During those years a massive amount of money came from the EU for infrastructures that was well invested and now we have one of the best roads and railways net of the world. Lots of grants from the BEI and money from investors was offered for health care projects. In 10 years from 2004 to 2012, 34 hospitals have been built hosting over 6.000 beds all overvthe Spanish geography. 18 under the financing systems of PPP, PFI or PPI, of different styles 8 of them include medical services, all finished and under operation. Since 2011, 6 of the others are stopped or delayed for economical reasons.

The Experience in Madrid

Madrid a region of 8 million inhabitants, on a total surface of 7.000 Sq km that in 2003 had 28 public hospitals totalizing 21.400 beds in 80 hospitals of which a 71% were public and 29% in private hospitals. Between 2004 and 2012, an important activity took place in the sector: 11 new public hospitals through PFI and PPP systems were built and that totalize 3.350 beds and 5 private that added another 540 beds to the total health care resources. This includes the new building for one of the most important hospitals of the region Puerta de Hierro of 460 beds then, that was moved from the city to the northern suburbs 10 km out of Madrid to a new building through a PFI totalizing 720 beds.

Simultaneously a process of creating a new building through a substitution process in its original site, for one of the large stand most prestigious, 12 of October Hospital 1.250 beds, was started and the two first phases of the three planed to be done between 2004 and 2014 (non stop). Further important enlargement and refurbishment took place simultaneously in an other four hospitals buildings of the region totalizing a total of another 900 beds. This program enlarged and modernized the total health care net of the region and added over 3.800 beds and affected another 2.000 beds.

New PPP Financing Procedure

The new procedure, that was already uses in Valencia with 5 hospitals including medical services, and two in Catalonia as non medical services spread all over the Spanish geography in a few years: PPI Public Private Investment o PFI Project Finance Investment; PPP Public Private Partnerships. This financing model is being implemented throughout the country, in a number of new hospitals: Hospital de Burgos; Hospital de Toledo; Hospital de Asturias; Hospital de Son Dureta en Palma de Mallorca; Hospital de Vigo. And, it is also beginning to be used for refurbishment and extension following the British example.

The different Models of the Financing System

7 hospitals with concessions that cover: construction; maintenance; cleaning; laundry; catering and restoration; administrative services; storage management; commercial spaces; all this under a 30 year management lease. Four other hospitals that also include medical services (Figure 1).

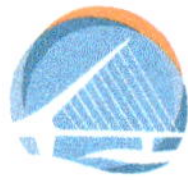

Time Frame for the Model's Development

Public competition for public building grants time limit: 56 days; construction contract award: 40 – 60 days; project development: 4 to 6 months; construction time frame: 18-24 months; total time frame from the start of the process to its operation: 26 - 30 months; except Majadahonda: 36 months. The total investment being more than 1.2 billions euros to be paid in 30 years.

Composition of Concessions Presented

They are temporary companies formed by: construction companies; supply services companies (usually owned by the construction companies).

Financed by an investment bank. In the case of Valdemoro: also introduces a medical insurance companies.

Consequences of the Application of the "New Financing Model" on Hospital Design

The decisions previously taken by the public administration, are now taken by suppliers of services and private investment managers. The concept of depreciation is replaced by the laws of return on investments that rule the private financial system.

The decisions that previously corresponded to the tertiary level, are now in the hands of the concessionary. The decisions at the secondary level, basically depend on the construction companies. The financiers manage the investment.

CONSEQUENCES OF THE CRISIS

Management Privatization

It will report an important reduction in costs, whether maintenance and cleaning etc. (grey gown) or sanitary services (white-gown). It is estimated that it will report a cost reduction of around 30%. Therefore the trend will be privatize even"more".

Refurbishment Instead of New Construction

In times of crisis, it would be better to fix what we have. Instead of introducing new hospitals lets fix the existing ones. These processes are more complex and require more experience. We must not forget that the patient is there. We must avoid risks we could be not sure about what they want but we are certainly sure about what they don't want. We should have enough knowledge to argue.

Surface Reduction

There is no doubt that surface programme and planning will be optimized. In the future it will require more constrained spaces. Europe has assumed that more than 150 m^2/bed is not acceptable "less is more". Number of beds will be also reduced, by doing "more with less".

Sustainable Technology

In the aim of finding a new technology oriented to reduce power consumption, the possibility of designing hospital buildings with an acceptable ecological footprint (and a BREEM classification) using a reasonable investment is a current trend.

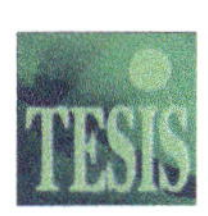

Staff Reduction

Planning and designing with the aim of reducing staff needs, will also be a current trend in these crisis times. It has already been applied systematically in private hospitals, therefore its application to public hospitals will be a consequence of its management privatization.

TENDENCIES AND TRENDS

Star Architects

The intervention of star architects can take us to "the Guggenheim effect". We cannot forget about Michel Foucault´s definition "L´hopital doit fonctionner comme una machine à guérir".

The Who Factor

In the end, a hospital has to be functional as a machine. It is very important: a hospital is one of the most important public investment, citizens must be awed.

Size Matters

The most sustainable sq. meter is the one we don't build because it's not needed. We must analyse and think before we start to Design and benchmark.

The functional programs and areas surface list should be revised and should be adapted to the new procedures.

The Silver Tsunami

Baby boom of the fifties is reaching their retirementage. Health care resources will be invaded in a short time by these citizens in their need for sanitary services.
They can collapse the health care system of all developed countries, are we ready for this avalanche? We need to move fast, increase the day procedures and use the available technology so people can be treated and healed at home. The telemedicine can change the needs of the hospitals.

Private sector transfer	Classic Model I	Mixed Model II	Partial concession contract II	Concession contract IV
Promotion	NO	NO	YES	YES
Majority Shareholder	NO	NO	YES	YES
Building industry	YES	YES	YES	YES
Infrastructure management	YES	YES	YES	YES
Catering Service	NO	YES	YES	YES
Healthcare Service management	NO	NO	NO	YES
Example Autonomous community	Andalucía	Asturias	Madrid 1	Valencia Madrid 2

Table 1. Changes in PPP model involvement.

The Biochemical Threat

We are seen more and more illness produced by very virulent viruses and bacterias, that can provoke pandemics that can spread all over the world. Viruses and bacterias, like ebola. This can become a new way off war, think of antrax… and a very uncontrolled and dangerous one. We must think our hospitals in a very secure way and be prepared to isolate wings or areas to comply P4 biosecurity procedures. Progressive tendency of including "private iniciative". Outsourcing is becoming more common every day. All hospital services such as laundry, catering, maintenance and sterilization will be progressively outsourced, under a leasing system.

Changes in PPP Model Involvement

Advantages for Politicians

It's obvious that one opens the hospital and gets the greetings and the next to come has to pay for it. They can see the results in a shorter period of time 3 to 4 years in hole against 6 to 8 years of the conventional model. The cost, of construction, the total cost of services for a long period and the time schedule is fixed.

Advantages for the citizens

The period in which they get access to the medical service is reduced considerably, and this for the citizens is crucial. The disadvantage is that we leave our sons to pay for it. Some say that is an advantage who uses the service, and the building pays for it, so it's generation logic, but we are leaving debts to the next generations to come.

Is This a Business

Of course it is!! For the service companies that increase their income and annual turnover for a long and fixed period of time with a fixed price. But mainly for institutional funds, investors and banks because they get a fixed and ensured return on investment for a long period of years.

New Management Models

Changes in PPP Model Involvement

Changes in management progressively shift to private management. The client shifts from being public entities and administrations, to being public companies and enterprises, to being a Public-Private Partnership to finally become a Health Services Provider. In the UK, where Public-Private Partnerships started to take place in the 80´s, it was said that the client shifted from "Prince to Cinderella" transferring the weight of the National Health Service (NHS) to maintenance and cleaning services companies (what we call "grey gowns").

The next step, which is to privatize the Health Services Providers, has already taken place in Spain and seems unfeasible. Changes in promotion and management systems reduce time. It has been reduced from 10 years in the 90´s to 24 months in total nowadays (project and construction of Torrejón-Hospital).

Too often this forecast completion periods transfer to political election deadlines. These shorter and strict deadlines will take their toll on the life span of the hospital.

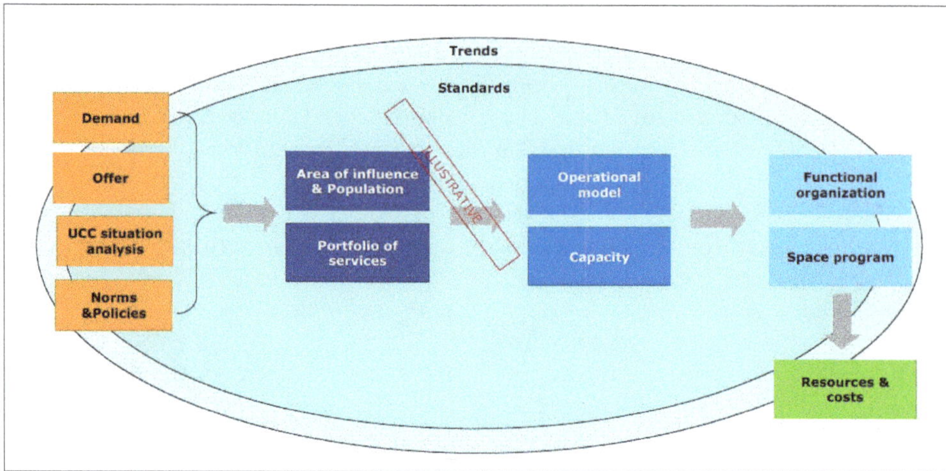

Figure 1. A functional program for a hospital has to reconsidered.

BIM ADVANTAGES

New generation of systems and processes, known today as Building Information Modelling (BIM) involve a conceptual revolution in the way we approach a project, and the way we design, develop build and manage the buildings during their lifetime process.

BIM involve different tools, processes and methodologies. Instead of designing a single drawing which would include a tag tool like CAD, BIM represents in a three- dimensional model a database which includes all the properties and parameters of every single element of the whole building (Figure 2).

For the technicians in the construction sector, BIM represents a completely new approach to the designing process.
Since 2007, Árgola produce and develop all of their architectural works with the programme Autodesk Revit Architecture. Árgola constitutes a paradigmatic successful case introducing BIM system in an architectural office. This is a cutting edge team where Revit has been used for more than 5 years already. Few of their members are indeed registered Autodesk trainers, faculty members of the 1st BIM Master IDESIE in Madrid, in designing, construction and building management by using BIM tools. BIM – proved benefits: 50% reduction in requested project information (RFI) 10% project cost reductions; 18% reduction in construction documentation production; 2-3% improvement on the material execution budget (Figure 3).

EDAC RESEARCHES ON EVIDENCE BASED DESIGN

Architectural design based on scientific evidence provides advantages in relation to patient care and medical professionals and staff satisfaction and performance.
This "scientific evidence" in the design of new hospital infrastructures has demonstrated that a good functional and operational plan has to take into account the factors shown in Table 2.

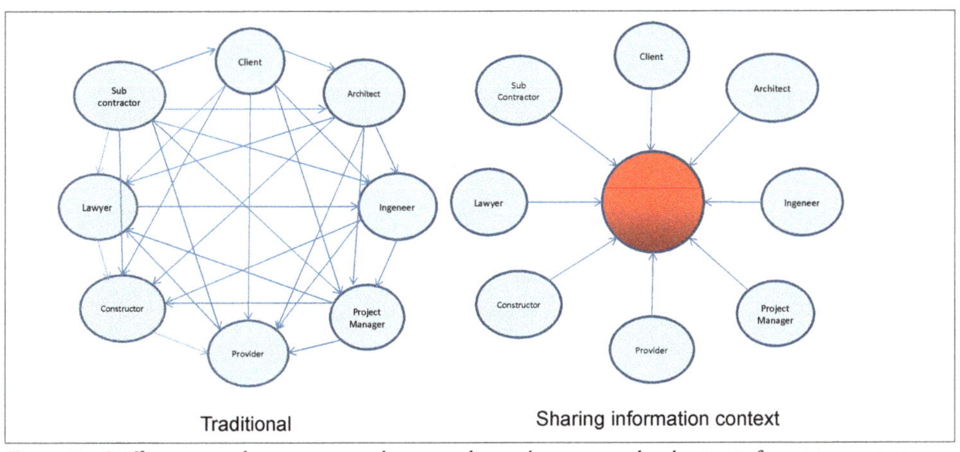

Figure 2. Differences on the process regarding a traditional context and a sharing information context.

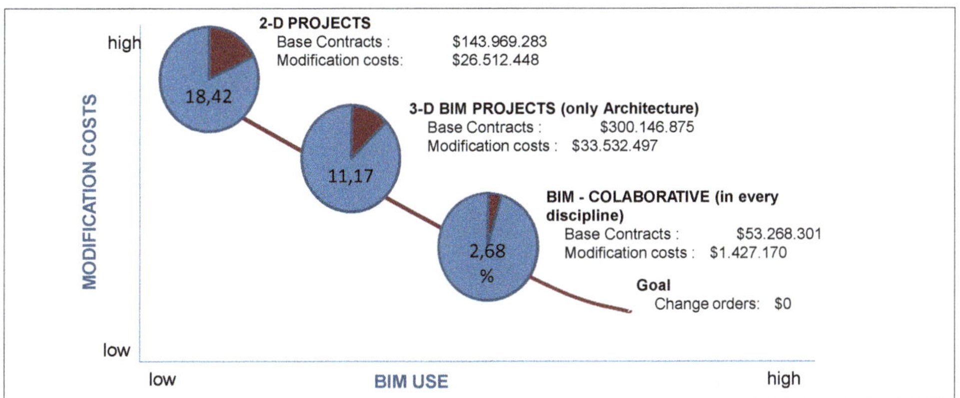

Figure 3. BIM advantages.

Healthcare Outcomes / Design Strategies or Environmental Interventions	Single-bed rooms	Access to daylight	Appropriate lighting	Views of nature	Family zone in patient rooms	Carpeting	Noise-reducing finishes	Ceiling lifts	Nursing floor layout	Decentralized supplies	Acuity-adaptable rooms
Reduced hospital-acquired infections	**										
Reduced medical errors	*		*				*				*
Reduced patient falls	*		*		*	*			*		*
Reduced pain		*	*	**			*				
Improved patient sleep	**	*	*				*				
Reduced patient stress	*	*	*	**	*		**				
Reduced depression		**	**	*	*						
Reduced length of stay		*	*	*							*
Improved patient privacy and confidentiality	**				*		*				
Improved communication with patients & family members	**				*		*				
Improved social support	*				*	*					
Increased patient satisfaction	**	*	*	*	*	*	*				
Decreased staff injuries								**			*
Decreased staff stress	*	*	*	*			*				
Increased staff effectiveness	*		*				*		*	*	*
Increased staff satisfaction	*	*	*	*			*				

Table 2. Summary of the relationships between design factors and healthcare outcomes.

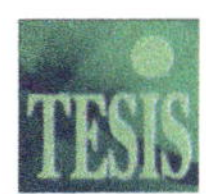

The on Going Research Proposal

Main goals: analyse the impact that design can have on an hospital on the organization and managements in its future; measure the satisfaction of the different groups involved in the health care system, such as patients, visitors, doctors, staff and managers. Look for evidence in how the different managing programs, procedures and systems are changing the hospital design and will do so much more in the future.
Architects are the only profession that can´t measure the satisfaction on their work after they have finished.
Secondary goals: identify common problems that have caused later modifications, in order to be revised in future projects; communicate to the different involved groups the advantages that the health institutions can offer to the designs, specially those that have proved an improvement on the organization and functionality, for an optimization of resources and the satisfaction of the infrastructure users.
Identify excellence practices to be disclosed in order to optimize the investments that are already done: by creating an observatory o good practices bank in each area of activity; by adopting the "benchmarking" as an improvement strategy including national and international experiences.

And finally, develop measurable indicators that prove the cost benefit of these innovations, as well as the good practices for the agents: authority and sanitary managers; medical and nursery staff; citizens, regarding activity, technical quality, professional and patient security and costs.

Why Spain?

The assessment "post" of the architectural hospital design is uncommon in our context.

This moment seems to be a propitious occasion to research for different reasons: existence of a huge amount of publication and analysis about the topic in other countries; the emergence of the hospital architecture based on a scientific evidence, which prove objective advantages in designs; high number of new construction hospitals developed in Spain in the last few years; multitude of formulations used for infrastructure funding including from the traditional ones (with a charge to public budgets) to the collaborative public-private formulations.
Different management models and provision of services which range from the classic administration, to foundations, public companies or concessions for the service management. Different types of project planning and modelization, without having any feed back. The need of architectural offices of measuring the levels of satisfaction that their work will cause in the different interest groups and their cost-effectiveness.

Selection of Institutions and Hospitals of the Target Universe

The selection of health institutions and hospitals to partecipate in the research will be done according to the following criteria: the size of the sample must be representative, to ensure the study validation and extrapolate the outcomes and the conclusions to the centre universe; the sample must include health

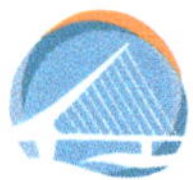

institutions which have replaced previous ones to assess the economical costs and the clinical aspects before and after; the selection should refer to a strategic analysis in order to identify those factors which can be convenient for their economical and clinical impact.

Stage 1. Areas Subject of Study

Areas selection, subject of study should have into account those which have higher impact: as a result of being the ones who solve more hospital cases, e.g. obstetrics or emergency; as a result of having a high impact in costs such as the critics areas or the surgical block; as a result of their impact in the client satisfaction, e.g the UTPR.

Stage 1. Tools Design

Tools will be used in order to know the advantages and the affectivity that different hospital designs present to different interest groups (Figure 4).

Stage 1. Tools Approval – Trial in 5 Centres - Including their Management Representative

The research team will present the assessment tools to a reduced endorsement team of Hospital managers, to gather their opinion and enrich the content of their contributions. We will proceed afterwards by the application "in situ" in a hospital, considered as pilot hospital. This pilot hospital would be a previous stage to then extent it to other hospitals: its utility and its practical application; the methodological inconsistencies detected in order to be revised. The most relevant actions in order to achieve the project goals and those that doesn't report any benefit in relation with the required effort. The acceptance and the comprehension by the different agents involved in the project. Changes as a result of the pilot hospitals will be incorporated by the research team. Assessment tools will be presented to the endorsement team for their final approval (Figure 5).

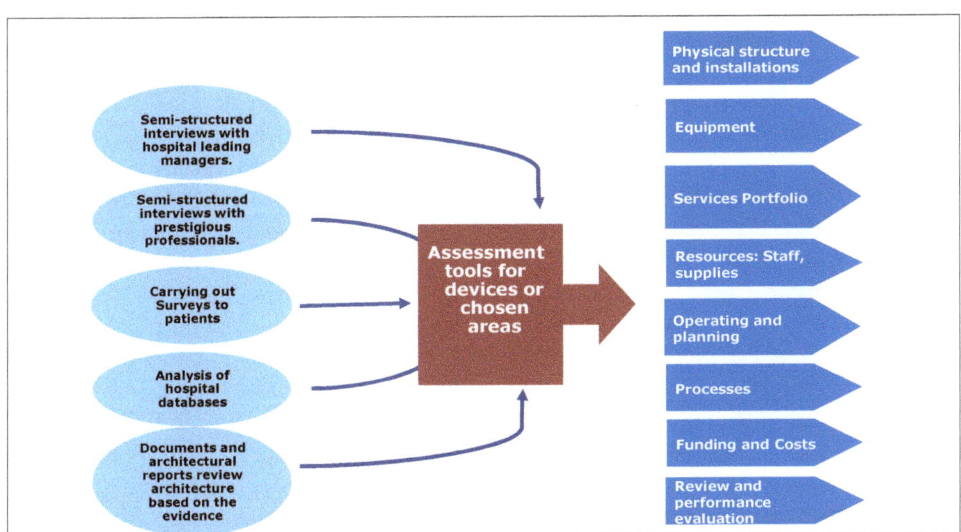

Figure 4. Stage 1. Tools design.

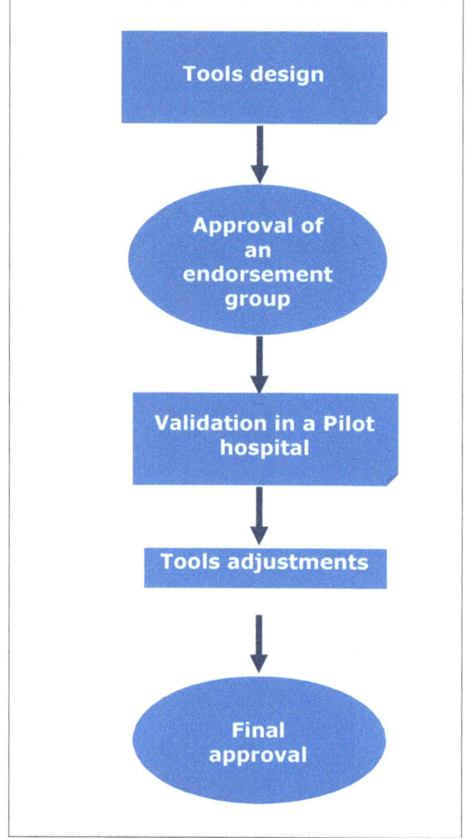

Figure 5. Stage 1. Tools approval – trial in 5 centres- including their management representative.

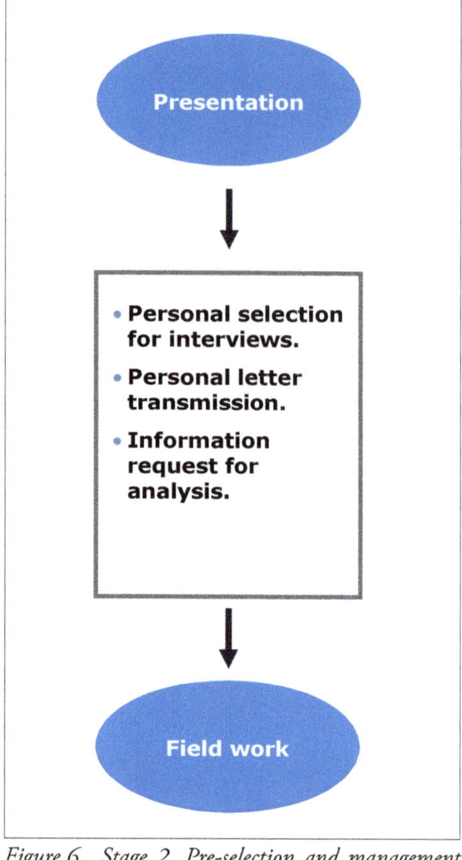

Figure 6. Stage 2. Pre-selection and management system analysis.

Stage 2. Pre-selection and Management System Analysis

Afterwards the research team will have meetings with every institution directors to specify the scope of the project, the planning and the action timeline in each hospital. A list with the selected people will be required for interviews and the centre staff for the selection of a surveyed group sample (Figure 6).

A covering letter will be sent to each of them before the interviews to require their collaboration and allow them to know the importance of the project.

An additional information enquiry for the analysis will be requested, forwarding a survey to every centre. An interview calendar will be programmed per institution, as well as meetings to ultimate the survey responses, and visits to the relevant centres, guessing the length-for each of them. A final report will be draft per hospital or institution, and a final objective assessment and an executive summary redacted by the research team will also be included. A final presentation with the final report will be done for each centre, once the process and the tools used for the study are over.

BENCHMARKING

A benchmarking will be developed between hospitals and recommendation will be elaborated through an analysis matrix that allows us to visualize:

- Advantages and disadvantages found in hospitals: common to every centre; the activity impact, cost reductions in quantitative terms, and quality improvement in the services they provide.
- The factors that can have caused these differences.
- The quantitative and qualitative indicators used for measurements and their results.

Cross-check of the Outcome with the Documental Data Basis

Founded data will be checked in the documental basis: to analyse their concordance with the scientific documental evidence; to identify additional innovations and their contribution in terms of higher level/price.
A suggestions proposal will be done for the following aspects development: of the own hospitals, analysed areas and the service provided; of the non-explored options and the need-to-improve aspects; of the gathered evidence (and advantages) diffusion and communication.

First Results

First Result of the Research: Torrejón's Hospital in Madrid 1 (a PPP including medical services):

- Patients Management Software System (Florence): best results in Madrid on the Pols of patients and citizens satisfaction 95%; biggest percentage of Day Surgery versus, they never needed or opened a 2 wards a 15 % of the programed number of beds; a 50% of the waiting areas can be saved in policlinics, emergencies, and all outpatients services; other areas are small due to the managements results like day surgery and day hospitals.
- Double corridors to separate external and internal flows: through measuring the frequency of the use in different corridors and sharing the results with the management team we got to the primary conclusion that a 25% of the surface designed for main circulations and general flows could have been safe.

FIRST CONCLUSIONS TO THE RESEARCH

With these two conclusions and adding the other under used spaces, due to the use of management system software, like the two wards that have neverbeen used. It will report a total surface reduction between 10 and 12%, from 4,200 to 4.800 m^2 these areas could be use for other purpose. Radiotherapy has already been increased 1.200 m^2.

Good and Bad News

Good news: the first result after only three months and only the first phase competed are very promising; a lot of issues can be analysed with the system that we are managing and results will flow and become evidence; we will then, with results, be able to establish benchmarking for the next designs.

Bad news: the study and its results will take longer than we expected and will need more resources; our fellow architects and engineers dislike other storevise their work. The collaboration of institutions and managers is slow and not too good. They are not interested in the possible comparison and the consequent benchmarking. As a conclusion we are facing resistence.

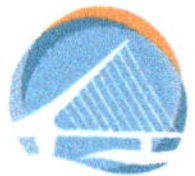

Two Hospitals in the South of Chile

Álvaro Prieto Lindholm

prietolindholm.arq@gmail.com
AARQHOS, Monjitas 251, Santiago, Chile

In the decades of 1960-1970 two similar hospitals in its conception, in two different southern cities in Chile are replaced by new buildings: one in the same area, using some of the existing building and the other in an entirely new place.

The growth of the first hospital doubled its surface and its execution lasted for seven years; in the case of the second, its size was quintupled due to multiple factors such as an increase of users, among others. Its execution will last almost 5 years.

Both new buildings have huge differences, despite the short time between the two. They share, however, design criteria and some features that still relate them.

Alvaro Prieto Lindholm. *Architect, Master in Architecture Pontificia Universidad Católica de Chile, 2004; Specialist in Hospital Architecture. Author of hospital Projects in Public and Private areas, with over one million square meters projected. Chilean architecture offices and foreign institutions advisor (Uruguay and Costa Rica). Scholarship holder in France, Sweden, Germany and USA to study his specialty. Assistant and / or speaker at International Conferences in Chile, Argentina, Mexico, Spain and Japan. Visiting Professor at Universities of: Chile, Spain, Argentina and Venezuela.*

Development

In the 1960s, it was needed to replace old hospitals in the cities of Osorno (built in 1939 and partially destroyed by an earthquake in 1960[1]) and Puerto Montt, located approximately 800 and 1,000 km away from Santiago to the south, respectively.

Therefore two projects were born in the late '60s and early '70s, they were similar projects in terms of morphology, criteria, functionality, size and aesthetics.

[1] *The largest recorded earthquake in the world.*

San José de Osorno New Hospital

Preliminary design: Alvaro Prieto Lindholm MSc Architect, Project Development: Gumucio Lührs & Asociados Arquitectos

Osorno's first hospital was called "Santos Cosme y Damián" in 1560-1568. It was one among five other hospitals at

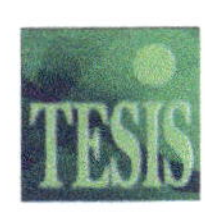

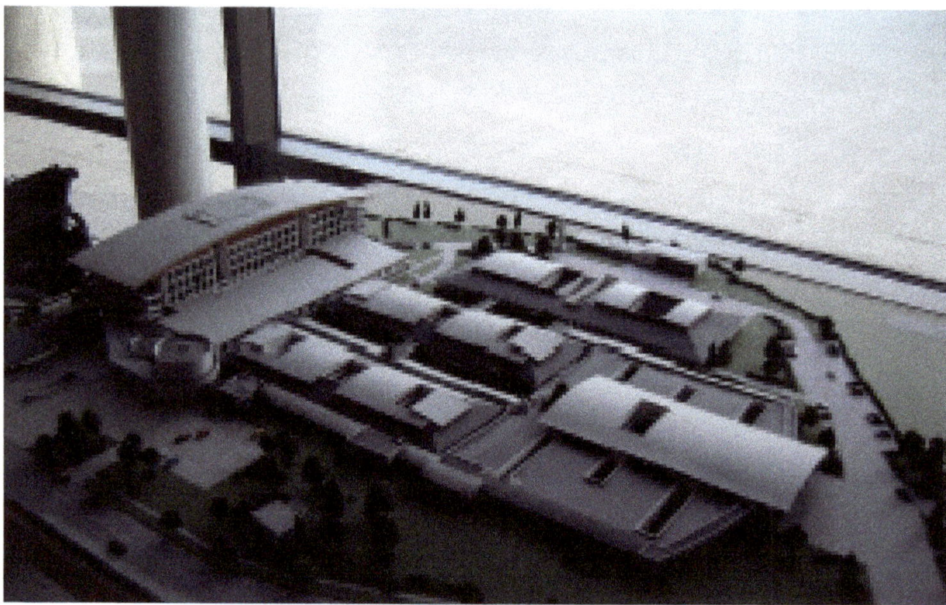

Figure 1. The new Hospital San José (Osorno), 2007- 2013.

times when Chile was recently discovered by the Spanish.
The city was devastated in 1604 and refunded in 1794[1]. A new hospital was built between 1886 and 1888; its name was San José. It had to be rebuilt in 1901 and in 1918, due to big, terrible fires. In 1939 a new San Jose hospital appeared.

In 2004, a Pre-investment Study (PSH) for the Hospital Standardization was entrusted for the hospital built between 1967 and 1971 (replacing the one in 1939). Some conclusions were: poor functionality, due to its inorganic growth and amendments of patient care areas and clinical support ones (mixtures of flows and qualitative and quantitative deficiencies). This building had 353 beds and 17,000 m^2.

The study also originated a new Architectural Medical Program (AMP) and three possible solutions or alternatives.

Construction of the new project started in 2006, with a capacity of 362 beds and approximately 45,000 m^2 of total area.

The proposal chosen for the hospital normalization, the best technical - economic one, separate internal flows (personnel, supplies and inpatients) and external flows (visits and outpatients) by creating a peripheral building surrounding the hospital. It involved the demolition of existing buildings (5,668 m^2) and the construction of new ones (30,800 m^2). There was also need to plan self-sufficient stages to be built or remodeled (12,424 m^2) gradually, without interfering with patients´ care and recovery.

[1] *Cfr: Bielefeldt, Germán, "History of San José Hospital of Osorno" p. 6 and below.*

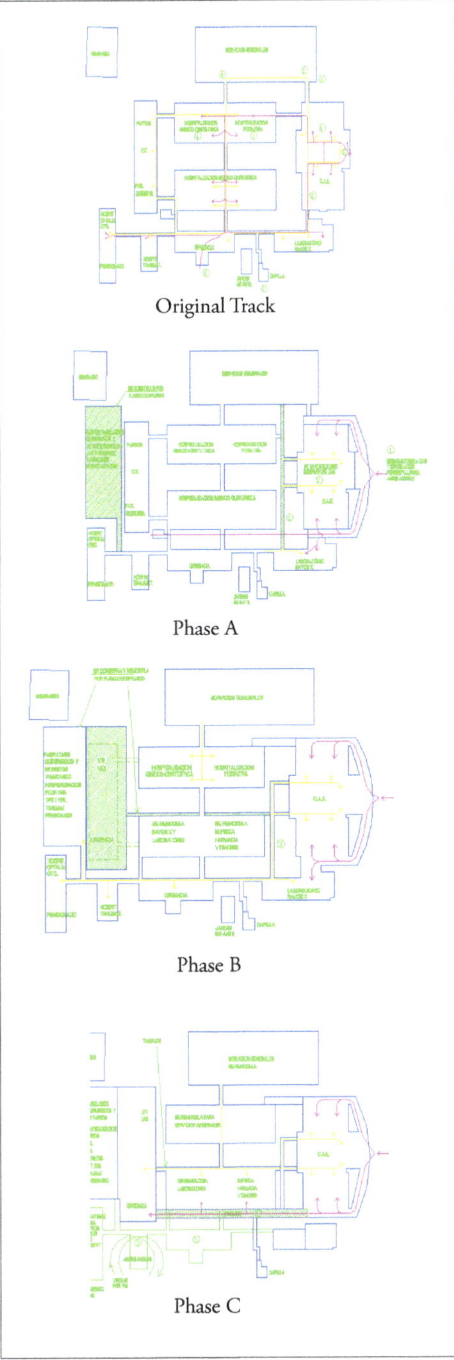

Figure 2. The new Hospital San José (Osorno), building program.

In an empty space, a 5-storey building, to surgical wards, Emergency, ICU, Neonatal ICU and was built; hospitalization (internment); spaces for piping and air conditioning equipment, with an heliport on the roof. It has elevators and stairs differentiated by type of user, separating the internal and public visits and flows.
A central corridor was built as an internal connection for the whole hospital.

For the construction of the different buildings, a series of movements were programmed, from the old facilities into the new ones. In this way we could demolish old parts leaving empty space for the new buildings.

Puerto Montt Hospital

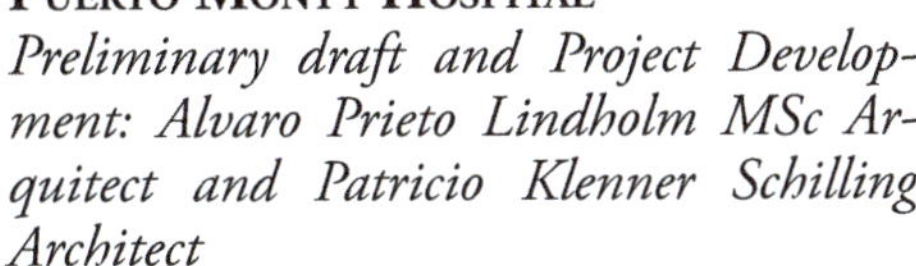

Preliminary draft and Project Development: Alvaro Prieto Lindholm MSc Arquitect and Patricio Klenner Schilling Architect

Puerto Montt, the region´s capital city since 1980, had its first "hospital", a small cottage, in 1853. It was in the beginning of the German colonization in the south of Chile.
In 1875 the "Hospital de la Caridad" appears, with 50 beds, run by the Sisters of the Immaculate Conception.

In 1882, it is renamed "Hospital Santa Maria". This building was replaced in 1938 by the "Hospital Regional" with 200 beds. The earthquake in 1960 forces to re study the situation of hospitals. In 1968 a new project is started, and in 1972, the new hospital was inaugurated, with 440 beds. Highly specialized services are added in 1984 and 1996, coming to have a building area of 25,608 m^2.

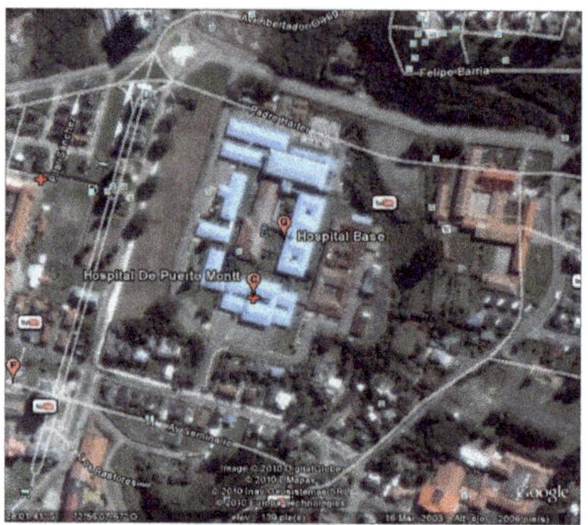

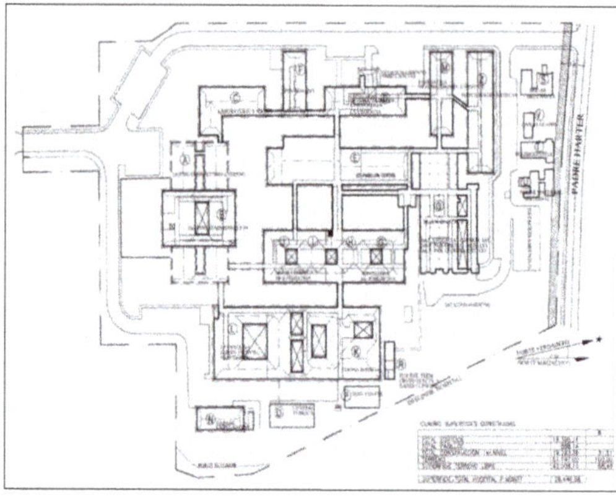

Figure 3. Puerto Montt Hospital, January 2010.

These important renewal and extensions, some inorganic ones due to the population growth as a regional new capital city, made it necessary in 2006 to have a Hospital Prefeasibility Study (HPS), for a complete standardization. This study, like the one in Osorno, yielded important data: defects and flaws, huge circulatory problems, clinical deficiencies in services and in the number of rooms. The new Medical Architectural Program raised the number of beds up to 525 and the surface to more than 110,000 m^2. Nevertheless there was vulnerability in the site. It was located in the middle of the city with difficult access and too far away from users of new urban areas.

After analyzing several alternatives, it was decided to move the high complexity establishment to a different area[1].

The site chosen after a selection of offers in a public bidding has an area of 8.02 hectares, and it is located in the northern entrance, within an area of urban expansion in a urban ratio. The ground is almost horizontal in the southern part and it rises slightly up in the north part.

The alternative for the new hospital (according to its topography, alignment, entrances and other hospital architecture criteria) is formed by 4 main buildings and 2 secondary ones:

- a building (A) for different specialties, ambulatory attention;

- a building (H) for admission and hospitalization. In between there is a roofed yard expanding the visitors' area;

- a building (Q) for imaging, emergency, endoscopies, mayor and ambulatory surgery, deliveries and neonatology.

Beneath these three buildings there is a parking lot and the entrance for the personnel and dressing rooms.

In a top level, a third level in a slope of the area there is building (S). We find here the industrial support and supplies services.

[1] *Among the reasons given are: a - actual field it is hard to access by being in the center of the city, with narrow streets; b - most beneficiaries come from outside (of the islands, and surrounding cities outside the core radius); c - vacant allow more expansion possibilities.*

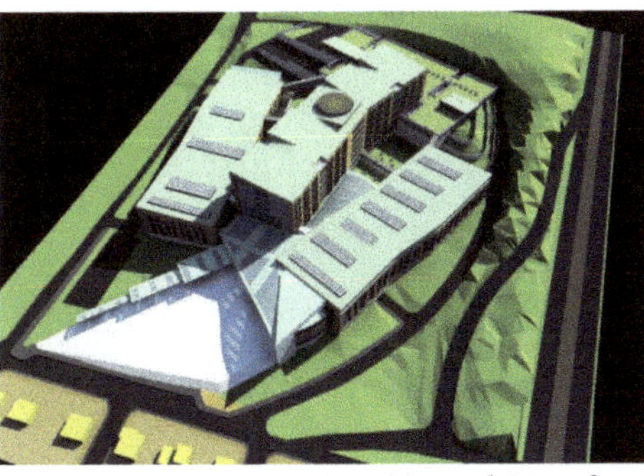
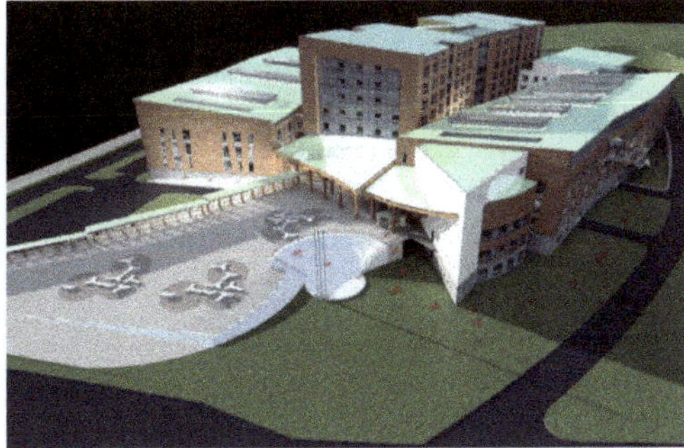

Figure 4. New Puerto Montt Hospital. View from the east.

Differences and Similarities

According major concepts and design criteria seen in these two works and following the Congress thematic line (Sustainability, Humanization, New places); there are differences and similarities between the two projects.
Although they had similar origins, today they have significant differences despite the short time between building one and the other. This can be seen in their recent inaugurations (2013 and 2014).
The most important difference is because Osorno hospital was raised on the grounds of the already existing hospital. Always trying to maintain, at all stages of the work, a functional continuity despite demolitions, excavations, air pollution, temporary and/or definite transfers. There were power, water, gas, telephone and medical gases cuts, new constructions, vibrations that a ltered instruments, surgical operations, etc. There were many functional restrictions. A period of 7 years of construction was planned.
The new hospital in Puerto Montt, built in a new field, was completed in one single step that took a little bit more than 4 years.
The other main differences occurred in sustainability, bioclimatic architecture and energy saving: only Puerto Montt incorporates the concepts of energy efficiency such as thermal envelope, ventilated facades, windows and glass type thermo low emissivity; low energy lighting equipment, and natural ventilation, sunlight and use of HVAC systems with energy recovery, building heat engines and machinery. It also includes geothermal energy.
The building contains two networks of cold water, one for dirty (or used) water called "gray water" for irrigation and toilets.
As it has been recently finished, there are not yet substantial studies to back-up the previously done studies on the use of economic resources vs. sustainability.
As a counterpart, Osorno Hospital used recycled resources from the existing buildings, which meant materials savings. Also, great importance was given to the orientation of the rooms.
Puerto Montt projected green covering on some terraces, but the idea was withdrawn by the authorities considering maintenance costs. However, big yards and roofed entrances for rain protection were accepted.
In Osorno planters were projected in front of each window in hospitalization areas. Unfortunately they cannot be used because of a project mistake.

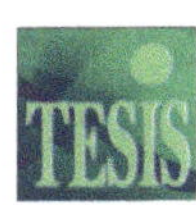

The draft Osorno had to use a module 7.00 m. In Puerto Montt was increased to 8.00 m, providing better fit and more versatility to the structure.

Hospital´s vulnerability; the hospital in case of disasters; the safe hospital. Both projects favor these design criteria in their structures and their non-structural elements and facilities. The two buildings have concrete walls, mainly in the body perimeter and inner parts of columns, slabs on each floor and steel roof structures. The idea is to continue working before, during and immediately after earthquakes.

For fire protection, active and passive containment (such as the buildings zoning) with fire walls and a humid and dry extinguishing network were set.

Osorno Hospital has evacuation ramps at both ends of the 5-storey building.

For humanization, "holistic approach to patient, new attention proposals respecting cultural diversity and patient-centered care" both projects include inpatient rooms (hospitalization) of no more than 3 beds, with a universal toilet inside. For universal accessibility, there are toilets suitable for people with all types of disabilities and / or accompanied (elderly; obese, children); access ramps with no steps, railings and banisters for young adults, older adults and children; tactile signaling suitable for people with visual disabilities.

Both projects include wood in coatings and some structural elements of the entrance and / or waiting rooms.

Showing respect for traditions and cultural diversity, both buildings have Ecumenical worship rooms. In Puerto Montt, the community composed of both Catholics and Christians of other denomination, requested to separate rooms. In both buildings the rooms can be used by patients, staff of the hospital and the public with separated entrances. Both projects share the functional hospital criterion. This means, among other concepts, an actual functionality of a health building such as good relations between critical services, differentiated flows and circulations, both vertical and horizontal, between the public and the staff. This has been respected as a sine qua non requirement and as a way to promote the efficient and friendly use of the building.

Conclusions

Hospitals in the future have to consider many changes occurring in a short time. Not only from the medical point of view (aging or increase of obese population), but also human (only Puerto Montt has integral delivery rooms or LDR rooms) and technologic ones.

Along with the incorporation of new criteria, Talca Hospital project, for example, was started almost along with Puerto Montt include, seismic isolators and energy dissipaters to alleviate the effect of an earthquake in non-structural elements (ceilings, walls, partitions, facilities, windows and glass, furniture, piping, etc.), reducing even the thickness of structural walls; geothermics for HVAC and sanitary hot water was included; organic green coverings, PVC windows that break the thermal bridge into the building.

An answer to the question posed by this Congress: "The changes in the design of hospitals and medical technology are the result of the patient´s needs or simply a consequence of technological developments? " You can say, both. But more than that, it is important to consider the extreme rapidity of changes.

New Paradigms on Public Health Architecture in Chile

Silvia Barbera, Jorge Batesteza, Cristóbal Tirado

info@bbats-tirado.com
Partners on BBATS+TIRADO architects,

We present the first hospital concession of Chile and the region (South America): El Carmen de Maipú Hospital (Dr. Luis Valentin Ferrada - Maipu - Santiago) and Clinical Metropolitan La Florida Hospital (Dr. Eloisa Diaz Insunza - La Florida - Santiago) both projects developed by BBATS Consulting & Projects SLP / Silvia Barbera, Jorge Batesteza, Cristobal Tirado (Barcelona, España) and Murtinho + Raby / Pedro Murtinho, Santiago Raby (Santiago, Chile). The new hospitals are defining a new paradigm on the way health architecture was being done in Chile, mainly because four facts:

- The new hospitals are concessioned, the first ones with this business model in South America where the concessionaire designs, builds and works the non-clinical hospital services.

- The international experience provided by BBATS Consulting & Projects SLP in the understanding of health architecture looks to improve the clinical performance, the welfare of the patient and the spatial orientation among others.

- The development of the concept of friendly hospital by incorporating green roofs, differentiated circulations, natural light, interior courtyards and a cultural and social component.

- Incorporation of seismic protection elements such as isolators, expansion joints and hospital vulnerability elements in order to ensure the functioning of the building after a disaster.

Silvia Barbera, Jorge Batesteza. *Architects Universidad de Buenos Aires 1976. Specialists on health architecture. CEOs BBATS Consulting & Projects Slp with main office in Barcelone Spain, and offices in Chile, Panama and Peru. Partners in BBATS+TIRADO architects (Chile). Advisors on Chile and Panama offices. Architects of health projects in Spain, Haiti, Panama, France, Chile and Nicaragua. Assistants and/or lecturers on international conferences in Spain, Tokio, Chile, Argentina and Panama.*

Cristóbal Tirado. *Architect Pontificia Universidad Católica de Chile 2005 and Master in Architecture Universidad Politécnica de Barcelona, Spain. During his early years worked with different Chilean architects, among them Smiljan Radic. Later worked and studied in Barcelona, Spain. In 2009 settled in Chile and established BBATS+Tirado architects, where he have developed different kinds of projects (health, culture, education, security, sports, housing, master plans, etc). In 2014 received the national award by the Architectural Association of Chile, as the best Chilean Architect under 35 years. Since 2010 he re-joined the School of Architecture of the Pontificia Universidad Católica de Chile as undergraduate teacher.*

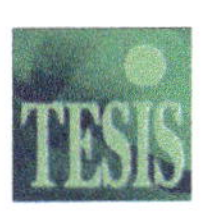

The new hospitals, El Carmen de Maipú and Clinical Metropolitan La Florida, have come to improve the health architecture scene in Chile, not just because of the new business model in which a private gets a concession and develops the design and construction, and after that runs the non-clinical business, but because the international experience on projects like this is very important. We worked on the conception of a new health architectural concept for Chile including good care for the different aspects of the project like ubication on the plot, volumetry, inner spatiality, urban image, and most important the patient wellness and clinical functionality.

This implied to BBATS, after two years of competition developed in Barcelona - Spain, to set up an office in Chile in late 2009 to conduct the project development and supervision of works of the hospital of Maipu and La Florida.

The construction of these hospitals was a strong break regarding the public health infrastructure in Chile, as they are projects of high standard, good quality in architecture, finishes and operation. We noted the advantage of working with a direct client -concessionaire- because it will be the institution operating the building over the next 15 years. There has been a concern for creating systems that reduce consumptions, operational and maintenance costs during the concession. This translates into a benefit of quality from the design approach.

As for international experience the main concept behind hospitals of this size, is the correct zoning of different areas of a complex program, because the programmatic relationships should prevail. Having found that setting and in response to the demands of the neighborhood, the terrain and the environment, a first volumetric proposal is defined and combined with a proposed imaginary. It was defined for both hospitals a specific order that takes into account the wellness on the patient and make easier the orientation and stay in the hospital. These characteristics, new in Chile, configure a new standard and help to understand the concept of friendly hospital.

We understand as a friendly hospital not just one where the stay is pleasant and it's overturned to the patient and the user, but one where the local culture is integrated in a new way. In order to the first fact we decided to include daylight in all enclosures, interior courtyards that articulates the different programs and public zones, waiting rooms and circulations that are exclusive for the visitors, an easy orientation system inside the building (clear signage) and in a special way the reposition of the terrain built surface with free access green roof plantations. Regarding the integration of culture, some elements of the Mapuche people are incorporated in both hospitals in different ways. First decision for both hospitals was to include them through signage and translations on Mapuche language Mapudungun, and second, by incorporating elements and concepts of Mapuche culture in the design of the buildings.

Finally remark that the incorporation of seismic protection elements such as elastomeric isolators, to secure the functioning of the building after a disaster, usual situation in Chile, especially in terms of earthquakes. This involves thinking buildings with a horizontal cut that divides the building in two parts, one that could be called the earthly building, traditionally founded in the earth and other called the heavenly building, which sits

on the isolators and moves over them. This means a special job in the development of complex expansion joints as it becomes necessary to counteract the dissimilar movements between the earthly and the heavenly building.
For both hospitals we describe below the individual project strategies used to address the particularities of each terrain and programmatic complexity, on a management model that we believe presents great challenges and opportunities for the development of public health infrastructure in the region.

HOSPITAL EL CARMEN, DR. LUIS VALENTÍN FERRADA - MAIPÚ - SANTIAGO

The El Carmen de Maipu Hospital has 70.301 m², 375 beds, 11 operating rooms and 6 delivery rooms, 125 medical consultations, 523 parking spots and 347 seismic isolators, to house 1,500 staff, in the most populous municipality in the country.

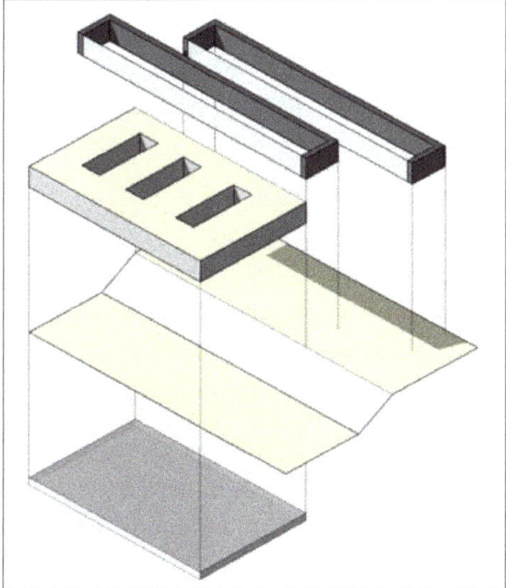

Figure 1. El Carmen de Maipú Hospital – Santiago, Chile: volumes scheme.

The hospital it's located in a plot of 250 m by 250 m (aprox 50,500 m²) with a considerable green prescence and with enough space to decide the position of the building in the site. However the difficulty it's given by the important difference in the ground level, - 10 m difference between the south entrance and the north access - , with a slope that make's a diagonal against the avenue of the project main facade.
This implied to develop the project in two different levels: a half buried plinth that builds de difference of the existing slope minimizing the earthworks, with the subsequent extension and recovery of the upper level (north access) that builds a green free access roof and articulates the lower level (plinth) and the upper level that's built as two parallel dislocated aerial hospitalization bars that rest above the natural ground and the green roof. The ubication of the hospitalization areas responds to a better orientation (north-west) and a better environment linked with the green roof and the park areas on the site.
The programmatic distribution is divided into three groups: two underground floors of parking and clinical support services grouped with the two levels on the plinth that house the heart of the hospital: emergency rooms, radiology, operating rooms and critically ill patients; a technical gallery on the green roof / park level and two upper floors for hospitalization units.
Looking for the best performance, the project is developed in a perfectly horizontal clinical organization, and has a fairly small urban scale in relation to the 70,000 m² built. This is seen in that - despite having 7 floor - this is not reflected in any of its facades.

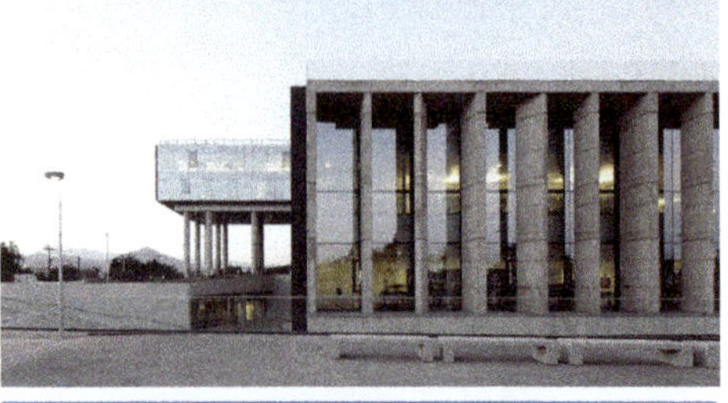

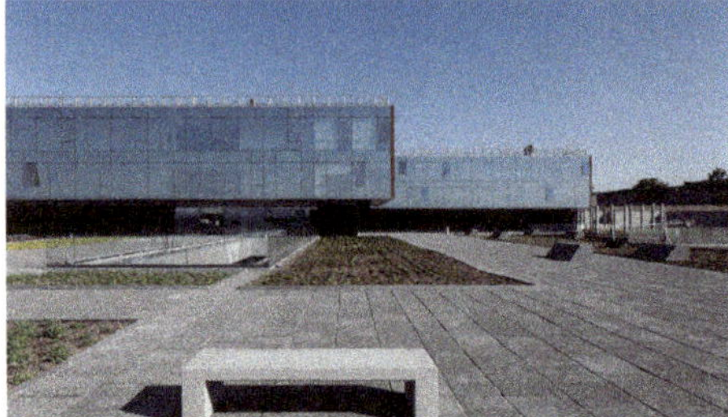

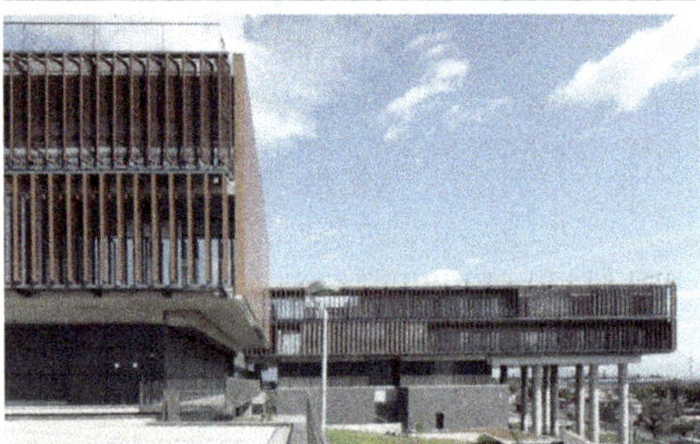

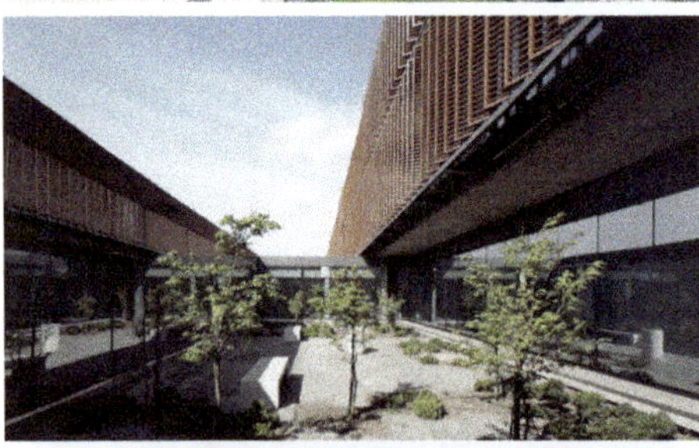

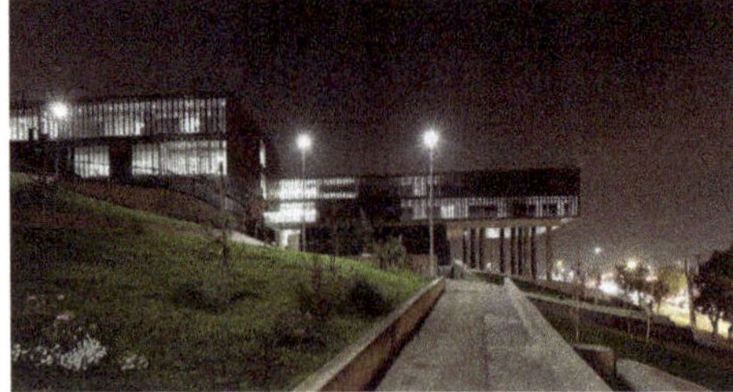

Figure 2. Hospital El Carmen de Maipú, Santiago Chile.

Hospital Clínico Metropolitano, Dra. Eloísa Díaz Insunza -La Florida-Santiago

The Metropolitan Clinical Hospital consists of 67,504 m², 391 beds, 17 operating rooms and 4 delivery rooms, 112 consultations and procedures, 555 parking spaces and 224 seismic isolators, to house 1,500 staff.

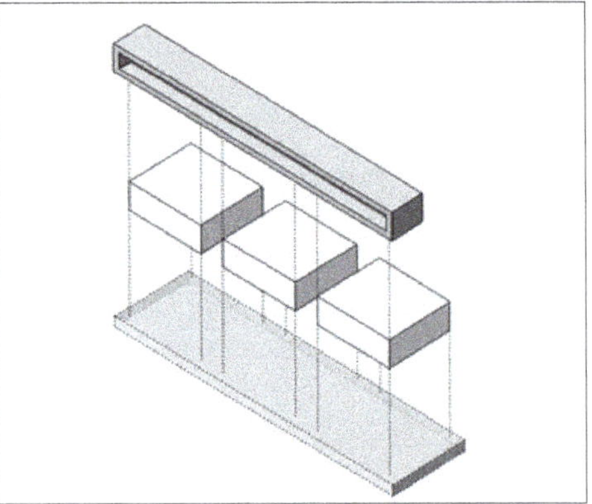

Figure 3. Clinical Metropolitan La Florida Hospital – Santiago, Chile.

The project it's located on a 16,800 m² plot with very unbalanced proportions: 350 m long and 50 m width in a ratio of 7 is 1. For this reason and in function to the complexity of the program, the occupation parameters, constructability and permitted height we decided to extreme the urban parameters looking to recover as much as ground level as we could on an on the green roof.

In response to the limitations of the land, we chose two strategies: programmatic clustering in volumetric boxes, with the aim of recovering the extent of the blocks, and setback of the facade, transforming the sidewalk into a public promenade, thus generating a prelude to building.

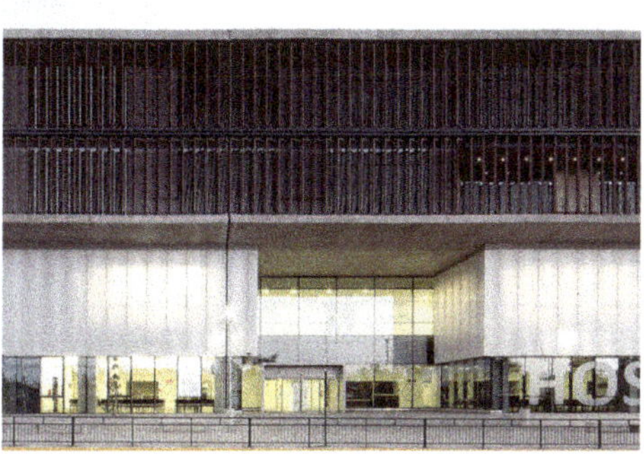

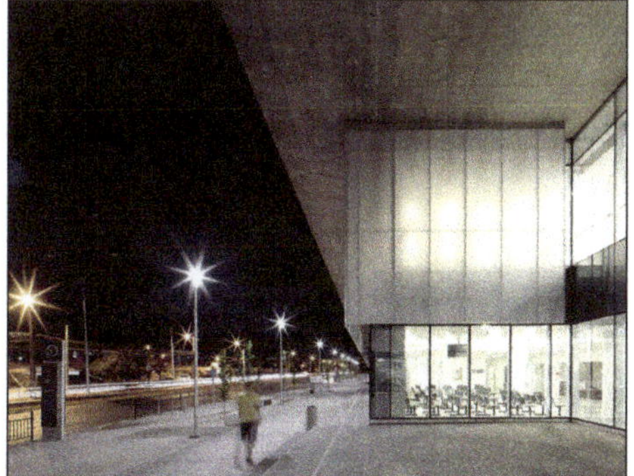

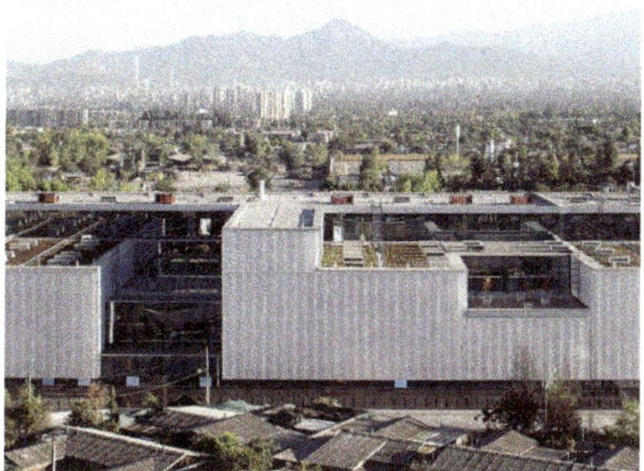

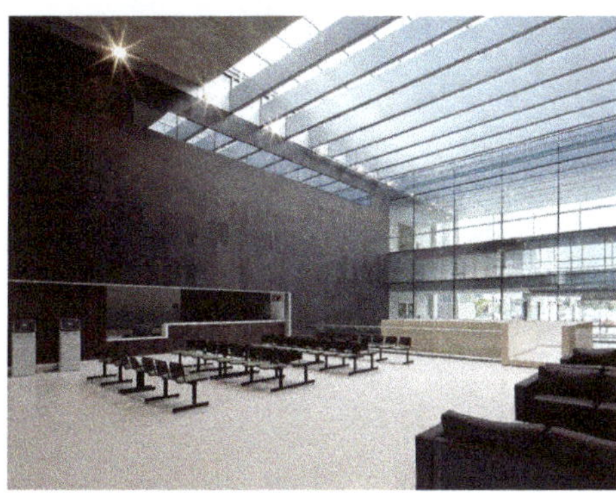

Figure 4. Clinical Metropolitan La Florida Hospital - Santiago, Chile."315

The first strategy is to generate the urban lecture of programmatic boxes (psychiatry, consultation, imaging, emergency) articulating the 350 m facade in four smaller volumes. Between the boxes are located the different access to the hospital. The boxes retrieve the measure of the blocks lost in the original plot.

The second strategy is the setback to the north of the first two floors of the building under the cantilevered body of hospitalization providing a more generous dimension to the sidewalk that runs parallel to the waiting rooms on the first floor. In that way we transform the sidewalk into a urban promenade which reinforces the character of the av. Froilan Lagos (ex "The Park") and is visually linked to the internal program of the building.

The coronation bar (3rd and 4th floor) build's all the 350 m facade, linking the lower boxes building a marquee to the promenade and houses the hospitalization areas. The perimetral concrete belt confines the programmatic volume giving unity to the facade. This element gives to the building the dimension of the 350 m terrain and transform it into an urban reference that can be seen from the distance, from the A. Vespucio highway and the elevated urban city rail (metro).

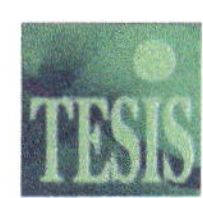

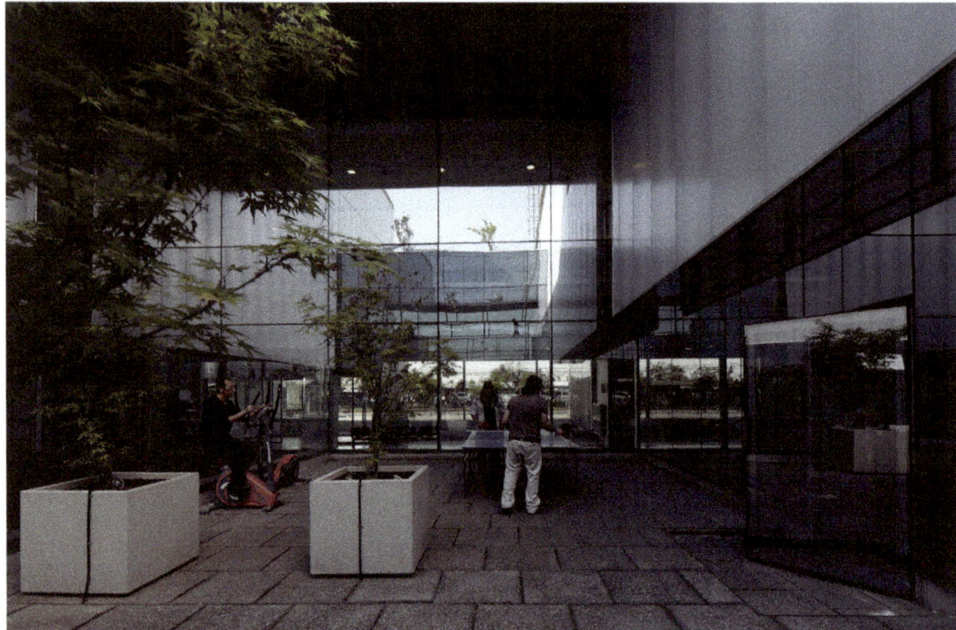

Figure 5. Clinical Metropolitan La Florida Hospital – Santiago, Chile.

The third floor terrace is intended as a green roof, planted with different species of sedum, with low water consumption and moderate maintenance. This is the natural extension of the south public circulation of the hospitalization bar, a place for rest and contemplation at the point where the views open to the Andes mountains, and the valley of Maipo.

Architecture, Health and Futures "Gender Vision"

Susana Miranda Ruiz[1], Luis Enrique López Cardiel[2]

smaesac@gmail.com
[1]Arch., President, Sociedad Mexicana de Arquitectos Especializados en Salud A. C.
[2]Arch., Past- President, Sociedad Mexicana de Arquitectos Especializados en Salud A. C.

Speaking about health infrastructure is approach to the strategic public policy, which are creating opportunities for the committed and visionary professionals who work in the health area. The interest in predict the technical and scientific futures becomes to begin exciting for designers who has ethical and aesthetic challenge in their specialty. They have to respond to current medical practices that are aimed to prevent and care the health of the population, live more years and live better than years ago. Nowadays, for woman is encouraging corroborate that programs with gender equity are priority in any politic initiatives; this inclusion will be beneficial to achieve universal coverage with effective quality and with the optimal infrastructure. The human progress has been changed through the evolution. Natural desires for advance in social, economic, and ecological aspects have incited collective changes, which provide positive stages for the attention for your health. Such as a short-term stage, in countries where health policy is fragmented, nowadays exist a goal to succeed health systems of universal character; this is the guarantee of rights of equality in the protection for health, including of course a gender prospective. One of the improvements in the health attention in the future is the implement of the basic hospital infrastructure which principal objective direct and guide prospective to prevent illnesses, on the contrary of the actual actions which take care of the illness. Nowadays the sustainable design is a great challenge for the creativity of building architecture of medical attention, which generates new international legislative, normative and regulatory topics. The scientific, technological, red integration in media communication and the inversions in biotechnology and more, present surprising expectative that widen the efectivity of the multidisciplinary reds.

Arch. ***Susana Miranda Ruiz*** *has a specialty in Planning and Design of Buildings for Health, she has a master in Valuation of Real State and Industrial Design; she also has a degree in Public Spaces and Safe Cities.*
She has been professor at the Architecture Faculty, UNAM for 8 years and adjunct coordinator of the degree "Architecture for Health Care Buildings", UNAM. She has worked around 23 years as a specialist business woman in Architectural Design Health, and she worked with the Government of the Mexico City, in the Urban Development Department for 9 years.

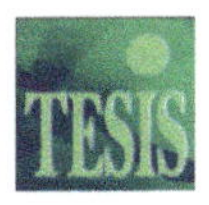

The diverse professionals and specialized technicians in the health sector, form a complex structure that promotes strategies for the optima growth in the medical practice. Without a doubt these movements are being favored with the presence and participation of the woman. In the superior education these days, the women exceeded in about 80% in presence of men, the goal for this woman is archive in the professional life. The United Nations for Development Program (PNUD) assures: "Empowering women gives an impulse to flourishing economies, productivity and growth". The hospital infrastructure of the future is aimed to be operated by multidisciplinary complex team composed by a great number of women. The women have to identify and position their relevant qualities to plan, design, construct, conserve and operate spaces for healthcare, of course they have more sensibility and they appreciate caring for someone else as them.

The stages for the years 2030 and 2050 are promising if taken in counter that each time exist human necessities which fortify individuals and society, presenting as a consequence the creation of vanguard builds dedicated to interest and focus in health.

Faced to the professional development of long term in Mexico, "SMAES" created a prospective vision for the year 2050, through 4 Anticipation Futures Nodes (NOA's for the Spanish acronym) which are structured by multi-disciplinary and trans-disciplinary teams integrated by experts and specialist on public policies health system. Each NOA-s studies and development holistic proposals on futures for the year 2050, under a sequential method of stages develop by the Center of Investigation and Development of Futures (CEIDFU for the Spanish acronym).

The planted prospective of short, medium and long term allowed us to explore strategic and point out carrier Future Agents for each fact, for seeing program stages between 5 and 15 years, projecting an extreme experience like visionary architects.

For the development of this exercise, in accord to the prioritization of challenges we selected four thematic blocks.

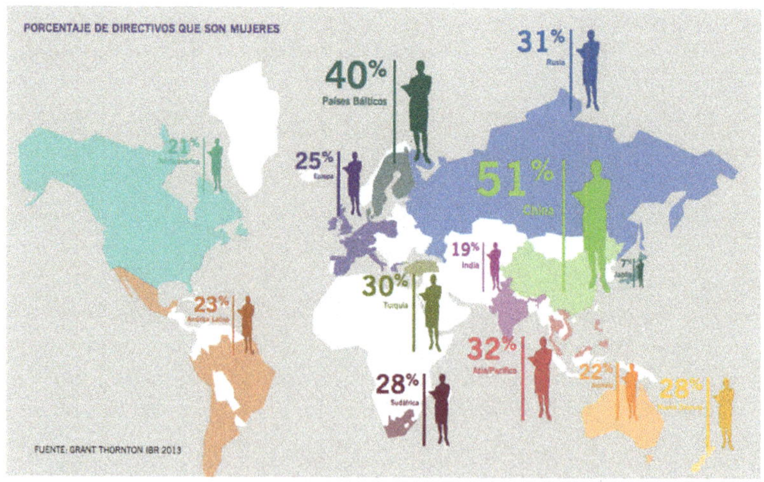

Figure 1. percentage of managers who are women.

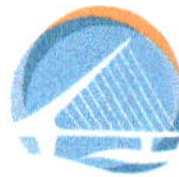

THEME 1. PERINATOLOGY ATTENTION BUILDINGS

Challenges. Incidence of the genomic in the forms of conception, gestation, and the new environments when born.
Year 2050-Prospective. The scientific and technological contributions achieve benefic process for health as the diagnostic illness by genomic test; with this accomplish the detection of future illness and the respective diagnostic to eradicate it.
Genetic engineering will have greater height in treatments for sicknesses added with the creation of new areas like the Genomic Microbial for the application of personalized and friendly pharmaceuticals for the individual. In perinatology we will be able to choose the characteristics of the embryo by the profound management of the DNA with the human genome.
La creation of Blood Banks of Cells, Ovules and Sperms Genetically Improved (BaSeCOEM for the Spanish acronym), will open the door to the individualize information with the genetic code corresponding to each human being. At the end one of the objectives is the guarantee of the improved health matter in the increase of life expectance greater than 150 years.
Gender vision. The experimentation is the fundamental key for the positive culmination of the forthcoming stages, here enters the role of the women derived of the preoccupation and desire of incrementing her professional stile of life, conserving their physical appearance, preventing previous wear, during and after the pregnancy but without losing the mother and child connection. The result is the new method of gestation outside of the human body that simulates natural conditions in the mother's womb (artificial womb).

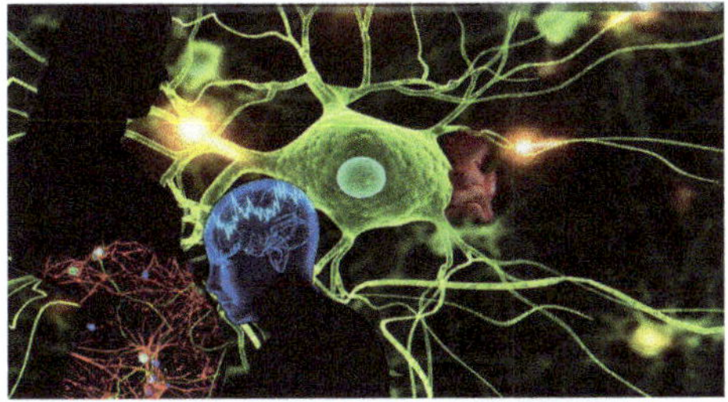

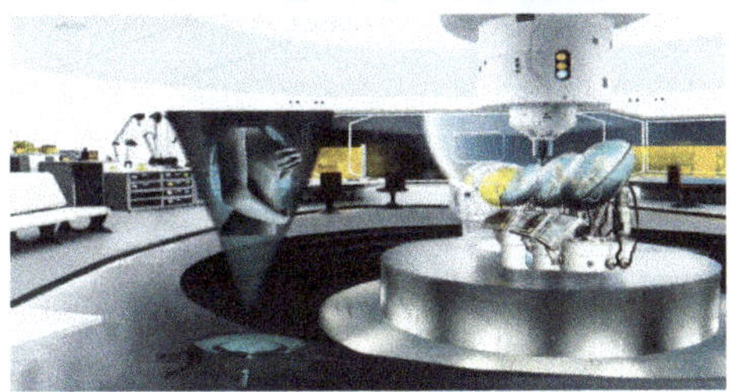

Figure 2. Theme 1, Perinatology attention buildings.

THEME 2. REMOTE SETTLEMENT ATTENTION BUILDINGS

Challenges. Prevalence of the extreme poverty in small towns under 2500 habitants and the coverage of health attention services in remote sites. This is the fundamental sustainable development objective. In social terms the people with economic limitations live in conditions that don't allow cover to their basic requirements and guide the deterioration of their health.
Year 2050- Prospective. One of the principal factors that affect the development is poverty, which is of much importance to consider improvement under holistic focus; in housing, transport, education and of course health. The continuous goal is to elevate the quality of life of the rural population or sub-urban and extinguish their sorrow. The infectious illnesses due to lack of hygiene will have disappeared just like geographic places forgotten and unknown.

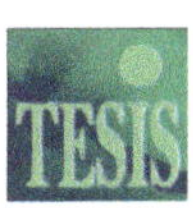

The development of alternative forms of energy adding with the technological advances will convert the traditional rural emergency spaces in the Digital Units of Robotic Health Attention (UDRA's for the Spanish acronym) and their location according to the new zone and distribution will respond to new parameters of accessibility and aero-space transport.
Gender vision. The social impact will consist of gender equality in the whole world, the prevented medicine will for part of academic education in all the institutions with the same objective, granting the deserved level of word wide attention to women, and the all the right to decide about their body without fear and risk to their health. On the rural communities the woman will participate in a decisive manner in projects in which the motor to impulse the economy will be the health centers. It wills impulse the restlessness of the creation about worldwide program of inversion destined to the remote settlements; it will fortify the infrastructure on the process development countries.

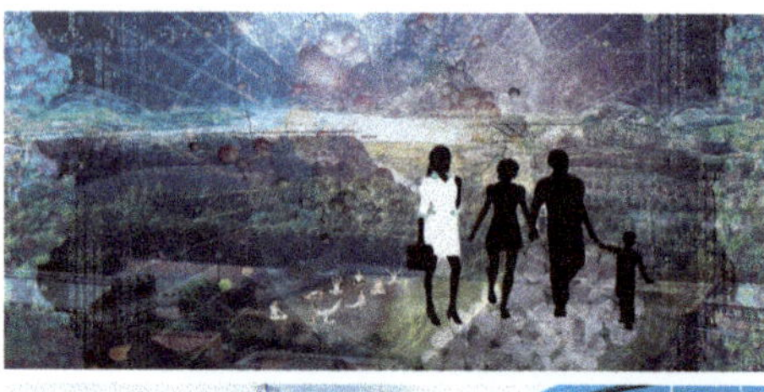

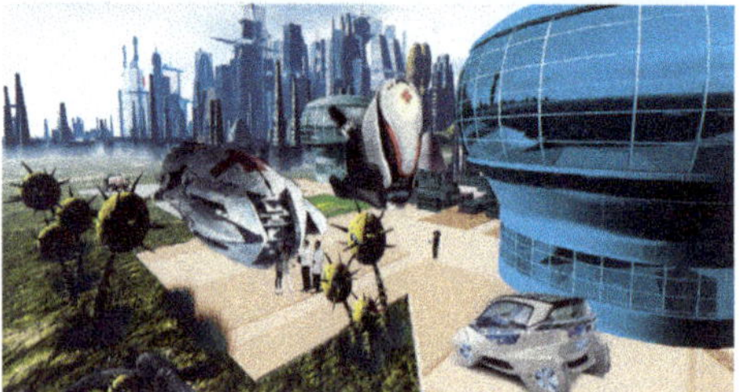

Figure 3. Theme 2, remote settlement attention buildings.

Theme 3. Pathological Depressive Attention Buildings

Challenges. Increment and no knowledge as pathology. It estimates the 1 and 4 persons have depression and the majority doesn't know (2010). The environmental stress, like the visual discordance, additive and inclusive contaminated air result intolerable to survive in urban environment. The stress is understood like a silence mortal illness... the depression.
Year 2050-Prospective. The design of the buildings for health take in counter elements of natural composition, artificial and mixed, just like additional volumes, patios, plazas, hallways, colors, textures, light, shadow, circulations and visual relations, both terrestrial environments like extra orbital's.

Coordinating the design for spaces dedicated to health, the technological advances circulate like the production of medicine to cure the sadness without hurting an organs in the body, we will establish protocols and identification of genetic motives, we will spread the realization of the trans-cranial stimulation and neuro–surgery, will we confection the individual fabrication of pharmaceutical that eliminate the generation of anomalies in neurotransmitters. The interpersonal relation of patients and therapists of high throughout constant monitors, it will be no discussion, just like the existence and relation of the Cyber Pharmacies the culmination of this space will be the extinction of depression, thanks to inter cranial devices, that will control the cause and the effect.
Gender vision. Depression affects both man like women however this have more probability of being diagnosed for this

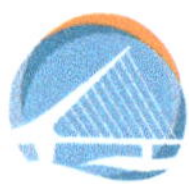

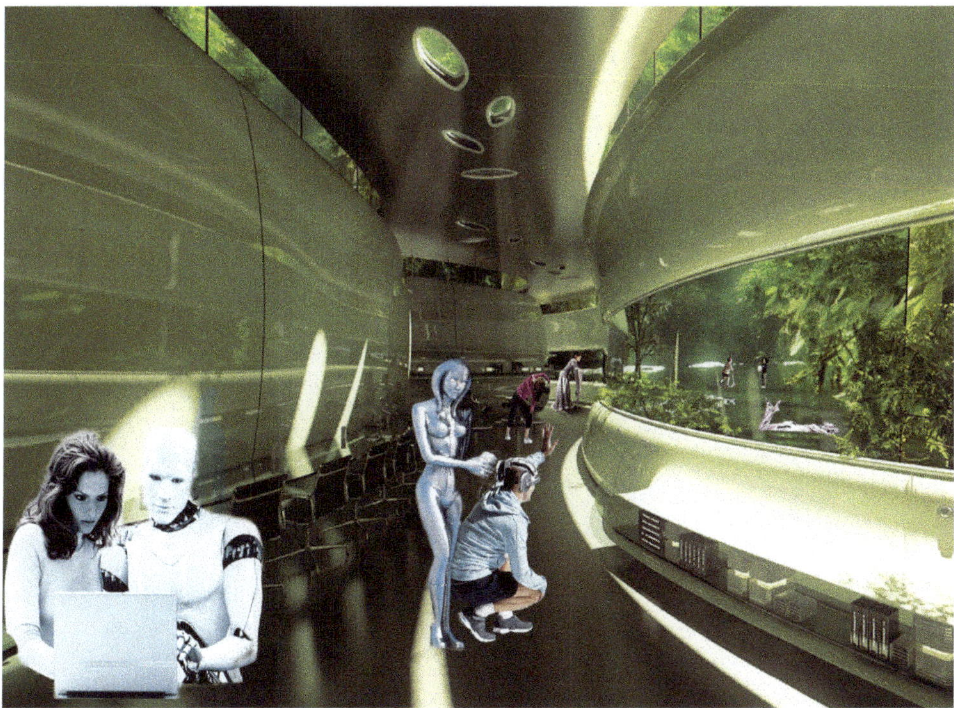

Figure 4. Theme 3, pathological depressive attention buildings.

illness in a determined year according to the Mental Health National Institute there are stages during a women's life that will detonate for the possible development of depression like puberty, the days before menstrual periods before, during and after a pregnancy, and the period of, before, and after menopause. The women will synthesize medicine that will module the female depression, of low budget and will create new applications with laser system to remove hormonal female disorders.

The new scientific conceptions of this pathology are the cost to achieve empowerment to women with hidden talents, elevating professionalism in the productivity on benefit of the family and social surrounding.

THEME 4. ELDERLY POPULATION BUILDINGS

Challenges. The longevity and chronic degenerated illnesses, the spaces to improve the quality of life. The tendency is that there will be a lack of geriatric specialists and few social programs of attention.

2050-Prospective. The positioning of the Elderly Health Medical Specialist Unit in the Elderly Health, (UMESAM´s for the Spanish acronym), will identify models and prototypes that count with open spaces and closed for its wellbeing. The Research Centers, Production and Organ Transplant (CelPROT´s for the Spanish acronym) will open the door to start to a "fourth age".

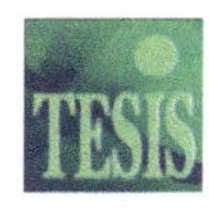

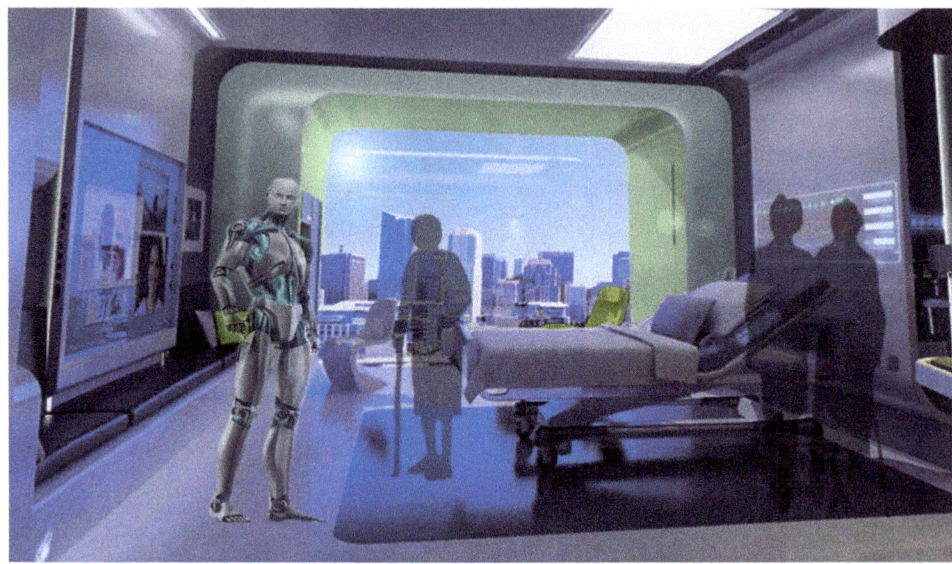

Figure 5. Theme 4, elderly population buildings.

Economic matter requires of greater impulse to public budget destined to wellbeing in attention to the elderly, focusing on the gender equality and age so that way with develop social economic culture around the third age, thanks to the timely boost budget focused on programs made for socio-economic culture favored the elderly with gender equity.

Gender vision. The natural sensibility of the women allows them plan appropriately projects and actions for the care and enjoyment about good quality of life style for elderly population and by consequence the family will be pleased with the results.

Health architectural spaces will be designed with special equipment for woman necessities, because women are physically and psychologically different from men.

Conclusions

As a final conclusion, the evolution is also destined to impact the actual architectonic language, the concept of "construction", unconsciously added to the permanent solitude like a value will disappeared and substituted for a greater passenger term which will manage the precise the mobility and adaptation to real time.
Men and women architects, far from being figures between engineers and special technicians will return their process of design more fluent and above all look for sociality of the technological advances from them the re-interpretation of the architecture and cities. The conceptual architecture, will experiment the transformation of being solid and static energy, it will be understood like a permanent transformation achieving the attention to the human being in physical and emotional health matter.

Physical Resources in Costa Rican Health: An Evolution in Design and Public Health System

Vania Ureña Fallas

Asociación Costarricense de Arquitectura e Ingeniería Hospitalaria (ACOAIH)

The universalization of health care in Costa Rica, through the Costa Rica Social Security Fund, has achieved a remarkable development in public hospital infrastructure, thus extending medical care to nearly all the national territory and favorably increasing the health care rate, both of which are key components in measuring a nation's development and welfare. These results prove the commitment of all the people involved in public health care to achieve stability and equity coverage which rely on a support network based on areas of specialization and, most importantly, the users' own needs. This presentation shows some of the projects that have been developed in recent years, all of which incorporate new strategies that allowed the evolution of architectural design and contributed to people's dignity and the humanization of the physical environment and its therapeutic and healing effects. The latter is considered essential to the development of health infrastructure in our country.

Vania Ureña Fallas. *Architecture graduate studies. Member of the Federated Association of Costa Rican Engineers and Architects (CFIA). Co-founder and President of the Costa Rican Association of Healthcare Engineers and Architects (ACOAIH), 2011-2014. Coordinator of the 1st and 2nd Congress of Healthcare Estates in Costa Rica. Healthcare Construction Training Workshops. Approximate area 4.000.00 sq.m, Design phase. CFIA-Registered Projects: new works at Hospital de Heredia, 40.000 sq.m, inspection. Revamping 15 operating theaters, Hospital San Juan de Dios, 2.400 sq.m. Nutrition, clothes room and passive archives building, Hospital Calderón Guardia, 5.000 sq.m, design and inspection. Renovating 6 operating theaters Torre Sur–Hospital Calderón Guardia, inspection. Refurbishing aqueduct Tanks, Hospital Calderón Guardia, inspection.*

Worldwide Evolution of Hospital Infrastructure

Throughout architectural history, healthcare building design has not been an important referent when it comes to morphological progress in the implementation of design concepts. At the beginning, this type of buildings operated exclusively for sanitary purposes, as places to keep the sick or to safeguard the healthy from epidemics derived

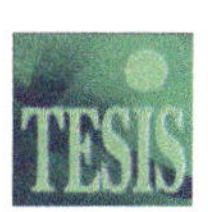

from hospital-acquired infections. These buildings were closely linked to the country's social, political, and economical background since they reflected the conditions of the society and the industrial and medical developments at that time.

In many cases, these aspects defined the typology of the healthcare centers, the flow of relationships between existing spaces, and the aseptic conditions. Such is the case of Pasteur's development in bacteriology, which led to the optional operation of future healthcare centers and the proper maintenance of the existent ones. According to Czajkowski and Rosenfeld's research, these healthcare centers continued to evolve into cloisters, wards, mono, bi, and poly bloc buildings, and systemic and basement blocs.

Some of these typologies derived not only from the required hygienic conditions but also from the development of construction, technological equipment, and all the supplies which are essential to healthcare centers. It is important to highlight that such typological changes, the ones based on the implementations cited before, "do not imply their disappearance but rather an evolutionary line, which, at times, becomes cyclical since, for indefinite causes, they tend to reappear. (Czajkowski, 2000).

The Evolution of Healthcare centers and the development of social security in Costa Rica.

In Costa Rica, the government's policy has been key to social development, improvement, and changes. Because of such view, the army was abolished on December 1st, 1948, after the Civil War and along the transition of the Governing Board led by José Figueres Ferrer. From then until now, Costa Rica has created several social welfare institutions and programs focused on health. This enabled authorities to go beyond and include, within this socio-political framework, the universalization of health care services.

Consequently, Costa Rica occupies one of the first positions in Latin America regarding nationwide healthcare coverage, closely following pioneering countries such as England and Chile. Because of our government's decisions and implemented measures over the years, by the two thousands, we have achieved the OMS goals, obtaining a health index similar to the one of developed countries, thus establishing a fundamental precedent towards continuous growth and development.

In this spirit of commitment towards security and health development, the Health Ministry and the Costa Rican Social Security Fund were created in 1922 and 1941 respectively, and the Law of the Universalization of Social Security was enacted in 1961, thus generalizing medical services throughout the national territory in less than 10 years.

From its beginnings, the Costa Rican Social Security Fund advocated for the centralization of the healthcare system and the definition of a tripartite fee from the employer, the employee, and the State, the latter supported by our Constitution as a social solidarity system to help finance this institution economically.

Beginning of Organized Hospital Facilities in Costa Rica Prior to the Creation of the Costa Rican Social Security Fund. First antecedent - San Juan de Dios Hospital - Province of San José

In 1855, the first hospital facility, San Juan de Dios Hospital, is officially established, which is administered by the Sisters of Charity. This healthcare center was designed by the Italian architects, Lorenzo Durinni and Francisco Tenca, and provided health coverage to the population in the southern region of the capital. It is currently one of the three specialized national hospitals. Its design reflected the ward typology with a neo-gothic architecture; its "L" shaped distribution was aimed at patient wards, medical, and support areas.

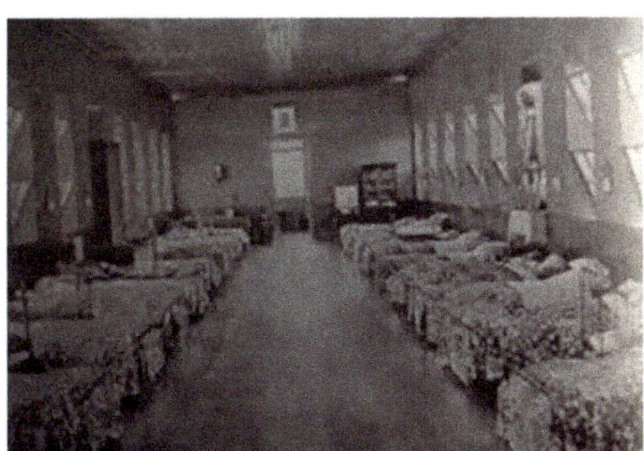

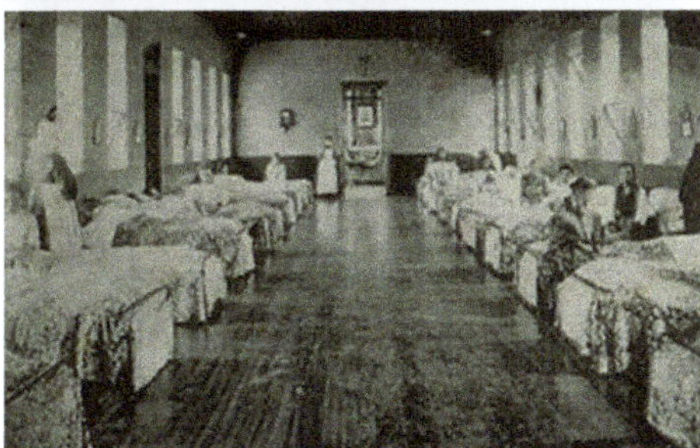

Figure 1. 1902 Photograph from the Women's Ward at San Juan de Dios Hospital. www.ccss.sa.cr.

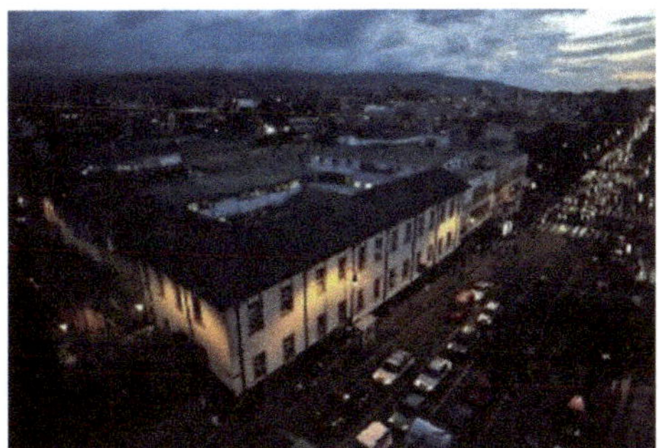

Figure 2. Taken from www.nacion.com.

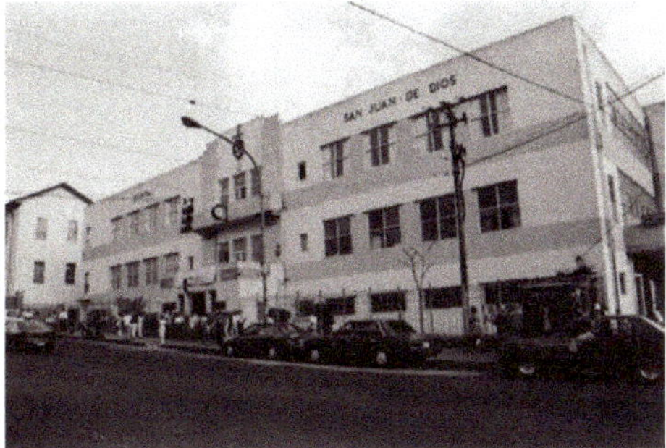

Figure 3. Pensión Echandi Building Photograph. Taken from www.asamblea.go.cr.

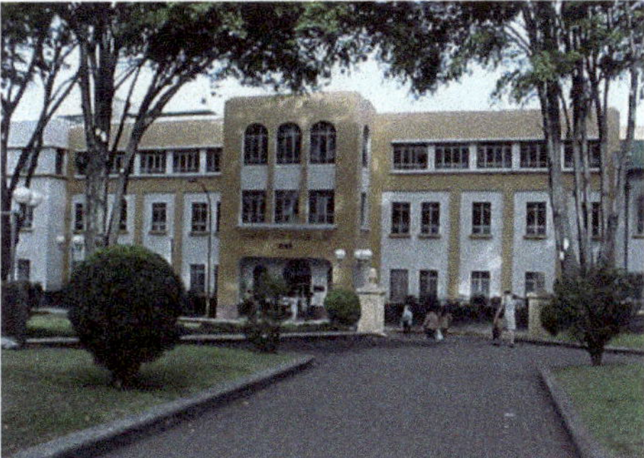

Figure 4. Medical Entrance Door Photograph. Taken from www.missmoveabroad.com.

Along its existence, the hospital has been remodeled several times to meet its growing demand, beginning from 1920 to 1930. In 1934, both the Echandi boarding room and the out-patient facilities were built. By the end of 2013, fifteen surgery rooms were equipped with the latest technological developments.

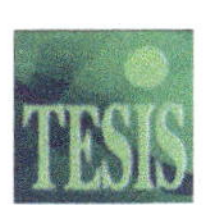

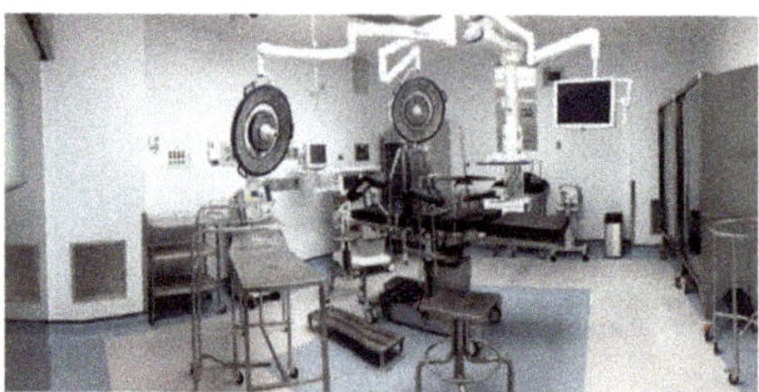

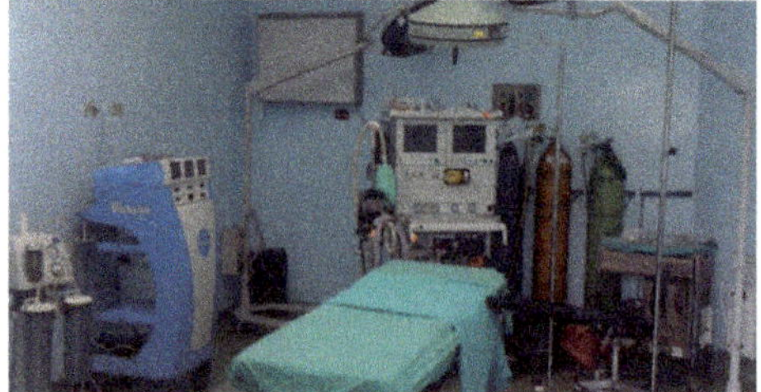

Figure 5. Operating Room at San Juan de Dios Hospital, 2013 Photograph.

National Psychiatric Hospital, Dr. Manuel Antonio Chapuí and Dr. Roberto Chacón Paut. A Specialized Vision on Hospital Infrastructure

One of the main concerns of the 1800's was the conditions of the mentally ill. As a result, in 1892, the first specialized medical facility for mentally ill patients, Hospital Nacional Insanos, was opened. Later, in 1896, it changed its name to Hospital Nacional Psiquiátrico Manuel Antonio Chapuí y Torres (National Psychiatric Hospital).

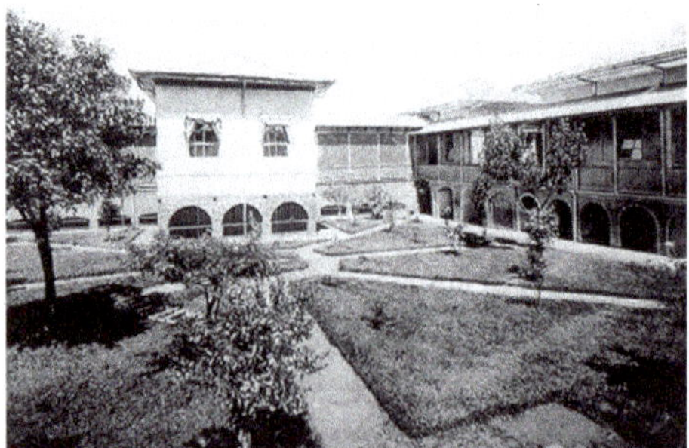

Figure 6. Taken from www.ccss.sa.cr.

Its distribution started from a central nave, largely occupied by the chapel which had a neo-gothic dome that can still be appreciated. From such nave, the wards were located to the sides; their distribution was very functional, and halls connected the whole building.

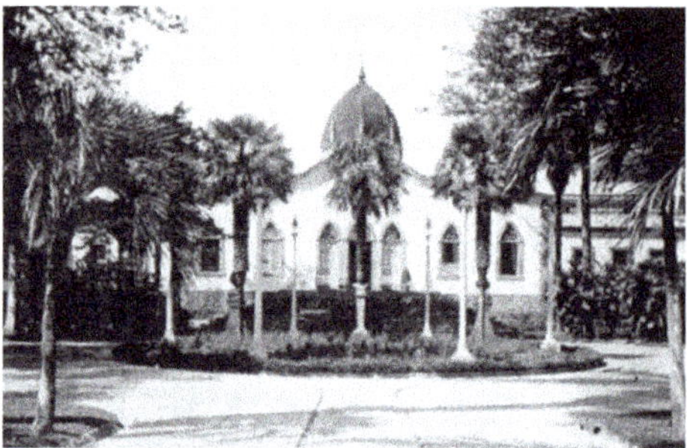

Figure 7. Taken from www.ccss.sa.cr.

By 1950, the facilities were insufficient to shelter all the patients; therefore, a building is acquired in the province of Cartago, tailored to meet the necessary conditions for 200 patients; thus, Dr. Robert Chacón Paut hospital is born.

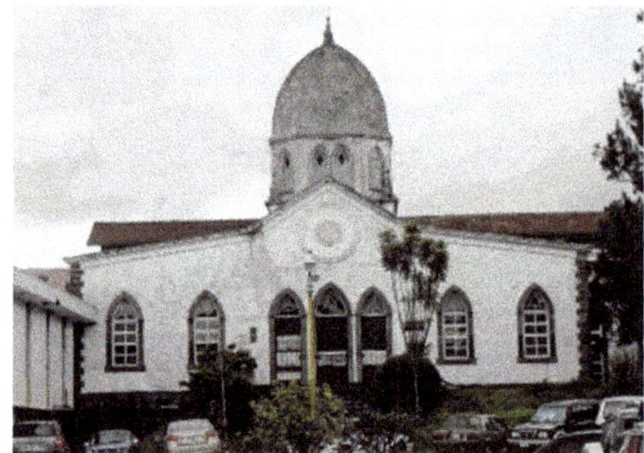

Figure 8. Taken from www.ccss.sa.cr.

This hospital is still operating. It is important to highlight that the buildings were designed for the General Adventist Conference; their space design allowed distributing patients in wards.

At the moment, it provides specialized psychiatric healthcare and psychosocial rehabilitation services following a holistic approach, and it also alternates community treatment. Its healthcare services range from prolonged stays to crisis intervention, daycare center, and residential-type structures.

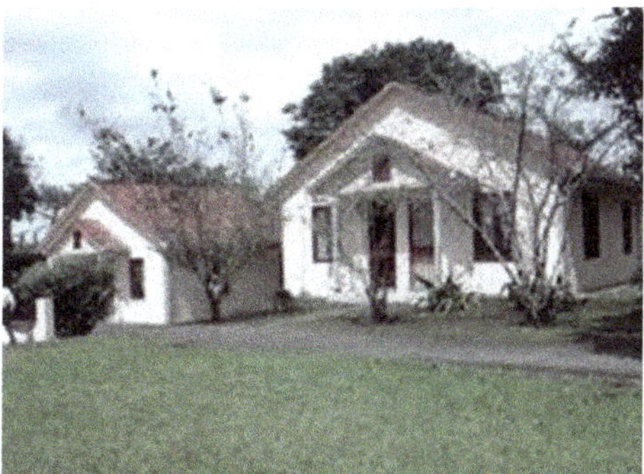

Figure 9. Taken from www.ccss.sa.cr.

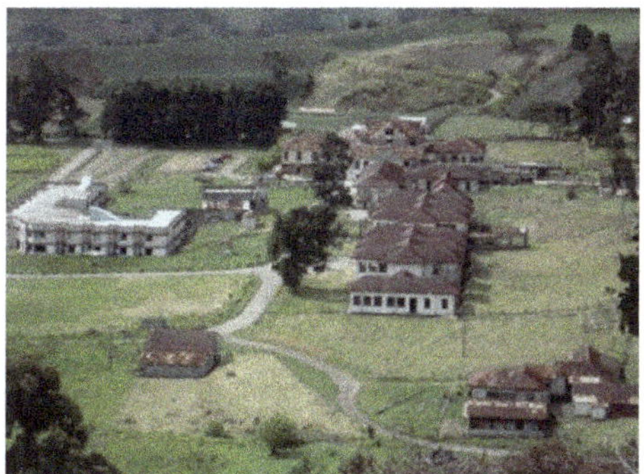

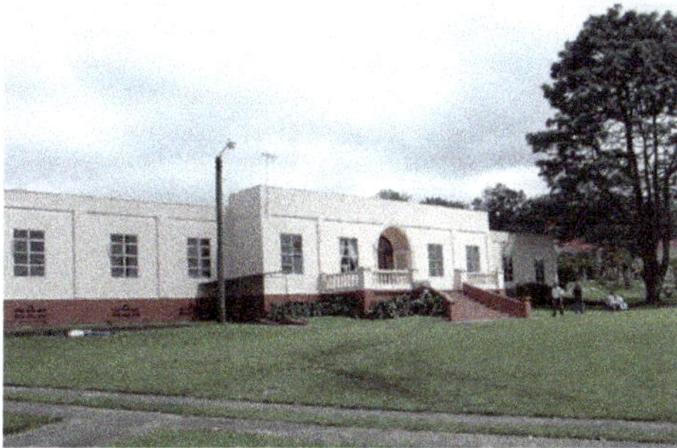

Figure 10. Photographs of Dr. Roberto Chacón Paut Hospital. Taken from www.ccss.sa.cr.

By 1974, the facilities of Dr. Manuel Antonio Chapuí and Torres National Psychiatric Hospital are opened; this hospital is located outside San José downtown. Its ward distribution allowed patient interaction with green areas as part of their therapeutic treatment.

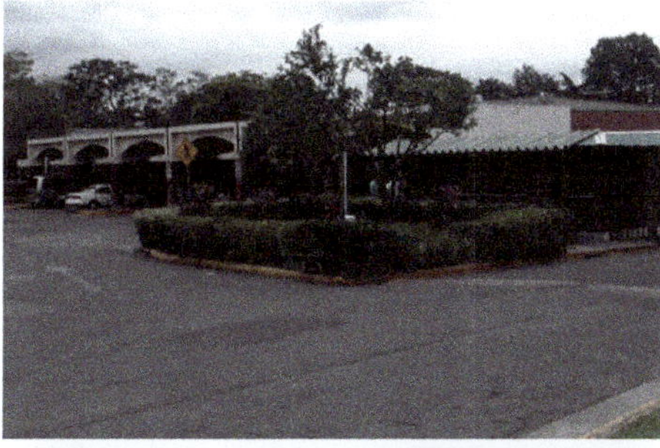

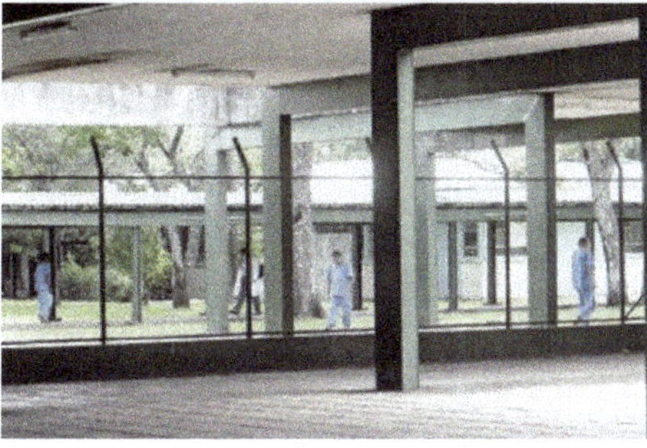

Figure 11. Dr. Manuel Antonio Chapuí National Psychiatric Hospital, www.ccss.sa.cr.

SAN RAFAEL HOSPITAL - PROVINCE OF ALAJUELA, FIRST HOSPITAL ENTIRELY BUILT BY THE COSTA RICAN SOCIAL SECURITY FUND

After building San Rafael Hospital in 1905, social security coverage extended from the northern part of the country to the metropolitan area, in the province of Alajuela. Its neo-classic style exhibited internal halls that favored cross-ventilation and invited doctors and patients to enjoy of a distracting and therapeutic environment.

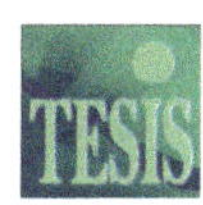

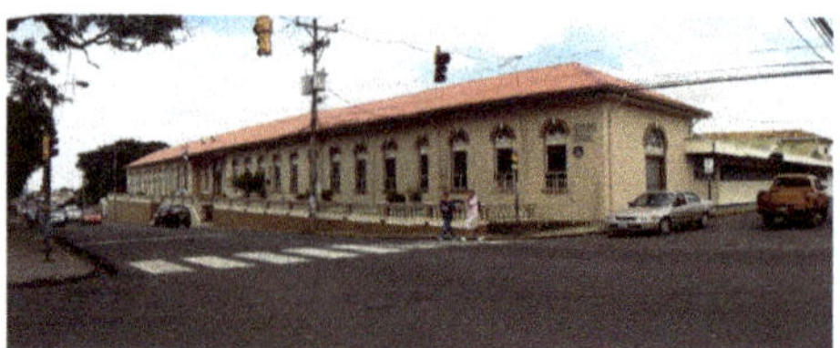

Figure 12. Old San Rafael Hospital founded in 1905.

In 2004, the new facilities of San Rafael Hospital were opened; a block basement typology can be appreciated, leaving the first floors for diagnostic and outpatient services, and internal medicine on the upper floors.

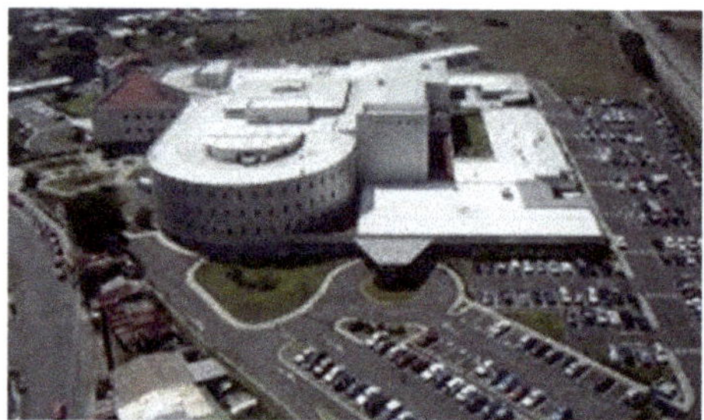

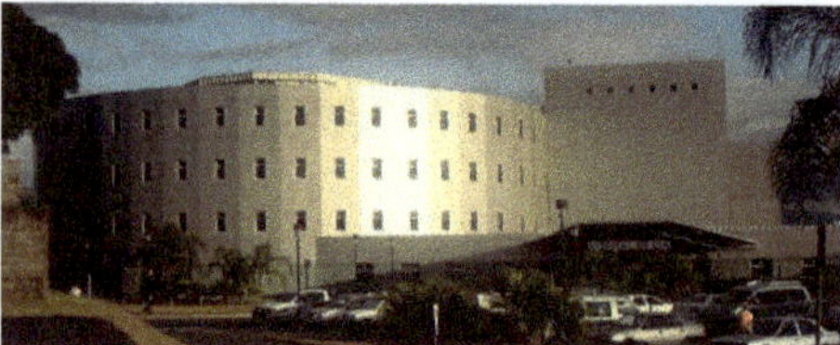

Figure 13. San Rafael Hospital - Alajuela.

DR. RAFAEL ÁNGEL CALDERÓN GUARDIA HOSPITAL: FIRST HOSPITAL WITH POLICLINIC INFRASTRUCTURE

At the beginning of 1938, the first facilities of the Policlinic were built. Initially, these facilities were designed to house a foster house as the government's response to the social situation. Once finished, it was designed to provide workers with medical care. This building has its own art deco language and was declared national heritage.

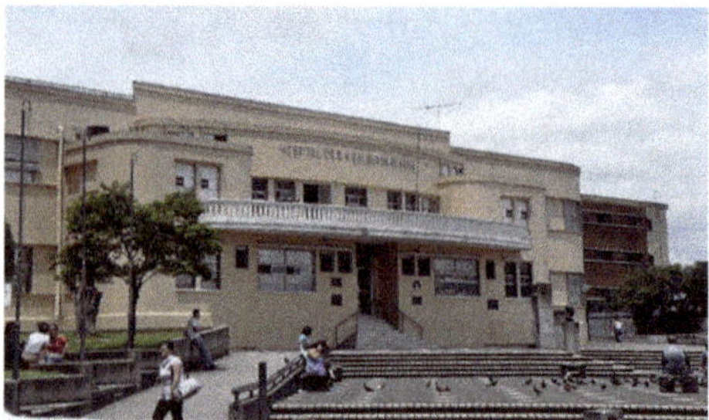

Figure 14. Polyclinic Building. Taken from: www.comons.wikimedia.org.

Once the Costa Rican Social Security Fund was consolidated, it was baptized as Calderón Guardia Hospital; this became a specialized medical facility that, throughout history and due to its increasing demand, has built several facilities at different times, all of which have been connected through halls. Since the facilities have been built in different periods, several architectural tendencies can be observed; however, the typology of these medical centers reflects a monobloc style, because of its geographical location.

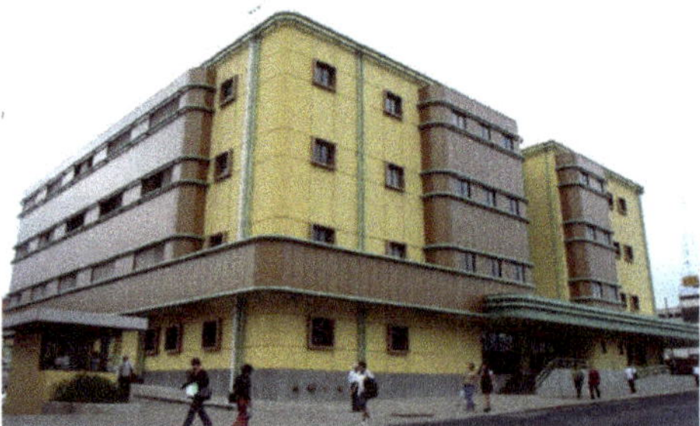

Figure 15. Emergency Building. Taken from: www.crhoy.com.

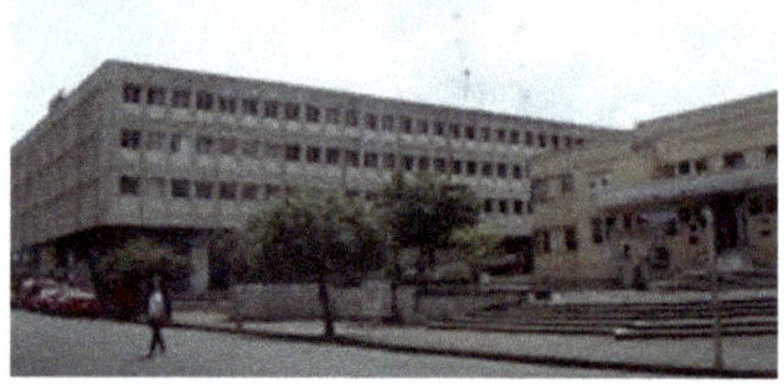

Figure 16. Surgical and Inpatient Building. Taken from: www.columbia.co.cr.

As part of the implemented improvement policies within the institution, on July 2014, six remodeled operating rooms from the emergency ward were handed over. At the moment, new technology and national and international protocols are still being established.

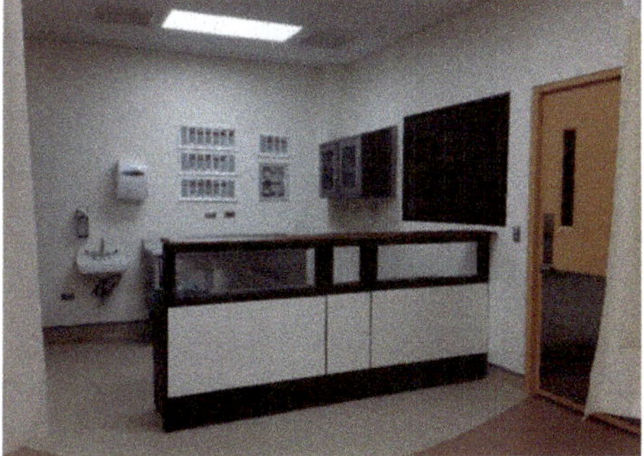

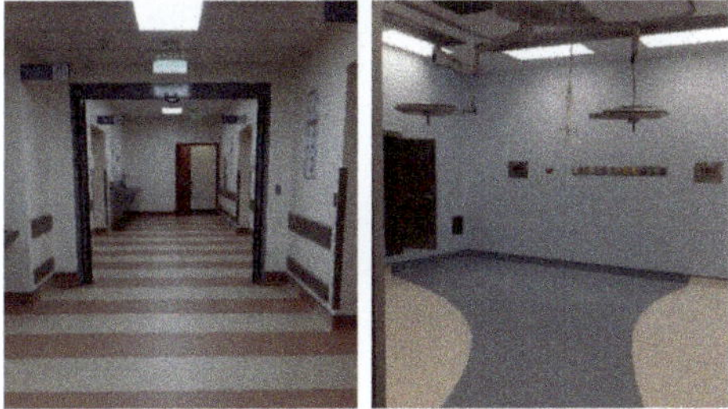

Figure 17. Photographs taken by Architect Vania Ureña Fallas.

At the moment, a facility to house the Nutrition, Clothing, and Passive Archive Units is still under construction; it is meant to have an area of 5,000 square meters.

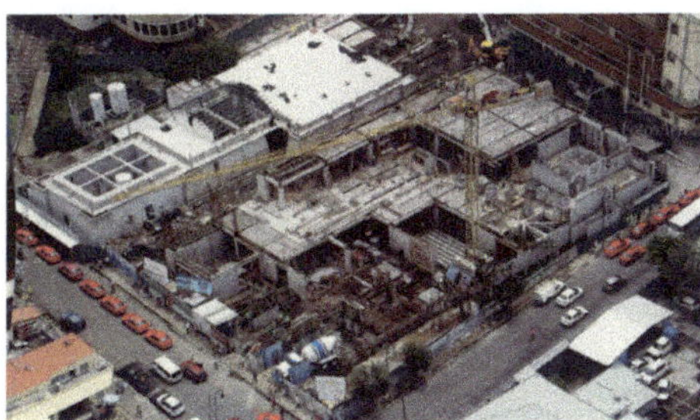

Figure 18. Photos: Photo Air. Courtesy Structures SA.

San Vicente de Paul Hospital - Province of Heredia. Last Hospital Built by the Costa Rican Social Security Fund

The opening of its new facilities was in 2010. With a capacity of 246 beds and 37,000 square meters of construction, this old structure dates back to 1890.

Its modernization consists of six modules linked together through halls that offer users a visual tour to the main entrance of the square, which is the one welcoming visitors. In this design, simplicity and majesty converge, applying to its concept of internal design, materials, textures, and colors that highlight a warm and pleasant image. The project was designed to meet social welfare standards to its full extent, leading to the lowest environmental impact, and taking into account all the existing national and international regulations.

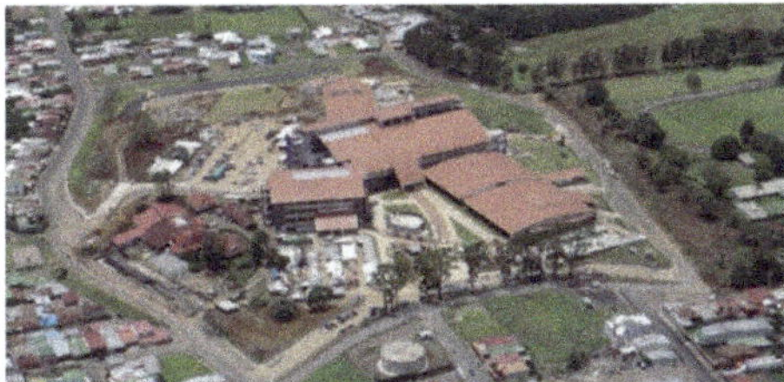

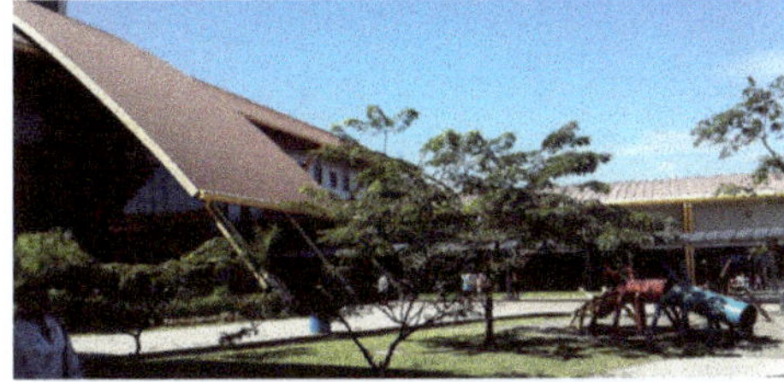

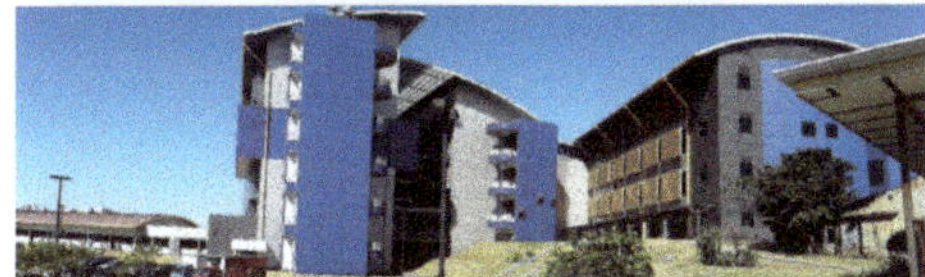

Figure 19. Photographs by Architect Vania Ureña Fallas.

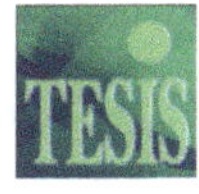

Outcomes of the Evolution of the Healthcare System

As confirmed by the Central American Bank for Economic Integration (BCIE) in its 2011 edition, today Costa Rica has one of the highest and more positive health indexes in Central America. According to this entity, the infant mortality rate is 9.5 deaths in one thousand while the mortality rate for 5 years is 11 deaths in one thousand.

This data contrast with the institution's current problems, which relate to patient care, life expectancy at birth, and changes in morbidity and mortality in diseases such as dengue and malaria.

The inclusion of the poorest is consistent with the implementation of a nationwide healthcare coverage system, where there are 455 inhabitants per physician and nearly a 100% births per qualified staff. Such figures allow Costa Rica to have a life expectancy level of 79.5 years, the highest in Central America by 2011, ranging from 77 for male to 81.9 for female; this in spite of its third world status. According to the U.N. Development Program (PNUD), in 2013, Costa Rica ranked in first among the Latin America countries with the highest life expectancy level, 79,4 years, which is considered a general standard in developed countries.[1]

The established healthcare model solves problems at three different levels. The main feature of this model is the complexity of its medical services. Thus, service is divided to avoid excessive demand in general and specialized medical units. Such is the case of the third level, which provides inpatient and therapeutic services requiring cutting-edge technology. The second healthcare level offers basic hospital and outpatient interventions such as General Surgery, Internal Medicine, and Pediatrics, thus leaving outpatient services for prevention, recovery, and rehabilitation to the first level.

The implementation of these three levels demonstrated the need to improve the first one, which was not given so much importance since the 1970's. Thus, this last level is reinforced, through a more social approach to healthcare and not merely as an indicator of success. To support this view, it was necessary to increase the number of support teams and comprehensive healthcare programs which guaranteed continuity of user service.

Some of the first and second level buildings that have been developed in different regions of the countries and have improved social services are: Centro de Atención Integral de Salud (CAIS), Integrated Health Center in Siquirres, which has its own concept based on its humid weather conditions.

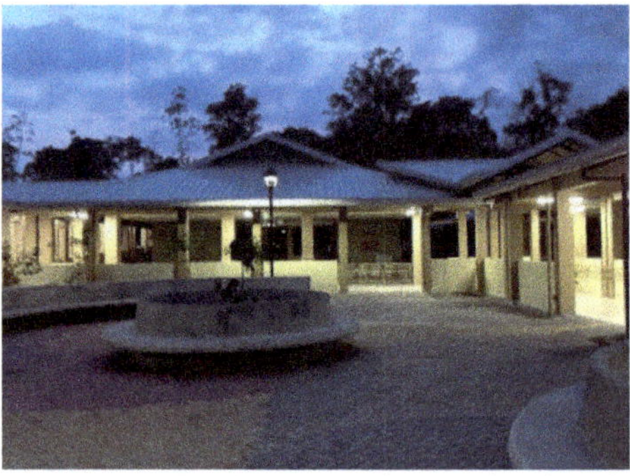

Figure 20. CAIS Siquirres. Photograph taken by Engineer Luis Orias.

[1] *Costa Rica Stastitical File, BCIE 2001. Human Development Report, 2013, the Emergence of the South, Human Progress in a Diverse World.*

This building consists of modules connected by halls that favor natural ventilation and user's views. By the end of 2010, CAIS Puriscal was opened, with a dimension of 5,400 square meters. Tomas Casas Hospital, located in the southern area of the country, follows a module concept which favors flexibility, and is incorporated in its environment as part of the patient's healing process.

Today's healthcare service network, which started back in 1845, consists of 2,313 first level buildings, 123 second level centers, and three public general hospitals, six specialized hospitals, and ten specialized centers which belong to the third level.

Certainly, our country is currently reaping the benefits of more than 70 years of evolution in its views, political reforms, and the impetus of the Costa Rican people to achieve something unthinkable for many Central American countries. It is a dream that must be kept in time. This social security ideology has become central to peace.

Proclaiming social healthcare a universal and compulsory right to all Costa Rican citizens has placed our country among the top healthcare countries. The increase in life expectancy and the decrease in infant mortality levels prove this.

In contrast, the increase in such indexes has proved that the age projection of the

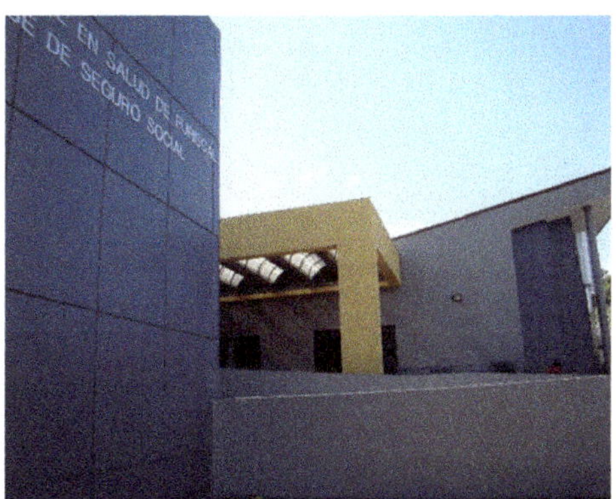

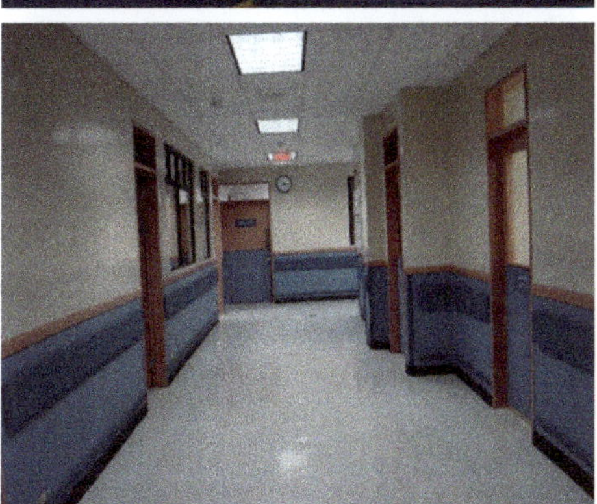

Figure 21. Integrated Health Center Puriscal. Photograph by Architect Jorge Abarca.

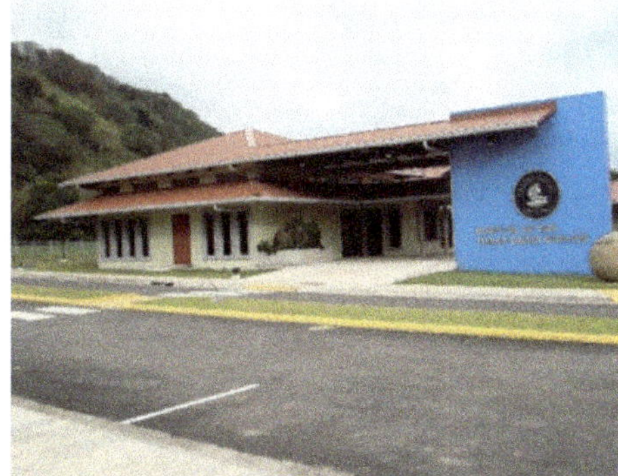

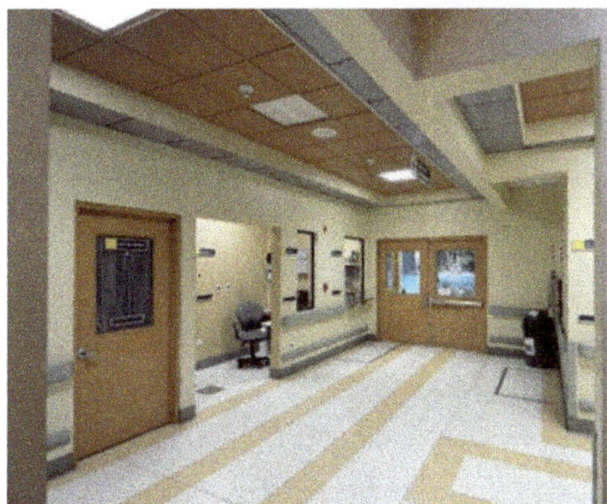

Figure 22. Tomas Casas Casajuz Hospital. Photograph taken by Architect Jorge Abarca A.

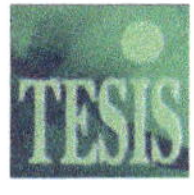

population is unstable when it comes to the number of people ages 15 through 64. This will cause an abrupt shift in the insurance holder's future medical service. These needs point at specialized services in geriatrics, diseases, and ailments.

This information is confirmed by the 2011 national census, which concludes that "the size of this population will triple in the next 40 years, increasing from 316,000 people in 2012 to more than a million people by 2050. With this increase, senior citizens will exceed 0-14 children after 2040."

The changes in life expectancy and medical developments have posed a challenge to all the professionals involved in planning and developing health centers through the care network; therefore, the institution has established policies to adapt the future projects to the new demands and thus provide service based on the existing needs.

Some of the projects under development are the East Tower of Calderon Guardia Hospital with 239 beds that will offer gineco-obstetric services, labor rooms, and inpatient and imaging services; the re-construction of Monseñor Sanabria Hospital in the province of Puntarenas with 500 beds, which was partially destroyed by the 2012 earthquake; Max Peralta Hospital in the province of Cartago; The National Center for Pain Management and Palliative Care, the Oncological Tower located in Calderon Guardia Hospital; alongside these structural projects, purchasing medical equipment is also being contemplated.
At the moment, the Inpatient Tower of the Annexation Hospital in the province of Guanacaste is under construction; this hospital will increase the capacity to 136 beds; The 5,000 square-meter building of the Nutrition and Clothing Units from the Calderon Guardia Hospital and others will improve the existing public health network in Costa Rica.

Development of Dutch Healthcare in Cure and Care

Douwe Kiestra

Dutch Association of Healthcare Engineering (NVTG), Netherlands

How do we design hospitals in the Netherlands, will it be the hospital of the future and does it still look like a hospital. Let us surprise you. The Netherlands is one of the most densely populated countries in the world. We would like to show how we ensure good elderly housing. Together with Jan Willem van Rijen of Deerns and Reimar von Meding, chief architect at KAW we take you with us to the future but also today. The NVTG is honoured to host the 24th Congress of the International Federation of Hospital Engineering in 2016. We intend to organise an interactive conference where professionals in the field of Healthcare Engineering and Architec-ture, from all over the world, will meet to exchange new ideas, case studies and experiences. We invite you visit the 24th congress of the IFHE in The Hague in the Netherlands.

President of the NVTG, Dutch association of healthcare engineering; 2nd Vice President and ExCo member of the IFHE. IFHE member advisory panel IFHE Digest. General Director Pranger-Rosier (installation company). Education: Higher professional education – building engineering and Master business administration.

About NVTG: founded in 1947. From 50 (1947) to 700 members today. IFHE member since 1970. Co-founder IFHE-Europe. Cooperation with governments and universities. National and regional activities.

Congress Theme IFHE 2016: "Healthcare Engineering creating effective and efficient care world-wide".

Congress Subjects: Architecture & Design, Healthcare Building Technology, Hygiene, Sustainability, Energy Efficiency, Facility Management, Maintenance, Biomedical Engineering, Safety.

Programme highlights: Active participation of IFHE-colleagues from member associations; International keynote speakers; Interactive workshops by IFHE members; Plenary and parallel sessions; Visits of (care and cure) institutions; Cultural excursions.

Participants: Representatives of IFHE member associations; Other interested professionals in Healthcare Engineering

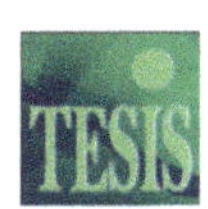

International, national and regional government representatives.

Supporting Organizations: Municipality of The Hague; Dutch Center for Health Assets-TNO; Nyenrode Business University; Kivi Niria, Dutch Engineers Association; ISSO, Dutch building services research institute; The Hague Convention Bureau.

Supporting WHO Objectives: With the exchange of knowledge we will pay specific attention to the objectives of the World Health Organisation. For many decades IFHE and WHO have been in intensive contact, with IFHE supporting the goals of WHO. WHO urges the healthcare engineering sector to apply its creativity and resources to support sustainable health sector development in low-income settings whilst maintaining safety, quality, effectiveness and efficiency of care. For the IFHE Congress 2016 in The Netherlands, this will be our challenge!

We like to invite you all to the 24th Congress of IFHE The Hague – The Netherlands.

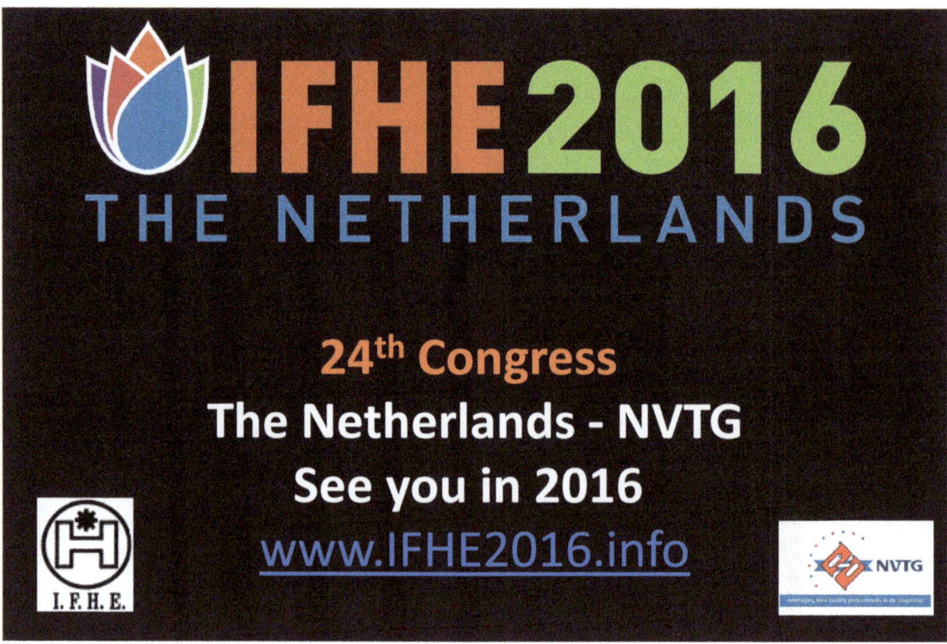

Your Hospital in 2040

JW van Rijen

Deerns Nederland B.V., Netherlands

As hospital buildings in general have a lyfespan of approximately 50 years and looking at the logistic and technical infrastructure we should look at least 50 years ahead during master planning and design. Taking into account changing and adapted building techniques and in general a midlife renovation our horizon is 2040. To include the consequences of demographic developments, the rapid changing medical techniques, technical devel-opments within and outside the healthcare this is a huge challenge. The biggest developments are to be expected in the field of ICT developments and the impact on the flexibility of the buildings in size and functionality. For example 24/7 monitoring of patients, possible due to increasing data-transmis-sion opportunities as well as the introduction of revolutionary "lab on chip "technology in diagnostics. Now a days already high risk patients are being monitored with minimal impact on the quality of their life and technical possibilities already available to prevent or warn the patient for potential dangers in their near surroundings. Also in the imaging techniques revolutionary changes are to be expected with big consequences for the buildings and technical infrastructure of healthcare institutions. The implementation of X-ray techniques to be used per-operative on existing operating theatres in frequent situations is impossible or at least has a very big impact on investments or changes. The same situation exists for imaging techniques in radiotherapy. Other developments are more technical or in the field of sustainability looking at a circular economy, diminishing emis-sions, all electric hospitals and the hospital as an healing building. The past could be the best Prophet ...
In this presentation we will shortly look back at the most important developments in the last 25 years, most recent spectacular developments and the prediction of the world in the following 30 years! Looking at what impact these will have on your building and technical infrastructure to be prepared on these developments!

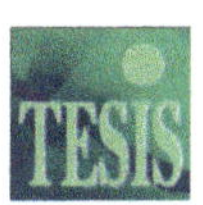

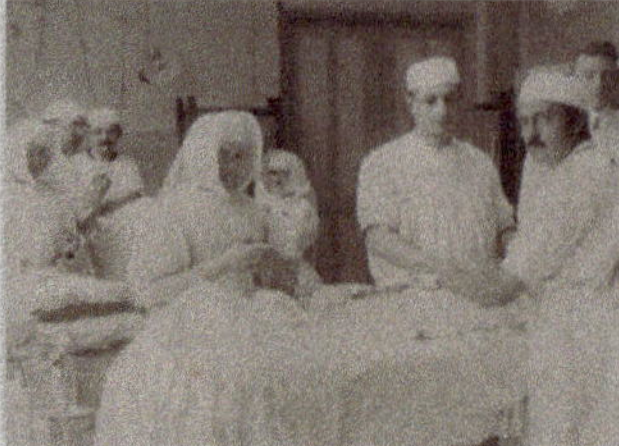
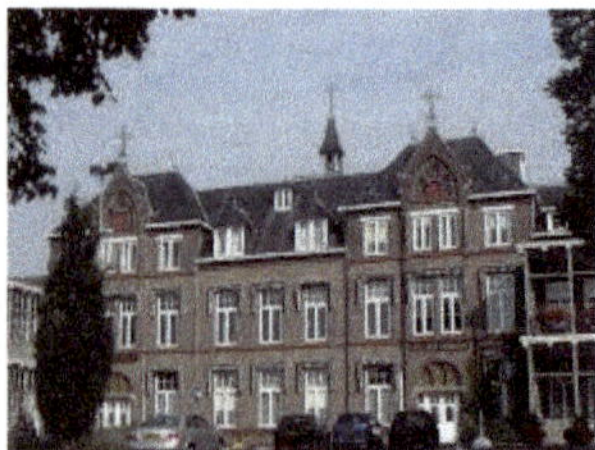

Figure 1. Past.

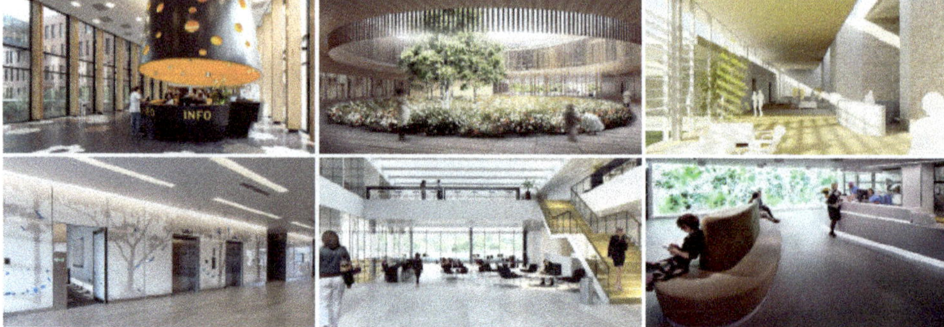

Figure 2. Present: functional differentiation of public areas.

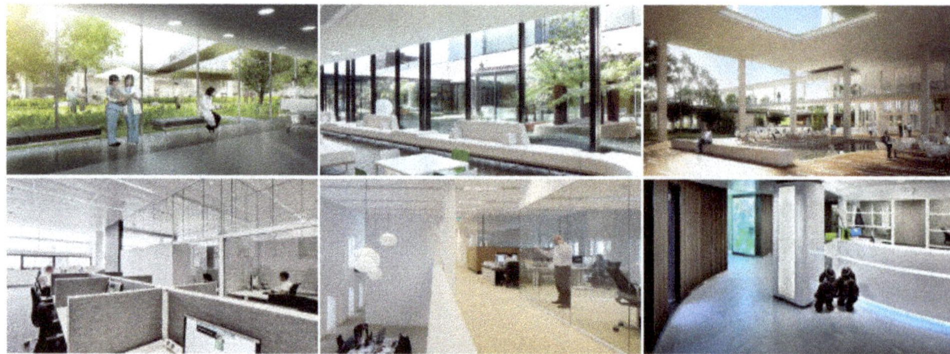

Figure 3. Present: functional differentiation of polyclinical areas and offices.

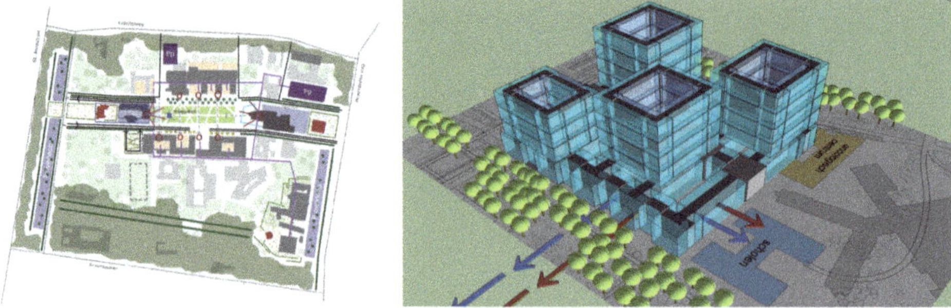

Figure 4. Future: integral sustainability for campus development and synergy.

Healthcare Architecture in the Cultural Diversity of Brazil

Fábio Bitencourt

Associação Brasileira para o Desenvolvimento do Edifício Hospitalar (ABDEH), Brazil

In the midst of many health assistance needs actually in Brazil, highlight the special need for healthcare buildings that can attend program commitments of the Ministry of Health to meet the diverse demands of this segment care. With a population of over 200 million inhabitants (IBGE Brazil, 2014), and 12% or the equivalent of 24 million people over 60 years, the country has 5,565 cities in its 8.5 million km², an area comparable to 47% of the entire area of South America In this context, the wide range of topics related to the healthcare activities has particular importance. With 468 785 beds and 6,426 hospitals built and running, Brazil still has a high demand, because according to the parameters of the World Health Organization (WHO) recommends 4 beds/1000 inhabitants, while the all the country still has only 2.45 beds/1000 inhabitants. It results in a deficit of more than 296,000 beds that will establish the need for distinct and fast solutions for healthcare in the basic, intermediary and high complexity buildings for healthcare. The regional diversity of occupation density in Brazilian territory has the same diversity and complexity of epide-miological characteristics of other countries in the Latin American community, each with its own characteristics and particularities. Health assistance in Brazil has a distinct opportunity to start your period of architectural qualification for the hospitals and other health buildings, appropriating his needs for climatic conditions and the sustainability requires for each region. Simultaneously it is time to provide security and human comfort to main users - health professionals and patients - in so far as the technology and expertise to new buildings are already available.

Fábio Bitencourt. *President ABDEH. Architect, professor, researcher. Doctorate in Sciences of Architecture, Master in environmental comfort. President of the Associação Brasileira para o Desenvolvimento do Edifício Hospitalar (ABDEH) - 2011/2014. Member of the Brazilian Academy of Hospital Administration (ABAH). Professor at postgraduate courses in architecture, ergonomics, human comfort and health care management. Author of various books and publications on hospital architecture, human comfort, healthcare environments and er-gonomics. Member of the Organización de Expertos Americanos en Tecnologías para la Salud (OEXAIS). Honorary Partner of the Asociación Chilena de Arquitectura y Especialidades Hospitalarias (AARKHOS). Works since 1993 with planning and design architecture, master plans, construction and management of health care buildings.*

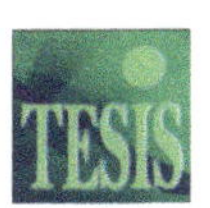

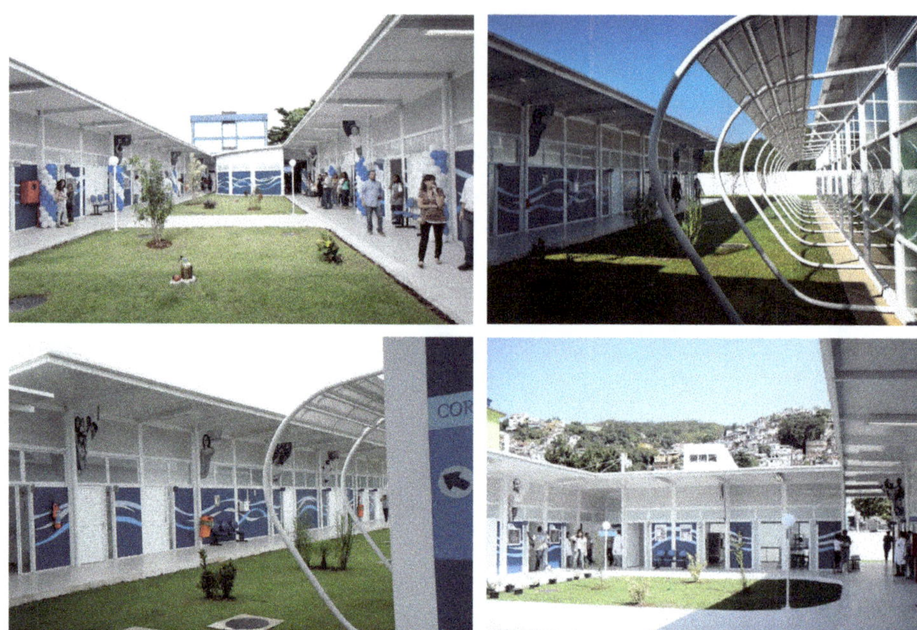

Figure 1. Family Health Clinics, Rio de Janeiro, RJ. Source: PMRJ, RioUrbe 2013.

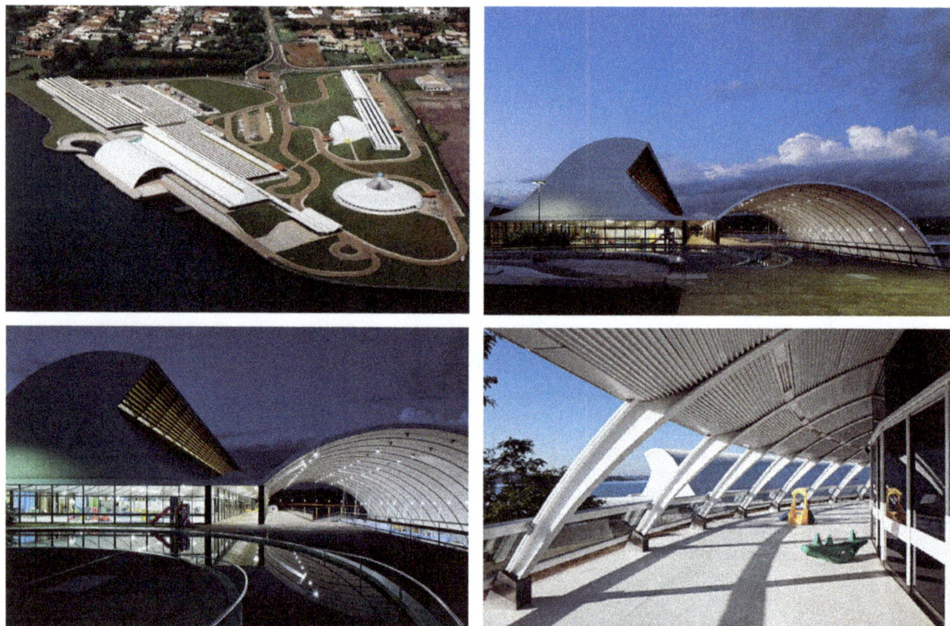

Figure 2. Sarah Hospital Group, architect João Filgueiras Lima (Lele) Unit Sarah Lago Sul, Brasilia. Source: Lele, 2012.

Guiding Principles for Projects of Hematology and Hemotherapy Units

Marcio Nascimiento de Oliveira

Associação Brasileira para o Desenvolvimento do Edifício Hospitalar (ABDEH), Brazil

In the past decade, the Brazilian Ministry of Health has been developing a series of publications and tools aimed at improving the processes of organization and overall quality of the infrastructure of the public healthcare network (SUS). Introduced in 2006, the SOMASUS - System of Support for Elaboration of Projects of Investment in the Healthcare Infrastructure - has quickly become the main source of information for technicians and projects managers who work in the field. Using a simple web-based interface, the system has made it easy for anyone to check the spatial requirements and configurations of more than 500 settings, providing crucial information such as workflow charts, layouts and lists of equipment and furniture, along with their basic description and specification. The Ministry has since been extending this database, in order to include services that were not covered initially, such as those related to the processing and distribution of blood and blood products. Conducted via a joint research with the Federal University of Rio de Janeiro, the results of this new expansion were published earlier this year, in the form of a Guide, which brings important information about the Blood Network's infrastructure, organized according to the level of complexity of the service, and including the characteristics of each physical setting, such as: commonly used equipment, human resources and waste generation. The Guide is an indispensable tool for those working on the adaptation of existing buildings or in new projects.

Marcio Nascimiento de Oliveira. *Architect (University of Brasilia - 1991), holds a Master's Degree (MgGill University, Montreal - 1997). Director of the Architectural Department at the Catholic University of Brasilia where he also coordinates of a graduate course on Healthcare Architecture. President of the ABDEH – Brazilian Association for the Development of the Hospital Build-ing. Currently works as a consultant for the General Coordination of Blood and Blood Products of the Brazilian Health Ministry.*

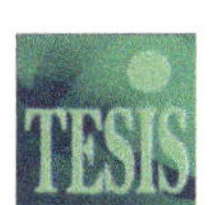

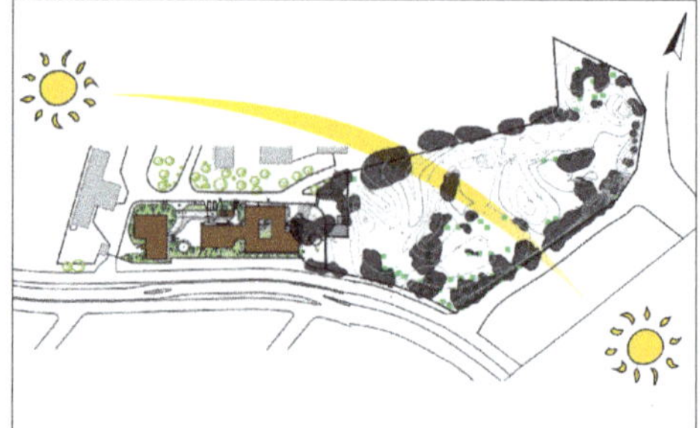

Figure 1. Hemocentro Coordenador - RS, orientation of the site and the apparent sun path.

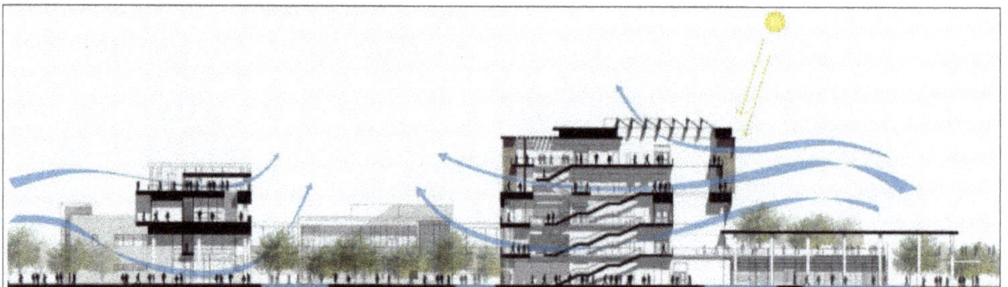

Figure 2. Sections.

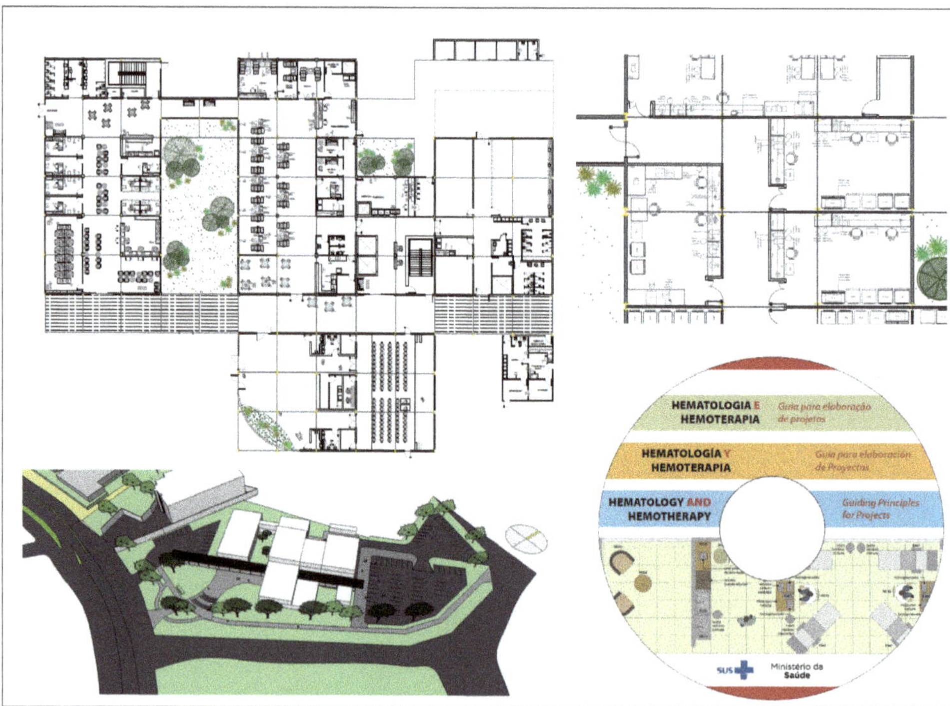

Figure 3. Hemocentro Coordenador - RS. Guiding Principles for Projects.

The Health Scenario in the State of São Paulo and Presentation of Pitangueiras Hospital in Jundiaí – SP

Ana Paula Naffah Perez Letaif

Associação Brasileira para o Desenvolvimento do Edifício Hospitalar (ABDEH), Brazil

The region of São Paulo in Brazil has actually approximately 44 million of inhabitants, almost 22% of the Brazilian population, being the most populous state of Brazil. Besides it, is today the unity of the federation with higher socio-economic development, accounting for 34% of the National GDP. São Paulo now has a total of approximately 900 hospital units and of this total, approximately 600 units are linked to health public system and 300 units are individually owned units, not directly serving users of the public assistance. These units add up to a total of 110.000 beds, and thus the region of São Paulo has a ratio of 2.5 beds per 1.000 population. In he Hospitals in which we work, the case of Pitangueiras Hospital, located in Jundiaí city, near São Paulo city, is an relevant case. Firstly because the Jundiaí city is the 7th largest in the region of São Paulo and because there are a very deficient health assistance services. The Hospital, which was designed and built in the 60s years, was built entirely of reinforced concrete, even their inside walls, what has always been a concept much criticized by unit managers, since all Hospital building suffers several changes during its use. With this, the directors of operator and the Health Plan opted for execute an extension for insertion of the most critical and required immediate expansion areas. By this way, in the expansion tower were placed, in addition to expanding the area of emergency care, inpatient floors of apartments with one bed, as well as the Intensive Care Unit and the expansion of the surgery center, with the migra-tion of high complexity rooms for this new block. Other major challenge was the unification of the facades of the unit, old block and new block, which was essential to modernizing the brand and beginning a new aesthetic standard for the Hospital and for the itself Health Plan which is owner of the unit. This project was completed in 2011 and all the building was completed in 2013.

Ana Paula Naffah Perez Letaif. *Architect graduated from the Faculty of Architecture and Urbanism at the Mackenzie University in 1993. Architect in the Leitner Arquitetura e Consultoria from 1993 to 1995. Project Manager Consulting and Architecture Bross Arquitetura e Consultoria from 1995 to 2005. Founder and Director of The C+A Arquitetura e Interiores, with participation of creating projects for residential, com-mercial, health and interior from 1998. Speaker Adh'2012 – Congresso Nacional de Arquitetura e Engenharia Hospitalar. Speaker of Medical Management Brazil in November 2013. Regional Director of the Sao Paulo ABDEH- Brazilian Association for Development of the Hospital building in 2011 until 2013. Executive President of the fifth ABDEH National Congress held in September 2012 in São Paulo. Vice President of Financial Management ABDEH in 2014-2017.*

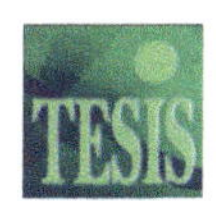

Some Features About São Paulo

São Paulo is the most populous unit of the federation. São Paulo is responsabile for generation 34% of GDP national. 5565 county of brazilian, 645 are in São Paulo, ie 11% of the county are in our state. São Paulo is a great reference in the national health sector.

The Health Care System in the Estate of São Paulo

In 2010, the state of São Paulo had 900 hospitals and more than 110 000 beds; this beds ares distributed in public hospitals ans related health care system and privated general and specialized hospitals; the state of São Paulo, 43% of the population is served by SUS system, contrasting with national media that is 26% of the population; the media of beds in the state of São Paulo is 2.50 beds per 1,000 inhabitants.

Examples of Primary Care

AME – Ambulatório Médico de Especialidades (Specialized Medical Ambulatory: 55 UNITS – 2014; 3,200 of medical specialists; 50 types of exams.

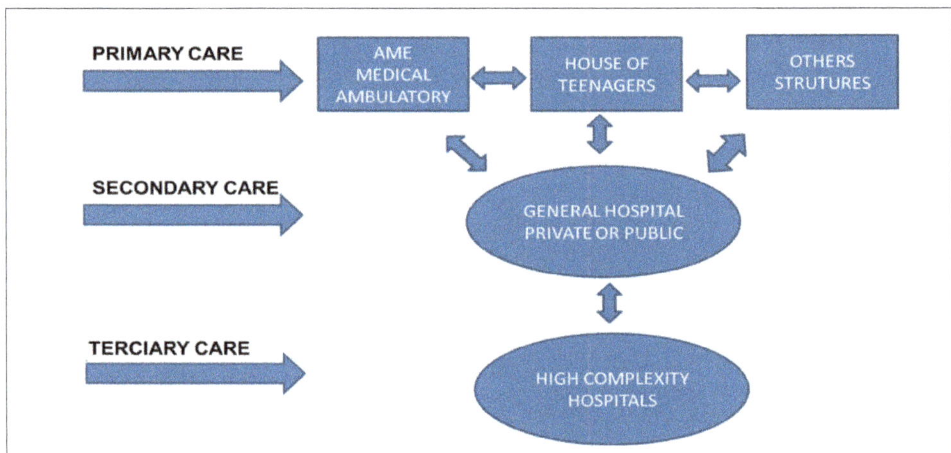

Figure 1. Struture of the healthcare system.

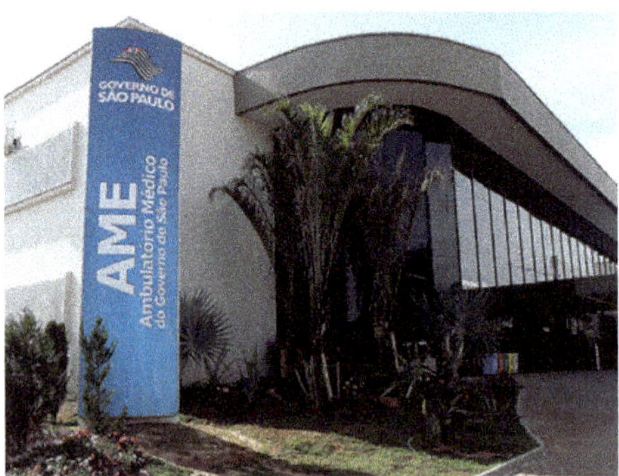

Figure 2. Amparo – SP.

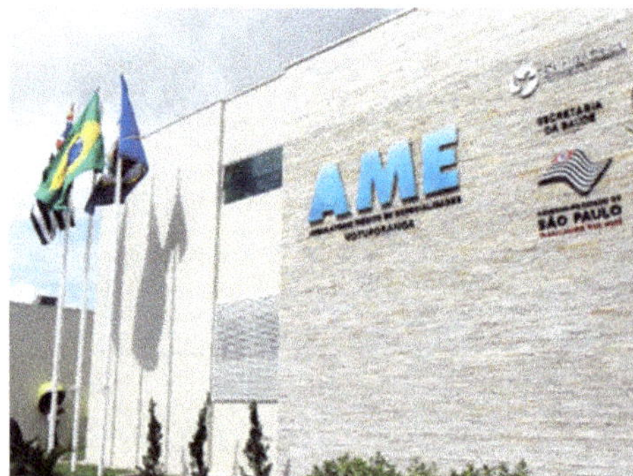

Figure 3. Votuporanga – SP.

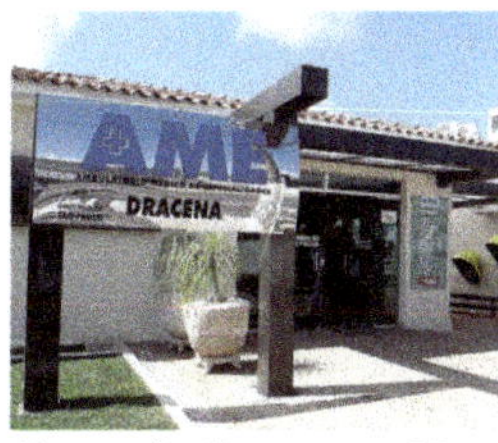

Figure 4. Dracena – SP.

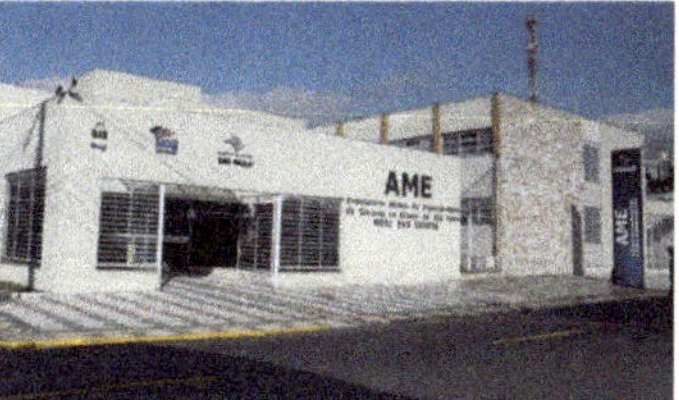

Figure 5. Mogi Das Cruzes – SP.

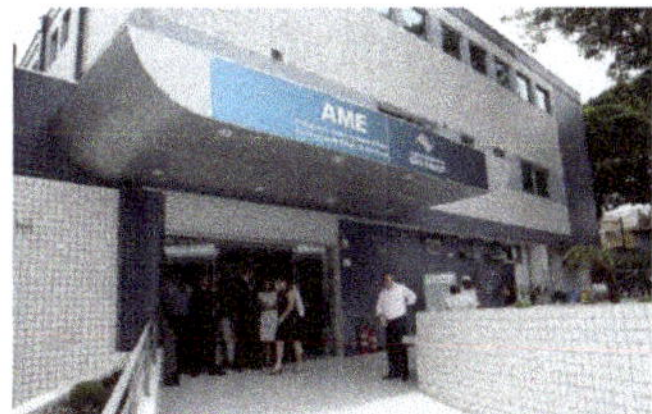

Figure 6. Sorocaba – SP.

THE ADOLESCENT'S HOUSE

Units provide medical, social and psychological free to youth through a team composed by professionals from different areas such as doctors, dentists, audiologist, social workers, nurses, teachers and psychologists.

Program "Adolescent Health", 20 years. 25 units distributed in the state of São Paulo. the houses of teenage also provide space for activities of interaction among youth, families and residents of the community, and further promote lectures on sexuality; language courses offer and culinary, dance classes and cultural workshops.

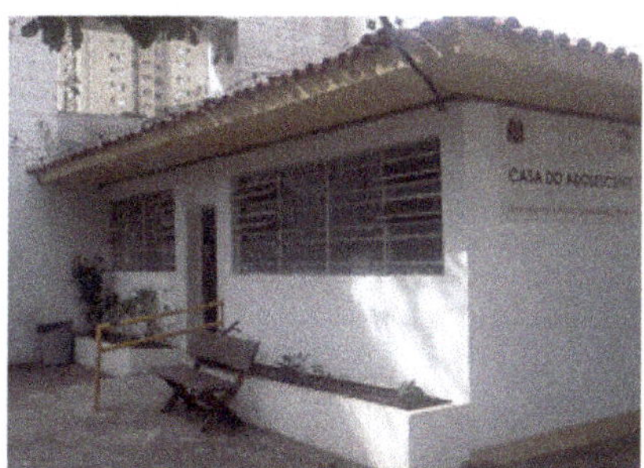

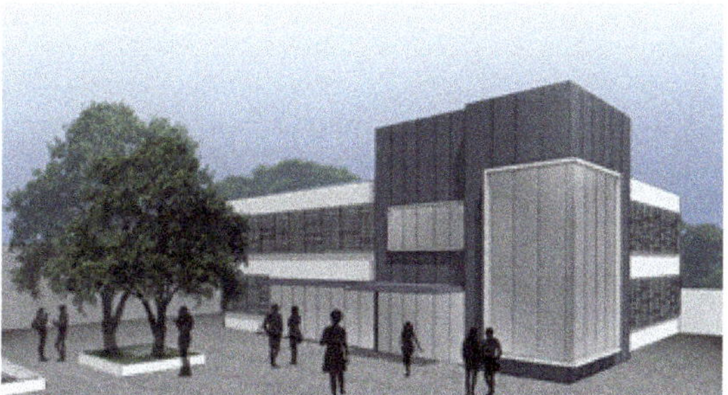

Figure 7. Pinheiros Unit São Paulo (left) and perspective of New Pinheiros Unit São Paulo (right), SP.

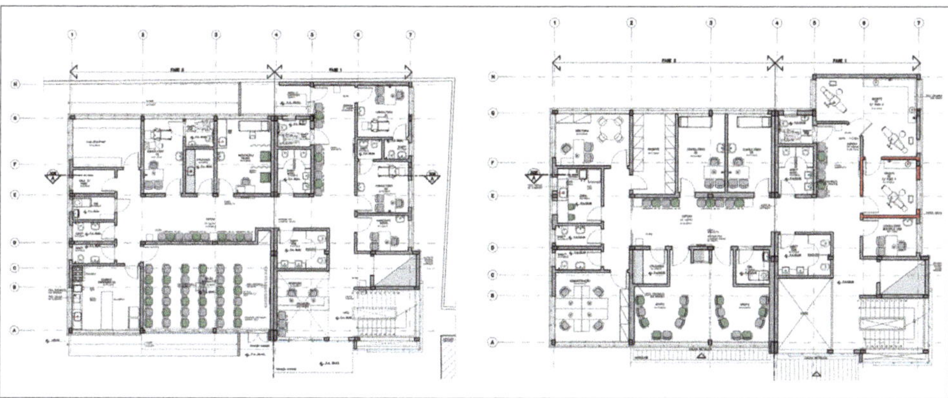

Figure 8. Main floor and second floor.

Program for Women Breast

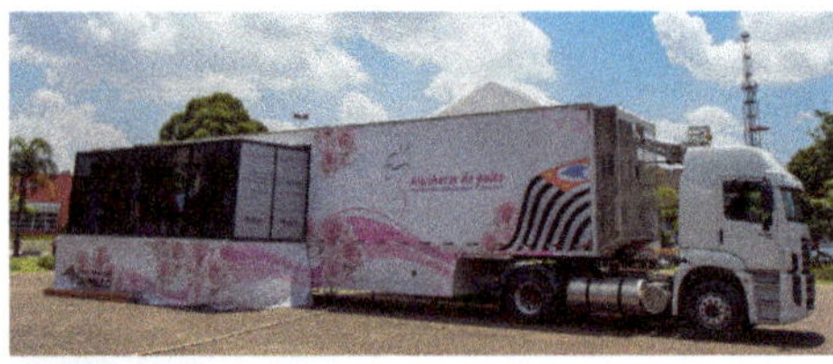

Goal - 5 trucks for outpatient care mastology and implementation of mammography interior of the state of Sao Paulo. 4 trucks in operation until now. Attendance - 60 mil mamoograms / year. Multidisciplinary team consist of technical radiology, auxiliary of nursing administrative officials and a sonograp.

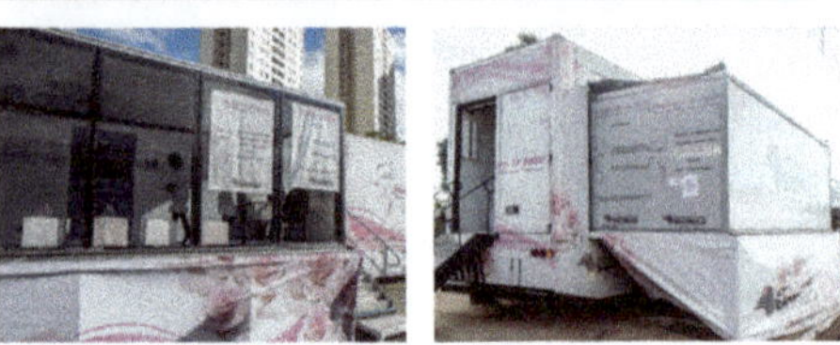

Figure 9. Program for women breast.

Examples of Private Secondary Care

Pitangueiras Hospital Sobam Group – Jundiaí

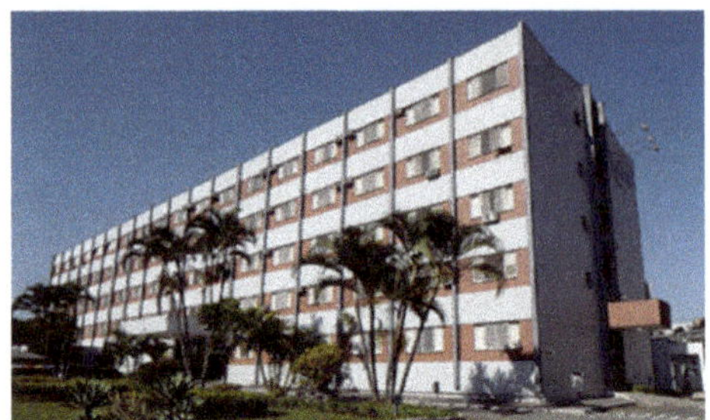

Designed in hospital 70s initial composition with 70 beds; locks of all existing building, foreign and home are concrete which hinders extension and modification of sectors. In 2011, after the execution of a master plan, we made plans to expand with a new block containing the expansion of sectors hospitalization of more complex sectors to this new block.

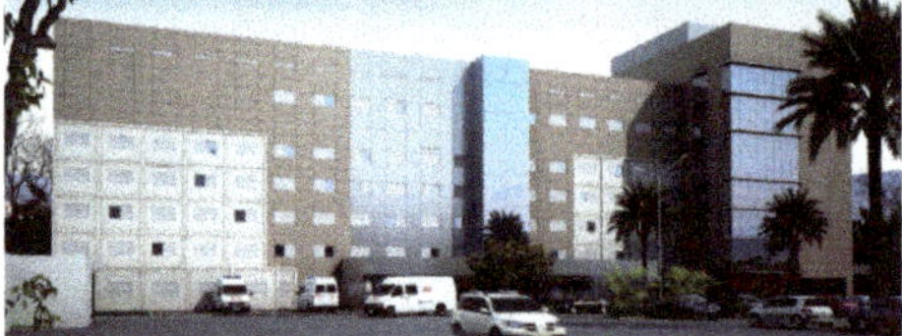

Figure 10. Pitangueiras Hospital Sobam Group – Jundiaí.

Examples of Public Terciary Care

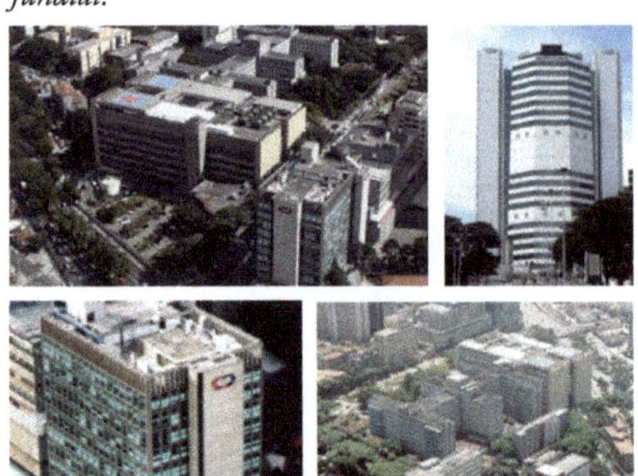

Figure 11. Clinicas hospital.

Reference in the treatment of diseases of high complexity. Biggest complex in Latin America - 378,000 sq ft built area (2012). 2.200 beds – distributed in 7 institutes. outpatient apointments more than 1.500.000/for year. Compound with some of hospitals in most important of Brazil - Institute Of Cancer, Heart Institute and Child Institute. Hospital College of Medicine of USP - internationally recognized in reference in teaching excellence. Pharmacotechniques – unit where drugs are developed and innovations for treatment of various diseases.

Strategic Planning: User Immovable Asset Management Plan for the Western Cape Government Health Department

Milné van Leeuwen

Milne.VanLeeuwen@westerncape.gov.za
Western Cape Government Health, South African Federation of Hospital Engineering, South Africa

In fulfilling its mandate to provide comprehensive health care in the Western Cape, theDepartment of Health has developed a User Asset Management Plan (U-AMP) in relation tothe immovable assets that it uses or intends to use. The Medium Term ExpenditureFramework (MTEF), which provides a three year view of the budgetary requirements, as wellas a 10 year and beyond vision of infrastructure requirements are incorporated in this plan. The MTEF forms the basis of the annual budget allocation for infrastructure as contained inthe annual Division of Revenue Act (DORA). Funding allocation will only be made by theNational Department of Health if a satisfactory U-AMP has been submitted by the pre-determined date. Future infrastructure funding to the Department will be subject toperformance based expenditure with resultant increased emphasis on better planning. This paper will explore the methodology behind the latest version of the U-AMP and considersome of the outcomes such as the extent of the property portfolio, the condition andutilization thereof and prioritisation plans related thereto. An overview of the proposedmethod to determine the placement of future ambulance stations will also be discussed. Theconclusion will include anticipated improvements to future U-AMPs.

Milné van Leeuwen. *Qualifications: BSc Quantity Surveying from University of the FreeState, South Africa. Masters in Property Science from the University of the Free State,South AfricaPast Chairperson of the Western Cape Association of South African Quantity Surveyors for 3years from 2006 - 2008Member of the South African Council of Quantity Surveyors for 4 years from 2010 - 2013Director: Infrastructure Planning at the Western Cape Government: Health from 2010 tocurrent dateProject Manager at ABSA Bank Corporate Investment from 2008 - 2010Director: Works General Buildings at the Western Cape Government: Transport and PublicWorks from 1996 - 2008*

Introduction

The Government Immovable Asset Management Act, Act 19 of 2007 (GIAMA) primarily regulates the acquisition, management and disposal of immovable assets and relates to all infrastructure that are held.

The strategic plan as contained in the User Asset Management Plan (U- AMP) is used to develop the Medium Term Expenditure Framework (MTEF) budget

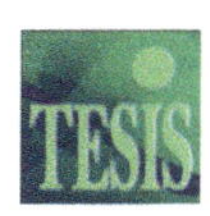

for a department. This MTEF budget provides a three year view of the budgetary requirements as well as a 10 year and beyond vision of infrastructure requirements. This forms the basis of the annual budget allocation for infrastructure as contained in the Division of Revenue Act (DORA) which is re-enacted annually. Future infrastructure funding to the Provincial Health Departments will be subject to performance based expenditure with resultant increased emphasis on better planning.

U-AMP in Practice

Informants to the U-AMP

The ultimate objective of the U-AMP of the Western Cape Government: Health (WCGH) is to ensure the optimal infrastructure delivery of provincial health facilities in the Western Cape, in support of the Provincial Government and aligned to the Department's strategic vision for health services delivery. Accordingly, linkages of National, Provincial and Departmental strategic documents are very important.

National Government

The National Infrastructure Plan outlines infrastructure projects that are of national strategic importance. National Department of Health: Negotiated Service Delivery Agreement (NSDA) outcome is: "Improve healthcare and life expectancy among all South Africans".

WCG

Provincial Strategic Plan – Delivering the open opportunity society for all Infrastructure Framework 2040.

WCGH

Western Cape Government Healthcare 2030 (Road to wellness) was developed against the background of a changing external environment.

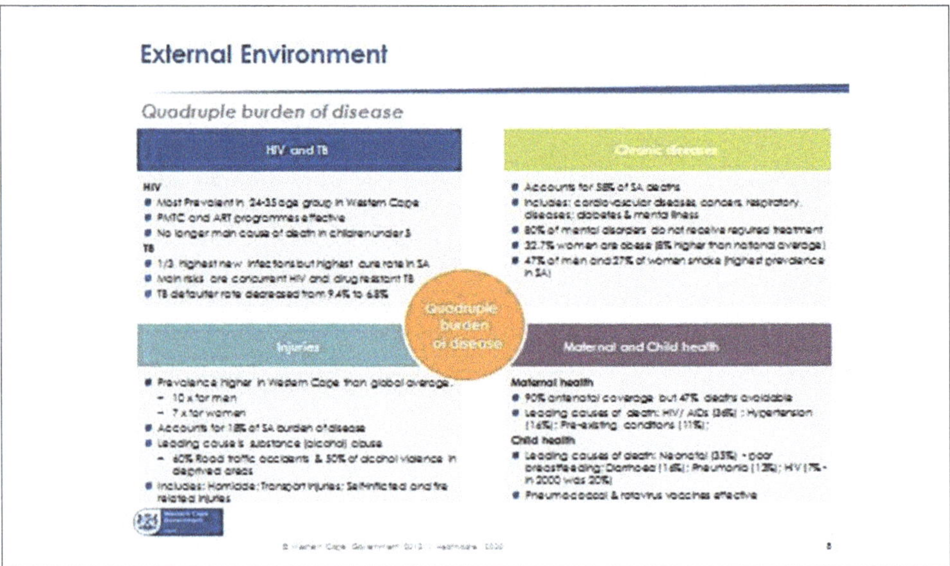

Figure 1. Factors influencing the Healthcare service delivery.

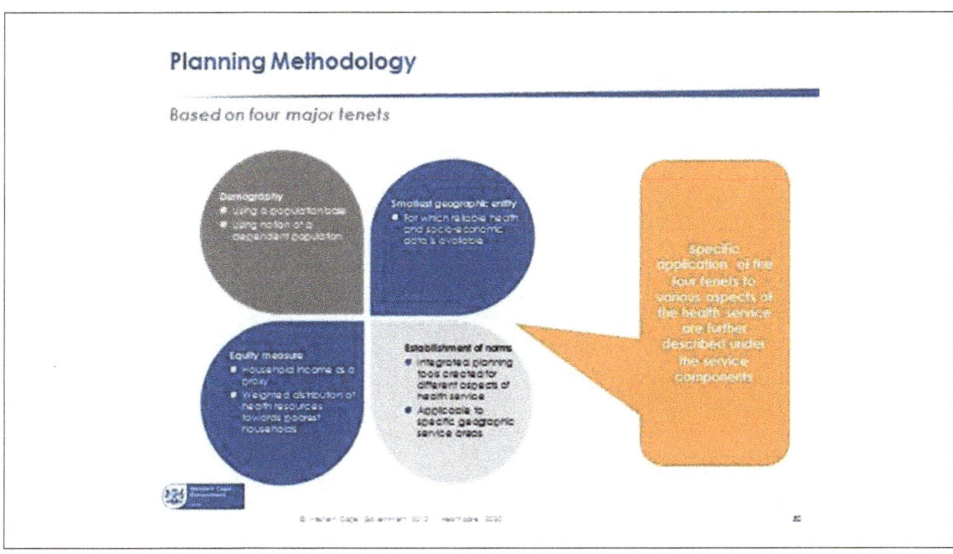

Figure 2. Planning methodology tenets.

The planning methodology behind the service delivery platform of 2030 has four major tenets:

i. Using a population base and dependent population;
ii. Using the smallest geographic entity for which reliable health and socio-economic data is available;
iii. Using an equity measure with household income as a proxy that weights the distribution of health resources towards the poorest households; and
iv. Establishing norms and creating planning tools for different aspects of the health service that allows for its application to specific geographic areas.

Demographics

Demographic information further acts as informants to the planning processes with South Africa census 2011 being the main source.

The process of town planning consists of two primary components namely land use management and spatial planning.

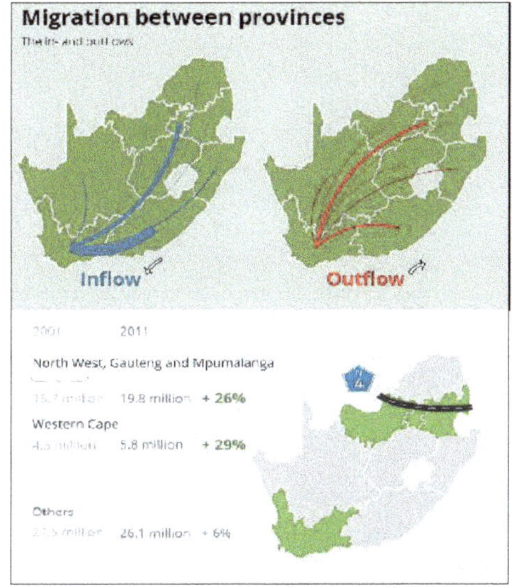

Figure 3. Population growth of 29% from 2001 to 2011 in the Western Cape with in migration being one of the main reasons.

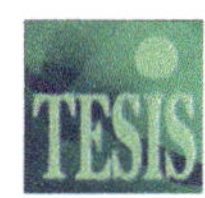

Finding the correct site for health facilities is a major contributor towards ensuring that appropriate urban forms are promoted to optimise the accessibility of facilities.

Immediate housing developments will impact on number of persons visiting current facilities and may result in over utilisation of current facilities or may indicate future demand. Figure 4 shows where housing developments have been approved for implementation.

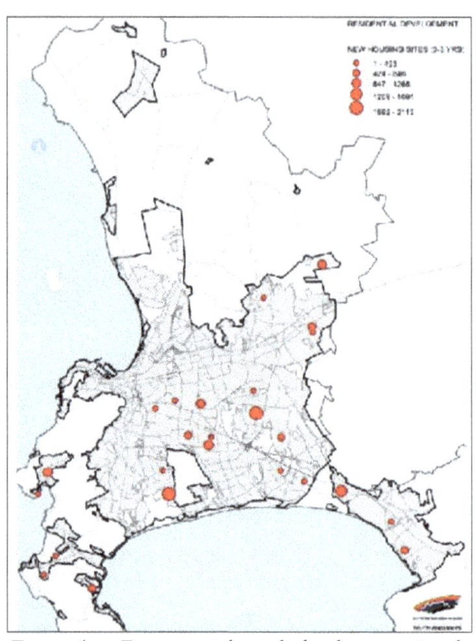

Figure 4. Future residential development in the City of Cape Town.

What health care facilities do we have?

Details of each facility has been gathered which include physical address, facility type, geographical details, size, details, GPS co-ordinates etc.

Health Facility Type	Total No.	No. WCG-owned / about to be transferred to WCG	No. leased facilities[1]
Tertiary Hospitals	3	3	
Primary Health	263	175	88
District Hospitals	34	34	
Psychiatric Hospitals	4	4	
Provincial Hospitals	5	5	
Rehabilitation Hospitals	1	1	
Emergency Medical Services	59	46	13
Forensic Pathology Laboratories	17	9	8
Regional Laundry and on-premises laundries	7	7	
Specialised Hospital	1	1	
TB Hospitals	6	6	
Nursing Colleges (Training facilities)	12	5	7
Workshops & other	4	4	
Nurses residential accommodation	12	11	1
Totals	454	334	120

Table 1. Accommodation currently occupied by WCGH.

[1] Inclusive of City of Cape Town facilities where WCG has a presence but excluding facilities only owned and operated by City.

How are we using it and how do we analyse the usage?

Based on information received from Western Cape Government: Transport and Public Works (WCTPW) and information gathered from the specific districts, each facility is analysed annually in terms of the condition with C5 being excellent and C1 being very poor, accessibility with A5 being optimum location and accessible and A1 where the location does not support the service delivery and usage. Facilities which experience a high level of pressure in providing services due to insufficient space are identified as well as any underutilisation. Service information provides the number of visits to the health care facilities and the overnight patient numbers. Performance ratings of P1 to P5 are allocated with P5 being highly sensitive facilities such as a hospital and P2 facilities which are providing essential support only for example a satellite clinic.

Condition

The overall overview of the condition assessment as attributed is summarized in the table below:

The average condition of all health infrastructure is rated "fair". The condition of all buildings is being improved by means of day-to-day and preventative maintenance, minor refurbishment, major upgrade and replacement with newly built facilities. All state-owned health facilities rated C1 are in the process of being replaced or are earmarked for upgrading.

Suitability Ratings

In order to arrive at a suitability rating the required performance standard and the accessibility rating is used to determine the suitability rating index with A being suitable, B meets the minimum suitability criteria for its function and C does not meet the required suitability criteria.

Operating Performance Index

The operating performance index is derived from the condition rating and the required performance standard with 1 exceeding its functional and operational requirements, 2 meets the functional and operational requirements and 3 does not meet the expected functional and operational requirements.

Condition Status	State-owned Health Facilities	Leased Health Facilities
C5	8%	
C4	29%	17%
C3	56%	67%
C2	7%	17%
C1	1%	

Table 2. Overall overview of condition assessment of state-owned facilities.

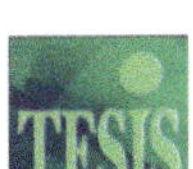

Required Performance Standard	Condition Rating				
	C1 (Very Poor)	C2 (Poor)	C3 (Fair)	C4 (Good)	C5 (Excellent)
P5	3	3	3	2	1
P4	3	3	2	1	1
P3	3	3	2	1	1
P2	3	2	1	1	1
P1	2	2	1	1	1

Table 3. Operating Performance Index.

3% of WCG-owned health facilities do not meet the expected operational requirements whilst 82% are rated "good" with 15% meeting expectation.

Functional Performance Index

The functional performance index leads us into the decision framework.

Suitability Index	Operating Performance Index		
	1 (Optimal)	2 (Minimum)	3 (Outside)
Optimal – A	A1	A2	A3
Minimum – B	B1	B2	B3
Outside – C	C1	C2	C3

Table 4. Functional Performance Index.

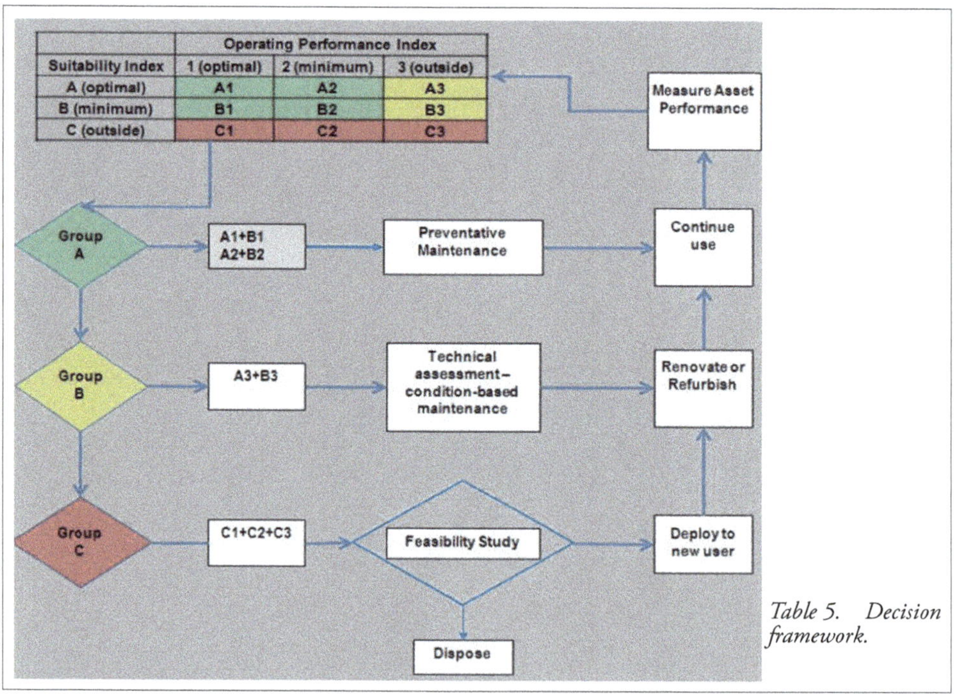

Table 5. Decision framework.

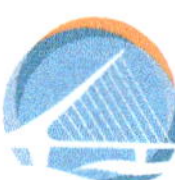

Analysis and implementation plan

Most of the facilities resorted in group A and B which indicated either continued maintenance or renovation of the facilities.

Where a facility resorted under group C further detailed investigations were required to determine the future of the facility. In addition individual assessments were made to cross-check the results. In the event that the result is to replace/extend further investigations must follow to strengthen the decision.

Utilisation Improvement Action to be taken	Provincial owned health facilities	Leased Health facilities
Extend	21%	7%
Maintain	61%	55%
Refurbish	0.3%	
Relinquish	0.1%	5%
Replace	7%	25%
Replace in future	6%	8%
Replace/Extend	0.1%	

Table 6. Utilisation Improvement Actions – Assessment Findings.

Financial Year	Estimated Value of New Buildings, Replacements, Renovations and Upgrading / Additions Required	Escalated Value of New Buildings & Replacements@ 10% p.a.	Actual Infrastructure Budget (Excluding Maintenance and Rehab)	Cumulative budget	Estimated Total Backlog (Backlog minus budget allocated per year)
2014/2015	15,000 000 000	15,000 000 000	222 220 000	222 220 000	14,777 780 000
2015/2016	14,777 780 000	16,255 558 000	272 750 000	494 970 000	15,982 808 000
2016/2017	15,982 808 000	17,581 088 800	416 382 000	911 352 000	17,164 706 800

Table 7. Infrastructure backlog.

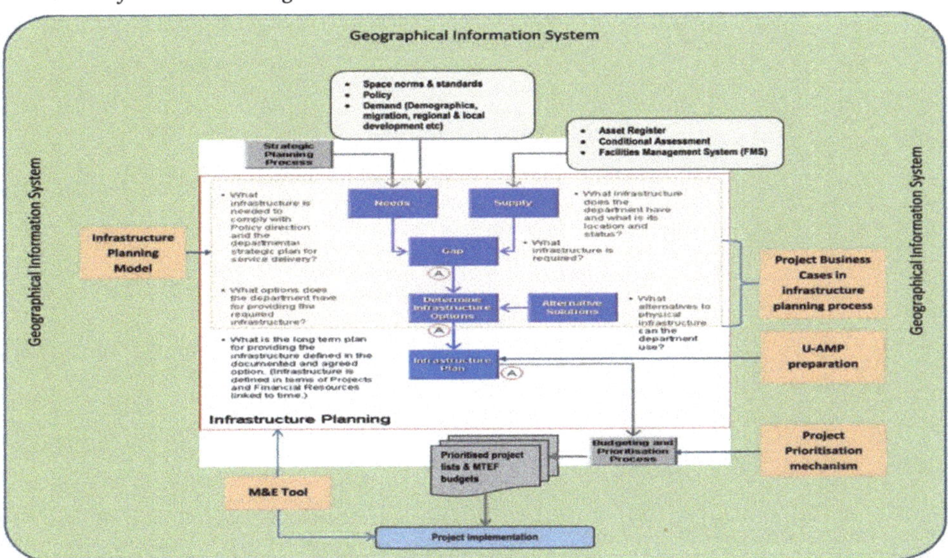

Figure 5. Overview of the Health Planning process.

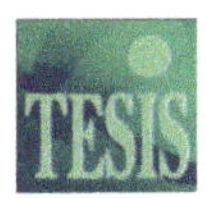

ANALYSIS OF THE PLACEMENT OF AMBULANCE STATIONS WITHIN THE WESTERN CAPE

Introduction

The placement of ambulance stations is crucial in terms of responding within the shortest possible time of being called out. Certain goals have been set for response times by the Emergency Management Services in the 2030 Healthcare document which have been used as norms in the Geographic Access analysis. The location of the existing facilities were plotted and the area that the ambulances are logically able to cover in eight minutes in urban areas (5 km) for Priority 1 call outs and fourty minutes in rural areas (40 km) was then plotted against the dependant population density background. The road network which was used provided a travel distance surface which is adjusted for topography and existing movement infrastructure thus providing a more accurate analysis layer than a simple straight line distance based analysis. The dependant population density was compiled with the South Africa Census 2011 information and utilising the concept of dependant population and highest density areas. The areas not covered and where the dependant population density is very high will thus determine the gap in the provision of services.

Results

Figures 6 and 7 respectively indicate the results for the Western Cape and for the City of Cape Town in particular. In interpreting the results of this analysis, it can be deducted that future ambulance stations will be required in the Strand area, Kraaifontein, R300, Heideveld and possibly midway between town centre and Atlantis on the N7. This analysis will be further refined in 2014. Analysis of the rural areas does not highlight any major gaps in terms of population density. Further work will indicate how we can specifically determine the best location for an ambulance station. This will facilitate finding the best potential sites and using the centroids of the surrounding towns and examining the distances and time travelled.

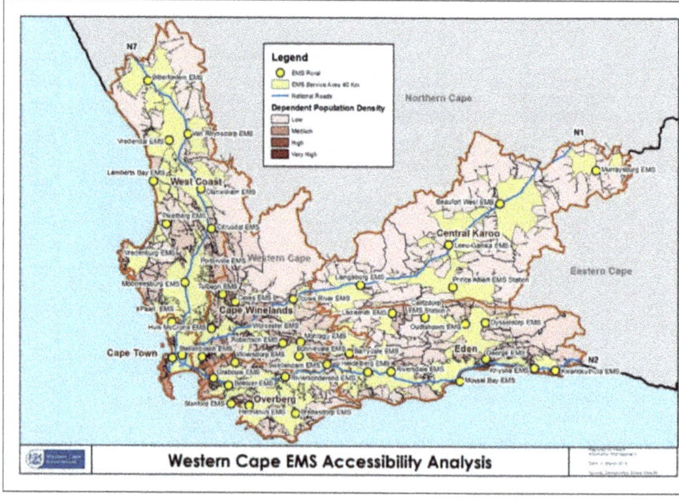

Figure 6. Analysis of 40km coverage of existing ambulance stations against the dependant population density for the Western Cape.

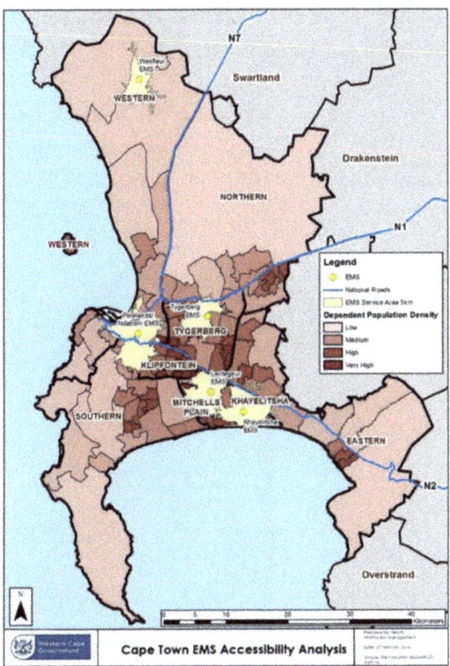

Figure 7. Analysis of 5km coverage of existing ambulance stations against the dependant population density for the City of Cape Town.

Conclusion of analysis

This approach enables backlogs to be geographically presented and communicated in order to prioritise the funding allocation for new ambulance stations where it will have the highest impact on the community.

FUTURE IMPROVEMENTS TO THE U-AMP DOCUMENT

Financial and human resources are limited and it is important to ensure that optimum utilization thereof is achieved. Infrastructure can be the tool to assist with the management of the service. It is thus very important that facilities are demographically and equitable dispersed throughout the Province in order to provide the optimum service. Historical placement of facilities by local government and some lack of integrated planning resulted that smaller than feasible facilities were being built in some instances. The analysis of the town of George below geographically indicates an overlap of facilities provided in terms of the service norms which is five kilometre radius.

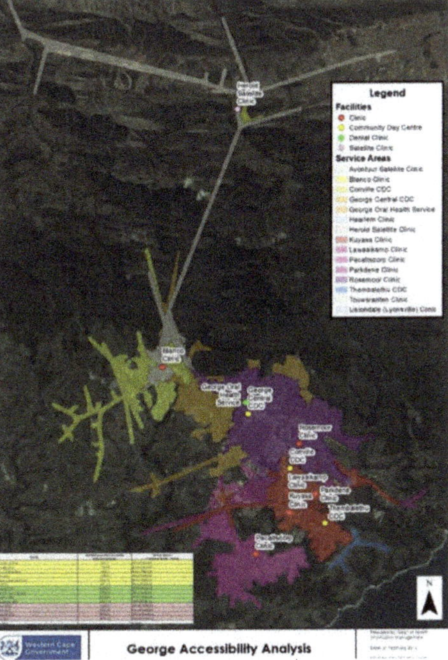

Figure 8. George accessibility analysis.

It is hoped that by such and similar analyses will lead to:

- Evidence-based decision support and support for planning;
- More accurate data will lead to information, then to Knowledge and from Action to Outcomes;

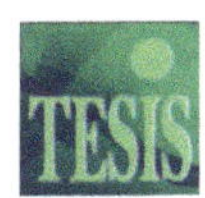

- Enhanced decision-making with better development results, monitoring and feedback and technical rigour.

The ultimate objective of the WCGH U-AMP is to ensure optimal delivery of provincial health infrastructure facilities in the Western Cape and to ensure that the greatest needs in the

Province are addressed as the highest priorities, whilst ensuring that optimum cost efficiency and affordability is achieved.

Shaping the Future: Re-Thinking Ancient Hospitals, a Current Challenge

Pier Francesco Cherchi

pfcherchi@unica.it
Architecture Assistant Professor, Cagliari, Italy

The issue of our proposal is about rethinking ancient hospitals and shaping the future through imagination and architectural design. It is a methodological research and a technical proposal on the restoration and rehabilitation to current hospital needs of ancient healthcare facilities. The research moves over starting from several questions. Is it possible to reconcile the requirements of the protection of historic buildings, with the technical and functional characteristics of a modern hospital? Is it feasible to upgrade ancient hospitals to modern standards of fire safety, insulation and accessibility by very careful work on the fabric, using all means to address deficiencies without damaging older materials, spaces or finishes? What future is possible to imagine for old hospitals, that for their function assume an important position in the memory of a community? The research addresses the complexity of the issue by analyzing related cases, already subjects of projects and realizations, and proposes answers to these questions by investigating a case study example, the hospital of San Giovanni di Dio in Cagliari (Italy).
The San Giovanni di Dio hospital, is an extraordinary nineteenth-century building, located in the oldest part of the city, designed by a master of neoclassical architecture, the architect Gaetano Cima. In 1842 Gaetano Cima imagined an innovative building designed as a place for wellness and health care of its citizens. He conceived it as a real urban device, able to relate to the city and determine subsequent developments. The hospital, which is gradually being disposed of, it was for more than 100 years the most important in Sardinia. The study is not intended to be exhaustive, nor is intended to define solutions universally applicable. Our intent is to foster a common sensibility towards practices of reuse of existing facilities and to promote debate about would should be the future of ancient hospitals, that in many cases have remarkable architectonic, cultural and historic qualities.

Pier Francesco Cherchi*, architect and engineer, is an assistant professor at University of Cagliari (Italy). Since 2004, he has been fostering teaching activity as a lecturer in the courses of Architecture Design. He develops academic research investigating the relationship between architectural design and construction of the city, paying particular attention to the issues of urban space reuse and recycling of existing buildings, as best practice of architectural sustainability. He is co-founder of C+C04STUDIO architecture office (www.cc04.net). As a professional, since 2000, has been developing several projects at different scales, working also on the design and construction of hospitals in Italy.*

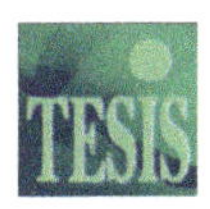

State of the Issue to B e Discussed

The issue of our proposal is about rethinking ancient hospitals and shaping the future through imagination and architectural design.

It is a study that is being conducted on both theoretical and technical fields, and that relates to the theme of restoration and rehabilitation to current requirements of ancient hospitals, now abandoned or partially used. The survey addresses the complexity of the issue starting from some questions. Is it possible to reconcile the demands of conservation and preservation of a historic building with the technical, functional and regulatory needs, typical of a modern health care facility? What future do we imagine for the ancient hospitals that have historically played an important role in the civic structure of a community and that for this reason contribute in forming the memory and identity of a society? The research addresses the complexity of the issue by analyzing related cases, already subjects of projects and realizations, and proposes answers to these questions by investigating a case study example, the hospital of San Giovanni di Dio in Cagliari (Italy).

Brief Background

The San Giovanni di Dio hospital, is an extraordinary nineteenth-century building, located in the oldest part of the city, designed by a master of neoclassical architecture, the architect Gaetano Cima. In 1842 Gaetano Cima imagined an innovative building designed as a place for health care of its citizens. He conceived it as a real urban device, able to relate to the city and determine subsequent developments. The hospital, which is gradually being disposed of, it was for more than 100 years the most important hospital in Sardinia. The solutions adopted by Cima were amazing if compared to what at that time was designed and built in Italy and in Europe.

It is a building that manages to combine the needs of wards division, with those arising from the need to rationalize the relationship between the parties, facilitating communication and orientation. Next to these aspects strictly related to the function, is the architect's ability to conceive an hospital not isolated from the city, not separated by a park or surrounded by a fence, but a piece of the city with urban characteristics closely. Top architect, in many ways revolutionary, Cima had envisioned an urban building, able to build a relationship with the city and its inhabitants. His intentions merged into a drawing that for simplicity we schematize as consisting of a stem aligned along the way, a real scenic backdrop and connection to the city, to which were attached a series of oblong bodies, harmoniously arranged in a simple radiocentric plan, the focus of which was made up of the chapel, visible from all wards, real generating center of the whole composition.

The destiny of Cagliari's ancient hospital is common to many others in Europe and in the world, made in the past with innovative type-morphological characteristics, outdated today. Between '60 and '80 of the past century, in Italy, as in the rest of Europe, many cities expansion were conceived planning the city referring to the "polycentric city", a model providing a core connected to peripheral nuclei. These were in some cases highly specialized structures, universities, research centers and hospitals. So in the '70s and in the years subsequent, Cagliari also equipped itself with new hospitals, located in the exterior of the city. The old hospital was dismantled and today there are few activities still housed inside. In this state of abandonment we must answer by imagining a new destination, a new life for the hospital and for the city.

The Approach

Cima's hospital is 19th century structure whose qualities are visually, architecturally, and historically remarkable. Of course the idea of a demolition is not only impracticable due to the legal protection applied on the building, but also it is not even imaginable a different destiny than restoration and reuse for such a building that contributes to raise the cultural identity of an entire community.

The approach must combine careful conservation with strong modern intervention into the fabric. Also, at the same time, it must challenge all the complexity of an intervention capable of a global rethinking of the building.

But the issue that must be addressed is that relating to the new role within the city. In the world there are several samples of best practices that through an "adaptive reuse" have introduced new features.

These interventions, which often provide for conversion into homes and shops, however, are a betrayal of the original function and the civic role that these ancient buildings had in the city. From these considerations, our research explores solutions that, combining the requirements of protection and conservation, are able to re-think a new civic role by inserting functions related to health and wellbeing and at the same time introducing new public functions.

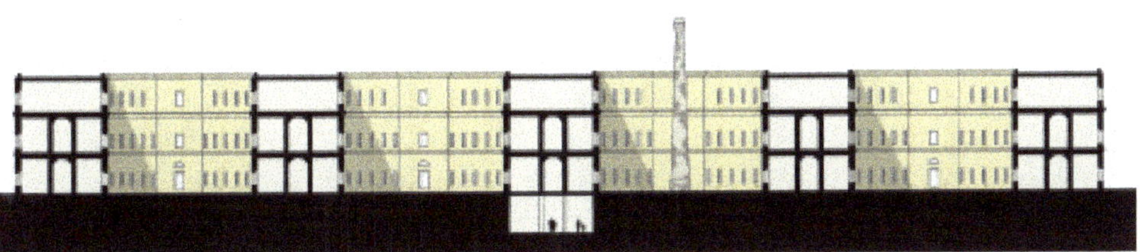

Figure 1. San Giovanni di Dio Hospital in Cagliari (Italy), section (current state).

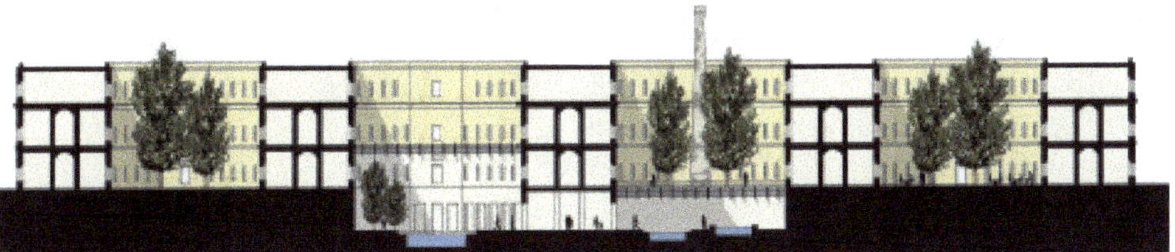

Figure 2. Section (modified state): rethinking courtyards and ground floor internal spaces as an extension of urban space.

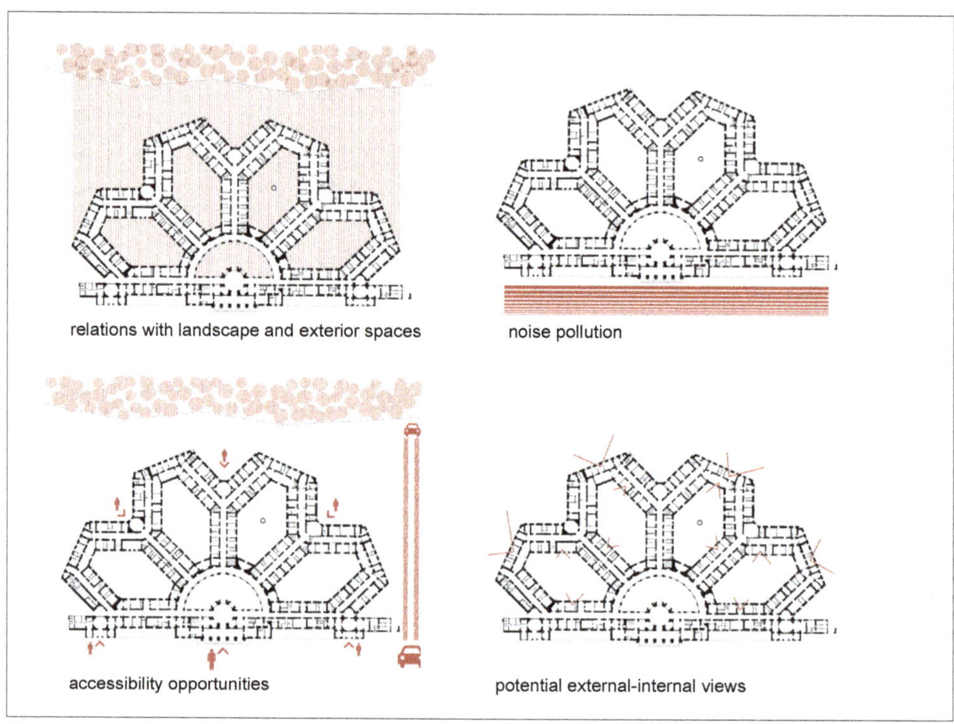

Figure 3. Analysis of the adaptive reuse potential.

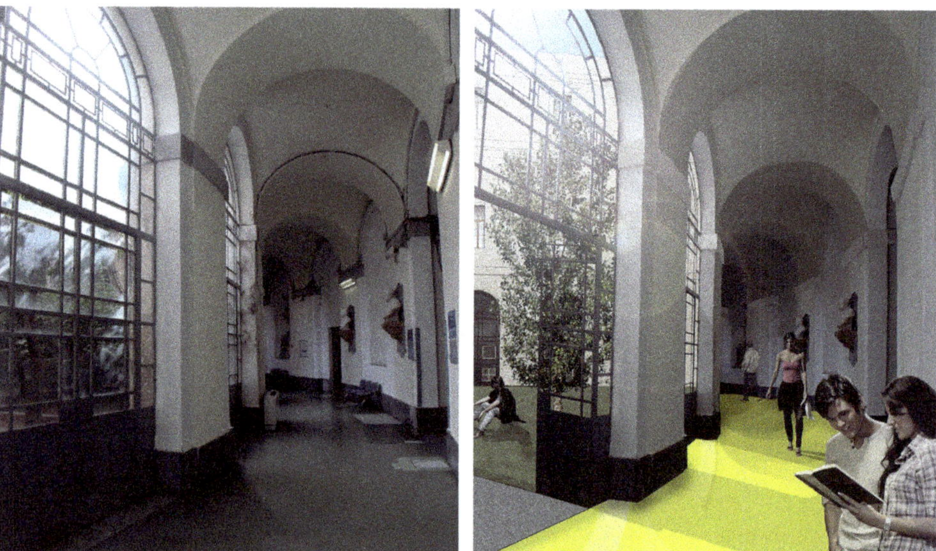

Figure 4. Starting from its original urban vocation (a place of healthcare for the entire city) design envisions to re-functionalize Cagliari's ancient hospital maintaining its soul, and at the same time introducing new features marked by character to create a civic landmark and a cultural and social meeting, not weakening its civic role and at the same time fostering dynamic relationships in citizens' lives.

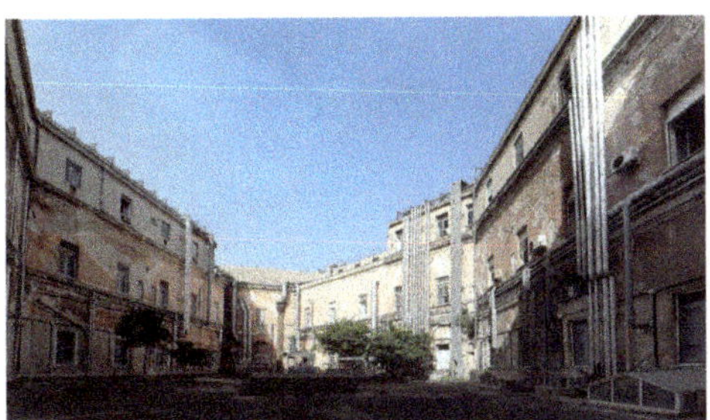
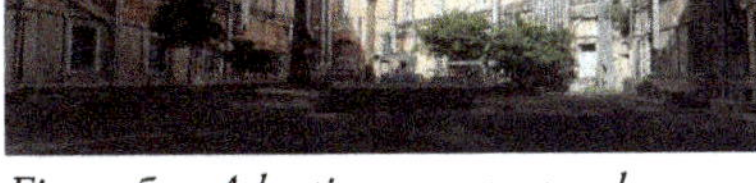
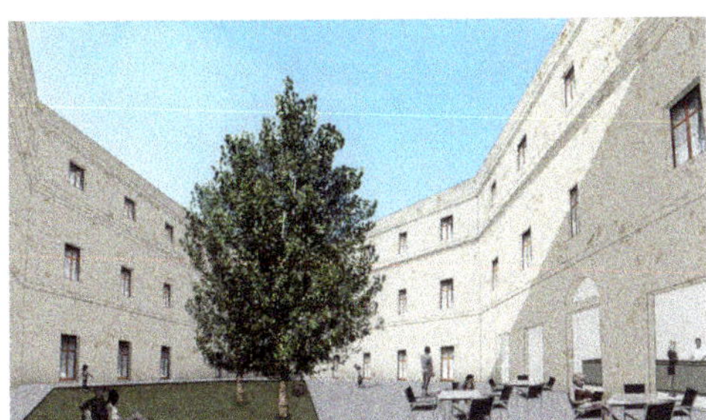

Figure 5. Adaptive reuse proposal.

The Idea

Starting from his original urban vocation, a place of healthcare for the entire city, we envisioned to re-functionalize Cagliari's ancient hospital maintaining his soul, and at the same time introducing new features marked by character to create a civic landmark and a cultural and social meeting, a gateway to the city, able to not weaken its civic character and at the same time to enable dynamic relationships in the lives of citizens.
One hypothesis of functional program could be divided into a central function, linked to healthcare and wellbeing, and in one or more satellite functions, marked with a civic character and able to connect the building with the City. The study could be split and divided as follows:
- central and main function: the redevelopment of a former hospital could be linked to the insertion of a central role for health and care related to well-being. Nowadays the Wellness and Wellbeing activities are very desirable activities, and are increasingly getting greater in people's lives. For this reason we decided to create a center for body and spirit care, containing different activities: training memorial, psychology and psychotherapy, hydrotherapy, foot massages, reflexology, shiatsu, tai chi, yoga, zero balancing, rolfing and others. At the same time, the building due to its large size could accommodate outpatient facilities or other charitable activities dedicated to the older segments of the population.
By placing these tasks in the new complex, its health vocation would retain unchanged.
- satellite function: the main function could combine to one linked to culture, society and traditions (temporary exhibitions, cultural events, arts and crafts etc.). These functions would have the role of connecting all citizens with the building, which could accommodate exhibitions, conferences, events and literals related to culture and local traditions.

Implications/outcomes

The implications are also related to the opportunities that each design choice determines. Upstream of each rethinking and reshaping of architectural and environmental heritage of a community is necessary and important to formulate the questions about the consequences of each choice. Is it right that a community invests resources to keep alive old artifacts whose conformation is often difficult to reconcile with the demands of the current needs of hospital organization? We believe that if faced with a historical monument, part of the historical and cultural heritage of a community, the primary purpose is the conservation and protection; thus, facing a monument that is also a place of healthcare, the ultimate goal is full restitution to the city of a monument, still able to contribute in improving safety, welfare and health. This study is not intended to be exhaustive, nor is intended to define universally applicable solutions. Our intent is to foster a common sensibility towards practices of reuse of existing facilities and to promote debate about what should be the future of ancient hospitals, that in most cases have remarkable architectonic, cultural and historic qualities.

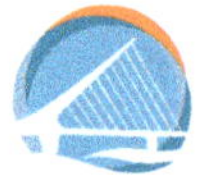

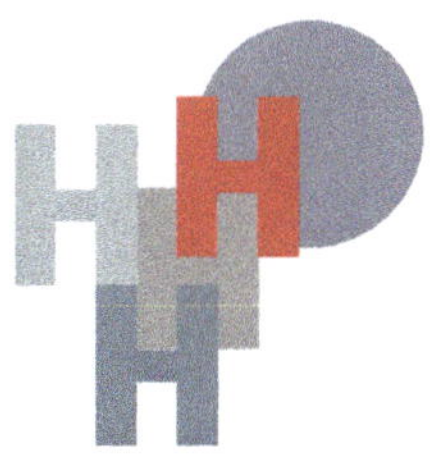

Masterplans, Projects and Works

Session Introduction

Designing a hospital ex novo or upgrading an existing hospital inevitably leads designers and planners to touch on issues of a dual nature: on the one hand all the design aspects related to the building, and on the other how the building integrates with the urban area and the infrastructure set up for the network of care facilities located throughout the region.

The need to concentrate care, research and education activities in one place means that healthcare facilities have become ever larger until they assume the form of an actual landmark. In the face of this phenomenon it is necessary to ask what is the right size in order for the hospital to be enjoyed by patients, relatives and staff, and for it to be considered human scale and remain, as far as possible, non-institutional and homely. At the same time, treatment in the design of a healing environment should be accompanied by the efficient programming of works and supported by the latest available technologies with high efficiency in terms of reducing hospitalization time. The need to optimize the flow of people and supplies forces reflection on the right balance to achieve in the relationship between the presence of vertical circulation and horizontal connections within the structure and the careful organization of pedestrian entrances and driveways.

It is imperative to plan the spatial relationships with the existing network of other healthcare facilities, and this means planning the infrastructure by linking the different focal points of the system.

The assessment of all these elements should also consider how to reduce the maintenance and operating costs of the facility, trying to find, in the preliminary stages of planning and programming, design solutions capable of ensuring economic benefits in the budgets over the long term.

Merging of Three Former Hospitals into a Single Entity, Oslo University Hospital

Per Christian Brynildsen

pcb@ratioark.no
Architect and partner, Ratio arkitekter AS

Oslo University Hospital is formed by the former National Hospital (Rikshospitalet), Ullevål sykehus, and Radiumhospitalet, Norway's most important cancer treatment hospital. The merging of three highly ambitious and prestigious hospitals into one entity has created unforeseen challenges in fields of organization, logistics, economics, procedures and patient politics. Although the hospitals are located very close, only a few kilometers apart, the organization seems to be unprepared and uncooperative facing obstacles which from an outside view seem small and petty. To meet the challenges of the future, this situation is sought solved through an hitherto unmatched ambitious project, the total remaking of a large part of Oslo outskirts into a large campus like area of research, treatment and education, in close proximity to Oslo University and various private and public research institutions.

Per Christian Brynildsen *born 1960 in Norway. Diploma from Oslo School of Architecture 1986. Partner I Ratio arkitekter AS(formerly Medplan arkitekter AS) since 2003. Selected works: Rikshospitalet, Oslo, Norway, 1992-1999. St. Olavs hospital, phase 1 and 2, Trondheim, Norway 2000-2006. Regional Hospital, Akershus, Norway, 2000, competition. Lasur Leprosy Hospital (with Jan Olav Jensen), Maharashtra, India 1983-1984. Stavanger Concert Hall, Stavanger, Norway, 1st prize international competition, 2003-2012. Awards: Aga Khan Award 1998, Leprosy Hospital, India; Norwegian Concrete Element Award 2012, Stavanger Concert Hall.*

Implications of this new medical facility far exceeds the program for treatment, research and education within the hospital itself, and works as a catalyst for a total renewal of the urban area. Issues to be addressed are:
traffic, the site adjoins the large ring road around Oslo metropolitan area, but will need better public transport than provided today;
urban, any development of this size will have ring effects on a wide area consisting of thousands of dwellings, workplaces, schools, kindergartens and other institutions;
commercial, the sheer size and number of employees in an institution of this size will have dire effects on the habits and opportunities of shops and service facilities in a wide proximity of the hospital;

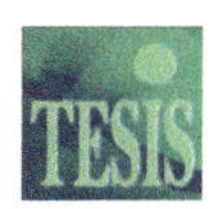

environmental, even in a relatively open and green environment like the Oslo suburbia, forces will attack any open space, any green unused plot, any continuous park like landscape, and the protection of these qualities must be guarded with zeal as well as understanding of the importance of keeping the milieu for future generations;
energy, as the buildings we make continue to be a large contributor to our carbon footprint, merely saving energy in the lifespan of the building is not enough, rather the construction and the demolition of the building must be taken into account as well;
economy, the benefit of merging and the possibilities of saving money by better coordination and allocation of resources must not be wasted on out-of-control mastodon like organizations with poor coherence and understanding of day-to-day work;
medical, the accumulation of knowhow and skill should be channeled into better treatment for the patient, and not spark internal rivalry or sub optimized flow of patients, goods and personnel in the institution;
architecturally, any building complex exceeding 500 thousand square meters will have a huge impact on the surroundings, and the building itself must support the philosophy of the Norwegian society, combined with state of the art treatment and spearhead research and development;
politically, namely from a, by and large, egalitarian society where very few are very rich or very poor, and where the public health system is the choice of treatment for almost everyone, and extremely high expectations of treatment of the highest standard possible.

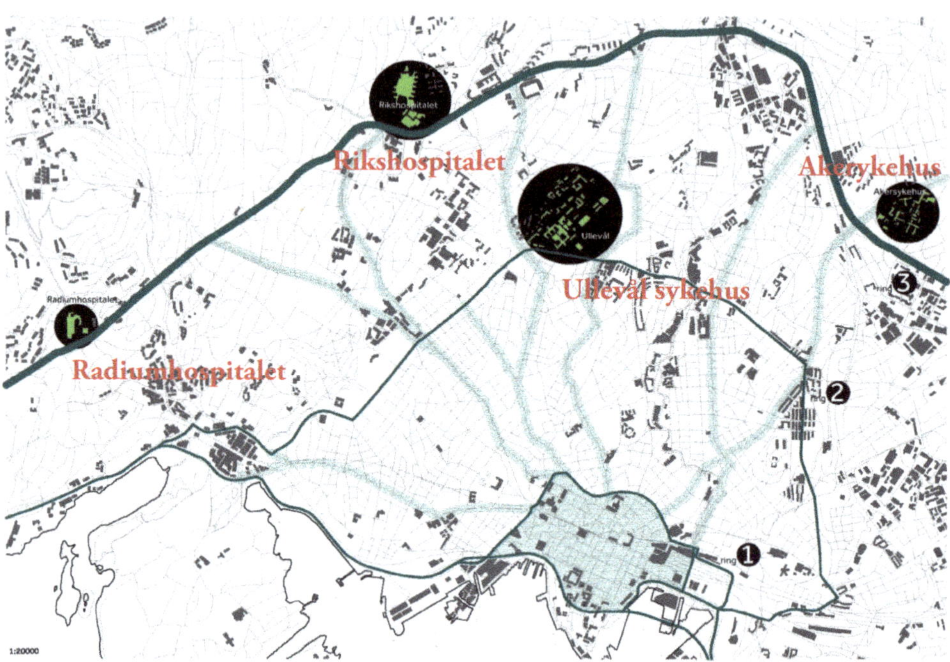

Figure 1. National Hospital (Rikshospitalet), Oslo's largest local hospital, Ullevål sykehus, and Radiumhospitalet.

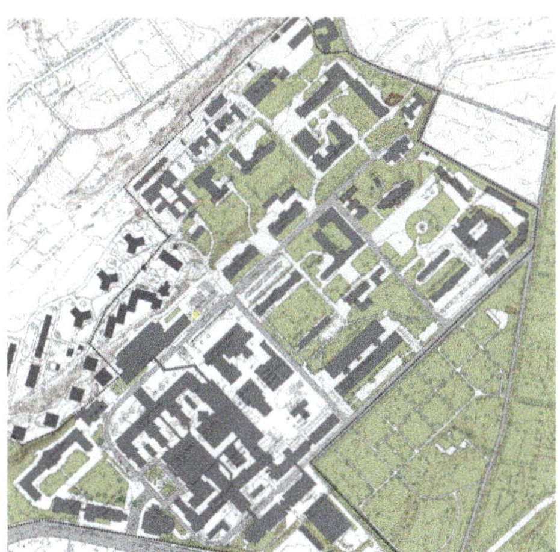

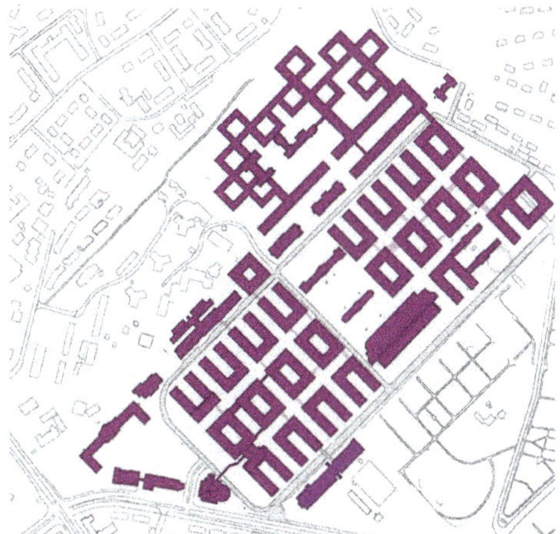

Figure 2. Ullevål, Oslo's largest local hospital, part of Oslo University Hospital (right) and full development at the Ullevål site (right).

For the thorough analysis of the challenges, the government has employed not only Ratio, but Nordic office of architecture and the Danish firm C.F. Møller to review and visualize the complex from a number of sides and with different approaches. All the firms have, through their experience and current portfolio, showed a very high standard of skill necessary to reach the goal, without spilling resources on blind alleys in the project. All this within a society which has benefited from an extremely lucky or beneficial economic situation as a petroleum lubricated rich economy, undented by the financial crisis of 2008 and a wage growth rate standing apart from every one of our neighbors in Europe. As a result giving both wealth and an extremely high cost of living, taking even the most unfortunate individuals in Norway up to new levels of prosperity as our egalitarian ideals pull even the poor to a middle class living standard, where poor children are defined by the lack of participation in recreational activities or the humiliation of not being able to bring gifts to birthday parties.

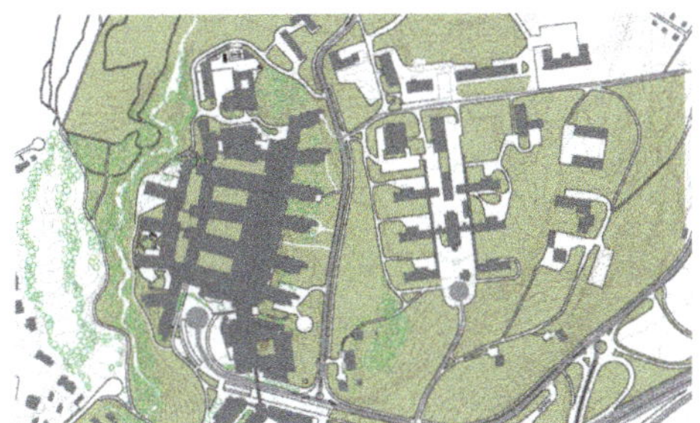

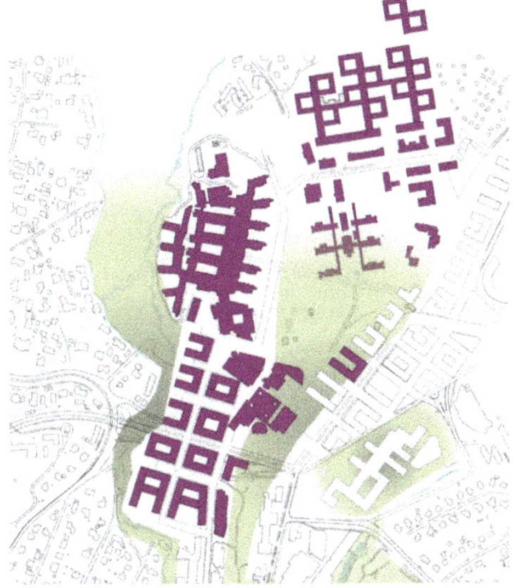

Figure 3. One of the different scenarios at at Gaustad.

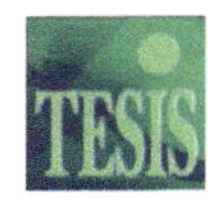

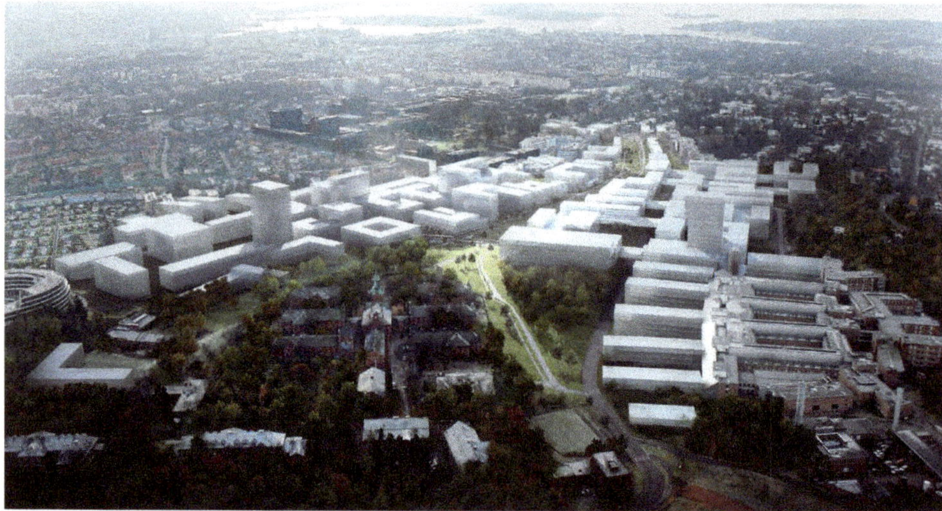

Figure 4. Campus Oslo, Gaustad - Blindern - Ullevål, project aerial view.

Paradoxically, the living standard makes even the simplest chores very expensive, and the lack of a poorly paid working class has supported both the Norwegian tradition of being a handy man, doing the job himself, and the necessity to import work force from other countries to take simple jobs such as cleaning, care and transport, as the Norwegians become higher and higher educated and "over skilled for manual labor".

From the outside, Norwegians can seem spoiled and unaware of the challenges present in many societies, struggling with urban decay, traffic congestion, air pollution, high population and migration. From the inside, the expectations drive us to provide the best treatment in the shortest possible time, to the vast majority of people, through modern, environmentally friendly facilities.

The Gaustad area in Oslo will, in the years to come, show if, in this time of our history, we can provide better than mediocre buildings, institutions and treatment facilities.

Parallel to our "noveau riche" possibilities of achieving quality, a risk averse culture has taken root, providing every job with a new set of paper work for quality control, born as it seems, out of a bureaucrats dream of streamlining and documentation of everything, from number of visits to the patient, through number of educational seminars per year for a doctor, to the correct in filling of check-boxes on any given control document. Ironically many believes that time spent on this control activity seem to take more time than the streamlining was intended to save.

Even more important, this regiment of control and checks seem to squeeze out the creative potential of projects in the Norwegian modern society. Whether or not the combined efforts of our highly motivated architectural firms can pass this obstacle will be followed closely by all involved; only time will show.

"Every hospital is too big, every hospital is too small"

The three hospitals forming the current Oslo University Hospital are:

- Rikshospitalet, or National Hospital, Serving the whole country in complex surgical fields such as organ transplantations, difficult cancer cases and rare syndromes.
- Radiumhospitalet, the Norwegian cancer hospital, famous in the country for its high quality treatment and respect and time for the individual, gaining a large amount of donations from both survivors of cancer and families of deceased every year.
- Ullevål sykehus, Oslo's largest local hospital, with large turnover, acute and trauma department, geriatric, pediatric medicine and laboratory functions for the metropolitan area.

The cultures of these hospitals are very different, each feeling threatened by becoming a "small" part of the new gigantic structure envisioned by the director. The financing system which lets money to a large extent follow the patient, adds to a sometimes bizarre situation of sending patients from one hospital to another a few kilometers away without being able to agree which hospital is the correct one to take care of the patient. This is of course a situation created by bureaucracy and stiff rules, and does not reflect the individual nurse or doctor's attitude to his or her fellow human beings.
Programming indicates a need for 650.000 square meters for a complete university hospital. When the National hospital was built, the philosophy was the "humanistic" hospital, meaning a patient and people oriented hospital with a small scale, short distances, friendly architectural spaces, extensive use of natural materials and mixed traffic of patients, staff and visitors. This implied a limit on its size not to grow too large and morph into a large factory for health, adding bits and pieces, filling in courtyards and extending technical plants wherever possible, a situation well known from similar hospitals all over the world. One crucial question is: Will the unique qualities of the less than fifteen years hospital survive such a massive growth? The cancer hospital has a special ring in every Norwegian's ears: There is a hardly a family in the country which has not had a relative in the hospital, successfully or unsuccessfully treated. The question for this hospital will be: Even if donations are funneled to research and treatment of cancer also in a merged hospital, will the public develop the same keen affection for a huge "superhospital", as for the old facility with its unbroken history on its site from the quaint listed original buildings in the leafy uptown suburb west of Oslo? And the local hospital, will it also lose some of its pride and identity as the people's hospital, running the risk of becoming a totally incomprehensible large conglomerate, consisting of innumerable city blocks with different names, long distances, shady and dark streets in between, or even if organized along a glazed street, so big that you will need more than twenty minutes to walk from one end to the other?

Specialized modern medical treatment require large and varied patient turnover to ensure high skill among doctors, and a vital environment for research and exchange of ideas between expert staff. This favors large hospitals. In Norway, with its five million inhabitants, you could argue that in many fields, one hospital is optimal to give the best treatment pos-

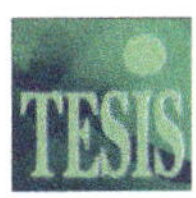

sible. In other words, most hospitals in Norway are simply too small.

Patients are people, and people consist of body and mind, or even spirit. What can a doctor or health ministry do if the patient does not mobilize his or her self-healing properties? I believe the answer is simple: Nothing. Norwegian health care was based on five health regions. Each had its university hospital at about 200.000 square meters. When merging the two regions with university hospitals in Oslo a giant was borne. The existing university hospital of 2.000.000 square meters are trying to solve the problem of giving its patients a feeling of identity by down scaling its building parts and easing the traffic routes between departments in different ways, but the public opinion all over is often the same: Most hospitals in Norway look too big!

No wonder then that the plans for the new gigantic hospital meets massive opposition among staff and patients organization, and has been forced through from the top, by hospital directors who live in the constant pressure between treating as many as possible and at the same time keeping costs down. Has the limit been reached? Is it possible to design a building of more than half a million square meters and at the same time achieve way-finding, small scale, human dimensions and a friendly and inspiring working environment for the staff?

For the time being, the staff has won a battle; the hospital is currently scaled down to 450.000 square meters. The urban, economic, political, infra structural and architectural implications remain to be solved.

How to Design and Build a Massive Urban Hospital: the Centre Hospitalier de l'Université de Montréal

Gustavo Lima

GLima@CannonDesign.com
AIA, OAQ, LEED AP, Montreal, Canada

Resulting from the fusion of three of the most important francophone hospitals in the city, the Centre Hospitalier de l'Université de Montréal (CHUM) is a state-of-the-art, 770 bed Medical Center, combining regional tertiary care, teaching and research. Anchoring the new Quartier de la Santé, the complex is an important link in the urban strategy of stitching the revitalized Vieux Port with the Plateau, one of the most livable urban neighborhoods in North America. Developed under a Public Private Partnership (P3), upon completion the CHUM complex will be one of the largest academic medical centers in the continent, with 220,000 square meters (2.5 million sf) over three city blocks, serving 345,000 ambulatory patients, 22,000 inpatients and 65,000 emergency patients each year. In addition to the 770 single-patient rooms, the CHUM will encompass ambulatory and diagnostic centers, surgery, intensive care, clinical laboratories and an adjoining research center. A large underground parking component, integration with the subway system, and LEED Silver design standards further improve convenience and quality of life. This presentation will introduce the principal design considerations and solutions implemented in the project, covering:

Part 1:

- *Public-private partnerships*
- *Architecture and urban design considerations*
- *Clinical planning and interior design*

Part 2:

- *Production tools & technology*
- *Construction*

Gustavo Lima. *A Principal at CannonDesign, Gustavo Lima has over 30 years of experience in architecture and construction management. Mr. Lima has an Architecture degree from the University of Buenos Aires, and a Masters of Architecture in Advanced Building Technologies from the University of New York at Buffalo. Mr. Lima is licensed in Buenos Aires, New York, and Québec, and is a LEED accredited professional. Gustavo Lima's area of interest resides at the intersection of design and construction, believing that both disciplines are essential components of a powerful client-centered architectural practice. Lima is CannonDesign's Project Director at the CHUM, a $1.8 Billion dollar medical center currently under construction in Montréal, Canada.*

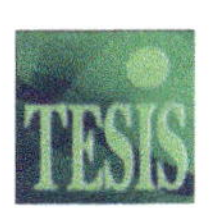

Part 1

Public Private Partnership (PPP)

A Public-Private Partnership is a financial and ownership arrangement between a public agency and a private company (usually a consortium), created with the purpose of allowing the public agency to develop a public-interest project by taking advantage of private expertise in the financial, design, construction and operational fields. In a PPP, the private entity designs, builds, finances and maintains and operates the facility, while the public entity provides the land and an annual payment, or lease, for an extended period of time, usually 25-30 years. At the end of the lease the facility reverts to the public agency.

At the CHUM, the consortium is made up of four firms: a healthcare development firm (Innisfree), a maintenance and operations firm (Dalkia), and two global construction companies (Obrascón Huarte Lain from Spain, and Laing O'Rourke from the UK). The integrated Design Team is comprised of architects CannonDesign[1] and NEUF Architect(e)s, mechanical and electrical engineers HH Angus and Roche, structural engineers Pasquin-St-Jean, and a long list of specialists, from IT, vertical transportation and civil and traffic engineers, to curtain wall, communications, landscape and food service specialists. The largest part of this team was co-located with the constructor in a single office in Montréal, but substantial work was also produced by remote offices accessing the BIM models over the internet.

Architecture and Urban Design considerations

Located at the intersection of two of Montréal's main arteries, the CHUM program promotes an active street life

[1] CannonDesign is an Ideas Based Practice, ranked among the leading international firms in planning and design for healthcare, science & technology, education, sports & recreation and government clients. At present, the firm employs a staff of 1,000, delivering services in 15 offices throughout North America, as well as in Shanghai, China, and Mumbai, India.

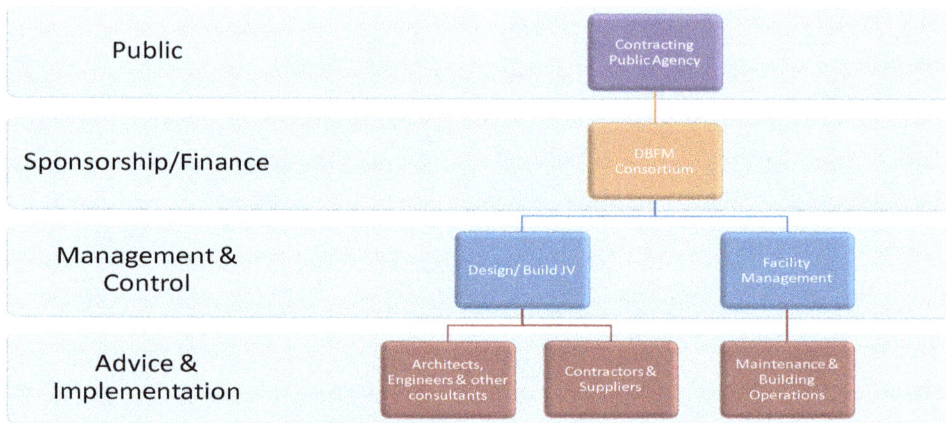

Figure 1. Public-private partnership (PPP).

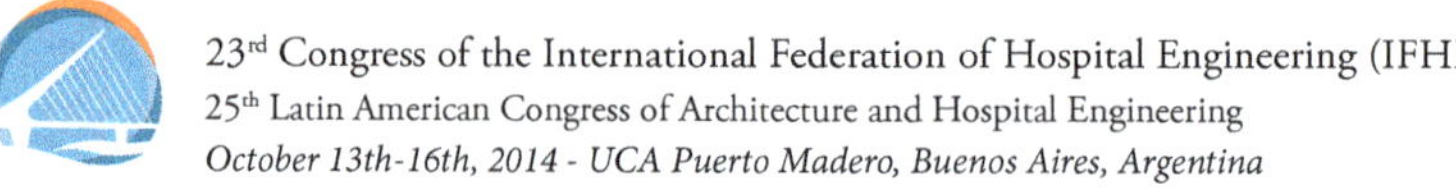

by harmonizing with the neighborhood context, re-establishing a link with old Montreal's historic quarter, and thoughtfully incorporating heritage buildings. A large underground parking component, integration with the subway system, plentiful open space, and LEED Silver design standards further improve convenience and quality of life for patients, physicians, and staff.

The indicative design provided with the RFP called for a two phase project, with only 55% of the entire complex to be completed in Phase 1 (Figure 2).

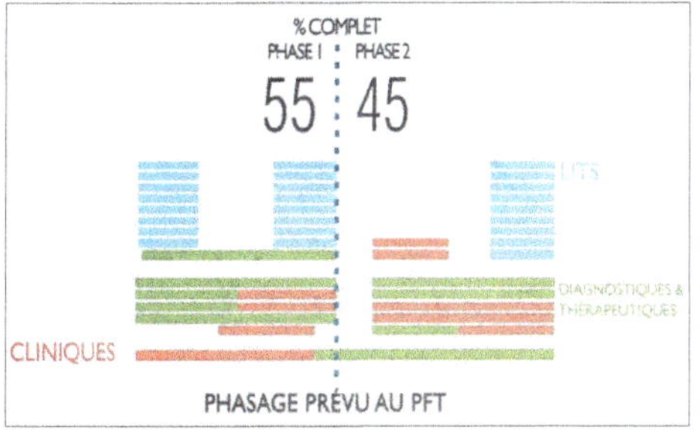

Figure 2. Two phase project.

This meant that only some of the Diagnostic and Treatment departments, 2/3 of the beds, and only a portion of the ambulatory clinics would be available by the end of Phase 1. The rest would have to wait until 2020. CannonDesign and NEUF Architect(e)s reinvented and reimagined the program, regrouping functions and departments into a completely different parti that provided 85% of the building in Phase 1 (Figure 3).

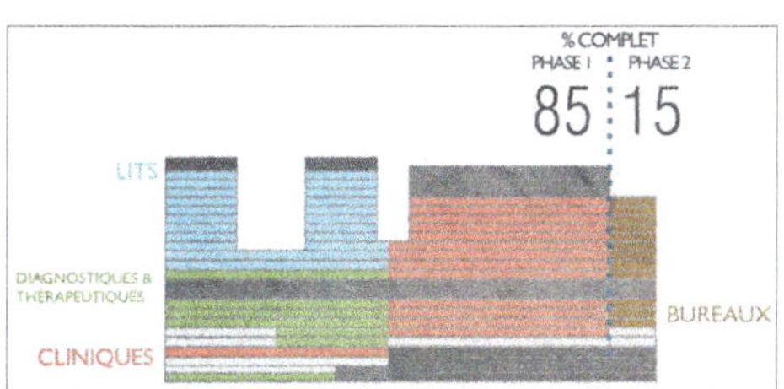

Figure 3. CannonDesign program.

This tour de force provided a fully functional hospital by 2016, all the beds, all the operating rooms, the entire diagnostic and treatment departments and 80% of the clinics, postponing only the offices, the auditorium and a portion of the parking, both of which could be easily accommodated off site until 2020. This parti, which took full advantage of the volume and height regulations in the City, resulted in a more efficient and economic construction, with a lower operational cost, giving the Collectif Santé Montréal consortium the necessary edge to win the competition.

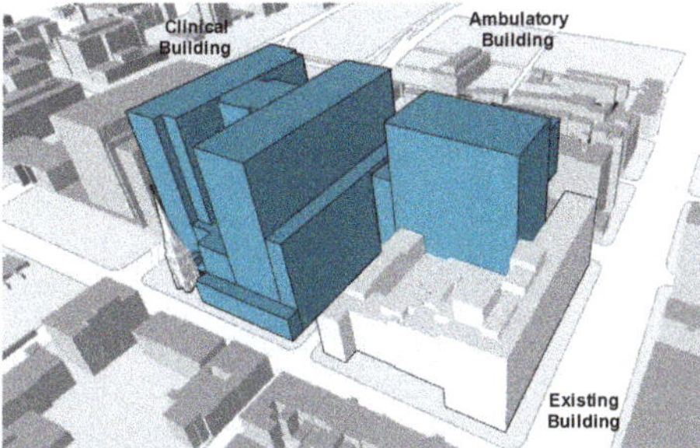

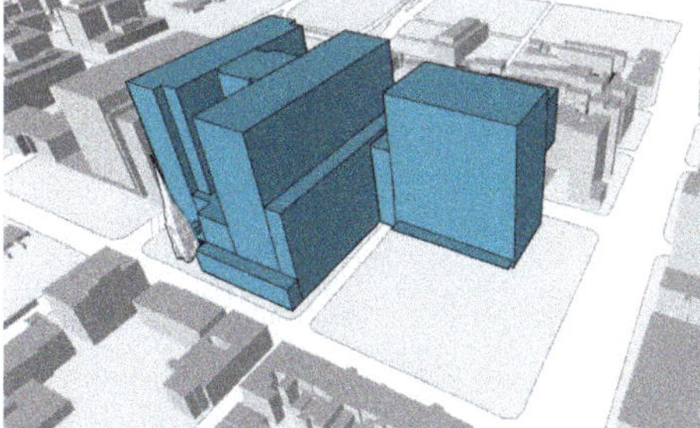

Figure 4. Phase I.

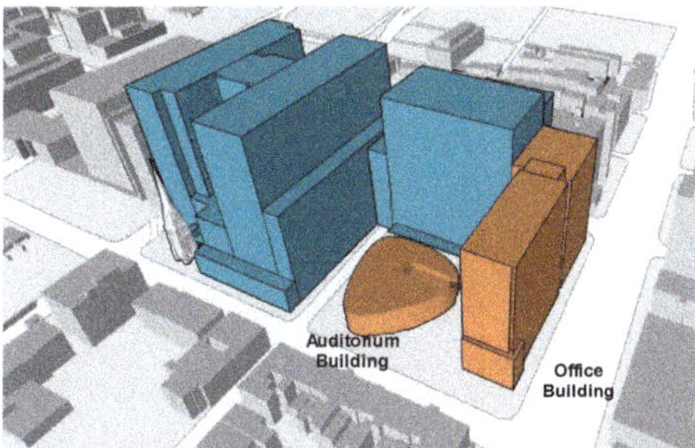

Figure 5. Phase II.

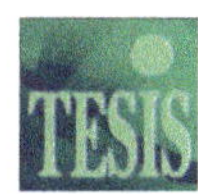

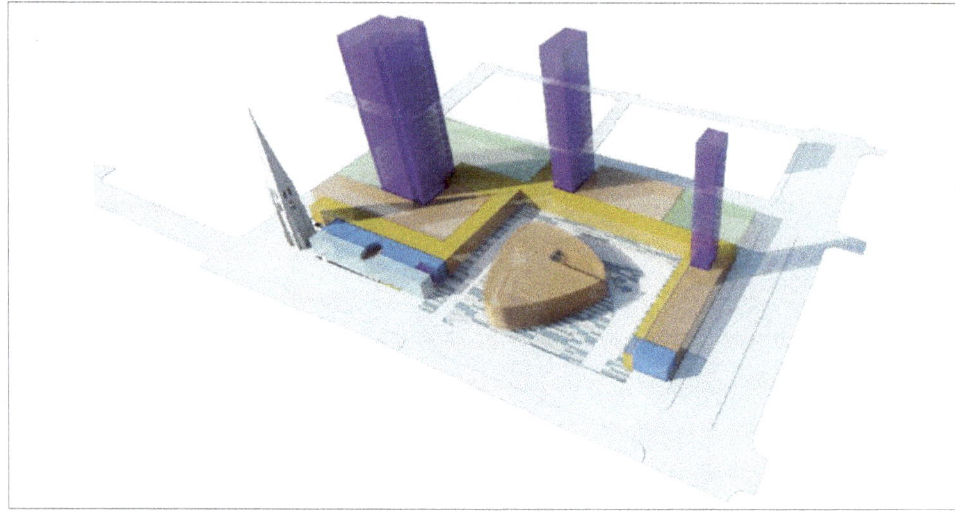

Figure 6. Wayfinding strategy.

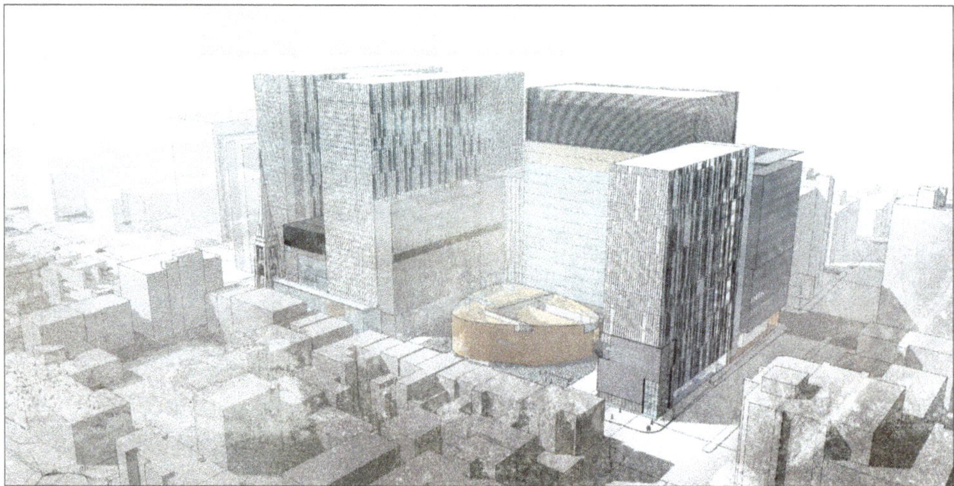

Figure 7. Configuration of the complex.

The parti incorporates an intuitive wayfinding strategy, with the public circulation always adjoining exterior views and light, allowing patients and staff to naturally orient themselves in the midst of a massive building.

This circulation then threads together the most important public spaces through the use of a common architectural language and detailing, providing natural clues and controlling the flow of people. Along this path, this common language, a sort of "device", stitches together all the public spaces in the complex: the Metro entrance, the historical remnants of the church which once stood on the site, the preserved Maison Garth, the Space of Contemplation, the lobbys, public entrances, elevators, library, cafe, pharmacy, plaza and auditorium.

Clinical Planning and Interior Design

One of the guiding principles of the clinical planning team was that of consistency and flexibility:
- all the patient rooms are identical (same handed, not mirrored);
- all the exam rooms are the same, across departments;
- the 39 Operating Rooms are virtually identical, and so are the MRI's and the LinAccs.

This reduces error on the part of the service providers, and allows flexibility in the future assignation of space.

Using the Technical Summary provided by the CHUM for each room type, the Design Team then embarked in the task of creating a series of template rooms, at 1:50 scale, that would be used across the entire complex.

Simultaneously, the Design Team was resolving, negotiating, and fine-tuning the department layouts at a 1:200 scale. When put together, after more than 33,000 man-hours of meetings, the template rooms populated the vast majority of the spaces in the building, effectively building the entire 12,000 + room complex from just a fraction of commonly developed and standardized rooms.

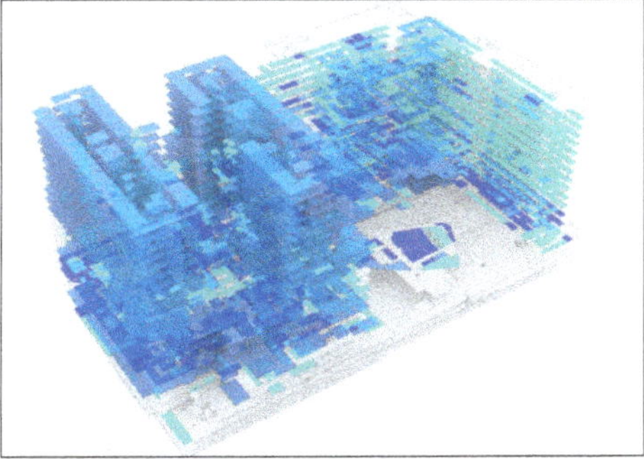

Figure 9. The distribution of the template rooms.

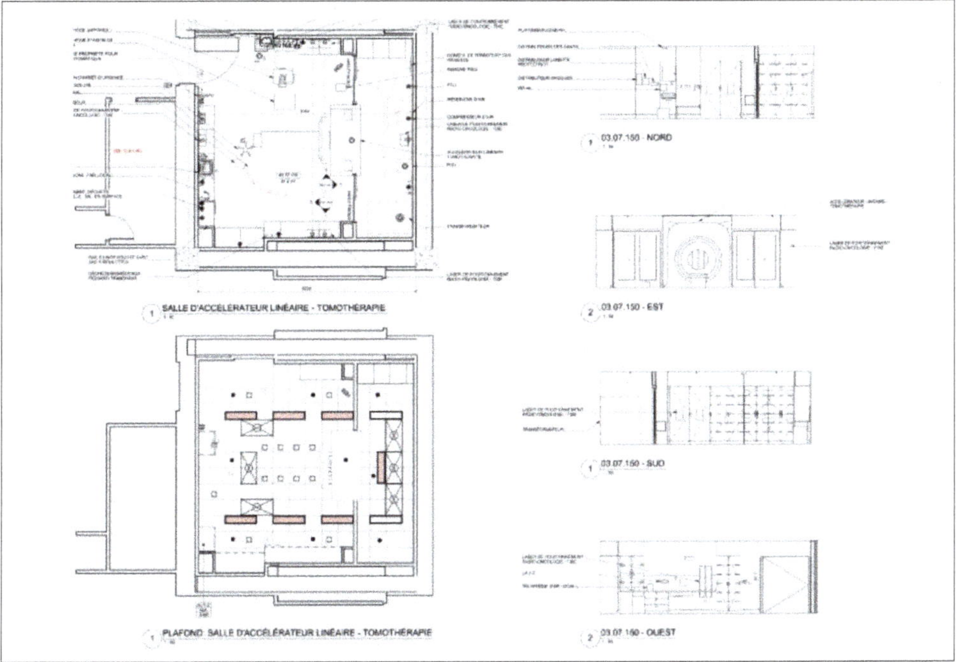

Figure 8. Template rooms.

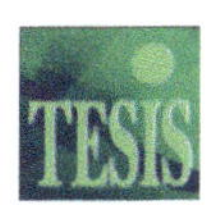

PART 2

Production Tools & Technology

A complex this massive, designed, documented and built in record time would be impossible without the use of powerful tools. The members of the Design and Construction teams agreed early on to use Revit as the common model developing tool.

While the consultants exchanged models every week (more than 100 models in total), the architectural team needed to work in a common model in real time. In order to accomplish this across a vast, transcontinental geography, CannonDesign deployed a Cloud 2.0 system, where powerful dedicated workstations, residing side by side in a proprietary Data Center, are accessed remotely via the internet.

Only keystrokes, mouse-clicks and images travel across the net, all the processing is done at the Data Center.

Medical Equipment is one of the most complex items in any hospital. CannonDesign was tasked with modeling and tracking the more than 150,000 individual pieces of equipment, ranging from MRI's to glove dispensers, through the evolution of the design and documentation process. For this purpose we used Codebook, a powerful database manager that integrates with Revit.

Other powerful tools used profusely in the project were Navisworks and BlueBeam PDF Revu, especially their Studio feature.

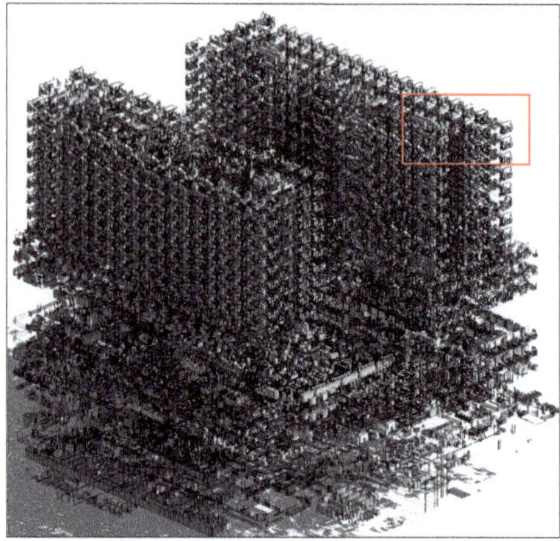

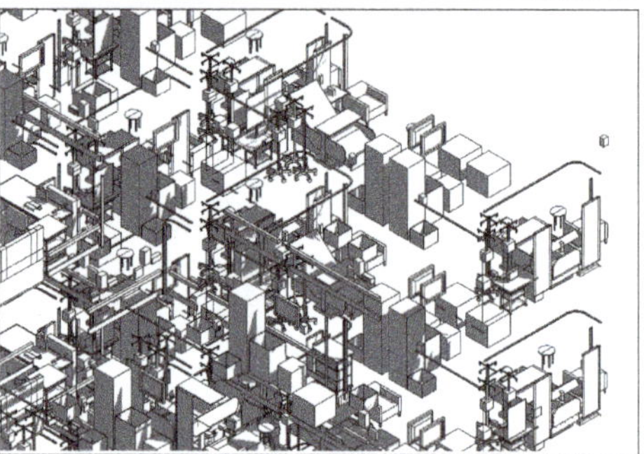

Figure 10. Codebook, a database manager integrated with Revit.

Construction

Some of the salient construction-related details of this project include:

- A load-bearing slurry wall perimeter foundation, socketed in rock, with temporary tiebacks and braced by the building slabs.

- A five level deep basement, which required blasting through more than 5 meters of solid rock.

- A seismically resistant "flat slab" concrete structure (this is a disaster-resistant building), rising to 22 stories about

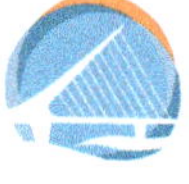

street level, and which will require about 150,000 cubic meters of trucked and pumped concrete.

- A unitized (panelized) curtain wall of more than 90,000 square meters in area, trucked from within the LEED-required 500 mile radius.

- Fully finished prefabricated bathrooms pods for all the 770 patient rooms will be trucked and lifted in place.

- At the peak, there will me more than 2,500 workers active at the site every day.

- Seven tower cranes are operational at the site, where three of the five buildings are under construction in Phase 1.

- A fully functional temporary power plant, built from scratch to feed the existing hospital during construction, and which will be completely dismantled in Phase 2.

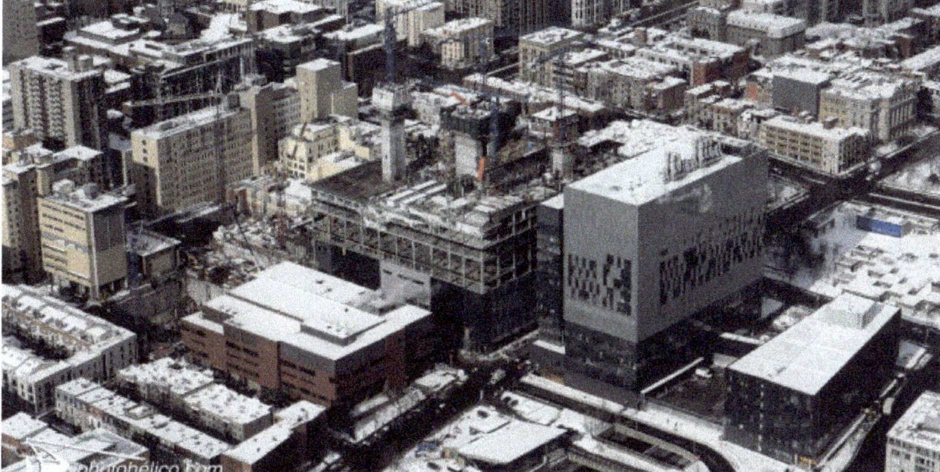

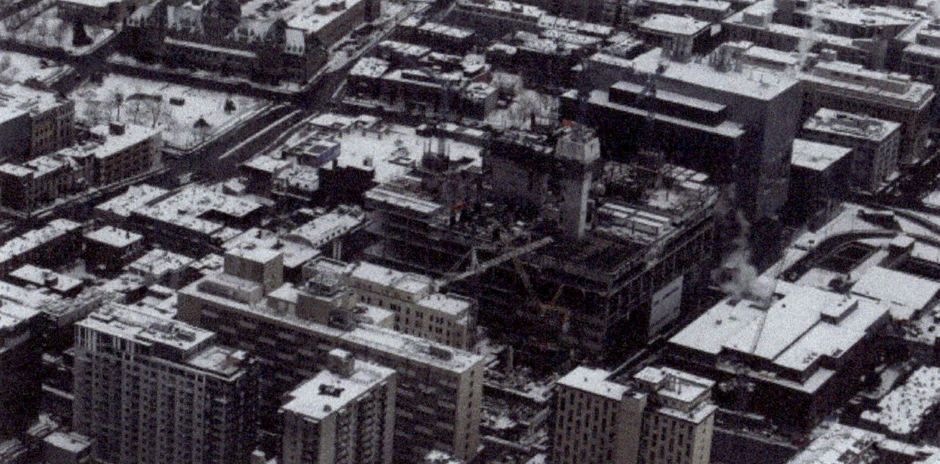

Figure 11. Construction phase.

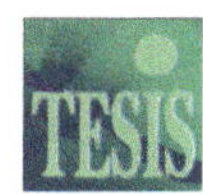

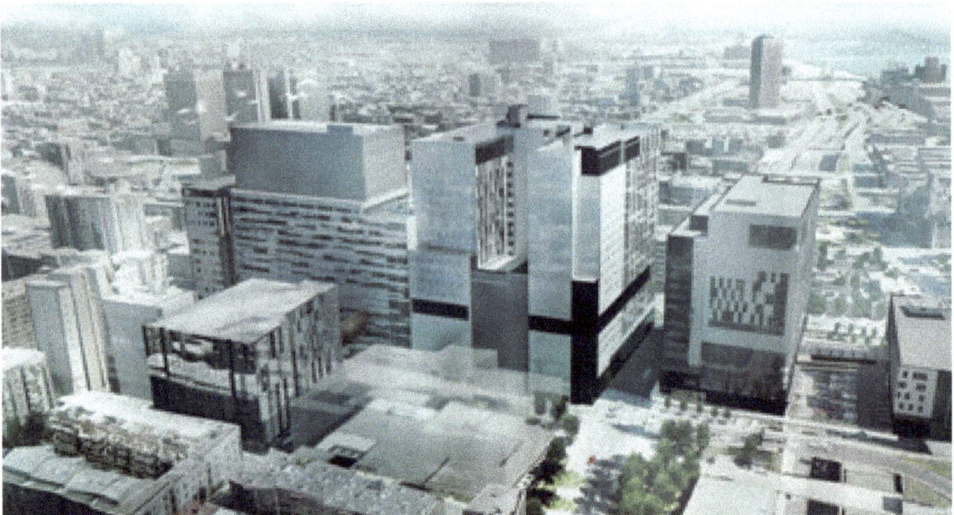

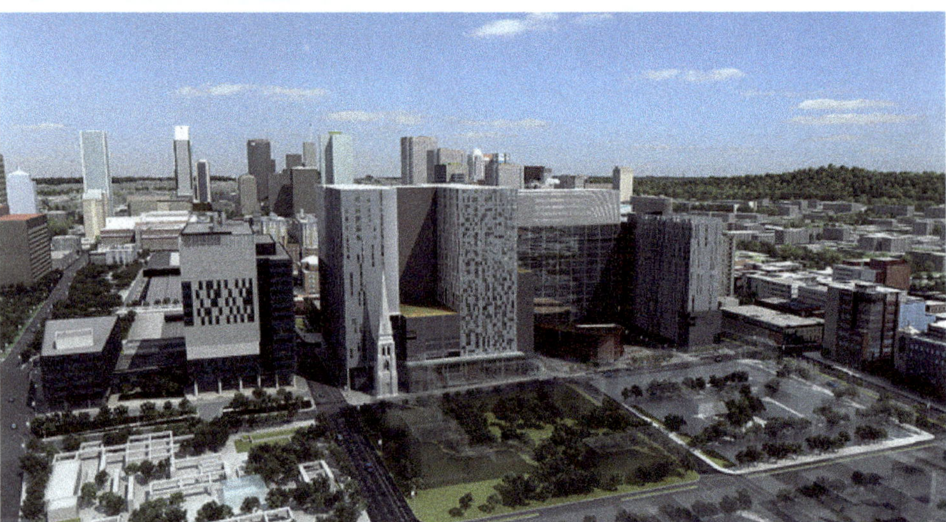

Figure 12. Centre Hospitalier de l'Université de Montréal.

Public-Private Partnerships are not without pitfalls, and require a high level of expertise, both on the Owner's side and on the Project Delivery Team's side.
But when done right, they are a powerful way to leverage the ingenuity, resources and initiative of private industry in order to obtain a building of a massive scope and size, completed in record time, which would have been virtually impossible under a traditional delivery process.

The New Integrated INCA Campus Design and the Radiotherapy Service Expansion Plan in SUS

Flávio Kelner, Salim Lamha

Associação Brasileira para o Desenvolvimento do Edifício Hospitalar (ABDEH), Brazil

The Brazilian national cancer care network has been the subject of a series of restructuring plans by the Health Department. In 2012 new investments were announced for the prevention and control of cancer in the country as part of a set of strategic actions to strengthen the prevention network, diagnosis and treatment of cervix and breast cancer, which includes the expansion of the offer of radiotherapy services with the allocation of resources in equipment and infrastructure, through the Plan Expansion of Radiotherapy in health system of Brazil denominated SUS.

The cancer incidence in Brazil, as well as throughout the world, has increased in recent decades, following the changing age profile of the population and the increasing exposure to risk factors.

Efforts to control cancer are developed around involving actions from preventive health linked to primary care, up to high technological density care, applied to diagnosis and treatment, this one related to high complexity.

So, by being cancer a disease of high magnitude, which requires timely attention, prolonged treatment and appropriate follow-up, given the possibility of recurrence, it requires a network of comprehensive and articulate assistance and effective regulation to ensure access to comprehensive healthcare, obtained by integration of specialized services (surgery, radiotherapy and chemotherapy).

In the city of Rio de Janeiro, the National Cancer Institute (INCA) is about to begin the construction of the most modern center of scientific development and innovation for cancer control in the country centralizing, in one place, the areas of research, care, education, prevention, surveillance and early disease detection.

Flávio Kelner. *Graduated in Architecture and Urban Planning at Santa Úrsula University on 1988, National President of Associação Brasileira para o Desenvolvimento do Edifício Hospitalar (ABDEH) from 2005 to 2008 and Member of the Academia Brasileira de Administração Hospitalar. Participation on several conferences as a speaker and attendee over the last 10 years. Performed technical visits to renomated health institutions in Europe and US, as well as the most important hospitals in Brazil. Invited as a Professor for conferences on MBA courses on the healthcare field. Now, runs RAF Arquitetura, a company with over 100 employees split on two units, one in Rio de Janeiro and one in São Paulo.*

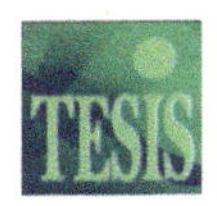

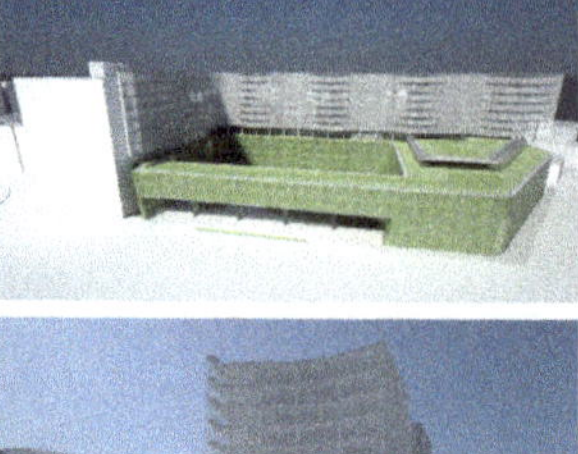
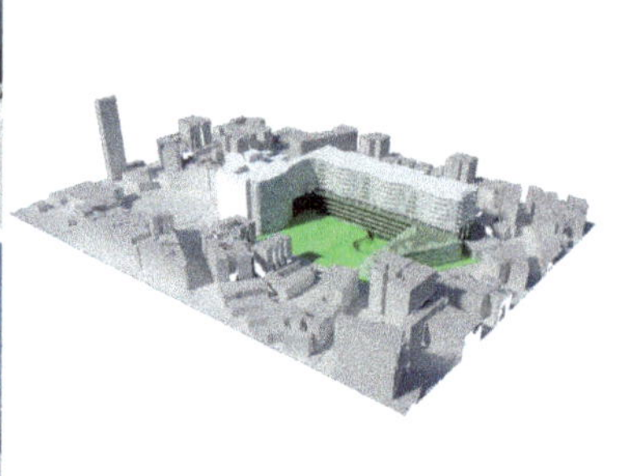

Figure 1. INCA concept.

Currently, INCA has scattered units in 18 buildings throughout the city. This project has the concept of bringing them all to the same place providing a unique environment of knowledge exchange.
The project includes the renovation of the existing building (HC1) and the construction of a new building complex, interconnected in a site with a total area of approximately 15.000 m². The total construction area is 140.000 m², distributed in four blocks, up to 12 stories each.

This challenge should be seen as an opportunity to improve the built environment and to create values with committing solutions through more efficient processes of design and construction.
The design of the new "Integrated Campus" was developed with the use, and for the use, of the highest technology and most modern architectural and construction concepts.
The implementation of this new building in a region protected by the Federal , State and Municipal Historical, Artistic and Cultural Preservation Agencies , required special attention to avoid any impacts that may cause damage to the heritage. This new insertion into the urban tissue should propose ways to maximize positive impacts toensure the economic and cultural revitalization of downtown activities, which is the goal of the city Hall of Rio de Janeiro and aspiration of all Cariocas.
Under the expansion plan of Radiotherapy in Brazil, RAF Architecture, in partnership with MHA Engenharia, faced the challenge of developing design solutions for 41 hospitals and for the expansion of 39 existing services, totaling 80 radiation therapy solutions, located in various regions of a country of continental dimensions.
This project will benefit all Brazilians from the public and private health system (both, SUS and non-SUS), since the majority of registered hospitals with SUS are not public, but provide services to both systems.

Finally, we conclude that several factors make these special projects and should be thought of as strategic for the country. The understanding of the urban developments and their relevance to society constraints, are key to ensuring the feasibility of their implementation, requiring special attention of public officials throughout the course of the process.

Grupo Oroño - Health Providers Since 1950 – A Tradition of Innovation

Andrés Haugh, Cristian Mander

mantego@sanatorioparque.com.ar
Grupo Oroño – Health Providers

The emblematic Oroño Boulevard was founded in 1862 as part of the Urban Program of Rosario Local Government. There, traditional families built mansions and small palaces of different styles that left a mark in terms of beauty and a style typical of Europe. Over time, a great part of this architectural treasure was demolished, thus, erasing a unique aesthetic component from the past. Grupo Oroño (GO) is the union of the most important care centers of Rosario city and its surroundings. It guarantees a direct access to an excellent medical care. Grupo Oroño is a synonym of high quality, competitive and accessible medical care. Each institution is a model in terms of experience, infrastructure and technology.

Andrés Haugh *was born in Rojas, Buenos Aires, Argentina in 1972. He Studied Architecture at Universidad Nacional de Rosario (UNR) and graduated in 1997. There, he received the first prize in a student's competition: ARQUISUR. From 1997 to 2000, he worked as a teaching assistant for the subject Architectural Project in charge of architect Anibal Moliné and also worked with renowned architects from Rosario City such as Caffaro Rossi Architects, Augusto Pantarotto and Gerardo Caballero. In mid-2000 he started working as Maintenance Supervisor in Sanatorio Parque. In 2004 he joined Grupo Oroño technical office participating in the development of Grupo Oroño projects.*

Development

Go Health Providers: Provides medical care service to prepaid medicine and private insurance systems; Performs scientific investigation programs related to health, through the structures of its institutions; Coordinates common activities and implements financing mechanisms to the activities of the institutions that integrate the society.
Go Management: Negotiation of arrangements and health services costs per capita; Financial management of purchases and contract of third-party services; Medical audit and legal issues services; Health services engineering; Incorporation of new practices to increase the financing of private insurance and prepaid medicine; Administration and management of primary attention outpatient network; Bioengineering development and incorporation of high cost / low frequency use technology, with common use between its institutions; Coordination of networked computer systems and communications.

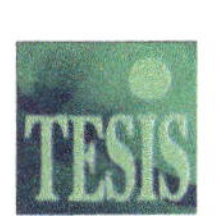

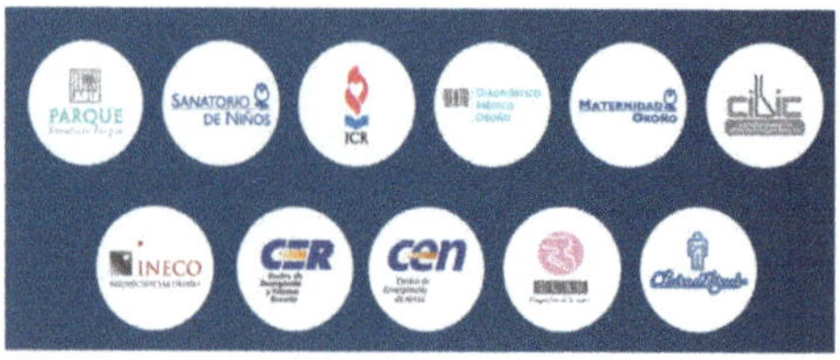

Figure 1. Go Institutions.

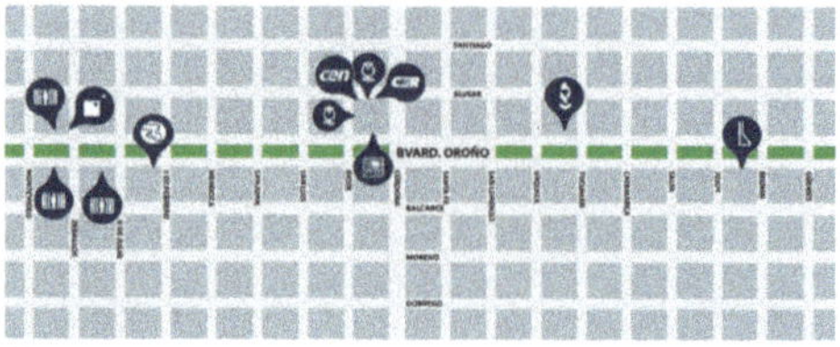

Figure 2. Go Location.

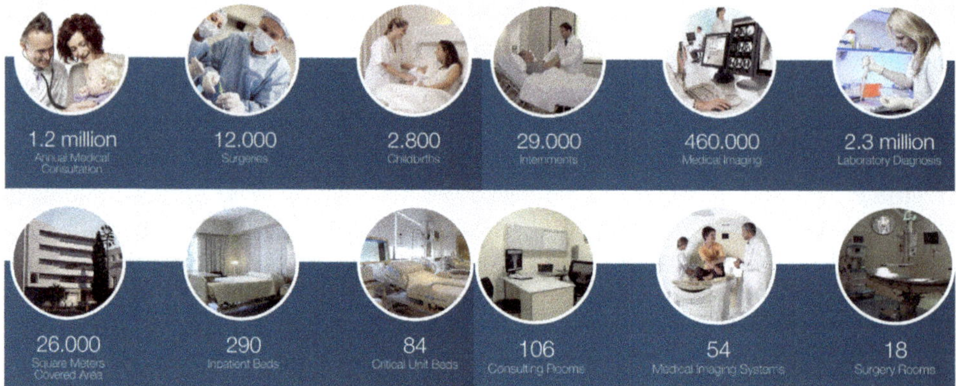

Figure 3. Go Numbers.

Go Financing: Medicina Esencial is the most important health insurance provider in the province of Santa Fe; It counts with more than 60.000 members who can choose between prepaid medicine and private insurance system; It provides to its associates its own health centers with direct health financing, offering a more accessible fee.

Director's Plan for the clinics Sanatorio Parque and Sanatorio de Niños

Physical resources vs. sustainability

Two icons of rationalist architecture from the 50s were designed by the renowned architect Jaime Roca and nowadays have to adapt to the constant growth of demand as well as to the technological, use, aesthetic and security needs.

They are a good example of Strategic Planning, where the adjusting of existing facilities is a real challenge in the development of each project. The decision of transferring the Maternity Unit of Sanatorio Parque was the most ambitious project of Grupo Oroño over the last years.

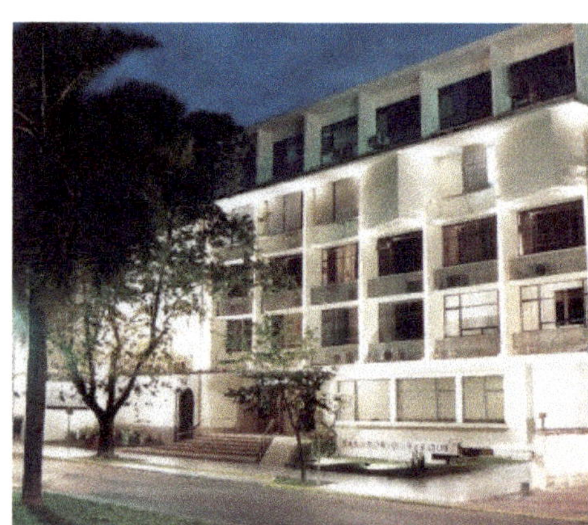

Figure 4. Sanatorio Parque.

Maternidad Oroño

The Maternity Unit has its façade and independent access in Rioja Street. The technical area is situated on the third floor, and there, all the patients are examined with monitoring and ultrasound. It has four Labor, Delivery and Recovery Rooms and two Operating Rooms that are exclusively used forobstetric surgeries.

The Labor, Delivery and Recovery Rooms have natural light. Each of them has a toilet and is equipped with beds which are adaptable to avoid moving and disturbing the patient during labor. In those rooms it is also possible to perform a C-Section if required. They are designed as operating rooms equipped with centralized monitoring system, special lamps, medicinal gases and critical care cribs.

The Neonatology Unit has 25 positions distributed in three sectors depending on complexity. It also has special room for the babies' families so that they can visit and see them without time restrictions, thus, facilitating the professionals performance, minimizing the risk of infections and lowering the level of anxiety of family members.

There is a connecting bridge that allows physicians to move and transfer patients to the critical care units and operating rooms of Sanatorio Parque. This represents a great advantage in case of emergencies.

The individual rooms are comfortable and are equipped with everything you may need to welcome family members without affecting the care and assistance of other patients.

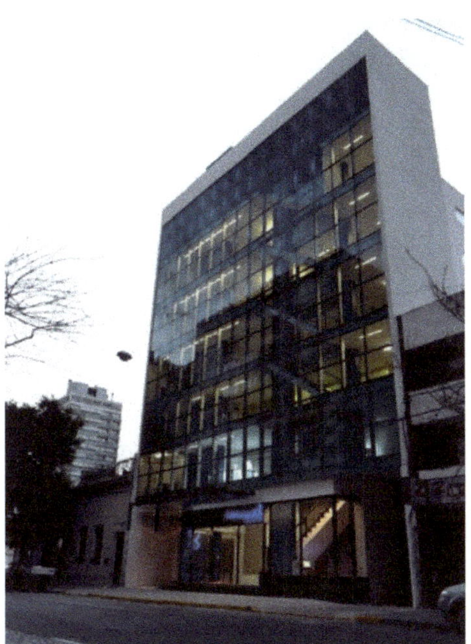

Figure 5. Maternidad Oroño.

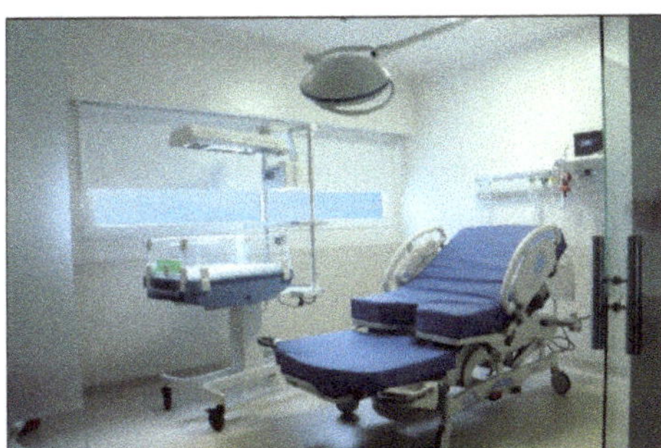

Figure 6. Delivery Room.

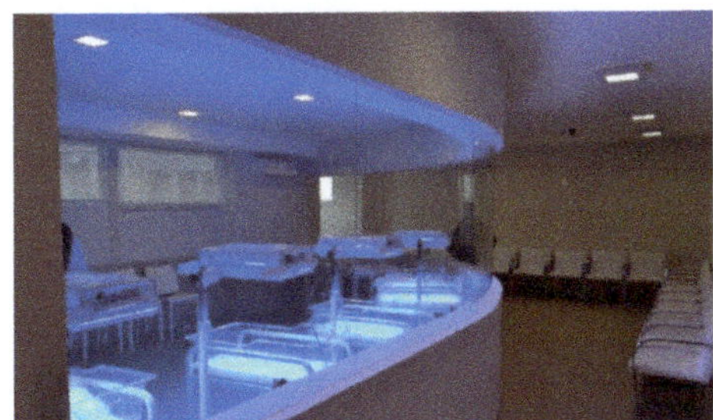

Figure 7. Neonatology Unit.

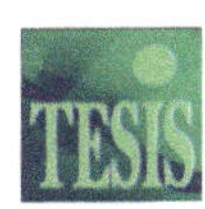

There are spacious waiting rooms ideal for companions and visitors to stay while the baby and its mother rest.
Different textures, colors, views inside the building and fantasies combine creatively with the natural light that prevails in the building.

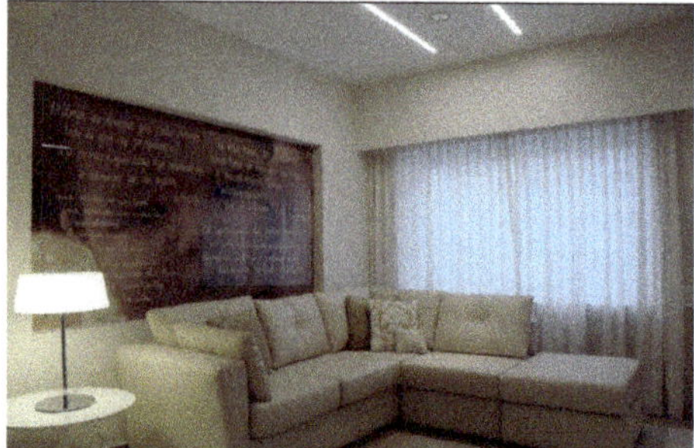

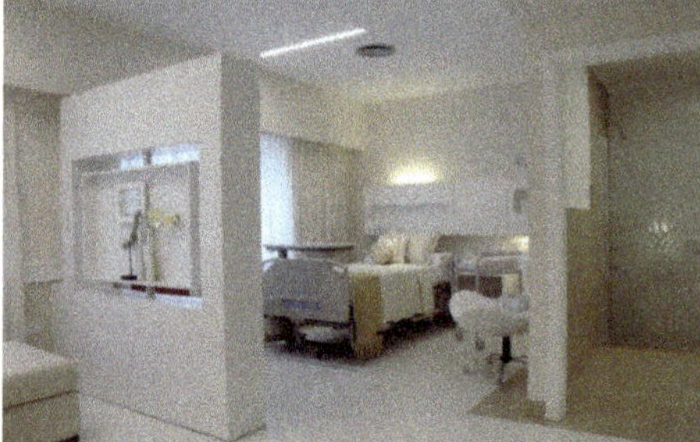

Figure 8. Waiting room (above) and private room (below).

Sanatorio Parque

The enlargement of the building in Alvear Street is a real challenge. Even though all the work is done in a single plot, it is necessary to work in the façade of the whole block that during a long time had a green opening area and an internal path used by the nearby residents that had nothing to do with the clinic; an inconceivable idea for nowadays.
On the other hand, it was necessary to design a new front view for Sanatorio Parque, whose Boulevard façade is a historical referent in the city.

It was also necessary to avoid the environmental impact when working near old cypresses and palms that have given name, identity and relevance to a prestigious institution during six decades.
The building had adjusted to these giants, as if it was asking for permission. But in the ground, there were signs that led the way, the architecture. It was there, it was only necessary to find it.
The position of the building line allows for a space of meeting, calm and tranquility: something which is not so common in the centers of our cities. It is also the space for pedestrian and vehicular access and also it allows access for suppliers.
This project was created from the need to enlarge Centro de Emergencias Rosario (CER) and transfer the Critical Care Units (UCC in spanish) and the Diagnostic Imaging Department where outpatients and in-patients circulate.

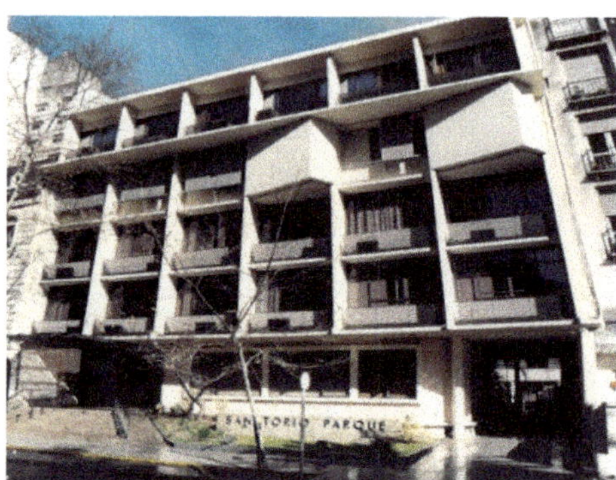

Figure 9. Sanatorio Parque.

The CER receives and derives patients in the ground floor. The Resonance Area is located underground, the Ultrasound Area is on the first floor, the Intensive Care Units and Operating Rooms are on the third floor and the Minimally Invasive Surgery Department is situated on the fourth floor.

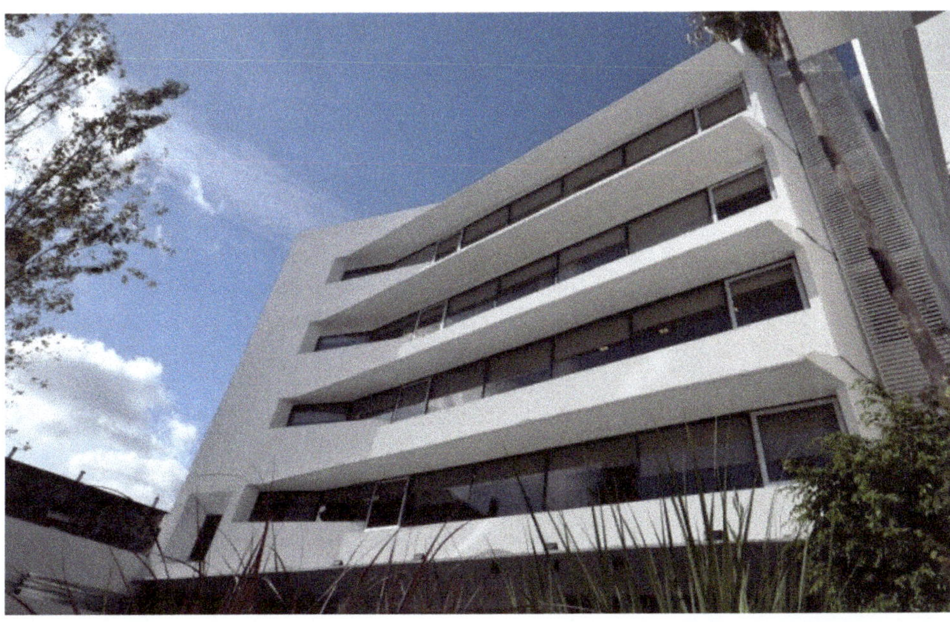

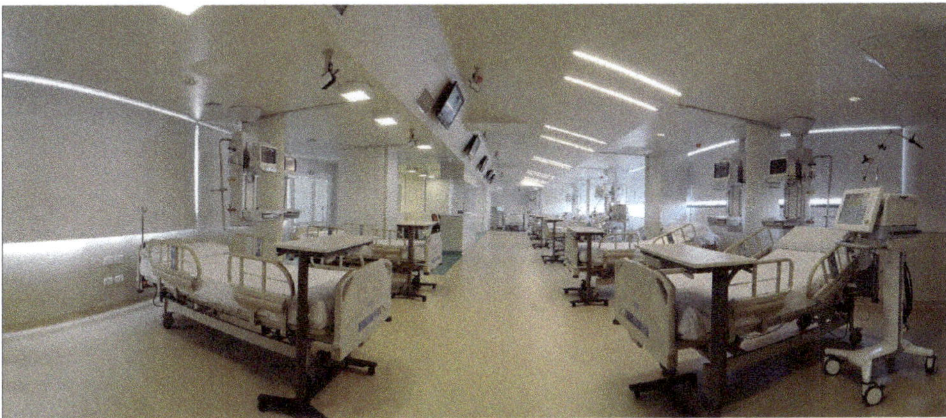

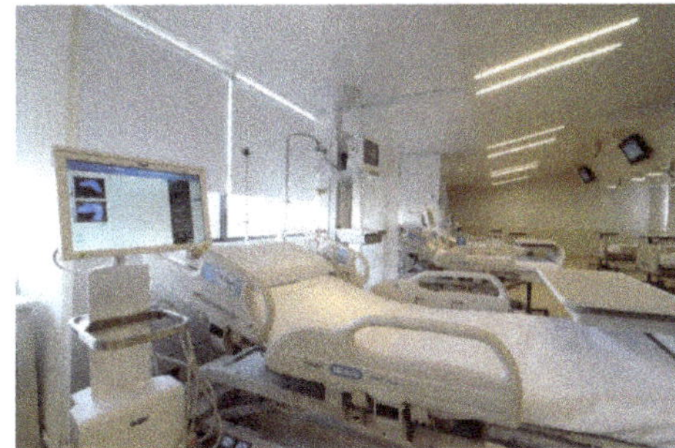

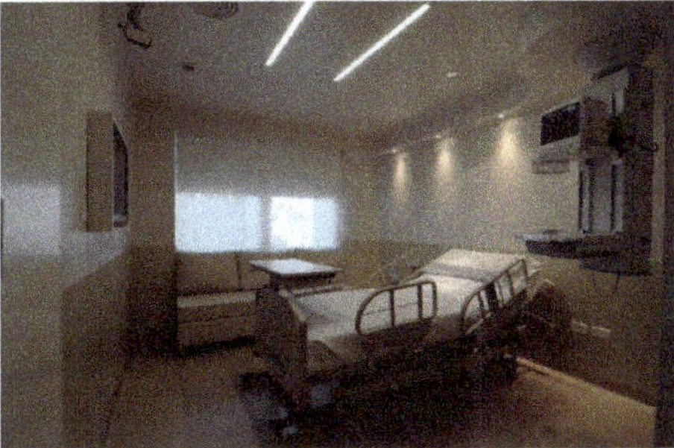

Figure 10. Centro de Emergencias Rosario (CER) and the Critical Care Units (UCC in spanish).

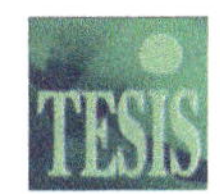

All the areas are connected through two elevators: one exclusive for in-patients and the other for out-patients.

The CER has a triage space, two doctor's offices for in-patients and eight doctor's offices for sporadic visits. It has ten positions for transitory in-patients, two doctor's offices for Traumatology and a plaster room. The Intensive Care Unit has three sectors for in-patients: the Coronary Care Unit with nine positions, the Intensive Care Unit with nine positions and six individual rooms with space for a companion.

The results in patients that receive Critical Care are really positive when they have the possibility to be in contact with the outside. So it the location in time and space is of crucial importance.

The main premise in the development of this project was that every patient must have a view to the outside and the spaces where they stay should receive natural light.

The exhaustive search and selection of technology was of vital importance to follow this concept. It was possible to avoid the interruption of the views and the complete darkening of the rooms; to allow for the circulation of patients, for the isolation of different areas of the building and for communication between all sectors; and to install emergency alarm systems and monitoring systems for all patients. Thanks to Architectural design, it was possible to develop and make the most of these facilities.

Space Management, a Good Habit for Successful Design Hospital Nacional Dr. Alejandro Posadas

Jose Ondarçuhu

jose@concretarsalud.msal.gov.ar
Ministerio De Salud De La Nación, Argentina

We are immersed in a universe in constant transformation, before this we aim to create strategies to generate favorable conditions that routed the change so we can arrive at the desired objectives. Under the development of complex projects, process management coupled with the correct calibration of the need and physical and technological response is one of the main conditions that allow the project to be successful and can last over time. We propose a planning mechanism that involves an analysis of operating costs and strengthens the spirit of simple, low cost of implementation and maintenance solutions. We looked for constructive, technological and image solutions related to the functions, processes, and implantation, we propose to analyse the intervention strategy of the master plan of the Dr. Alejandro Posadas Hospital. In 1957 the Thoracic Surgery Clinic was born in a 56.000 m² building, 7 floors and a design which met the requirements that at these time were essential to the care of chronic lung disease patients, open spaces and balconies oriented to permit the sun baths. With the passage of time more complexity is added, most services have developed excellent features and complexity, transforming the establishment as a regional referral center adult - pediatric, this technological and operational developments were not accompanied by architectural planning, areas designed to meet the new requirements were developed organically, this process coupled with increased demand result in dramatic role conflict, loss of functioning and less quality of care.

José Ondarçuhu. *Architect, Healthcare design Specialist, Master of Urban Planning. General Coordinator of the Health Facilities and Biomedical Technology unit, Ministry of Health. He has served as Program Coordinator of International Cooperation, Ministry of Health, Consultant of the Pan American Health Organization (PAHO) and the Ibero-American Consultant Social Security Organization (ISSO). Has participated in the development of more than 50 projects of health planning, hospital architecture and technology in the national and international level. He currently teaches at ISALUD University. Author of various articles of health planning, has given many lectures and workshops on health architecture and technology management. Member of the Argentine Association of Hospital Architecture and Engineering (AADAIH).*

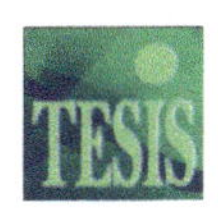

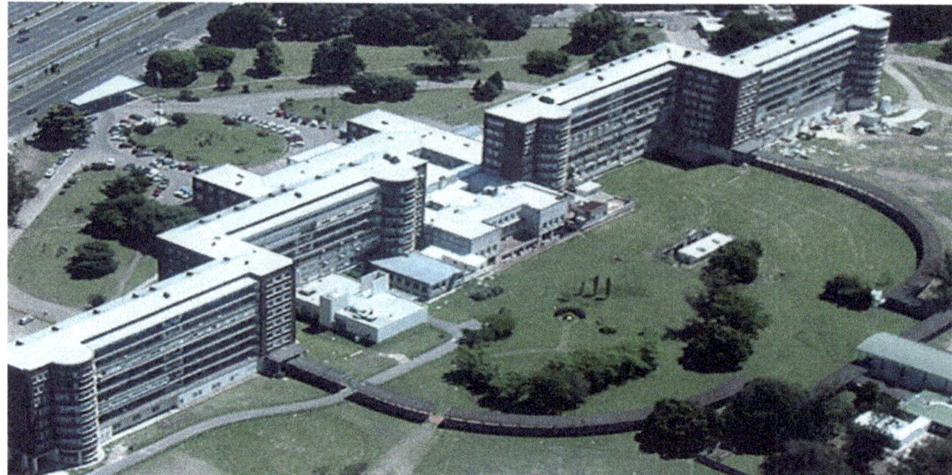

Figure 1. National Hospital Prof. Dr. Alejandro Posadas.

In this situation a master plan was developed from the strength of the institution, high technical quality and a strategic location with a 3 million people influence area. A new operational structure and role for the Hospital were defined.
We propose a programming process, since under current conditions the Hospital has a design more focused on staff than on patients.

To respond to the new requirements some areas were relocated and redesigned and other new areas were created. The objective of the proposed functional organization is to reorganize the existing capacity of the Hospital, adapting to the demands and needs to satisfy. Projects meet production criteria, functionality, technological rationality, biosafety, humanization of health care with high spatial quality and respecting the original historic facade that is part of the social memory.

The challenge was to expand and optimize the production without interrupting the operation of the Hospital, discouraging some processes of low complexity and high traffic of patients and companions as ambulatory care and fostering the development of high complexity. We considered generate a new parallel building to the current block, consisting of a basement, ground floor and three floors. This new volume staying low complexity processes and complementary (ambulatory care, maintenance, information, teaching and research and administration). It joins the existing block by public or technical connectors.
On the body of the second level of the existing building , the more complex services are built, (Surgical Center, Multi organ bank and Histocompatibility Laboratory).
The set is complemented by two major services towers that have gases, power, air conditioning, hot and cold water.

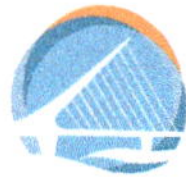

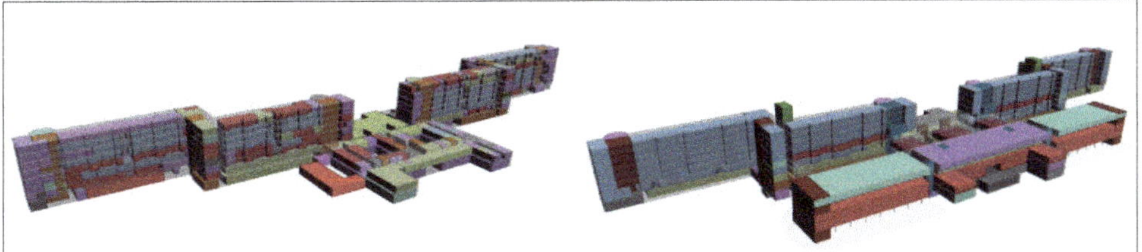

Figure 2. Current building diagram (left) and future building diagram (right).

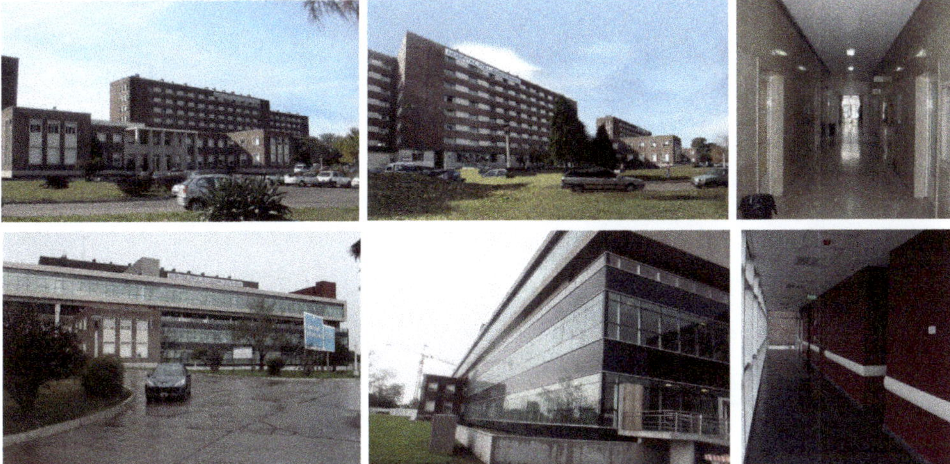

Figure 3. Images current building.

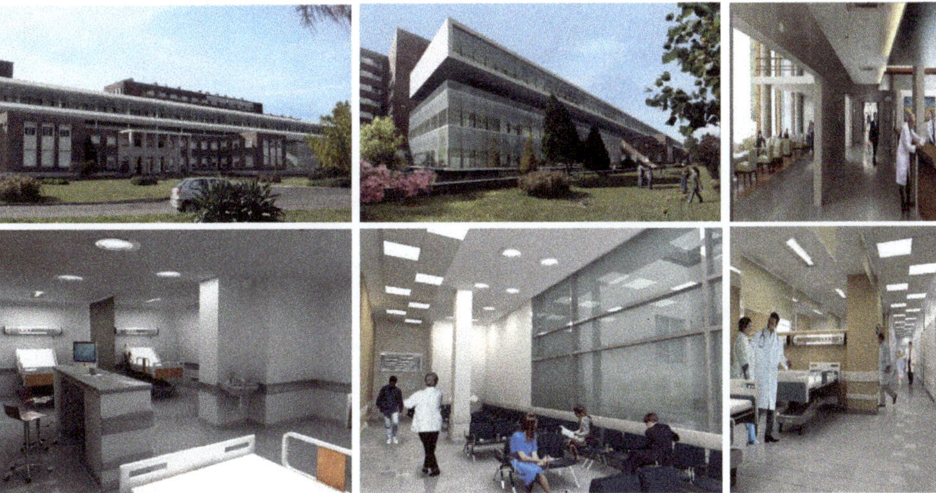

Figure 4. Images future building.

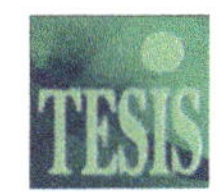

The rest of the activities are remodelations or adaptations of existing sectors, according to the Master Plan. The architectural proposal for the first phase of work will impact a total area of about 21.800 m^2, 16.200 m^2 of new floor area and 5.600 m^2 existing. The product is a set of steps which forms one of the most important public health projects in Argentina that tends to position Dr. Alejandro Posadas Hospital as one of the best hospitals in the country.

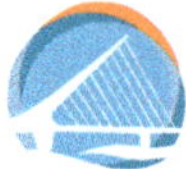

Remodeling and Extension of SMI Hospital

Pedro Francisco Elzaurdia

pelzaurdia@hospitec.com.uy
Sociedad Uruguaya de Arquitectura e Ingeniería Hospitalaria (SUAIH), Uruguay

The presentation will focus on the project for remodeling and extension of one of the most relevant hospitals in Uruguay, which has the highest technology within the private sector and reach the major prestige and quality standards of attention in the health field. The original building, constructed in 1948 for the high-level private healtcare and with only 50 beds.

Pedro Francisco Elzaurdia *CEO of Hospitec Ltda, Specialized Consultant Company in Health and Alimentation Projects. Previous experience: Ex – CEO of the Architectural Department in "Hospital de Clínicas, Dr. Manuel Quintela." Ex - CEO of the Architectural Department in "Hospital Militar Central de las FFAA" Managing projects with more than 400.000 m² in Health and Alimentary areas. Prized in multiple Architecture and Medicine contests Speaker in local, regional and international conferences related to health field. Ex IFHE EXCO member SUAIH secretary Author or co-author of multiples audited research works and Books related to health topics.*

The building changed through several extension in a new functional structure composed by 258 beds and giving as result the following arrangement:

Minimal Care beds (MC): Adults Beds 195; b. Children beds 13.
Intensive Care Units beds (ICU): Adults ICU Medical 18; Specialized Neurological ICU care 5; Cardiology ICU 9; Childcare's ICU 12; Isolation Medulla Transplant 6.
Surgical Suites: Cardiology Surgical Suites 1; General Surgical Suites 4.
Imagenology services: X -ray equipment 1; TAC 1; RNM 2; Cardiological Angiographs 3; Neurological Angiographs 1; SPEC 1.
Ambulatory services: Emergency Department; External consult services; Physiotherapy.
General services: Kitchen; Laundry; Sterilizing services; Boiler Room; Traditional services Medical Files.

The project classify the total of 375 beds in minimal, moderate and intensive care, following the arrangement below:

Minimal Care beds (MC): Adults Beds 273; Children Beds 24.
Intensive Care Units beds (ICU):

Adults ICU Medical 22; Specialized Neurological ICU care 8; Cardiology ICU 16; Childcare's ICU 22; Medulla Transplant Isolation 10.
Surgical Suites: Cardiological Surgical Suite 1; Hybrid Surgical Suite 1; General Surgical Suites 6.
Imagenology services: X-ray equipment 1; TAC 1; RNM 2; Cardiological Angiographs 3; Neurological Angiographs 1; SPEC- CT 1.
Ambulatory services: Emergency Department double capacity; External services consult triple capacity; Physiotherapy external services;
General services: Kitchen; Laundry; Sterilizing services; Boiler room; Parking Area with 200 places.

The output of energy power (Gas, Oil Gas and electricity) and potable water supply, generate an annual expenditure of over $ 2.000.000,00, through the following systems: 2 Steam Boilers 2TV / h @ 10 kg/cm^2; 3 Points of electricity supply in 6kV and 400 Volts; More than 100 Split or VRV units of air conditioners; 80 m^3 of water storage without firewater reserve.

The resulting conformation aims to achieve the elements which are detailed below:

In the area of functional structure, the following changes will be made: Reorganization of admission units to determine a clear circulation system and defining the different areas through a logical grouping; The concentration in the same level of high-tech services; Establishing an emergency area with a degree of correlation with the outpatient public and the rest of the health care floor in accordance with regulatory requirements; The construction of parking areas within the building limits and its proximity areas; The remodeling of the laundry, kitchen, and other attending services.

In the energy area the following changes are being made: unifying different power inputs (220 volts, 400 volts, 6Kv) at a single point in 20 Kv; setting-up a single point of emergency power generation; gradual removal and replacement of all secondary and tertiary systems, Split, VRV, secondary Chillers, etc, to create a single generating point of industrial refrigeration through cold compressors with high levels of heat recovery for HVAC systems and consumption; generate solar energy through hot water panels; remodeling of steam generating systems, back to the original situation, based on different sources of generation.

The expected result of the whole proposition aims to achieve the following goals:

Project goals in the functional area: a significant increase in the efficiency of the areas, allowing better use of existing staff, being able to meet the growth of patients with a minimal increase of staff; increase the quality of care, giving better conditions of security benefits; minimize in-hospital infections, through the incorporation of new systems, related to the functional design of the areas.

Project goals in the energy sector: significantly increase the electrical efficiency, allowing the growth of almost 100 % of the building results in an increase of no more than 20 % in electricity; changing the heat generation layout, according with the current legislation, through the incorporation of solar energy and heat recovery of the refrigeration systems, avoiding the increase of the current fuel oil consumption; the substantial change in the refrigeration system, in order to assure the optimization of the high-efficiency systems, which will generate heat and minimize the electric energy consumption per m^2.

In order to establish a control of the goals, the following elements will be implemented: a unit of register and control of the energy inputs, monitoring since January 2011 date and place; a unit of register of significant events in the area of quality indicators linked to the development of the works; a system of control of personnel and the results on the building complex; an analysis system of the care goals achievements.

FINAL SUMMARY AND EXPECTED RESULTS

It is expected that the results of this project may become standard goals for buildings of this type in the Uruguayan healthcare field.

According to our experience in the Uruguayan market, this would be the first health building whose objective is, not only the functional design, but also, as an added value to the building, the optimization of the energy and operative systems.

It is our pride as an organization that these experiences had a great influence in the healthcare market, by the direct influence on other health buildings in planning stages, which are designed to establish themselves as models in their area of specialty.

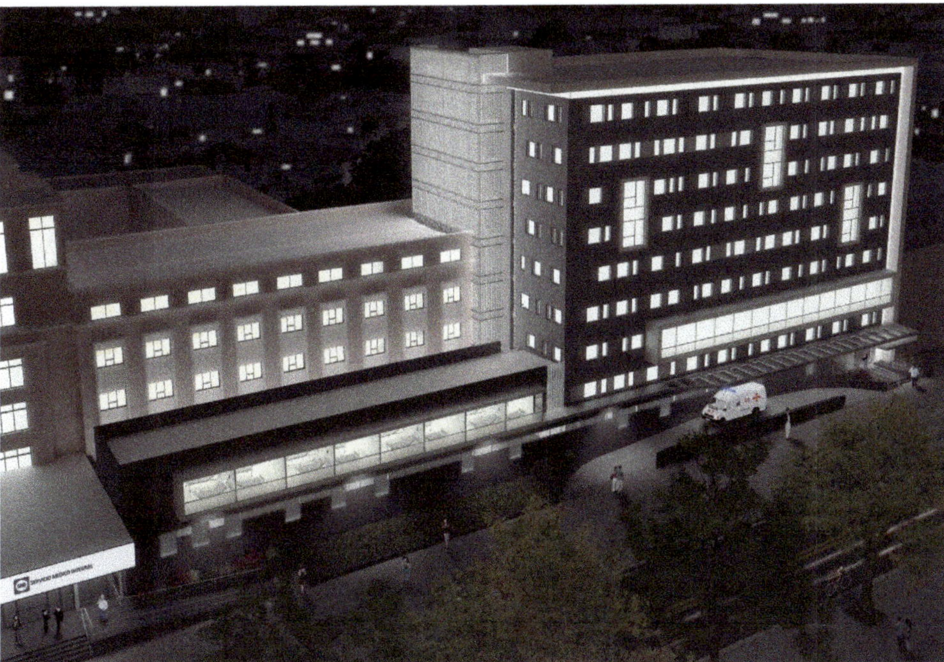

Figure 1. Rendering project.

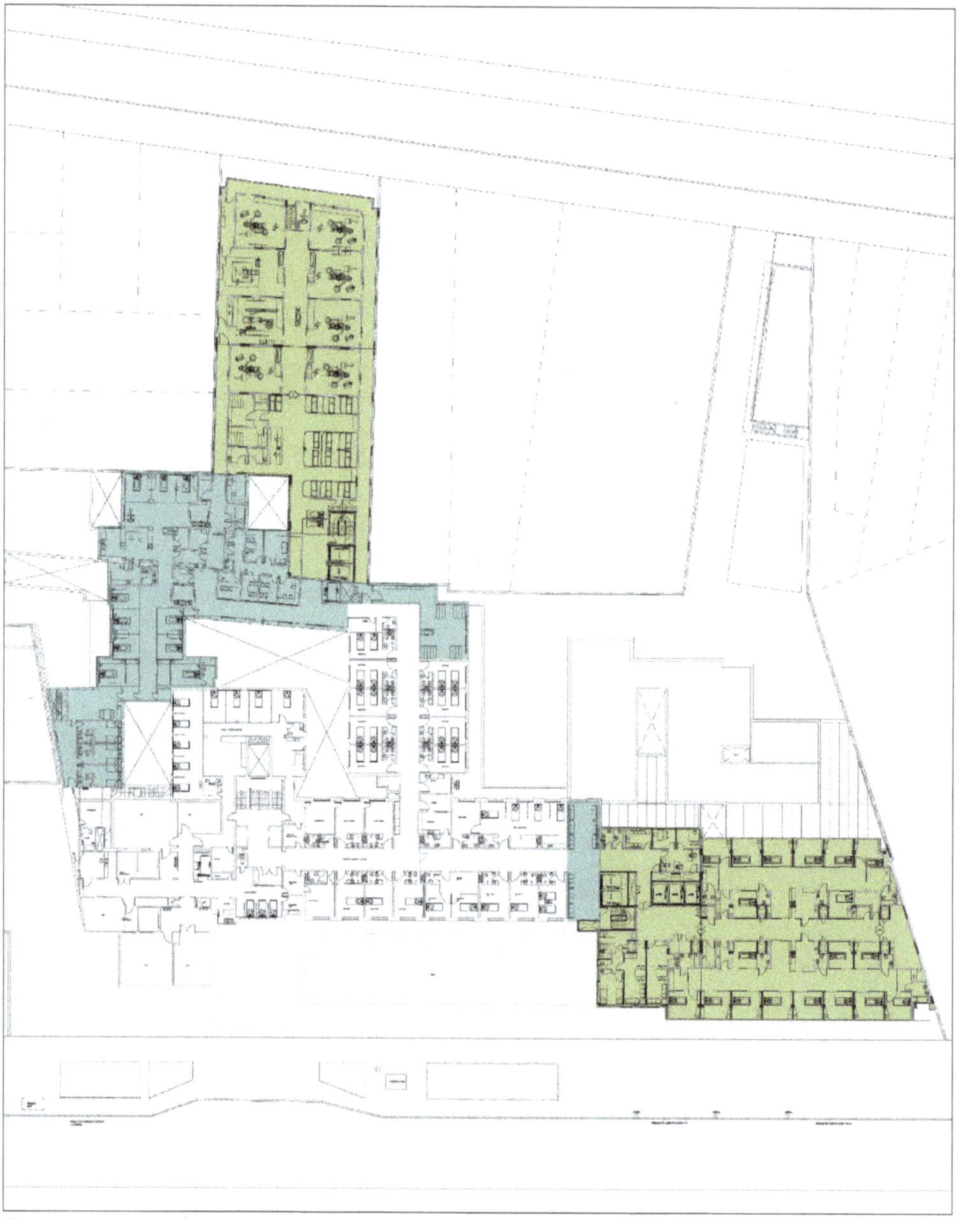

Figure 2. Project plant.

Health building in Uruguay is growing substantially as a result of state policies, and it is expected that new plants can improve their effectiveness and efficiency, producing substantial savings in energy and operational resources and ultimately in achieving the prestationals goals established by the MSP.

Polo Hospitalario del NEA, Inter City Hospital Evita. City of Formosa

José Luis Decima[1], Osvaldo Mario Donato[2]

arqomd@fibertel.com.ar
[1]Dr., Minister of Human Development
[2]Architect, Donato Osvaldo Mario And Associates, Health Consultants

The Government of the Province of Formosa, managed the creation of a Regional Hospital Polo, with the aim of structuring a core of specific hospitals with an integrated and networked operation. The proposed new Inter City Hospital Formosa, constitutes the apex of the System Health Care in the NEA region. Versatile general acute, outpatient and inpatient care by progressive undifferentiated surgical delivery medium risk, with medium complexity within the system of reference and counter, interacting with the High Complexity Hospital Pte. J. D. Perón. The program area of the hospital complex, covers the entire province of Formosa, northern Chaco, western Misiones and areas bordering Paraguay. The receptivity of the different ethnic and Aboriginal communities and the weather, were the main design guidelines, completing the Polo with future Hospital of Obstetrics and Pediatrics Hospital. The architecture of Evita Inter-City Hospital ensures sustainable development to the expansion of the frontier of innovative new technologies of diagnosis and treatment, bringing new concepts in functional organization through an interdisciplinary architectural medical program, with more complex alternatives.

***Osvaldo Mario Donato.** 1973 Architect. Specialist in Hospital Architecture and Engineering. Founding Member and former President of AADAIH. UNDP International Consultant, United Nations Program for Development. Managing Director of Architect Osvaldo Mario Donato and Associates, Consultant in Health. Managing director of TECNO BRAS SA. former Professor of Design from 1975 to 1985 FAU-UBA. Provincial Hospital Planning Consultant Formosa Province. Scientific Research, Graduate IIPC.*
***José Luis Décima** Doctor. Minister of Human Development of Formosa Province.*

Introduction

The Government of the Province of Formosa, managed the creation of a Regional Hospital Polo, unique in Argentina, with the objective of structuring a central core of specific hospitals in order to build hospital matrix network in the province, with an integrated network operation, constituting the apex of the Health Care System. The province covers an area of 72,066 km^2, with about 640,000 inhabitants, the urban population is about 78%. The capital, which has the same name as the province, with approximately 320,000 inhabitants, has a rapid population

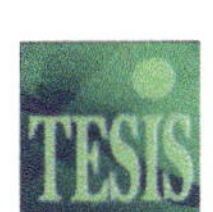

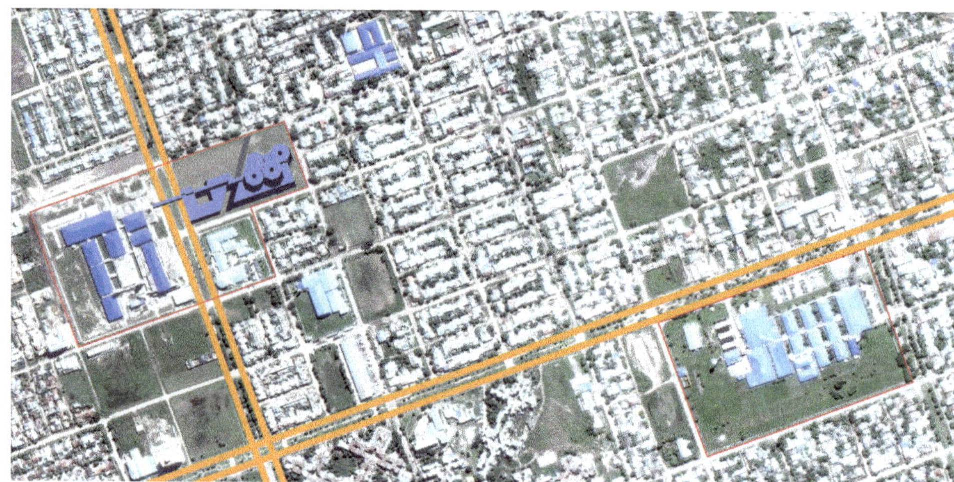

Figure 1. Province of Formosa, managed the creation of a Regional Hospital Polo.

growth, including population centers of Paraguayan origin with access to health services and education provided by the province.

A new operating paradigm arises in healthcare field, generating a provincial health system to adequately cope with the growth in the demand for the next 20- 25 years in the region of the NEA, approximately 1,200,000 inhabitants.

Shaping the Hospital Polo

HAC: High Complexity Hospital. Surface Area: 17,200 m^2; surface extension: 8120 m^2; beds: 150.

HIEF: Evita Interdistrict Hospital - City of Formosa. Surface: 18,000 m^2; beds: 175.

Hospital Dentistry. Surface: 3400 m^2; dental chairs: 33; auditorium.

Hospital of Obstetrics. Surface: 5000 m^2; beds: 80.

Hospital of Pediatrics. Surface: 8000 m^2; beds: 70; neonatology: 60 Cribs.

Regional Center of Hemotherapy. Surface: 1300 m^2.

Location

Metropolitan Area, City of Formosa. Avenue José de Luca Barbieris between Street Coronel Bogado and Street Obispo P. Scozzina.

Medical Assistance Program

It will be launched as a general-purpose Interdistrict establishment of acute patients of medium complexity, with major clinical and surgical specialties medium level risk of hospitalization and practices to medium complexity including outpatient and excluding maternal and child component.

Provide response to the present and future population of the program area: the districts of the capital of Formosa, also becoming the benchmark for District hospitals in the province and their areas of influence in Northeast Argentina. Inter act with High Complexity Hospital and other hospitals that comprise the Hospital Polo.

Management Model

The proposed new Interdistrict Evita Hospital of the City of Formosa, constitutes the apex of the Health Care System in the NEA Region. General versatile of acute patients, outpatient and hospitalization by progressive undifferentiated care, medium risk surgical provision, with medium complexity, within the Reference System and counter-reference, interacting with the High Complexity Hospital Pte. JD Perón.

The program area of the hospital complex, covers the whole province of Formosa, northern Chaco, western Misiones and areas bordering Paraguay. The receptivity of the different ethnic and Aboriginal communities and the weather, were the main design guidelines, completing the Polo Hospital with the future Obstetrics and Pediatrics Hospitals. The architecture of the Evita Interdistrict Hospital, prioritizes a sustainable development to the expansion of the innovative forefront of new technologies for diagnosis and medical treatment, providing new concepts in functional organization through an interdisciplinary architectural medical program, with more complex alternatives.

The project is based on the application of a number of policy guidelines with a new care model, structuring an increased use of hospital resources by incorporating a "progressive patient care" reducing traditional hospitalization. The incorporation of caring modes, also reducing waiting times for diagnostic and surgical procedures, as well as the further development of ambulatory surgery and reducing hospitalization times, will shift most of the patients to he new provisional areas.

The system of the will Day Hospital, will only incorporate patients requiring brief treatments, solving a significant amount of demand.

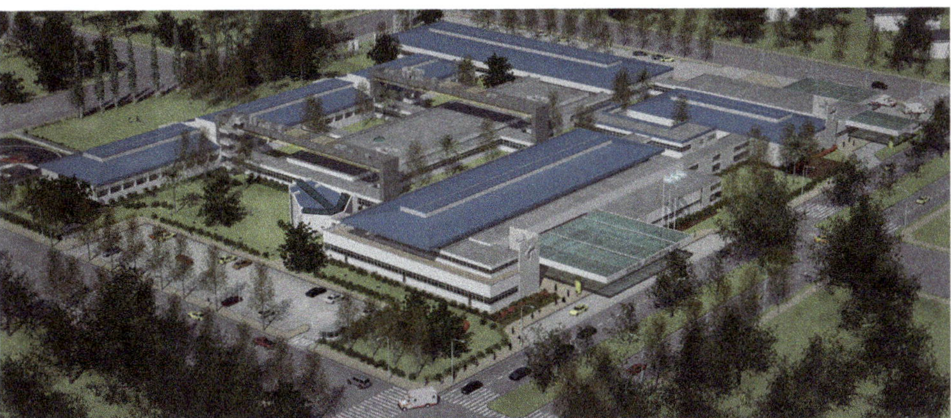

Figure 2. HIEF.

Medical Architectural Program

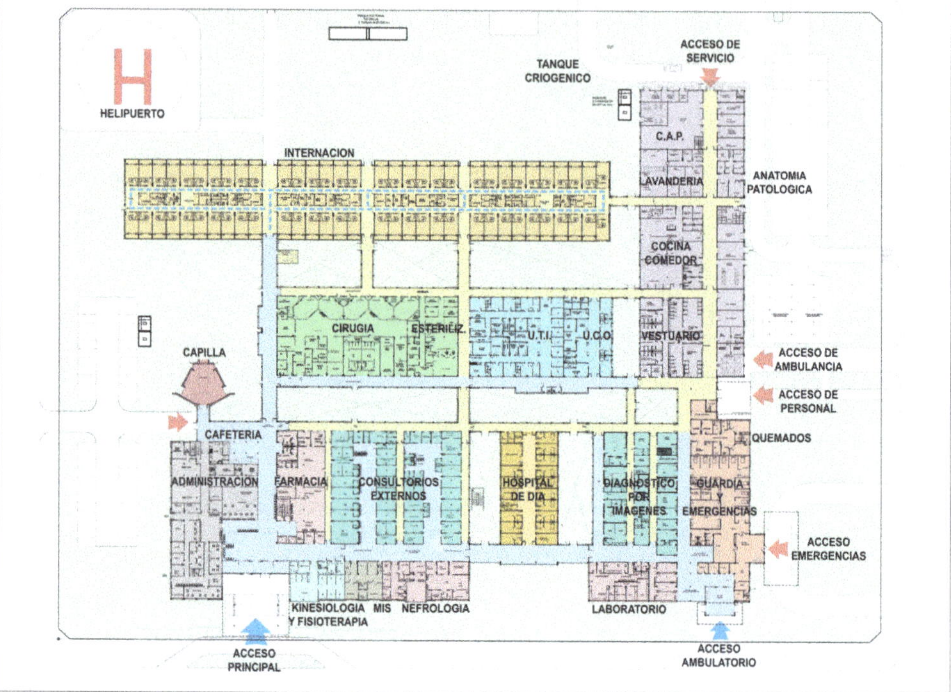

Figure 3. Ground floor.

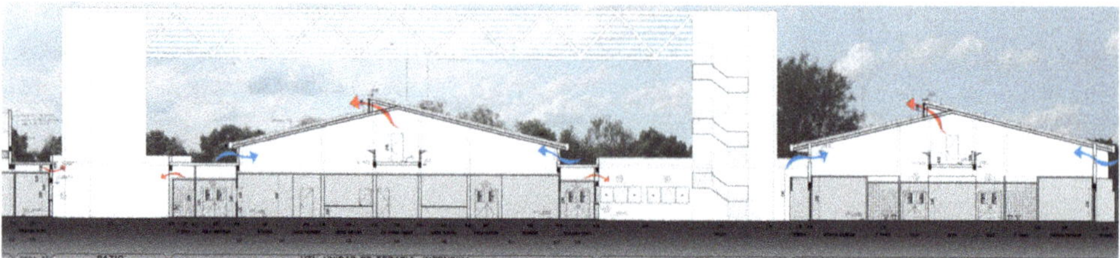

Figure 4. The bridge.

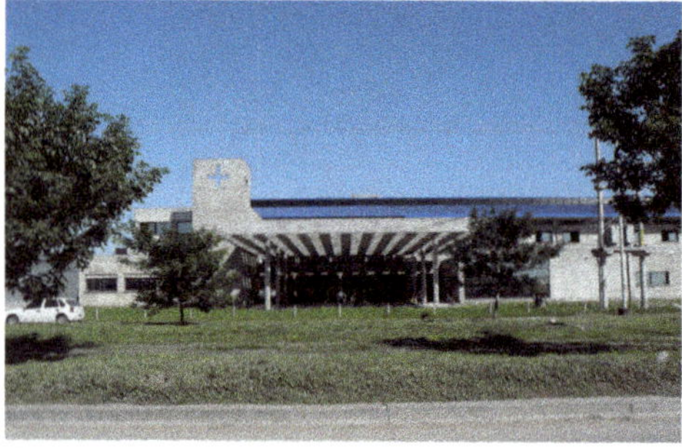

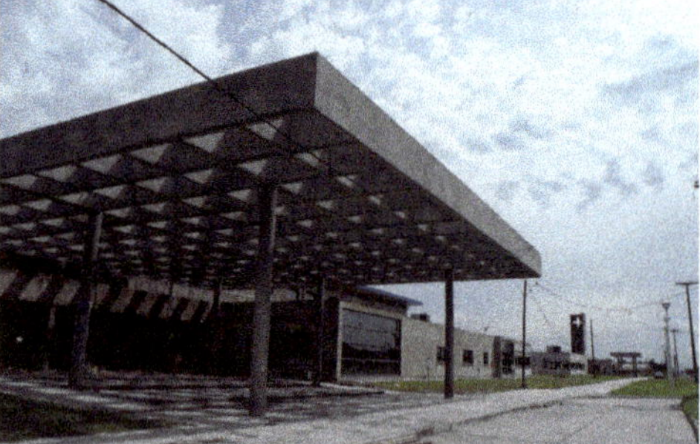

Figure 5. HIEF.

Conduction Sector, General Management and Administration: Directions, Admission and Administration Unit.
Technical Services Sector: Statistics, Social Service, Coordination.
Scheduled Ambulatory Care Sector: 28 outpatient clinics and complementary areas.
Unscheduled Ambulatory Care / Emergency Sector: 6 consulting rooms, 2 curing rooms, 3 Shock Rooms, 11 Observation Boxes and complementary areas.
Sector Hospital Day - Ambulatory Surgery: 9 single bedded rooms, 5 bedrooms with 1 sofa chair and complementary areas. 1 Operating Room, 1 Recovery Multifunctional Room and complementary areas.
Hospitalization Sector: 148 beds (20 Adult Intensive Care beds and 128 beds for Adult Care General and Intermediate).
Diagnosis and Treatment Sector: Surgical center with 5 operating rooms and complementary areas.
Clinical Laboratory: Hemotherapy; Imaging Diagnostics1 tomogrphy room, 1 serigraphy room, 1 X-Ray Room, 1 Ultrasound Room, 1 Endoscopy and complementary areas.
Physical Medicine and Rehabilitation: 1 Gymnasium, 6 Boxes for physiotherapy and kinesiology and complementary areas.
Pathological Anatomy: 1 Histopathology Laboratory, 1 Microbiology Room, 1 Autopsy Room and complementary areas.
Central Supply and Processing Sector: Warehouse, Laundry Room, Sterilization, Pharmacy, Kitchen and complementary areas. General unisex Dressing Rooms.
Complementary Services Sector: Library, Meeting Room, Dining Room, Chapel, Telephone Central Office, Dressing Rooms, Premises for Teaching Staff. Heliport. Parking lot for 100 vehicles.
Residents Accommodation Sector: 6 units of 2 bedrooms with 2 beds, bathroom and kitchen, each.

Typology- General Acute Patient Medicine Hospital

Network Complexity with HAC. Coverage Area: 17,181 m^2. Total beds: hospitalization 128; ICU / CCU 20; Day Hospital 14; Burned 4; Observation Guard 9. Total 175. All the care and hospitalization areas, are developed in a single plant. The areas of Conduction, Teaching and Medical Residency were designed on the First Floor. Architectural Party - Differentiation of Functional Pavilions, linked together by a pedestrian network which is strongly hierarchical and balanced by the sectors it connects. Architectural language of simple institutional identification, integrated into the city's plot. Urbanistically is the " Health Center Polo", characterizing the main access roads and link with other hospitals, as Emergency Roads, through a green light synchronization of traffic lights.

Hospital Concept

Differentiation of large areas: Hospitalization; High Complexity; Welfare Medicine - Outpatient – Diagnosis; Supply and Processes; Conduction – Administration; Teaching and Medical Residency. Prioritization of the immediate environment, in the hospitalization sector, in the Rooms – Exterior Parking Area relation. Improved environmental qualities. Residential Image "Non hospital like"; climate control with natural resources and minimum contribution of air conditioning. Acoustic isolation of the hospital system.

Surgical Center - Intensive Care - Sterilization

Maximize compactness, perimeter reduction, functional organization with differential circulations. Prioritization in composition of Operating Rooms, articulating main areas with secondary support areas, making surgery rooms highly flexible with two wing corridors free of crossings, which expand the surgical space itself.

Ambulatory Care Center and Access to the system: The clear differentiation between hospitalization and the outpatient population, generates a concentration of services, organized along Avenue Barbieris, forming the main front of the Hospital. Access is simple and straight forward, recognizing the main entrance, the entrance to the medical ward and laterally the Emergency access. This sector was planned systemically with circulation differentiation, and a system of care services, from the main entrance to the guard, considering the "Risk Patient" and the flux system, linking physical spaces with the number of patients and frequency of stay.

Supply and Processes Centre: All of the annexed areas, locker rooms, dining room, laundry room, power station, warehouses and workshops, are grouped along a side street, with straight access to supplies deliveries and waste disposal. The strategic location of this pavilion allows a simple and direct supply of the other two sectors. The modular system and constructive, proposes economical principles as a concept in the concentration and simplification of areas, all organized on the ground floor, with horizontal movements only.

Conduction Area - Teaching - Medical Residency: While all these activities are located on first floor, its formation in the physical plant, allows its functional and circulatory differentiation. The Conduction area is organized in the double height of the main entrance, integrating it around in its own surround space. The set of classrooms and resident rooms, although they have vertical circulations that link them directly to the care areas, situated along a second level, allows complete isolation of its activities from the rest of the hospital.

Design Methodology: Health System Global Planning; Strategic Planning - Programmatic depending on the different services; Physical Analysis of the environment and the proposed site; Process - Programming – Predimensioning; Decision Making based on internal and external relationships. Functional and Spatial organization: Synthesis Process; Grouping of large sectors. Modulation and Technologies. Realization - image – Facilities.

Conceptual Sustainability Era: Global Economy Principle in response to social and environmental problems. Avoid building vulnerability by early degradation, allowing the original conditions are maintained for a long time. Reconciling environmental sustainability of natural resources and ecosystems, with technological and social development that will generate the hospital, redefining the system of life. Passive Refreshment, channeling existing winds that sweep wet areas, nocturnal ventilation, air conditioning minimum contribution, ventilated covers. Photovoltaic panels with optimum slopes and orientation, independent of the structure of the hospital. Development in a single plant, synthesizing circulations and maximizing compactness with perimeter reductions in the healthcare sector. Concept of complete isolation as an extreme, thermal, hydraulic and acoustic conditioning, laying shades. Design and Technology as hospital infection control, with positive effects on the community.

Design Focused on the Patient of the Hematologic Oncologic Garrahan Hospital – Garrahan Foundation

Angélica Bonnahon, Laura Tonelli

arqsbt@yahoo.com.ar
Architecture firm ARQSBT, Argentina

The building and health care project implies to enlarge the operation for the outpatient care and hospitalization of patients with hematologic/oncologic pathologies. It implies substantial changes in patients' inter nosocomial care circuits to improve the high quality human and technical care response. The construction of 4,800 m² is developed in two levels: on the ground floor, a 2,400 m² building for care purposes which increases the hospital's care capability with 90 beds, and other 2,400 m² on the first floor intended as a mezzanine for technical support. A future enlargement of 2400 m² on the same area is foreseen, on a second floor.

***Angelica Bonnahon**, Licensed Architect. Physical Planner/Paris, France. Founder member of AADAIHi (Argentine Association of Hospitalarian Architecture and Engineering) Lecturer at OPS (Panamerican Health Organization)/OMS (World Health Organization) Consultant with BID (Interamerican Development Bank) **Laura Tonelli**, Licensed Architect. Master in Health Policies and Procedures, Europe/ Latin America, UNIBO (Università di Bologne, Italy).*

Development

The Paediatric Hospital "Dr. Juan P. Garrahan" is a public health institution, of national jurisdiction, of high complexity and is a South American model. Location of the work: Brasil Ave. No. 2150, City of Buenos Aires, Argentina. Commissioning Party: Garrahan Foundation, a non governmental entity, which contributes to the development of the Hospital as of 1988.
The Architecture firm ARQSBT has made the project of the new work, coordinated all facilities, elaborated the technical specifications, assessed on the call to public tender, evaluated the costs of offerors, and is in charge of the Project Management of the long term oncologic hospitalization and Day Hospital.
The Project comprises the elaboration of the medical/architectonic program with the needs proposed by the Medical Management and by physicians of oncologic, clinical and bone marrow transplantation services.
The needs of the child and his family are focused. Accessibility, sectorization of consulting, diagnosis and treatment areas are given priority, as well as to long-term or 24 hour hospitalizations.
A modular scheme (built and free) of the existing hospital was maintained. Examples of already built areas are the

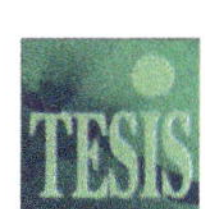

maintenance of structural intervals, the modulation of openings and services; the connection with the existing building, the circulation flows (public and technical) and the connection of different assistance sectors. Free spaces were laid out with modules of internal yards and gardens that render priority to the patient's view and recreation.

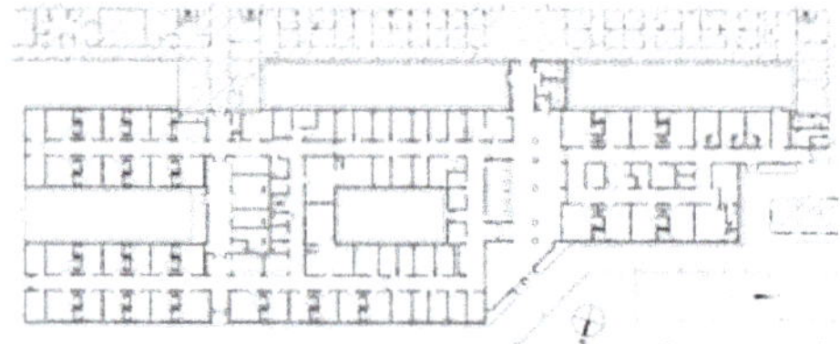

Figure 1. Ground floor and mezzanine.

Management and steps of the work: it was planned in two stages. The first stage consisted in making the reinforced concrete structure.

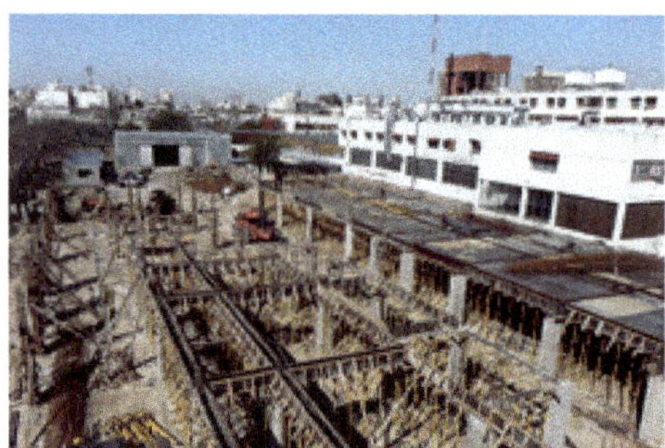

Figure 2. Partial views while constructing the structure.

The schedule of 1st Stage included the obtention of the administrative approval before the intervening entities, the award of the bid and the execution of the work (earthmoving and reinforced concrete structure).

The 2nd Stage of architecture and facilities involves the conditions of the project that foresee the use of materials (similar to those existing at the hospital) with the inclusion of new technologies. As far as the criterium adopted for masonry, it was decided to use "Retak" type bricks for these are of durable material and of quick assembly. Floors, similar to the existing ones, include sanitary baseboards. The foreseen facilities are: sanitary (cold/hot water will be directly connected to the hospital with the aid of present technology; drains and sewage will be built with new lines). The rest of the facilities will be developed on the technical mezzanine. This mezzanine is located on the first level and is exclusive, throughout its surface, to the lines of facilities which will later also be available at the second level. The technical infrastructure consists of: fire, electrical, electric radiant underfloor heating, thermomechanic, weak current facilities (data network, fire detection and alarm, control of accesses, LAN data network for telecommunications, cable telecommunication system, emergency notifiers and cardiac arrest alarms) as well as facilities for medical gases.

The schedule to begin the 2nd. Stage was fixed for March 5, 2014. The duration of the work is established in 14 months.

Working team:

Project and Work Management: Architecture firm ARQSBT, Bonnahon – Tonelli. Representantive of Project Management: Architect Hugo Sánchez. Digitalization: Architect Cecilia López Magliolo. Assesorors of Project Facilites: Sanitary and fire facilities: Architect Jorge Carelli; Thermomechanic facilities: Engineer Carlos Grinberg; Weak current facilities: Engineer Hugo Pandolfi and System Manager, Lic. ii (Bachellor Degree) Gustavo Carolo; Electric nd Medical Gases Facilities, Hospital Maintenance Management Engineer Gabriel Pettinari. Construction company: BRICONS S.A. Translation: Lic. Ana G. Piskulic, Sworn Translator.

Hospital Antonio Lorena – Cusco

Guillermo Turza Arevalo, Mario Jara Dueñas, Eduardo Dextre Morimoto

turjimsa@yahoo.es
Guillermo Turza Arévalo, Consulting Architect, Perù

The Hospital Antonio Lorena is located in the city of Cusco, Santiago district, province and department of Cusco. Its story goes back to the year 1689, when it began operations under the name of "La Almudena ". It operated for a century as part of the Convent of the Bethlehemites. In 1930, the Benevolent Society took over management of the hospital, as a charitable hospital with 500 beds capacity, providing four basic services. It is located in the Protected Historical Center of Cusco; however, the lot of land is located on the boundary of the area, so construction of the hospital was completely allowed.
The architectural proposal presented the image of a clear, identifiable, and sophisticated building carefully integrated into its scenic surroundings, thus assuming the role that a hospital of its kind would have not only in the repertoire of urban landmarks for the city of Santiago-Cusco, but also for the entire Cusco region. We also carefully considered pedestrian traffic and its relationship with the surroundings and landscaping in order to provide the most relaxing possible access to the hospital.

Guillermo Andrés Turza Arévalo*. Architect graduated from the Ricardo Palma University, a specialist in hospital infrastructure, project management, independent consultant on issues of health, an active member of Peruvian Association of hospitals; Representative of the Organization of American experts in Technologies for Health. Founding Member of Peruvian Association of Architects specializing in Health (APAES). Co-author of norm of Health Infrastructure MINSA (1994-2006).*

Development

The architectural proposal posed a building, which respects and adapts to the topography of the building's terrain. There is a slope of 15.42 m, between Avenida Grau and Calle Plazoleto de Belen, which has been used to produce a building "floating" on this survey line, starting at the lowest level, i.e., by Avenida Grau. The second dimension corresponds to access at Avenida Antonio Lorena, and the third dimension corresponds to the access at Calle Callo. The building has parking areas with 315 parking spaces for staff, visitors, and general emergency services. The total area, newly built, is 43,413.51 m^2.

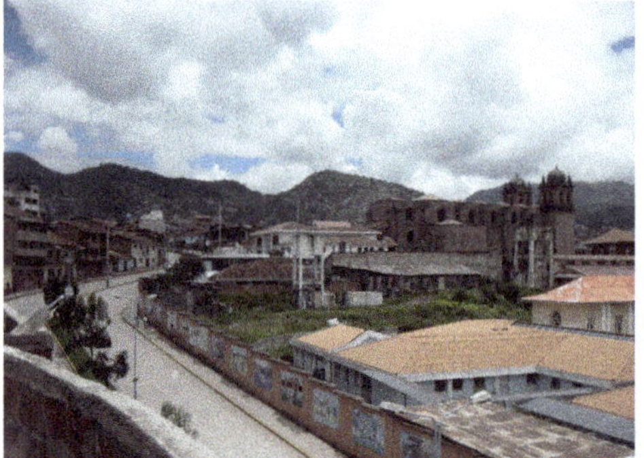

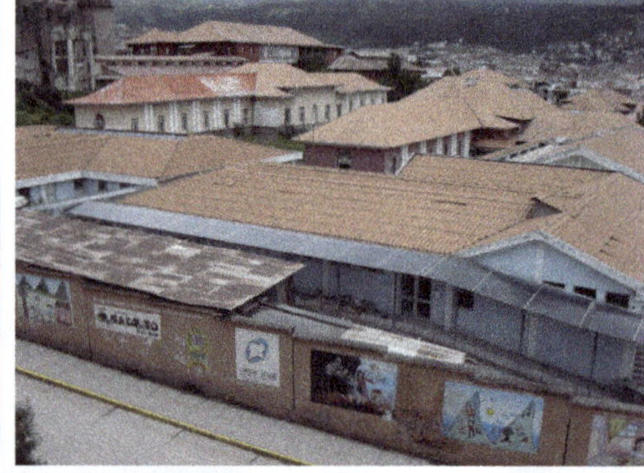

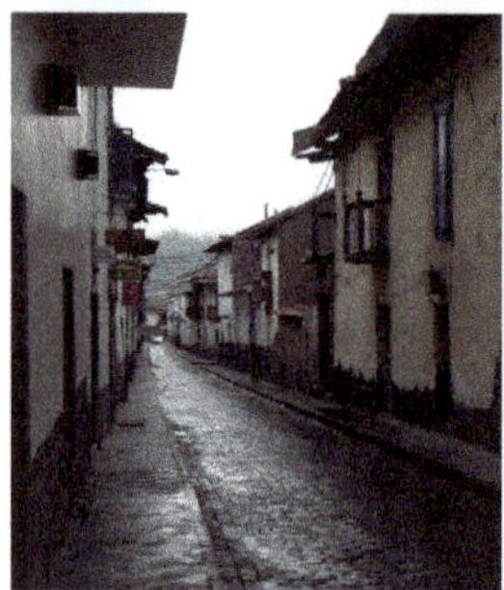

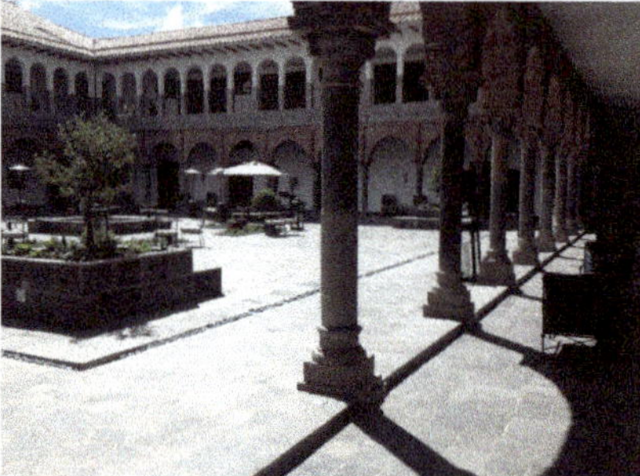

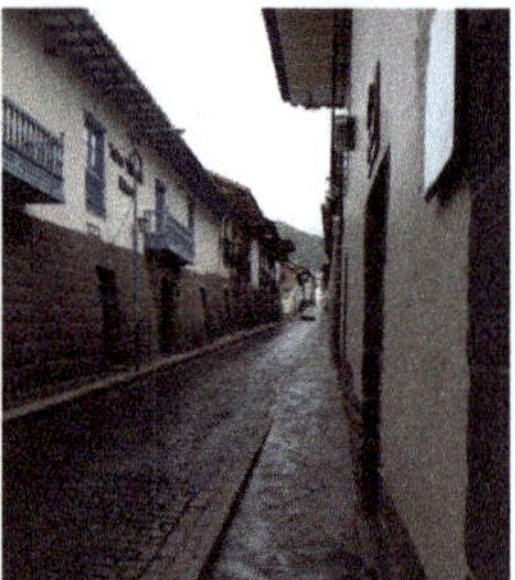

Figure 1. Hospital Antonio Lorena - Cuzco.

The architectural design seeks to integrate the volume of the hospital building within the surrounding space, through the greater integration with the landscape and the natural environment of the area. Architecturally the project meets the definition of a horizontal and vertical hospital, although its size has been carefully refined to obtain a balance of the routes and horizontal-vertical relationships (Figure 1).

The resulting architecture has no problem being implemented, since the very conditions of commitment to this project with the environmental conditions and active and passive response to these conditions, will give constructive solutions which in themselves resolve and define the shape of this project.

The execution implies a realization of a long-term investment, because most of its elements are fixed (permanent), and not going to change during the useful life of the building.

The new Hospital Antonio Lorena building has been designed on the basis of constructive premises for a hospital of the XXI century, incorporating respect for the environment and sustainability as one of the fundamentals of design, minimizing environmental impact, and with the use of appropriate technology to reducing power consumption, maximizing the efficiency of the construction process and subsequent operation. For this reason, this facility was designed using techniques for active and passive energy conservation and the use thereof.

We started from the premise of technology: the model of a hospital cannot be "born old", it must incorporate the latest trends and technologies in order that during its useful life it will not become outdated. This means that facilities should be the servants of the building and not the dominant motive of the scheme.

The development of architectural design adopted the criteria proposed in the Functional Program and the Medical Architectural Program. The new concept of service integration allows the Hospital to perform the activities set out in the Functional Plan, solving malfunctions or anomalies of the current hospital building, while providing capacity and features needed to meet future demands. The project radically posited an architecture that is affordable and healthy in all aspects. In a literal sense, it has its own utility, but it has to respect the perceptions and cultures of its users.

In this sense, we have avoided all that is symbolic in institutional architecture, which considers the user as a passive spectator, with consequent connotations of repressive architectures, and chose to investigate and propose an architecture that understands the user, and in which an establishment such as this exalts everything which is familiar and accessible. For this we reduced on the one hand compositional effects (main façade, access routes, symmetries, etc.) and on the other hand, increased certain functions and complementary features which categorize domestic aspects of the program (cafeteria, plants and gardens, extensive use of natural sunlight), not only in the workplace but in those areas for receiv-

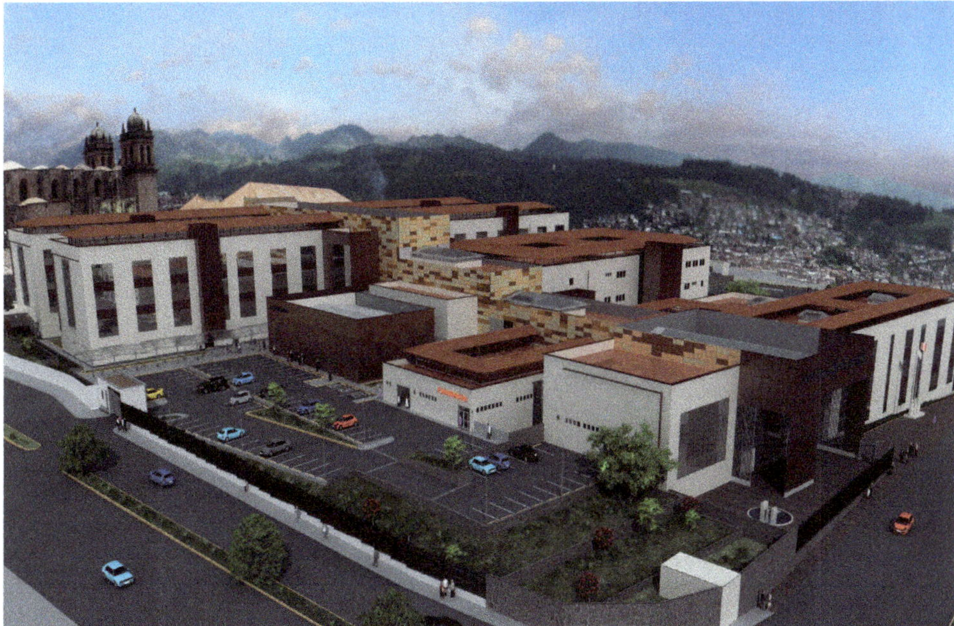

Figure 2. Aerial view of the hospital project.

ing patients, provided the architectural composition permitted.
The project realized the transformation and modernization of Hospital Antonio Lorena, and was guided by criteria guidelines of the proposed re-dimensioning of physical infrastructure as a whole.
The entire hospital is zoned for services as described in the sheets forming part of this study. In them, the location of each proposed service is listed and the box with corresponding areas is presented.

The sizing has been resolved with a concept of a flexible and integrated structural system, considering the flows of services, people and materials.

It also provides for the ability to adapt to future changes, and the possibility of changes in order to prevent rapid obsolescence. The maximum performance and the use of natural lighting and ventilation was considered, with balanced growth in the future and the possibility of restructures or internal reforms for adjustment with equipment installation.

Access to this establishment is through an entranceway, which gives access to the public hall where the lobby with elevators and staircase is located, and from which waiting rooms of different services located in the front and center of the building may be accessed. The patient access to the second and third level is reached from the staircase and lobby where two elevators are located. On the inside were designed two cores for stretchers mounted lifts and two staircases. One set of lift and stairway corresponds to the direct communication between emergency and critical areas as well as the different services (exclusively for medical staff - patients use); the other set is intended for services.

The retreats and the size of the architectural complex located in the central part of the field allow you to create a curtain of privacy with regard to the environment, giving the parking area a feeling of more space.

The design details, both for architecture and facilities, seek to provide maximum comfort to users of the building. The structure is of reinforced concrete, antiseismic, following the concept of "the safe Hospital".

We have designed the following types of accesses:

- Emergency Exits;
- Vertical Circulations;
- Horizontal Circulations;
- Secondary Circulations.

Pedestrian access is defined within the architectural complex, and the hospital entrance at the front provides alternative access points to services of higher demand. There is an avenue in front with optimal characteristics with respect to accessibility to mass transit, personnel and public pedestrian entrances, and to parking, emergency services, and ambulance, personal and general services.

With respect to internal circulation for people, there has been a systematic arrangement of circulation, searching for the minimum interference between different sorts of users, in pursuit of greater efficiency and convenience in the movement of physicians and technicians, and considering the convenience of visitors and suppliers.

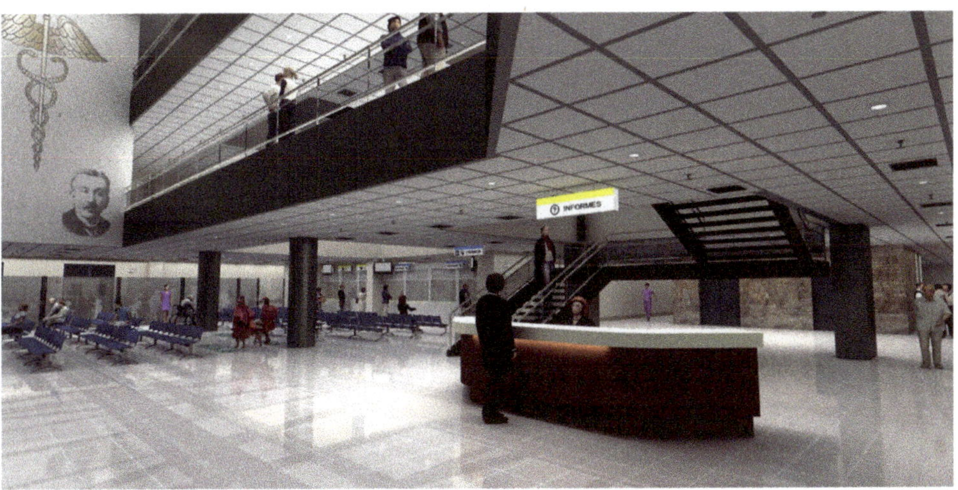

Figure 3. Atrium.

It also considered secondary circulations for interconnecting services between functional areas at different levels comprising the hospital building.

The use of differential circulations allows us to identify spatial types such as public, private, clean, dirty, etc. These functional spatial relations allow an ordering of the structure of the hospital, unlike the current hospital that has conflicts in most areas.

In the first level, with an area of +3,394 m^2, are Outpatient Sectors, Admission, SIS/SOAT, References and Cross-References, Diagnostic Aid (Blood Bank, Pharmacy), Physical Medicine and Rehabilitation. This level has concentrated and spatially arranged physical blocks associated with the largest number of users in the activities of the hospital.

Of the land area allocated for the new Hospital Antonio Lorena, the building's infrastructure at this level is 14,998.78 m^2, representing 39.40 % of total land area allocated, with an open area representing 23,065.15 m^2, equivalent to 60.60 %.

In the open area of 23,065.15 m^2, parking space for 315 vehicles for use by the public, patients, staff and services takes 8,318.21 m^2; gardens and pathways areas occupy 5,122.06 m^2; and sidewalks and ramps occupy an area of 9,624.88 m^2.

The location of the busiest sectors, areas of high public volume such as the areas, services and environments for public circulation and management, are most useful in the first level, with a logical distribution with respect to the flow of public to be treated according to the functional medical program, taking into account their vulnerability, axes of evacuation, and risk to the internal hospital.

At the second level, +3,398.22 m^2, fronting on Avenida Grau, there is space for external consultations, the Imaging and Laboratory Clinic, the Hemodialysis Center, and the Cafeteria.

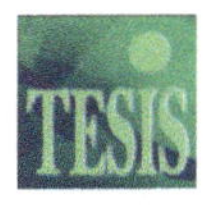

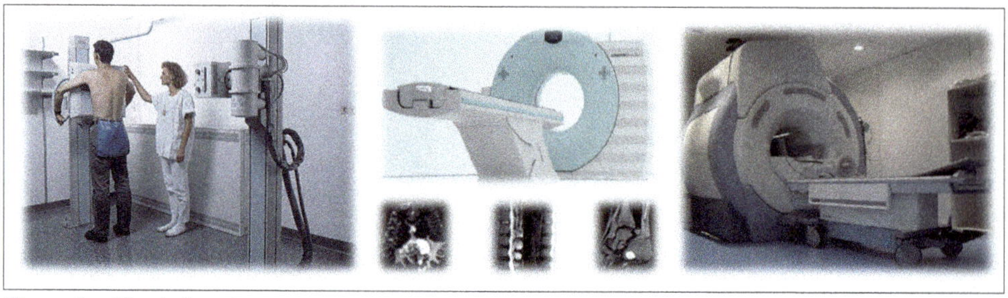

Figure 4. Hospital equipment.

These spaces are adjacent to the areas for Emergency Service, General Services and Power Generators, Electrical Sub-Station, Medical Gases, Maintenance, Hospital Waste Treatment and Storage Tanks areas.
From the access from Avenida Antonio Lorena are spaces for medical Confort (Instructional Classrooms, Auditorium), as well as entrances for patients and visitors to Oncology Services and Radiation Therapy. There is also access to the area of the Pharmacy and for patients in Hemodialysis Service.

From Calle Manuel Callo, where access for ambulances and patients to emergency service is located, one can also reach General Services (Nutrition-Dietetics, Laundry, Storage, Maintenance, Medical Gases, Tanks and Sewage Treatment) by different routes. The roofed area occupied by the infrastructure at this level is 14,892.73 m^2.
At a third level + 3,402.44 m^2, fronting on Avenida Grau, facilities for the administration of the hospital are located; from this level administrators communicate with the different services of the hospital. Under Emergency Services are located the Pavilion for Critical Patients (Intensive Care Unit - ICU), ICU Adults (Safe Zone), and the Procedures and Day Surgery cabinets.
In the Teaching/Instructional area, space has been provided for the Employees' Union and for Child & Nursery Care. From the public hall one can reach the medical services comfort facilities (Library, Teaching, and Residents' Quarters with a capacity of 50 beds), as well as three blocks of 70 inpatient beds for Gynecological- Obstetrics services and 34 beds for pediatric service. The roofed area occupied by the infrastructure at this level is 10,526.50 m^2.
At the fourth level, +3,406.66, in the central zone are located the Sterilization Center, Obstetric Center and Surgery Center. At the back of the building, blocks of both Inpatient Medicine (01 block 35 beds) and Surgery (03 Blocks of 35 beds each) are located. The roofed area occupied by the infrastructure at this level is 7,726.96 m^2.

At the fifth level, +3,410.88 m^2, at the back of the building are two blocks of Inpatient Medicine (02 Blocks of 35 beds each) and services of the Neonatal Intensive Care Unit and the Pediatric Intensive and intermediate Care Unit.
The roofed area occupied by the infrastructure at this level is 5,355.82 m^2.

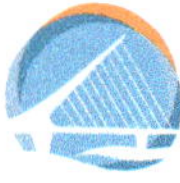

Think Before Acting: The Importance of Planning as Facilitator Element of Success

Maria Teresa Alonso, Lourdes Cillero, Mar Elvira, Carolina Muñoz

mtalonso@uniquehealth.com.es
Unique, Custom-Built Health Solutions, Spain

The current economic situation in developed countries (European Community, USA) has precipitated the need to contain costs in health infrastructure or at least to make the same expenditure contribute to improve the health outcomes. It is the responsibility of all of us to make optimization exercises in health infrastructures, what allow to obtain buildings that ensure quality care at a lower cost. Planning and previous studies represent less than 1% of the total cost of a complete project (project-construction-equipment) but its impact affects over 90% of the total planned investment and significantly defines the future operating costs of the hospital. This proposal is aimed to evaluate projects or infrastructures under construction that are necessary for the population but need to be "re-evaluated". Or for new initiatives (institutions, private companies, equity and venture investors) that haven't been sufficiently analyzed or defined during the pre-project phase and that could risk their viability and sustainability in the operation phase (for a lack of resources, personnel demand, etc.).

Maria Teresa Alonso. *Architect by the Facultad de Arquitectura of Buenos Aires (Argentina), Postgraduate in Environmental Intervention by the Universitat Politecnica de Catalunya and Postgraduate in Project Management. More than 20 years experience in project management and multi- disciplinary technical teams in public and private healthcare sector. Specialist in work teams management, functional diagnostics, master plans, transfer/ move plans and start-up processes of hospitals. Founding partner of Unique, a Healthcare Consulting with a multidisciplinary team (doctors, economists, architects ...), extensive experience in the health sector and that has developed among others, projects in Spain, Portugal, Honduras, Mexico, Guatemala, Peru, Colombia, Chile, Vietnam and Indonesia.*

Initial Needs

In a typical process of a new building analyzing or upgrading of an existing hospital, needs to be evaluated: the demand, the level of complexity of the center (portfolio of services and procedures) and therefore provide solutions which response to this identified demand. However, at present the options aren't to define "what size building meets my needs" but to wonder what changes are needed in the infrastructure that we projected / built to provide more and

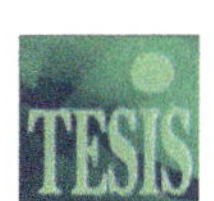

better use of the space we already have.
Individuals, private companies, governments, municipalities, etc. every day decide how to invest or how to start a project.
The starting point is to define what I have: An idea? Resources? A need? And from this point to begin to raise even more questions. Are the objectives clear? Who are the customers? Has been chosen the location? How much it costs? Do I have the resources or the ability to obtain them? How much time is needed for the implementation? Do I have this time ... or not?

Main Steps

The route of a project-construction works-equipment-opening hospital is often a simplification that ignores a fundamental group of works that could be very important to determine which hospital we will design.
The previous studies (definition of the scope, feasibility plan, cost estimation, project profile, expected activity, ...) and functional plan (determining service portfolio and sizing, proximity matrix, circulations and functional relationships, functional plan ...) are the basis for the technical teams to start the project.

Traditionally public administrations/ health providers have defined these criteria before ordering their projects. But it is increasingly nowadays to find that these parameters haven't been defined (for example we have found applications for just "xx beds hospital or xxx m^2 surface hospital" without identifying concerning specialties, complexity, portfolio services). And sometimes it is required to the project teams to take strategic decisions on matters beyond the classical scope of a project (for example, medical specialties to provide, number and type of doctors' offices, operating rooms, inpatient units, etc.).
The same is applied to the definition phase of the plan of hospital medical equipment: it is increasingly left to the suppliers themselves determining the equipment plan, regardless of whether it fits specialties and portfolio hospital services, or the needs of professionals and their patients.
And finally during the construction phase it is common to "forget" the coordination with the works of supply logistics equipment. And even worse, the work connected with the planning of the opening and operation of the hospital (what is the main reason of the whole process: to make available the projected health center to the population).

Main Steps ... and its Economic Impact

The entire process associated to an investment of this type, analyzed for a hospital of 350 beds and approximately 90,000 m^2, results in figures in which: construction works + equipment are nearly 90% of the investment. However project + construction management do not reach values of one digit... and planning, which is what defined that investment is less than 1% (Figure 1). And more importantly: if we think that operating costs represent annually the equivalent to 80-90% of the investment costs, means that the decisions we have taken in the early stages of the project (that have a meaning less 1% of the investment) are the ones which really are defining a very important part of the expenses during 20-25-30 years.

PHASE	% within Investment
Preliminary Studies	0,17%
Functional Plan	0,04%
Project design	3,14%
Site and Project Management	2,07%
Construction works (60,14%)	60,14%
Equipment (34,35%)	34,35%
Start-up process (0,08%)	0,08%
TOTAL	100,00%

Figure 1. Percentage within investment for each phase.

ANALYZING AND PLANNING

Everything seems to reinforce so therefore the idea of the importance of "planning before acting"- to think before take decisions- assess alternatives before committing (the resources of a government, an institution, a country) for many years. It is proposed therefore a sequence of analysis in which the variables associated with the Organization, Infrastructure and Equipment in phases are (Figure 2):

a. problem identification;
b. opportunities analysis;
c. proposal and evaluation of alternatives;
d. accompanying during decision.

a. Problem identification: to identify the key problems that could affect the project's viability or its adaptation to the requirements or baseline issues (clinical aspects, functionality, equipment and infrastructure).

Regarding the organization should be defined aspects like: what hospital we want? For whom? Adequate sizing. Has the integration of services been assessed with other centers or care levels? Is there any future underutilized healthcare structure?

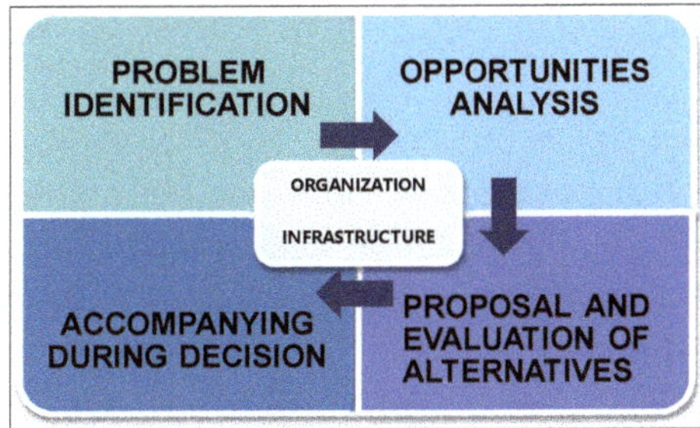

Figure 2. Equipment in phases.

The infrastructure suggests questions such as: does the functional organization contribute to an efficient time management? Are we facing an infrastructure with high maintenance costs? Is our building consuming more energy than necessary? Have you taken into account the energy savings?

And concerning the Equipment: does the defined technological level suit to the portfolio of services and complexity of the hospital? Have we taken into account the integration capacity of the equipment? Have we provided equipment that should not be included as an endowment? (supply duplication). Have been considered additional costs for consumables, maintenance, upgrades, etc.?

b. Opportunities analysis: It should be managed from a triple perspective: Functional (quality and quantity of services, functionality of the solutions), Economic (project costs, cost improvements as a result of the functional improvements) and Operational (reduce of delays, easiness of integration of project improvements). The analysis should allow the identification of those elements that may involve qualitative improvements in the final result.

Organization: to size a center depending on the needs of the area, taking into account available resources, partnerships, etc."Rethinking "the model of care (ICTs as drivers of innovation, impulse of effective relationships with other agents, self-care strategies , etc.). Infrastructure: to propose reorganization of circuits, functional areas, relationships, etc. To update and/or to introduce certain infrastructures to reduce energy consumption of the building, etc.

Equipment: to adjust the equipment to the complexity and service portfolio. Evaluate the cost associated with non-technological integration of computers. Identify difficulties related to non-standardization of equipment (cost, training, etc.). To analyze the costs associated with the operation of the equipment: spare parts, upgrade, renewals, etc.

c. *Proposal and evaluation of alternatives:* after having identified the problems and opportunities for improvement, we identify those initiatives or proposals that will allow us to achieve the objectives that have been proposed. Proposals should be evaluated taking into account both the improvement of critical factors, as well as their strategic adequacy.

Organization: Determination of costs underutilized or unused resources. To promote a more intensive use of those ones (high productivity). To size correctly the different areas according to objective variables (demand, profile, productivity, schedules, partnerships, etc.). To promote figures development that help to minimize the abuse in the use of resources.
Infrastructure: Functional and uses redefine. To redefine constructive solutions to optimize costs. To suggest sector divisions within the building in order to improve its efficiency. To optimize its built area.
Equipment: Analysis of equipment to be purchased: sizing, technological level, quality, quantity, level of integration of equipment, etc. Identification of procurement options appropriate to the type of equipment (purchase, sale, etc.). Proposal of equipment packs optimization, suppliers of reference, model acquisition and maintenance contract, guarantees, etc.

d. Accompanying during decision: For the considered alternatives, the decision is accompanied incorporating a methodology of matrix analysis that allows to prioritize the implementation of the various initiatives, based on the key factors for taking of decisions (estimated cost of the investment, impact on the quality care, volume of affected population, possibilities of care, etc..), and other variables that we decide to consider.

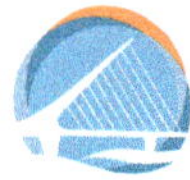

Results

1. Center profile (service portfolio, technological and healthcare level) suitable to the activity and target audience.
2. Strategic options (use of resources, care model, organization) being clearly defined from the start.
3. Sizing (installed capacity, surface area, resources) according to the expected profile of the center.
4. Estimation needs according to the needs of the investment promoter of the idea/need.
5. Usage of occupancy and operating data of *better efficiency.*
6. Possibility to incorporate from the start, elements that *increased care capacity*, and safety of both patients and professionals.
7. Customized solution, adapted to the local conditions / client (social, economics, etc..) that allow the adaptation to care changes or management.
8. Optimized operating costs, and adapted to the objective capacity and resources of the client.

Conclusions

Focus on working collaboratively with all the actors involved in the design of a health center work always adds value to the final result. There should be used tools to ensure *objectivity* in the design, taking into account all the relevant variables (service to be provided, population to be served, technology used etc.) in order to ensure that the work done has solved the existing needs of the users.

Our proposals must be based on the following principles: *to plan before acting, define goals or objectives and seek balance.*

And we are fully convinced that the optimization of investment in health infrastructures and better organization of their resources can:

offer more *(increasing service portfolio)*
reach more *(patients)*
and ***in the best conditions*** *(research and technology)*

TESIS Inter-University Research Centre
Systems and Technologies for Social and Healthcare Facilities
University of Florence, Italy

TESIS

www.ingramcontent.com/pod-product-compliance
Lightning Source LLC
Chambersburg PA
CBHW061230150426
42812CB00054BA/2553

* 9 7 8 8 8 9 0 7 8 7 2 6 3 *